D1246711

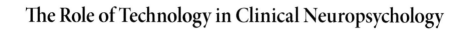

The Role of Technology in Clinical Neuropsychology

# The Role of Technology
# in Clinical Neuropsychology

Edited by Robert L. Kane and Thomas D. Parsons

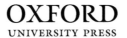

OXFORD
UNIVERSITY PRESS

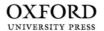

Oxford University Press is a department of the University of Oxford. It furthers
the University's objective of excellence in research, scholarship, and education
by publishing worldwide. Oxford is a registered trade mark of Oxford University
Press in the UK and certain other countries.

Published in the United States of America by Oxford University Press
198 Madison Avenue, New York, NY 10016, United States of America.

© Oxford University Press 2017

Library of Congress Cataloging-in-Publication Data
Names: Kane, Robert L., 1940- editor. | Parsons, Thomas D., editor.
Title: The role of technology in clinical neuropsychology /
edited by Robert L. Kane and Thomas D. Parsons.
Description: New York, NY : Oxford University Press, 2017. |
Includes bibliographical references and index.
Identifiers: LCCN 2016045478 (print) | LCCN 2016045653 (ebook) |
ISBN 9780190234737 (hardcover : alk. paper) | ISBN 9780190234744 (UPDF) |
ISBN 9780190668976 (EPUB)
Subjects: LCSH: Clinical neuropsychology. | Technology.
Classification: LCC RC386.6.N48 R65 2017 (print) | LCC RC386.6.N48 (ebook) |
DDC 616.8—dc23
LC record available at https://lccn.loc.gov/2016045478

1 3 5 7 9 8 6 4 2

Printed by Sheridan Books, Inc., United States of America

To Nan for enriching my life. To mentors and colleagues
for what they have taught me.

Robert Kane

This book is dedicated to my family, mentors,
and students—my greatest gifts.

Thomas D. Parsons, PhD

# { CONTENTS }

# { CONTRIBUTORS }

**Michael Barnett**
Department of Psychology
University of North Texas
Denton, Texas, USA

**Erin D. Bigler**
Department of Psychology and
    Neuroscience Center
Brigham Young University
Provo, Utah, USA

**Deborah Binder**
VA Northern California Health
    Care System
Martinez, California, USA;
Helen Willis Neuroscience
    Institute
University of California, Berkeley
Berkeley, California, USA;
San Francisco VA Medical Center
Department of Neurology
University of California
San Francisco, California, USA

**Laura Brattain**
Bioengineering Systems and
    Technology
MIT Lincoln Laboratory
Lexington, Massachusetts, USA

**Shane S. Bush**
Long Island Neuropsychology, P.C.
Lake Ronkonkoma, New York, USA

**Anthony J.-W. Chen**
VA Northern California Health
    Care System
Martinez, California, USA;
Helen Willis Neuroscience Institute
University of California, Berkeley
Berkeley, California, USA;
San Francisco VA Medical Center
Department of Neurology
University of California
San Francisco, California, USA

**Diane J. Cook**
School of Electrical Engineering and
    Computer Science
Washington State University
Pullman, Washington, USA

**C. Munro Cullum**
Psychology Division
University of Texas Southwestern
    Medical Center
Dallas, Texas, USA

**Prafulla Dawadi**
School of Electrical Engineering and
    Computer Science
Washington State University
Pullman, Washington, USA

**Unai Díaz-Orueta**
School of Nursing and Human Sciences
Dublin City University
Dublin, Ireland

**Matthew Doiron**
Department of Psychology
Drexel University
Philadelphia, Pennsylvania, USA

**Marianna Eddy**
Cognitive Science team
US Army Natick Soldier
  Research Development and
  Engineering Center
Natick, Massachusetts, USA

**Joe Edwards**
Department of Behavioral Health
Fort Wainwright, Alaska, USA

**Kristin Heaton**
US Army Research Institute of
  Environmental Medicine
Natick, Massachusetts, USA;
Department of Environmental Health,
  School of Public Health
Boston University
Boston, Massachusetts, USA

**Brian Helfer**
Bioengineering Systems and
  Technology
MIT Lincoln Laboratory
Lexington, Massachusetts, USA

**Diana Jovanovski**
Department of Psychology
University of Toronto Scarborough
Toronto, Ontario, Canada

**Robert L. Kane**
Cognitive Consults and
  Technology LLC
Washington, DC, USA

**Fred Loya**
VA Northern California Health
  Care System
Martinez, California, USA;
Helen Willis Neuroscience Institute
University of California, Berkeley
Berkeley, California, USA;
San Francisco VA Medical Center
Department of Neurology
University of California
San Francisco, California, USA

**Timothy McMahan**
Computational Neuropsychology and
  Simulation (CNS) Lab
Department of Psychology
University of North Texas
Denton, Texas, USA

**Daryush Mehta**
Bioengineering Systems and Technology
MIT Lincoln Laboratory
Lexington, Massachusetts, USA;
Center for Laryngeal Surgery and
  Voice Rehabilitation
Massachusetts General Hospital
Boston, Massachusetts, USA;
Department of Surgery
Harvard Medical School
Boston, Massachusetts, USA;
School of Health and Rehabilitation
  Sciences
MGH Institute of Health
  Professions
Charlestown, Massachusetts, USA

**Patrick Melugin**
Department of Psychology
University of North Texas
Denton, Texas, USA

**Joseph Moran**
Cognitive Science team
US Army Natick Soldier Research
  Development and Engineering
  Center
Natick, Massachusetts, USA

**Jeffrey Palmer**
Bioengineering Systems and
  Technology
MIT Lincoln Laboratory
Lexington, Massachusetts, USA

**Thomas D. Parsons**
Computational Neuropsychology and
  Simulation (CNS) Lab
Department of Psychology
University of North Texas
Denton, Texas, USA

**Tejash Patel**
Bioengineering Systems and
  Technology
MIT Lincoln Laboratory
Lexington, Massachusetts, USA

**Joey Perricone**
Bioengineering Systems and
  Technology
MIT Lincoln Laboratory
Lexington, Massachusetts, USA

**Pascale Piolino**
Memory and Cognition Laboratory
Center of Psychiatry and
  Neurosciences
University Paris Descartes
INSERM
Paris, France

**Gaën Plancher**
Memory and Cognition Laboratory
Center of Psychiatry and
  Neurosciences
University Paris Descartes
INSERM
Paris, France;
Cognitive Mechanisms Research
  Laboratory
Université Lumière Lyon
Bron, France

**Thomas Quatieri**
Bioengineering Systems and
  Technology
MIT Lincoln Laboratory
Lexington, Massachusetts, USA;
Harvard-MIT Division of Health
  Sciences and Technology, Speech
  and Hearing Bioscience and
  Technology
Massachusetts Institute of Technology
Cambridge, Massachusetts, USA

**Philip Schatz**
Department of Psychology
Saint Joseph's University
Philadelphia, Pennsylvania, USA

**Maureen Schmitter-Edgecombe**
Department of Psychology
Washington State University
Pullman, Washington, USA

**Maria T. Schultheis**
Department of Psychology
Drexel University
Philadelphia, Pennsylvania, USA

Christopher J. Smalt
Bioengineering Systems and
  Technology
MIT Lincoln Laboratory
Lexington, Massachusetts, USA

Joyce W. Tam
Department of Psychology
Washington State University
Pullman, Washington, USA

Alyssa Weakley
Department of Psychology
Washington State University
Pullman, Washington, USA

James R. Williamson
Bioengineering Systems and Technology
MIT Lincoln Laboratory
Lexington, Massachusetts, USA

Konstantine K. Zakzanis
Department of Psychology
University of Toronto Scarborough
Toronto, Ontario, Canada

{ PART I }

# Introduction

# Introduction to Neuropsychology and Technology

Robert L. Kane and Thomas D. Parsons

The word *disruptive* has become associated with the age of technology. The connotations of this term have changed drastically from years ago, when in schools it was associated with the type of behavior that would result in a trip to the principal's office. In the 21st century, "disruptive" often refers to changes that markedly affect and reshape the way things are done, opening up new approaches that change the way we live and function. Computers in various forms, from desktop systems to handheld devices and mobile phones, have played a large role in changing the way we live and work. Researchers no longer spend days at computer centers running study statistics and now can accomplish far more sophisticated analyses using notebook computers. Despite the dramatic changes technology has made in most phases of life, its impact on the practice of clinical neuropsychology has been minimal. It is fair to say that neuropsychologists have increased their use of computers for patient assessment and that some traditional test measures have been adopted for computers, simplifying the administration and scoring process. A number of tests have been developed and designed for computer administration. While computer use has increased especially in specific areas, such as aviation, pharmaceutical studies, and in evaluating concussion both in sports and in the military, the potential use of computers and other technologies to augment assessment has barely been exploited. The goal of this volume is to present ideas and accomplished work demonstrating the use of technology to augment the neuropsychological assessment of patients. Some of the ideas presented in the introduction are forward thinking, incorporate the use of advanced technology, and are potentially disruptive. Others represent incremental changes, but changes that take obvious advantage of using technology to modernize and streamline the assessment process. The introduction reviews the current state of technology in neuropsychology and sets the stage for the succeeding chapters.

## History of Computerized Testing

Neither employing computerized testing to assess cognitive functioning, nor the attempt to delineate, or at least inform, standards for computerized testing is new. In the 1970s, the microcomputer became available to the average person and shortly thereafter clinicians and researchers began exploiting the potential of the device for enhancing the cognitive assessment process. The brief overview of the history of computerized testing in neuropsychology provided here is not meant to be a comprehensive and inclusive review of available test batteries. Rather, the objective is to provide a selective review focusing on examples that illustrate the advancing technology.

Early efforts to make use of the microcomputer as a testing platform in neuropsychology focused on clinical assessment, toxicology, epidemiology, and performance assessment. Many of these early endeavors were reviewed in previous publications (Kane & Kay, 1992, 1997; Kane & Reeves, 1997). Some of the early batteries have evolved and are still in use. Others, many of which had the potential to make a significant contribution to assessment, had brief life spans and for different reasons didn't gain traction and disappeared from view. In addition, since the publication of the earlier reviews by Kane and colleagues, new computerized test batteries have emerged. The computerized test batteries and systems that are mentioned here were selected to highlight salient points regarding the history, development, uses, and future directions of computerized assessment in neuropsychology.

A compelling and obvious use for computerized testing is to study at-risk populations. A specific example of this was the interest of the World Health Organization (WHO) in assessing the effects of environmental toxins. The Neurobehavioral Evaluation System 2 (NES 2; Letz & Baker, 1988) was created to address this need. The NES 2 system was developed in the mid-1980s and its authors contributed to the WHO's recommendations for core neurobehavioral measures to study occupational hazards. Tests for the NES 2 were consistent with these recommendations and were designed to assess a broad range of CNS functions. Similar to other computerized batteries then and now, it allowed for flexible test selection and was translated into multiple languages (Kane & Kay, 1992). The NES 2 was a pioneering effort, and the subsequent NES 3 was one of the first to incorporate spoken test instructions to facilitate test administration. This early innovation, and one that arguably could increase the reliability of both group and individual test administration, has yet to be widely adopted, although it will be an option with the new release of CogScreen (Kay, 1995), which is discussed below.

Another early use of computerized testing was to assess the effects and side effects of pharmaceuticals on cognition. The Memory Assessment Clinics system (MAC; Larrabee & Crook, 1988) was developed for use in pharmaceutical studies and also to study age-associated memory changes. While a number of computerized tests and batteries have been, and are, employed in pharmaceutical studies, the MAC tests are mentioned here because they represent an early attempt to use technology to present tests designed to be ecologically relevant that would not have been possible using traditional testing methods. The MAC employed a microcomputer connected to a touchscreen and CD-ROM to present subjects with simulated tasks of everyday memory. The original MAC battery had eight test forms and was available in seven languages. While it predated the use of virtual reality and scenario-based assessment, it was an early, creative, and forward-thinking approach to use technology to capture cognitive performance in an ecologically relevant context. The MAC was used in studies of aging and in pharmaceutical research (Kane & Kay, 1992).

The need to test subjects multiple times is not limited to pharmaceutical studies. Repeated-measures assessment is important when studying the effects of other treatment interventions, as well as when studying the effects of environmental stressors, such as temperature, altitude, fatigue, and emotional stress, on performance. The need to assess performance under various conditions and to monitor the effect of drugs on performance drove the development of computerized testing within the Department of Defense (DoD), with laboratories in the Army, Navy, and Air Force producing test systems in the 1980s (Kane & Kay, 1992). In many ways, these systems set standards for subsequent efforts to develop computerized tests. They were designed from the beginning for repeated test administration, with the ability to create alternate forms. More importantly, the developers of the DoD systems understood the strengths and limitations of the computer systems they were using and implemented ways to simplify the user interface and to achieve adequate response timing, combining hardware timers with programming that accounted for factors like computer monitor refresh rates. This early work laid the foundation for standards in computerized testing (discussed below). Also worth noting was an early attempt to develop a standard test system that could be used by all the military services in various research programs. This test system, referred to as the Unified Tri-services Cognitive Performance Assessment Battery (UTCPAB; Kane & Kay, 1992), was developed by a tri-service working group and was initially designed to provide standardized cognitive assessment in a multistage drug evaluation program. The program included the evaluation of drugs that might prove useful as antidotes to toxic substances employed in chemical warfare. The UTCPAB system was first specified in 1985 (Hegge, Reeves, Poole, & Thorne, 1985). Various supporting documents then followed that included literature reviews pertinent to the 25 tests that had originally been chosen for inclusion (Englund et al., 1987; Perez, Masline, Ramsey, & Urban, 1987). Technical and funding issues eventually resulted in the UTCPAB's never reaching its full capabilities. However, it represented the first attempt to develop a consistent system across the DoD and was based on standards that addressed both psychometric and technical issues in computerized testing.

DoD's initial contributions to computerized testing stemmed from individuals working in different laboratories whose goal was to use a new technology to solve a problem: the need to test subjects on multiple occasions in order to assess the effects of various factors on human performance. Hence, the developing technologies within DoD were not visible to many potential users. A test battery that was developed within DoD and that is currently available is the Automated Neuropsychological Assessment Metrics (ANAM) system (Reeves, Winter, Bleiberg, & Kane, 2007). The ANAM system began as an effort to take work done within the DoD to assess performance and to implement the measures in the clinical arena (Kane & Kay, 1992). This effort became possible with the advent of software-based timing that got around the limitations in accuracy that resulted when just using the computer's clock to time responses. The use of software timers, along with a mouse interface, eliminated the need to rely on desktop computers with add-in lab cards and permitted testing to be done on a laptop computer without additional equipment. Advances in technology that permitted more precise response timing without additional hardware made it possible for neuropsychologists to develop computerized assessment batteries using off-the-shelf equipment, thus making more test batteries available to a larger number of potential users. Nevertheless, how different computerized test systems deal with timing issues varies. (This topic is discussed in greater detail in the section below dealing with standards.) That said, the transition from systems that required desktop computers (and in some cases add-in cards or external manipulanda) to more portable notebook computers, expanded the uses of computerized testing. Currently, computer-administered cognitive tests are used extensively in sports medicine, for military applications, and in aviation and spaceflight, and have been incorporated into clinical settings. The ImPACT test battery has been used extensively in sports medicine to assess the effects of concussion (https://impact-test.com/research/). In 1988, Congress mandated cognitive baseline testing for all deploying military Service members. The National Defense Authorization Act of 2008 (HR 4986; Section 1618) called for: "The development and deployment of evidence-based means of assessing traumatic brain injury, posttraumatic stress disorder, and other mental health conditions in members of the Armed Forces, including a system of pre-deployment and post-deployment screenings of cognitive ability in members for the detection of cognitive impairment" (US Congress, 2008). Except in the case of Special Forces, tests from the ANAM system were implemented for this purpose. As of this writing, baseline testing has been accomplished on 1,140,445 service members and the database of individuals tested includes test data on over two million assessments (D. Marion, personal communication, May 16, 2016). Updated norms for ANAM tests used for this purpose will be based on approximately one million baseline tests. Such an accomplishment would not have been achievable using traditional approaches to testing. NASA has flown the Spaceflight Cognitive Assessment Tool for Windows (WinSCAT; Kane, Short, Sipes, & Flynn, 2005) during all expeditions to the International Space Station (ISS). WinSCAT is composed of test measures from the ANAM system. The ability to implement computerized testing in orbit has permitted the monitoring of astronauts' cognitive status on ISS expeditions. At the time of this writing, WinSCAT has been used on 47 ISS expeditions (K. A. Seaton, personal communication, May 16, 2016). CogScreen (Kay, 1995) was developed in conjunction with the Federal Aviation Administration (FAA). It was initially designed to be used to screen for cognitive difficulties in aviators, and, while it is still used for this purpose, a number of airlines also use it to aid in pilot selection. When first developed, CogScreen required a lightpen and a touchscreen monitor (Kane & Kay, 1992). A later release replaced the lightpen with a stylus. While the new release will support the use of a touchscreen monitor, it will also run on certain tablet devices, expanding the settings where it can be employed (G. G. Kay, personal communication, August 29, 2015). These developments in sports medicine, DoD, and aviation were all made possible by employing computers to open up new and important avenues of assessment.

While a number of test systems were developed specifically for automated administration, traditional stand-alone measures have also been adapted for the computer. The original Halstead Category Test (Reitan & Wolfson, 1985) made use of a slide projector and a large wooden box with attached switches. At present, the Category Test is frequently given in booklet form or on computer. The Wisconsin Card Sorting Test (Heaton, 2003) is often given on computer. Changing the format of a test can raise questions about whether the automated version assesses the same aspects of performance as the traditional test and the extent to which previous norms apply. However, giving the Wisconsin Card Sorting Test on computer, in addition to simplifying the administration, likely reduces scoring errors. Continuous performance tests are available using stand-alone equipment. However, it is now more common to administer such tests on computers that can also be used for other purposes, including the administration of other tests. Recently, Pearson, with the Q-Interactive system (http://www.helloq.com), has moved toward implementing a number of traditional test measures using a tablet to replace multiple paper booklets and forms. While replacing paper booklets with tablet-based systems would seem desirable, the changes have been controversial, as evidenced by discussions and comments on neuropsychology list services, although a significant part of the controversy seems to be related to cost considerations and to the potential need to develop new norms, rather than to the merits of modernizing the testing process. Independent of issues surrounding any particular system, Q-Interactive represents a concept that was long overdue. Many traditional tests used in neuropsychology combine proven utility with archaic administration and scoring. Test materials used for traditional neuropsychological assessment are bulky and subject to wear. Many tests use flip cards that are difficult to manipulate, especially when trying to present stimuli at precise intervals, as required by the test instructions. Tests and test forms also take up space, requiring file cabinets and shelving. For neuropsychologists who test in more than one location, traditional test booklets and equipment tend to be more luggable than portable. Hence, a move in the direction of modernizing test administration should have long-term benefits. Test publishers have also been moving toward online administration of questionnaire-based tests, along with online scoring and report generation. Examples include Pearson's Q-global (http://www.helloq.com) and Psychological Assessment Resources' iConnect (https://www.pariconnect.com).

The goal of developing consistent metrics and databases to standardize the collection of cognitive data and to facilitate comparisons among studies of various disorders has been a recurring theme in science in general, including neuropsychology. NIH's Toolbox (Weintraub et al., 2014) is a recent attempt to establish a standard set of tools for this purpose and includes a set of cognitive measures designed to be administered across the life span. It was originally normed using notebook computers running Windows 7, but it has been transitioned to the iPAD. According to the NIH Toolbox help desk, equivalency studies are in process to verify that data from the iPAD are consistent with data obtained from the standard Internet-based system (personal communication, NIH Toolbox Assessment Center, May 31, 2016). In developing the Toolbox, NIH deliberately chose to stay away from proprietary tests, making the Toolbox vendor independent. Nevertheless, the system now costs $499.99 for a year's license that can be used in conjunction with up to 10 iPads (http://www.nihtoolbox. org). The need to charge for tests developed using public funding was predictable. Persons experienced in the development of computerized testing appreciate that keeping a system viable requires continued development in order to stay current with changing technology. Changes in technology add capabilities and open up possibilities, but the changes also produce challenges for test developers. Adapting test systems to operating systems and test platforms can be expensive and is especially challenging for tests that try to capture highly accurate response times. Other systems developed with government funding, such as ANAM and CogScreen, went through a process of technology transfer into the private sector and have been able to adapt to changes in technology as a result. Historically, government has been able to play a key role in developing technology but does not market it or commit to providing ongoing development funds. Hence, the concept of free public-domain software, while attractive, is not realistic.

One long-talked-about capability of computerized testing is the implementation of adaptive testing. Tests can be adaptive in two ways. One way is to use item-response theory to make the administration of a specific test shorter and more efficient. A second way is to employ decision algorithms that make use of an individual's performance on one or more tests to automatically select follow-up test measures. An interesting feature of the NIH Toolbox is its implementation of item-response theory to shorten the length of some of its test measures and to increase measurement efficiency (Weintraub et al., 2014). Computerized batteries that make use of a select and selectable series of short tests have minimized their need to incorporate item-response theory to shorten individual tests. Systems that use an individual's performance to select tests diagnostically to follow up on areas of interest have yet to be developed.

Another area that has received insufficient attention is Internet-based testing, which is discussed in more detail in chapter five, on teleneuropsychology. Here, it is worth noting the initial forays into this area made by Erlanger and his associates (Erlanger et al., 2002) in developing the Headminders system, as well as Psychological Assessment Resources' iConnect (already mentioned above). Headminders was developed specifically as a neurocognitive assessment instrument, geared toward remote assessment, that could be administered over the Internet. While according to its website it is no longer available, it is significant in that it was a forward-thinking effort to accomplish cognitive assessment remotely. The iConnect system has a broader capability for administering some tests via the Internet as well as scoring tests given traditionally using Internet-based software. iConnect is not specifically focused on neuropsychology or remote cognitive assessment, but some of its instruments have neuropsychological relevance and the system provides an option for examiners.

The computerized tests and batteries currently available to researchers and clinicians were developed in both the public and private sectors and in various countries. The growth of computerized testing has led to the need for published standards. In addition, the availability of automated measures has raised questions about their role in assessment and the additional value they offer over the traditional tests that have served neuropsychology well and that helped it to grow as a respected profession within the healthcare arena. The next section of this chapter reviews the potential uses and advantages of computerized tests. A discussion of standards follows.

## Advantages and Disadvantages of Computerized Testing

Some early efforts to develop computerized test measures arose out of a natural desire to take advantage of new technology. Others were focused on using new capabilities to address specific assessment problems. Some of the obvious advantages of computerized testing included the ability to precisely measure response times and to assess processing speed in various ways, and not just through measures that also assessed motor speed and visual scanning. With computers, it was possible to measure response efficiency during the administration of various cognitive tasks. Computers facilitated the development of tests with multiple forms for repeated administration (Kane & Kay, 1992). There was also the expectation that an automated test would reduce examiner error in both administration and scoring and would enhance standardization. Another anticipated advantage was that computers would permit the implementation of tasks and test paradigms that were potentially important but hard to implement through traditional means. Neuropsychologists typically don't measure divided attention and mistakenly refer to tests that have a set-shifting component, such as Part B of the Trail Making Test, as a divided attention test. With computers, test takers can be presented with two or more tasks simultaneously, creating the need for the persons doing the test to coordinate their responses between or among the different measures. A classic early example of a divided attention test was Tim Elsmore's SynWork test (Kane & Kay, 1992), which allowed for up to four tests to be presented at once. Individuals both earned and lost points on each test and had to implement effective divided attention and resource allocation strategies. The test also produced a single overall score. Hence, with computers it was possible to administer a true divided attention test.

A number of complex problem-solving tasks have also been implemented on computer that were not possible using paper and pencil. One of the early DoD batteries was the Complex Cognitive Assessment Battery (Kane & Kay, 1992), which was composed of several such test measures. Furthermore, integrating the computer with external devices has the potential to enhance the information obtained from more traditional measures. How someone draws or writes can be assessed by devices attached to a computer that is running software that can capture various parameters not measured with traditional paper-and-pencil writing and drawing tasks. Finger tapping can be measured by looking at tap-by-tap intervals, generating various scores in addition to the total number of taps produced within a specified time. Also, as noted earlier, computerized measures can facilitate group testing, not only by standardizing task administration but also through enhanced data management.

As computerized tests were being developed, it was apparent to researchers that test performance metrics could be synced with various physiological recording devices, permitting the simultaneous monitoring of behavioral responses and various physiological parameters. For example, eye movements or quantitative EEG measures can be recorded and correlated with cognitive task performance. While a number of researchers have simultaneously captured performance and physiological measures, this capability has not been generally integrated into clinical assessment approaches.

In addition to the potential advantages of computerized testing, there are also limitations. Computerized tests began to appear before computers and smartphones became part of everyday life. To some potential test takers, computers were new and unfamiliar devices, and published studies have shown that familiarity with computers affects performance (Iverson, Brooks, Ashton, Johnson, & Gualtieri, 2009; Johnson & Mihal, 1973). A major limitation for neuropsychology is that currently available systems don't capture spoken language; the assessment of language skills and verbal memory is an important part of a clinical neuropsychological evaluation. The most important thing a neuropsychological test battery has to do is to help the clinician answer the referral question. In most cases, addressing referral issues requires an assessment of skills involving language. While the issues of device familiarity and language assessment are important, the extent to which they will remain limitations for computerized testing will diminish with time. Today, computers in various forms are integrated into our day-to-day lives, and the generation growing up will likely expect that things be done by computer and would be somewhat surprised if someone put a blindfold on them and asked them to do the Tactual Performance Test. The integration of language into computerized testing is likely to occur sooner rather than later, with improved speech recognition engines and developing technologies surrounding virtual reality.

Nevertheless, one can anticipate that humans will be central to the assessment process for a long time. The clinical interview is still a critical aspect of the neuropsychological evaluation, and at present, the human is still the best expert system for putting the pieces together and developing the clinical impressions needed to address referral issues. Also, the issue of computerized versus traditional assessment does not have to be an either/or proposition; the two methods can augment each other. However, it seems reasonable to say that, until now, computers have been underutilized with respect to their potential contribution to neuropsychology. Computers have the potential to streamline the basic clerical tasks associated with test administration as well as substantially enhance the information than can be obtained during the process of patient assessment.

## Standards for Computerized Testing

Over time, standards for using computers to assess cognitive functioning have appeared. The standards have fallen into two general categories: specifying requirements related to the standardization and implementation of specific test systems, and providing general principles related to the use of computers in assessment. While there are a number of core principles, standards are not static and need to evolve with technology.

In the 1980s, as computerized testing was developing within DoD, it became evident that computers had both advantages and limitations as testing devices. While using computers opened up a range of possibilities in the types of tests that could be administered and for the development of alternate forms, a number of technical issues had to be addressed, especially for achieving highly accurate response timing at the millisecond level. Adding a delay loop into the program did not produce highly accurate timing and early computer clocks were not always reliable. Requirements emerged within DoD laboratories, not as formal documents, but as a means to both standardize administration and also to achieve accurate response time measurement. These informal efforts coalesced with the work done to develop the UTCPAB (discussed above) and were spelled out in detail by a NATO working group whose goal was to increase the comparability of data collected at various research laboratories (Kane & Kay, 1992). The working group, the Advisory Group for Aerospace Research and Development, produced a monograph describing a carefully selected set of measures, along with details related to stimulus characteristics and device parameters, subject orientation and placement, psychometric properties for individual test measures, experimental design, and data management (Santucci et al., 1989). The tests developed by the group were called the AGARD-STRES (Advisory Group for Aerospace Research and Development-Standardized Test for Research with Environmental Stressor) battery, and the specific standards that were developed applied to the seven tests that made up the system. While aspects of the standards were specific to a particular group of tests, this was one of the first times, if not the first time, specific technical and administration standards were applied for a computerized test battery to be adopted across different research laboratories.

With the development of computerized testing instruments, suggested standards for their use began to appear (Green, Bock, Humphreys, Linn, & Reckase, 1984; Groth-Mamat & Schumaker, 1989; Hofer, 1985). The most recent publication of standards for computerized testing was a joint American Academy of Clinical Neuropsychology and National Academy of Neuropsychology (AACN-NAN) position statement that was published in the *Archives of Clinical Neuropsychology* (Bauer et al., 2012). The various standards addressed common areas of concern. In part, the proposed standards underscored the concept that tests, no matter how they are administered, must meet requirements for reliability and validity. The other areas addressed included the requirement that test manuals provide information regarding the intended use of the test along and user qualifications. The standards also noted the fact that tests may change when the mode of administration or the platform on which it operates changes, and that there may need to be either separate norms or evidence of equivalency that support the use of previously collected norms. Standards required that the appropriateness and usability of the interface between the patient and the testing device be addressed, along with the robustness of the system and issues of test and data security.

Kane and Kay (1992), while not delineating standards as such, outlined an approach to reviewing computerized tests. They noted that there were two fundamental categories of information that needed to be addressed when assessing computerized instruments: psychometric and technical. The tests and batteries included in their paper were reviewed under the following headings: Background; Hardware Requirements and Subject Interface; Tasks Included; Test Administration; Test Presentation, Parameter Modification, and Alternate Forms; Data Output; Norms; and Validity Studies. They included in their review how tests approached issues of capturing response times, controlling stimulus presentation, and the use of peripheral devices. Cernich and colleagues (Cernich, Brennana, Baker, & Bleiberg, 2007), in updating the issues addressed by Kane and Kay (1992), also discussed issues related to Internet based test systems and the effect of operating systems. Patient privacy issues, underscored by HIPAA, demand strict attention to data security. The core point relating to standards was made by Kane and Kay in 1992: computerized tests have to be evaluated technically as well as psychometrically. Test developers have to appreciate technical issues in developing their test systems, understand the capabilities and limitations of their systems, and communicate them clearly to the user.

## Emerging Trends in Neuropsychological Assessment and Technology

Neuropsychologists have made much less progress than would be expected in comparison to other clinical neuroscientists in adopting technology. Decades ago, Meehl (1987) called for clinical psychologists to embrace the technological advances prevalent in our society. A decade after Meehl, Sternberg (1997) described the discrepancy between progress in cognitive assessment measures like the Wechsler scales and progress in other areas of technology. Sternberg Sternberg noted that the standardized tests in use when he wrote his paper had changed only slightly from when they were originally developed and contrasted the lack of development in testing to the dramatic changes in technology that had occurred in other areas. He observed that psychology was using measures whose origins were from the era of the black-and-white television, vinyl records, rotary-dial telephones, and the first commercial computers made in the United States (i.e. UNIVAC I).

At the same time that Sternberg was describing the discrepancy between progress in cognitive assessment measures and progress in other areas of technology, Dodrill (1997) was contending that neuropsychologists had made much less progress than would be expected in both absolute terms and in comparison with the progress made in other clinical neurosciences. Clinical neuropsychologists still use many of the same tests that they used 50 years ago. (If neuroradiologists were this slow in technological development, then they would still be limited to pneumo-encephalograms and radioisotope brain scans—procedures that are considered primeval by current neuroradiological standards.) Furthermore, advances in neuropsychological assessment have resulted in new tests that are by no means conceptually or substantively better than the old ones. The full scope of issues raised by Dodrill (1997) became more pronounced when he compared progress in clinical neuropsychology to that in other neurosciences. For example, clinical neuropsychologists have historically been called upon to identify focal brain lesions. When one compares clinical neuropsychology's progress with that of clinical neurology, it is apparent that, while the difference may not have been that great prior the appearance of computerized tomographic (CT) scanning (in the 1970s), the advances since then (e.g., magnetic resonance imaging) have given clinical neurologists a dramatic edge.

## CHANGING ROLE OF NEUROPSYCHOLOGISTS

In addition to serving as an example of progress in neurology and the clinical neurosciences, neuroimaging changed the referral questions that clinical neuropsychologists were asked. By the 1990s, neuropsychologists experienced a shift in referrals from lesion localization to assessment of everyday functioning (Sbordone & Long, 1996). With the advent and development of advanced technologies in the clinical neurosciences, there was decreased need for neuropsychological assessments to localize lesions and an increased need for neuropsychologists to describe behavioral manifestations of neurological disorders. Clinical neuropsychologists were increasingly being asked to make prescriptive statements about everyday functioning (Sbordone & Long, 1996).

## ECOLOGICAL VALIDITY

The changing role of neuropsychologists has also resulted in increased emphasis upon the ecological validity of neuropsychological instruments (Franzen & Wilhelm, 1996). An unfortunate limitation for neuropsychologists interested in assessing everyday functioning has been the lack of definitional specificity of the term *ecological validity* (Franzen & Wilhelm, 1996). Early attempts to define ecological validity for neuropsychological assessment emphasized the functional and predictive relation between a patient's performance on a set of neuropsychological tests and the patient's behavior in everyday life. Hence, an ecologically valid neuropsychological measure has characteristics similar to a naturally occurring behavior and can predict everyday function (Sbordone, 1996). Franzen and Wilhelm (1996) refined the definition of ecological validity for neuropsychological assessment through an emphasis upon two requirements: 1) veridicality, which means the participant's performance on a construct-driven measure should predict some feature(s) of the participant's day-to-day functioning (e.g., vocational status); and 2) verisimilitude, which means the requirements of a neuropsychological measure and the testing conditions resemble requirements found in a participant's activities of daily living.

### Verisimilitude

According to Franzen and Wilhelm (1996), a neuropsychological test with verisimilitude is one with task demands and testing conditions that resemble the demands found in a person's everyday activities. Verisimilitude is similar to face validity, in that it describes the "topographical similarity" (i.e., theoretical relation) between the neuropsychological test and the skills required for successful praxes in the natural environment (Franzen, 2000). While the task demands of learning and recalling a word list has "theoretical" similarity to the sorts of tasks that people perform in their everyday lives, the actual activities found in neuropsychological testing may be more representative of laboratory experiments than everyday activities. Moreover, most neuropsychological assessments present stimuli (e.g., words, numbers, and colors) at a controlled rate in a setting that is typically free from distractions. Also, patients often have repeated opportunities to learn the target stimuli (e.g., learning wordlists on the California Verbal Learning Test [CVLT]). While this level of administrative control results in reliability and internal validity, it may underestimate the impact of a patient's cognitive difficulties in everyday life or overestimate functional difficulties (e.g., the patient may use compensatory strategies in everyday life). Verisimilitude means that the measure resembles a task the patient performs in everyday life and that the test maintains the relationship between task demands and the prediction of real-world behavior (Spooner & Pachana, 2006). Early discussions of verisimilitude in neuropsychology emphasized that the technologies current to the time could not replicate the environment in which the behavior of interest would ultimately take place (Goldstein, 1996).

Most neuropsychological assessments in use today have not yet been validated with respect to real-world functioning (Rabin, Burton, & Barr, 2007). There are a few examples of neuropsychological assessments that emphasize verisimilitude in approximating cognitive constructs: attention (e.g., the Test of Everyday Attention; Robertson, Ward, Ridgeway, & Nimmo-Smith, 1996), executive function (e.g., the Behavioral Assessment of the Dysexecutive Syndrome; Wilson, Alderman, Burgess, Emslie, & Evans, 1996), memory (e.g., the Rivermead Behavioral Memory Test; Wilson, Cockburn, & Baddeley, 1985), and prospective memory (e.g., Cambridge Test of Prospective Memory; Wilson et al., 2005). While these tests were developed with ecological validity in mind, they are construct-driven tests used for identifying "functional" abilities that do not directly assess behavior in more life-like contexts. (Chaytor & Schmitter-Edgecombe, 2003).

## Veridicality

Franzen and Wilhelm (1996) also emphasized veridicality, which is the need to develop and administer tests in a way that the person's performance predicts some aspect of everyday functioning. Unfortunately, little is known about how well neuropsychological tests predict everyday behaviors. Moreover, logging a person's everyday functioning in a psychometrically reliable and valid manner presents difficulties. That said, there have been studies that are more correlational (Dunn, Searight, Grisso, Margolis, & Gibbons, 1990). These studies have found weak to moderate relations between neuropsychological test data and self-report information. Wen, Boone, and Kim (2006) reported a "weak" association between neuropsychological test performance and work capacity. According to Guilmette and Kastner (1996), underperformance on neuropsychological assessments is a modest predictor of vocational functioning in clinical groups. While deficits noted in test performance may relate to work failure, strengths identified during testing have a weaker association with occupational success.

While these correlational approaches offer some insight into everyday functioning, direct parallels between the demands found on neuropsychological tests and functional performance are often not evident (Makatura, Lam, Leahy, Castillo, & Kalpakjian, 1999; Wilson, 1993; Wilson, Cockburn, Baddeley, & Hiorns, 1989).

### VIRTUAL REALITY FOR NEUROPSYCHOLOGICAL ASSESSMENT

Virtual environments (VEs) are increasingly considered as potential aids in enhancing the ecological validity of neuropsychological assessments (Campbell et al., 2009; Parsons, 2011, 2015; Parsons, Carlew, Magtoto, & Stonecipher, 2015; Renison, Ponsford, Testa, Richardson, & Brownfield, 2012; Schultheis, Himelstein, & Rizzo, 2002). Given that VEs represent a special case of computerized neuropsychological assessment devices (Bauer et al., 2012; Schatz & Browndyke, 2002), they have enhanced computational capacities for administration efficiency, stimulus presentation, automated logging of responses, and data analytic processing. Since VEs allow for precise presentation and control of dynamic perceptual stimuli, they can provide ecologically valid assessments that combine the control and rigor of laboratory measures with a simulation that reflects real-life situations (Bohil, Alicea, & Biocca, 2011). Additionally, the enhanced computation power allows for increased accuracy in the recording of neurobehavioral responses in a perceptual environmental that systematically presents complex stimuli. Such simulation technology appears to be distinctively suited for the development of ecologically valid environments, in which three-dimensional objects are presented in a consistent and precise manner (Schultheis et al., 2002). VE-based neuropsychological assessments can provide a balance between naturalistic observation and the need for exacting control over key variables (Campbell et al., 2009). Importantly, the development of virtual environments is not meant to replace neuropsychologist involvement, but rather to augment the neuropsychological assessment to enhance predictive ability. To dismiss the neuropsychologist from the neuropsychological assessment would be to sacrifice valuable qualitative observations. In summary, VE-based neuropsychological assessments allow for real-time measurement of multiple neuropsychological abilities in order to assess complex sets of skills and behaviors that may more closely resemble real-world functional abilities (Matheis et al., 2007).

## Computerized Testing and the FDA

In 2011, the Food and Drug Administration (FDA) indicated its intention to view computer-administered neurocognitive tests as medical devices. Tests developed for computer or adapted for computer with specific computer-enhanced capabilities are to be considered Class II devices. The implications of this viewpoint going forward are not, as yet, entirely clear. In one sense, it is not surprising that the FDA would be concerned about computerized cognitive tests. Many people are capable of programming tasks and then marketing them as tests to assess, or as methods to improve, brain function. However, the same can be said of tasks that are administered through traditional means, and the burden remains on the test developer to adhere to psychometric standards and to address technical standards and limitations regarding their products with or without the FDA. Nevertheless, the ease of distributing various computer programs to the public over the Internet likely requires some mechanism for the regulation and control of computerized neurocognitive assessment software. It is not possible to ascertain the number of test publishers who have made application to the FDA for approval of their automated testing devices. However, as of this writing, the ANAM battery used by DoD has attained FDA clearance through the 510(k) process as an instrument for assessing cognitive functioning (https://www.accessdata.fda.gov/cdrh_docs/pdf15/K150154.pdf). The Defense Automated Neurobehavioral Assessment (DANA) received FDA 510(k) clearance as a system for assessing reaction time (http://www.accessdata.fda.gov/cdrh_docs/pdf14/k141865.pdf). Cognivue's Cognitive Assessment Tool received FDA de novo clearance as a computerized cognitive assessment aid http://www.accessdata.fda.gov/cdrh_docs/pdf13/den130033.pdf. How the FDA approaches its definition of automated neuropsychological tests as medical devices and the response of developers and users will affect the implementation and development of computerized testing in the future. It is important that the legitimate concerns of the FDA do not impede the ability to modernize and enhance testing approaches, because modernization is needed to augment the information that can be obtained from testing and to keep pace with rapidly changing technology.

## Computational Neuropsychology and Machine Learning

In addition to augmenting test administration, technology also has a large role to play in enhancing test interpretation and the predictions that can be made from test data related to a patient's clinical presentation and functional capabilities. Many terms and methods are related to the concept of enhancing classification and prediction by defining patterns identified from large data sets. The methods for doing this can be highly structured, making use of various statistical relationships, or involve unstructured data mining aimed at identifying underlying patterns. In many cases, neuropsychologists are not asked to make medical or neurological diagnoses but to provide data about a patient's neurocognitive status. In other cases, the pattern of deficits obtained during a neuropsychological evaluation, along with historical data, may make some types of underlying neurological conditions more likely than others. Neuropsychologists are also asked to make predictions from their test data about what an individual can and cannot do. The ability of neuropsychologists to identify patterns related to diagnoses and the prediction of important aspects of day-to-day function would be substantially enhanced by emulating efforts in other fields to systematically compile large data sets and to apply modern data analytic and machine-learning methods to enhance both diagnosis and prediction. Such data sets might also help in addressing vexing issues like how to control for cultural influences on test data so as not to overdiagnose potential problem areas or to miss impairment that may be present. Efforts have been put in place to aggregate data. The Alzheimer's Disease Neuroimaging Initiative (ADNI) collects standardized cognitive test scores along with neuroimaging and other data. The NIH has established Common Data Elements to allow data to be compiled for comparison across studies. Unfortunately, the effort needed to bring modern data analysis methods to neuropsychology has yet to be undertaken.

## Plan for Book and Chapter Summaries

This book discusses the benefits of technological adaptation in neuropsychological assessment. A common theme among neuropsychologists reflecting on the state of the discipline is that neuropsychologists have been slow to adjust to the impact of technology on their profession (Bigler, 2013; Bilder, 2011; Dodrill, 1999). Although neuropsychologists are ardent when emphasizing neuropsychology's role as a science, its technology is not progressing in pace with other science-based technologies. Instead, neuropsychological test developers tend to make cosmetic changes to paper-and-pencil assessments and emphasize improved psychometric properties (e.g., updated norms, improved subtest and composite reliability). An unfortunate limitation is that, without the technological advances found in neuroinformatics and computer-adaptive testing, neuropsychological test developers updating their instruments fail to account for back-compatibility issues that may invalidate clinical interpretations (Loring & Bauer, 2010).

Part I, Beyond Paper-and-Pencil Assessment, discusses the movement beyond paper-and-pencil testing to more technologically advanced platforms. First, Phillip Schatz offers an overview of the move from paper-based to computer-based assessments of human cognitive performance. He describes a need for validation research as we move to the new frontier of tablet-based assessment. In the next chapter, Maria Schultheis discusses various technologies that can be used for functionally relevant neuropsychological assessment. This is followed by a chapter describing a study by Diana Jovanovski and Konstantine Zakzanis in which they assessed whether a novel virtual reality task of executive functioning can be used as an appropriate outcome measure of the effectiveness and generalization of an executive function treatment program. Part I concludes with Robert Kane and Munroe Cullum's discussion of teleneuropsychology's potential for Internet-based assessment and home-based care.

Part II, Domain- and Scenario-Based Assessment, covers novel approaches that allow neuropsychologists to assess patients using innovative technologies. First, Unai Diaz describes advances in neuropsychological assessment of attention and a move from computerized continuous performance tests to a virtual classroom environment. Specific focus is placed upon validation of this novel approach. In the next two chapters, Parsons and colleagues discuss the development of virtual shopping tasks and their potential for assessment of multitasking and prospective memory. This is followed by a discussion of relevant military virtual environments for neuropsychological assessment. The next chapter covers Gaen Plancher and Pascale Piolino's novel work using virtual reality environments for assessment of episodic memory in normal and pathological aging. Finally, two chapters from Maureen Schmitter-Edgecombe's lab review smart environment technologies for monitoring and assessing everyday functioning.

Part III, Integrating Cognitive Assessment with Biological Metrics, examines how metrics from neuropsychological assessment can be combined with neurobiological metrics. In the first chapter, Anthony Chen looks at the use of neuroimaging data and computer games in neuropsychological rehabilitation. Next, Erin Bigler's chapter discusses the ways in which neuroimaging data can be incorporated into neuropsychological measures. Thomas Quartierri's chapter on multimodal assessment of neuropsychiatric disorders explores the use of interactive classifiers. Part III concludes with Michael Posner's chapter on the integration of technologies into the study of attentional networks.

Part IV, Conclusions, contains a discussion of the ethical and methodological considerations needed for adopting advanced technologies for neuropsychological assessment. The chapter by Shane Bush and Phillip Schatz focuses on the ethical implications. In the final chapter, Thomas Parsons and Robert Kane discuss the prospects for computational neuropsychology and the importance of integrating technology into neuropsychology.

## References

Bauer, R. M., Iverson, G. L., Cernich, A. N., Binder, L. M., Ruff, R. M., & Naugle, R. I. (2012). Computerized neuropsychological assessment devices: Joint position paper of the American Academy of Clinical Neuropsychology and the National Academy of Neuropsychology. *Archives of Clinical Neuropsychology, 27*, 362–373.

Bigler, E. D. (2013). Neuroimaging biomarkers in mild traumatic head injury (mTBI). *Neuropsychology Review, 23*(3), 169–209.

Bilder, R. M. (2011). Neuropsychology 3.0: Evidence-based science and practice. *Journal of the International Neuropsychological Society, 17*(1), 7–13.

Bohil, C. J., Alicea, B., & Biocca, F. A. (2011). Virtual reality in neuroscience research and therapy. *National Review of Neurosciences, 12*(12), 752–762. doi:10.1038/nrn3122.

Campbell, Z., Zakzanis, K. K., Jovanovski, D., Joordens, S., Marz, R., & Graham, S. J. (2009). Utilising virtual reality to improve the ecological validity of clinical neuropsychology: An fMRI case study elucidating the neural basis of planning by comparing the Tower of London with a three-dimensional navigation task. *Applied Neuropsychology, 16,* 295–306.

Cernich, A. N., Brennana, D. M., Baker, L. M., & Bleiberg, J. (2007). Sources of error in computerized neuropsychological assessment. *Archives of Clinical Neuropsychology, 22S,* S39–S48.

Chaytor, N., & Schmitter-Edgecombe, M. (2003). The ecological validity of neuropsychological tests: A review of the literature on everyday cognitive skills. *Neuropsychology Review, 13*(4), 181–197.

Dodrill, C. B. (1997). Myths of neuropsychology. *The Clinical Neuropsychologist, 11,* 1–17.

Dodrill, C. B. (1999). Myths of neuropsychology: Further considerations. *The Clinical Neuropsychologist, 13*(4), 562–572.

Dunn, E. J., Searight, H. R., Grisso, T., Margolis, R. B., & Gibbons, J. L. (1990). The relation of the Halstead-Reitan Neuropsychological Battery to functional daily living skills in geriatric patients. *Archives of Clinical Neuropsychology, 5*(2), 103–117.

Englund, C. E., Reeves, D. L., Shingledecker, C. A., Thorne, D. R., Wilson, K. P., & Hegge, F. W. (1987). *The Unified Tri-Service Cognitive Performance Assessment Battery (UTC-PAB): I. Design and specification of the battery* (Report No. NHRC-TR-87-10). Naval Health Research Center, San Diego, CA.

Erlanger, D., Kaushik, T., Broshek, D., Freeman, J., Feldman, D., & Festa, J. (2002). Development and validation of a web-based screening tool for monitoring cognitive status. *Journal of Head Trauma Rehabilitation, 17*(5), 458–476.

Franzen, M. D. (2000). *Reliability and validity in neuropsychological assessment.* New York: Springer.

Franzen, M. D., & Wilhelm, K. L. (1996). Conceptual foundations of ecological validity in neuropsychological assessment. In R. J. Sbordone & C. J. Long (Eds.), *Ecological validity of neuropsychological testing* (pp. 91–112). Delray Beach, FL: Gr Press/St. Lucie Press, Inc.

Goldstein, G. (1996). Functional considerations in neuropsychology. In R. J. Sbordone & C. J. Long (Eds.), *Ecological validity of neuropsychological testing* (pp. 75–89). Delray Beach, FL: Gr Press/St. Lucie Press, Inc.

Green, B. F., Bock, R. D., Humphreys, L. G., Linn, R. L., & Reckase, M. D. (1984). Technical guidelines for assessing computerized adaptive tests. *Journal of Educational Measurement, 21*(4), 347–360.

Groth-Mamat, G., & Schumaker, J. (1989). Computer-based psychological testing: Issues and guidelines. *American Journal of Orthopsychiatry, 59*(2), 257–263.

Guilmette, T. J., & Kastner, M. P. (1996). The prediction of vocational functioning from neuropsychological data. In R. J. Sbordone & C. J. Long (Eds.), *Ecological validity of neuropsychological testing* (pp. 387–411). Delray Beach, FL: Gr Press/St. Lucie Press, Inc.

Heaton, R. K. (2003). *Wisconsin Card Sorting Test computer version 4.0.* Odessa, FL: Psychological Assessment Resources.

Hegge, F. W., Reeves, D. L., Poole, D. P., & Thorne, D. R. (1985). *The Unified Tri-Service Cognitive Performance Assessment Battery (UTC-PAB), II: Hardware/software design and specification.* Ft. Detrick, MD: Medical Research and Development Command.

Hofer, P. J. (1985). Developing standards for computerized psychological testing. *Computers in Human Behavior, 1,* 301–315.

ImPact https://impacttest.com/research/.

Iverson, G. L., Brooks, B. L., Ashton, V. L., Johnson, L. G., & Gualtieri, C. T. (2009). Does familiarity with computers affect computeized neuropsychological test performance? *Journal of Clinical and Experimental Neuropsychology, 31,* 594–604.

Johnson, J. H., & Mihal, W. L. (1973). The performance of blacks and whites in computerized versus manual testing enviroments. *American Psychologist, 28,* 694–699.

Kane, R. L., & Kay, G. G. (1992). Computerized assessment in neuropsychology: A review of tests and test batteries. *Neuropsychol Review, 3*(1), 1–117.

Kane, R., & Kay, G. G. (1997). Computer applications in neuropsychological assessment. In G. Goldstein & T. Incagnoli (Eds.), *Contemporary approaches to neuropsychological assessment* (Vol. 1, pp. 359–392). New York: Plenum.

Kane, R. L., & Reeves, D. L. (1997). Computerized test batteries. In A. M. Horton, D. Wedding, & J. Webster (Eds.), *The neuropsychology handbook* (2nd ed., Vol. 1). New York: Springer: New York.

Kane, R. L., Short, P., Sipes, W., & Flynn, C. F. (2005). Development and validation of the Spaceflight Cognitive Assessment Tool for Windows (WinSCAT). *Aviat Space Environ Med, 76*(6, Suppl.), B183–B191.

Kay, G. G. (1995). *CogScreen: Aeromedical edition.* St. Petersburg: Cognitive Research, Inc.

Larrabee, G. J., & Crook, T. (1988). A computerized everyday memory battery for assessing treatment effects. *Psychopharmacology Bulletin, 24*(4), 695–697.

Letz, R., & Baker, E. L. (1988). *Neurobehavioral Evaluation System 2: Users manual (Version 4.2).* Winchester, MA: Neurobehavioral Systems.

Loring, D. W., & Bauer, R. M. (2010). Testing the limits: Cautions and concerns regarding the new Wechsler IQ and memory scales. *Neurology, 74*(8), 685–690.

Makatura, T. J., Lam, C. S., Leahy, B. J., Castillo, M. T., & Kalpakjian, C. Z. (1999). Standardized memory tests and the appraisal of everyday memory. *Brain Injury, 13*(5), 355–367.

Matheis, R. J., Schultheis, M. T., Tiersky, L. A., DeLuca, J., Milis, S. R., & Rizzo, A. (2007). Is learning and memory different in a virtual environment? *Clinical Neuropsychology, 21,* 146–161.

Meehl, P. E. (1987). Theory and practice: reflections of an academic clinician. In E. F. Bourg, R. J. Bent, J. E. Callan, N. F. Jones, J. McHolland, G. Stricker (Eds.), Standards and evaluation in the education and training of professional psychologists: Knowledge, attitudes, and skills (pp. 7–23). Transcript Press, ix, 163 pp.

PAR, https://www.pariconnect.com/.

Parsons, T. D. (2011). Neuropsychological assessments using virtual environments: Enhanced assessment technology for improving ecological validity. *Advanced computational intelligence paradigms in healthcare* (Vol. 6, pp. 271–289). Berlin: Springer.

Parsons, T. D. (2015). Virtual reality for enhanced ecological validity and experimental control in clinical, affective, and social neurosciences. *Frontiers in Human Neuroscience, 9,* 1–19.

Parsons, T. D., Carlew, A. R., Magtoto, J., & Stonecipher, K. (2015). The potential of function-led virtual environments for ecologically valid measures of executive function
in experimental and clinical neuropsychology. *Neuropsychological Rehabilitation,*
*11,* 1–31.

Pearson, Q-Interactive & Q-Global, http://www.helloq.com/.

Perez, W. A., Masline, P. J., Ramsey, E. G., & Urban, K. E. (1987). *Unified Tri-Services*
*Cognitive Performance Assessment Battery: Review and methodology* (AAMRL-TR-
87-007). Armstrong Aerospace Medical Research Laboratory, Wright-Patterson Air
Force Base, Dayton, OH.

Rabin, L. A., Burton, L. A., & Barr, W. B. (2007). Utilization rates of ecologically oriented
instruments among clinical neuropsychologists. *The Clinical Neuropsychologist,*
*21*(5), 727–743.

Reeves, D.L, Winter, K., Bleiberg J, & Kane R.L. (2007). ANAM Genogram: Historical perspectives, description, and current endeavors. *Archives of Clinical Neuropsychology,*
*22S,* S15–S37.

Reitan, R. M., & Wolfson, D. (1985). *The Halstead-Reitan Neuropsychological Test*
*Battery: Theory and clinical interpretation.* Tucson, AZ: Neuropsychology Press.

Renison, B., Ponsford, J., Testa, R., Richardson, B., & Brownfield, K. (2012). The ecological and construct validity of a newly developed measure of executive function: The
Virtual Library Task. *Journal of the International Neuropsychological Society, 18,*
440–450.

Robertson, I. H., Ward, T., Ridgeway, V., & Nimmo-Smith, I. A. N. (1996). The structure of
normal human attention: The Test of Everyday Attention. *Journal of the International*
*Neuropsychological Society, 2*(6), 525–534.

Santucci, G., Farmer, E., Grissett, J., Wetherell, A., Boer, L., Gotters, K., . . . Wilson, G. (1989).
*AGARDograph #308, human performance assessment methods* (92-835-0510-7).
North Atlantic Treaty Organization Advisory Group for Aerospace Research and
Development, Working Group 12, Seine, France.

Sbordone, R. J. (1996). Some critical isses for the neuropsychologist. In R. J. Sbordone &
C. J. Long (Eds.), *Ecological validity of neuropsychological testing* (pp. 15–41). Delray
Beach, FL: Gr Press/ St Lucie Press.

Sbordone, R. J., & Long, C. J. (Eds.). (1996). *Ecological validity of neuropsychological testing.*
Gr. Press/St Lucie Press.

Schatz, P., & Browndyke, J. (2002). Applications of computer-based neuropsychological
assessment. *Journal of Head Trauma Rehabilitation, 17,* 395–410.

Schultheis, M. T., Himelstein, J., & Rizzo, A. A. (2002). Virtual reality and neuropsychology: Upgrading the current tools. *Journal of Head Trauma Rehabilitation, 17,* 378–394.

Spooner, D. M., & Pachana, N. A. (2006). Ecological validity in neuropsychological
assessment: A case for greater consideration in research with neurologically intact
populations. *Archives of Clinical Neuropsychology, 21*(4), 327–337.

Sternberg, R. J. (1997). Intelligence and lifelong learning: What's new and how can we use
it? *American Psychologist, 52,* 1134–1139.

Toolbox, N. (n/d). Retrieved from http://www.nihtoolbox.org/

Weintraub, S., Dickmen, S. S., Heaton, R. K., Tulsky, D. S., Zelazo, P. D., Slotkin, J., . . .
Gershon, R. (2014). The cognition battery of the NIH Toolbox for assessment of

neurological and behavioral function: Validation in an adult sample. *Journal of the International Neuropsychological Society, 20*(6), 567–578.

Wen, J. H., Boone, K., & Kim, K. (2006). Ecological validity of neuropsychological assessment and perceived employability. *Journal of Clinical and Experimental Neuropsychology, 28*(8), 1423–1434.

Wilson, B. A. (1993). Ecological validity of neuropsychological assessment: Do neuropsychological indexes predict performance in everyday activities? *Applied and Preventive Psychology, 2*(4), 209–215.

Wilson, B. A., Alderman, N., Burgess, P. W., Emslie, H., & Evans, J. (1996). *Behavioural Assessment of the Dysexecutive Syndrome.* Bury St. Edmunds: Thames Valley Test Company, London.

Wilson, B. A., Cockburn, J., & Baddeley, A. (1985). *The Rivermead Behavioural Memory Test.* Titchfield, UK: Thames Valley Test Company.

Wilson, B. A., Cockburn, J., Baddeley, A., & Hiorns, R. (1989). The development and validation of a test battery for detecting and monitoring everyday memory problems. *Journal of Clinical and Experimental Neuropsychology, 11,* 855–870.

Wilson, B. A., Shiel, A., Foley, J., Emslie, H., Groot, Y., Hawkins, K., & Watson, P. (2005). *Cambridge Test of Prospective Memory (CAMPROMPT).* San Antonio: Pearson Assessment.

# PART II

# Beyond Paper-and-Pencil Assessment

# Computer-Based Assessment: Current Status and Next Steps

Philip Schatz

Since the 1950s, academic and researchers have examined artificial intelligence and the use of computers for assistance with, or automation of, data collection (Schatz & Browndyke, 2002). In the ensuing 60+ years, considerable technological growth has occurred. Perhaps most influential in the field of clinical psychology was the introduction of the personal computer in the 1980s, which allowed individuals to have computing devices in the home and/or office. Over the past 30 years, the percentage of U.S. households with a computer has dramatically increased, from 8.2% in 1984, to 42% in 1998, to 52% in 2000, to 84% in 2013 (File & Ryan, 2014; Newburger, 2001). As of 2014, approximately 50% of households have a tablet device (such as an iPad) or an e-reader (such as a Kindle or Nook) and approximately 28% of adults age 18 and older have read an e-book in the past year (up from 17% in 2011) (Zickuhr & Rainie, 2014).

However, despite widespread ownership of computing devices, in clinical practice, use of technology is not as commonplace. While the vast majority of clinical psychologists have used e-mail or Internet searches in their clinical practice, in a 2009 survey, only 47% had used computerized test administration software, 60% had used a computerized test-scoring software, and 54% had used a computerized test interpretation software (McMinn, Bearse, Heyne, Smithberg, & Erb, 2011), and only 20% (test administration), 29% (test scoring), and 22% (test interpretation) had used these technologies "fairly often" or "very often." Even as recently as 2009, in a report of an American Psychological Association (APA) Presidential Task Force on Technology, discussion of the role of technology in the future of psychology practice was limited to the use of electronic health records (in the context of documenting service delivery and reimbursement), expanding ways for streamlining assessments and service delivery, and training psychologists to use and integrate technologies (APA, 2009). Moreover, the most recent (2010) version the APA Ethics Code (APA, 2010) does not specifically mention the term *computer(s)* but does clarify that the Code applies to "activities across a variety of contexts, such as . . . Internet, and other electronic transmissions" (Introduction), and that "psychologists planning to provide services, teach, or conduct research involving . . . techniques or technologies new to them undertake relevant education, training, supervised experience, consultation, or study" (2.01, Boundaries of Competence).

This chapter reviews the history and current status of computer-based assessment, focusing on the growth of computer-based assessment, the introduction of Internet-based and tablet-based assessment systems, issues related to timing accuracy, and the ongoing need for validation and updated norming for technology-based assessment devices.

## The Growth of Computer-Based Assessment

The computerization of existing neuropsychological assessment measures is not a new phenomenon, with automated/computer-based versions of the Peabody Picture Vocabulary Test and Raven's Progressive Matrices first appearing in the 1970s (Space, 1975; Waterfall, 1979). With the Category Test and Wisconsin Card Sorting Test following suit, the APA convened a task force and ultimately published/established guidelines for computer-based tests and interpretation (APA, 1986). The guidelines distinguished among test developers, users, takers, and administrators, with test users being characterized by the choice of the test and interpretation of the results and test administrators being those who actually administer or supervise interaction with the test materials. Guidelines specific to developers focused on the degree of feedback provided about what would be expected in traditional testing formats (e.g., correct and incorrect responses, where appropriate) and on ensuring the accuracy of scoring, as well as on psychometric equivalence between computer-based and traditional versions.

Benefits of computer-based assessment include the ability to capture and engage the interest of the client, automated data collection and storage, the ability to measure multiple dimensions of performance (e.g., response latency) with greater accuracy than with a human observer (e.g., milliseconds), automated randomization of stimuli/trails, improved task efficiency (e.g., rapid change of font size for reading tasks, rapid modification of graphic materials), the ability to assess groups of individuals simultaneously, and decreased costs in terms of materials and personnel. These potential benefits are offset by limitations, in the form of decreased (or absence of) face-to-face interaction between the clinician and examinee, non-equivalent modes of assessment (as compared to traditional administration forms), limiting data collection to mouse or keyboard clicks, inability to present and/or collect information through verbal modalities, and the inability to easily terminate or modify the assessment.

## The Introduction of Internet-Based Measures

By the early 2000s, computers were used by approximately only 10% of clinical psychologists for the purposes of scoring test results, 4% for test administration, and 4% for interpretation (Camara, Nathan, & Puente, 2000). Forensic assessments appeared to be a specific application for computer-based test development, with the introduction of forced-choice symptom validity tests, such as the Test of Memory Malingering (TOMM), Victoria Symptom Validity Test (VSVT), Computerized Assessment of Response Bias (CARB), and the Word Memory Test (WMT), utilizing computer-based administration. During this same time period, commensurate with the increased popularity of the Internet, psychological testing administration began to take place via web-based assessment, with applications for assessment of concussion (Schatz & Zillmer, 2003) as well as general neuropsychological functioning (Gur et al., 2001). At that same time, the APA created an Internet Task Force, which ultimately reported on "Psychological Testing on the Internet: New Problems, Old Issues" (Naglieri et al., 2004), identifying issues related to test reliability, validity, administration, item security, and test-taker confidentiality, as well as making the distinction between the stand-alone administration of a "psychological test" and a more comprehensive "psychological assessment." Remote administration through Internet-based testing was recognized as violating a long-standing practice of not allowing patients to complete psychological test measures at home. In addition, variation in hardware configurations (computer age, monitor size) could affect accuracy of stimulus presentation and response-timing accuracy, as well as input accuracy (e.g., mouse versus trackball versus trackpad).

Despite the reservations about, and limitations of, computer-based and Internet-based assessment, there has been a rapid increase in the development of Internet-based measures, and the conversion of traditional paper-based measures to Internet-based measures. In the last few years, major test developers and publishers have released Internet-based portals providing access to widely used measures. Pearson's Q-Global system (Pearson, 2013a) is a web-based platform for test administration, scoring, and reporting. PAR's iConnect (PAR, 2012) is an online testing platform used to assign and administer assessments, to score results, to provide interpretive reports, and to track client data. MHS Online (MHS, 2015) provides an online platform that allows clinicians to administer, score, and generate reports. Together, these three services provide access to a variety of clinical assessment measures (see Box 2.1), for which there is a paucity of research establishing the equivalency of psychometric properties in comparison with their traditional forms.

BOX 2.1  Available Internet-Based Assessment Measures

**PEARSON Q-GLOBAL**

16PF® Fifth Edition

Basic Achievement Skills Inventory (BASI™)

Battery for Health Improvement 2 (BHI™ 2)

Beck Anxiety Inventory® (BAI®)

Beck Depression Inventory®–II (BDI®–II)

Beck Hopelessness Scale® (BHS®)

Beck Scale for Suicide Ideation® (BSS®)

Behavior Assessment System for Children, Second Edition (BASC-2™)

Brief Battery for Health Improvement 2 (BBHI™ 2)

Brief Symptom Inventory (BSI®)

Bruininks Motor Ability Test (BMAT)

Bruininks-Oseretsky Test of Motor Proficiency, Second Edition (BOT-2)

Career Assessment Inventory™

Campbell™ Interest and Skill Survey (CISS®)

Clinical Evaluation of Language Fundamentals®–Fifth Edition (CELF®-5)

Delis-Rating of Executive Function (D-REF)

Developmental Indicators for the Assessment of Learning™, Fourth Edition (DIAL™-4)

Expressive Vocabulary Test, Second Edition (EVT™-2)

General Ability Measure for Adults (GAMA®)

Kaufman Assessment Battery for Children, Second Edition (KABC™-II)

Millon® Adolescent Clinical Inventory (MACI™)

Millon® Adolescent Personality Inventory (MAPI™)

Millon® Behavioral Medicine Diagnostic (MBMD™)

Millon® Clinical Multiaxial Inventory-III (MCMI-III™)

Millon® Index of Personality Styles Revised (MIPS® Revised)

Millon® Pre-Adolescent Clinical Inventory (M-PACI™)

Minnesota Multiphasic Personality Inventory-2-RF® (MMPI-2-RF®)

Minnesota Multiphasic Personality Inventory®-Adolescent (MMPI®-A)

Pain Patient Profile (P-3®)

Parenting Relationship Questionnaire (PRQ)

Peabody Picture Vocabulary Test, Fourth Edition (PPVT™-4)

Sensory Profile™ 2

Symptom Checklist-90-Revised (SCL-90-R®)

Validity Indicator Profile (VIP®)

Wechsler Individual Achievement Test®–Third Edition (WIAT®-III)

Wechsler Intelligence Scale for Children®-Fifth Edition (WISC®-V)

Wechsler Preschool and Primary Scale of Intelligence™–Fourth Edition (WPPSI™-IV)

Woodcock Reading Mastery Tests, Third Edition (WRMT™-III)

**PARiCONNECT**

Adolescent Psychopathology Scale™ (APS™)

Behavior Rating Inventory of Executive Function® (BRIEF®)
Child and Adolescent Memory Profile™ (ChAMP™)
Clinical Assessment of Behavior™ (CAB™)
Clinical Assessment of Behavior™ Parent Extended Form (CAB™-PX)
Clinical Assessment of Depression™ (CAD™)
Eating Disorder Inventory™ (EDI-3™)
Emotional Disturbance Decision Tree™ (EDDT™)
Emotional Disturbance Decision Tree™–Parent Form (EDDT™-PF)
Eyberg Child Behavior Inventory™ (ECBI™)
Frontal Systems Behavior Scale™ (FrSBe™)
NEO™ Five Factor Inventory-3 (NEO™-FFI-3)
NEO™ Personality Inventory-3 (NEO™-PI-3)
Pediatric Behavior Rating Scale™ (PBRS™)
Personality Assessment Inventory™ (PAI®)
Reynolds Adaptable Intelligence Test™ (RAIT™)
Reynolds Adolescent Depression Scale, Second Edition (RADS-2™)
Reynolds Child Depression Scale™–Second Edition (RCDS™-2)
State-Trait Anger Expression Inventory-2™ (STAXI-2™)
Structured Inventory of Malingered Symptomatology™ (SIMS™)
Test of General Reasoning Ability™ (TOGRA™)
Vocabulary Assessment Scales–Expressive® (VAS-E®)
Vocabulary Assessment Scales–Receptive® (VAS-R®)

**MHS ONLINE**

Anger Regulation and Expression Scale™ (ARES™)
Autism Spectrum Rating Scales® (ASRS®)
Behavior Intervention Monitoring Assessment System™ (BIMAS™)
Comprehensive Executive Function Inventory™ (CEFI®)
Children's Depression Inventory, Second Edition® (CDI 2®)
Children's Organization Skills Scale™ (COSS™)
Conners 3rd Edition® (Conners 3®)
Conners Comprehensive Behavior Rating Scales® (Conners CBRS®)
Conners Early Childhood ™ (Conners EC™)
Emotional Quotient Inventory: Youth Version™ (EQ-i:YV™)
Family Assessment Measure–III™ (FAM-III™)
Jesness Inventory-Revised™ (JI-R™)
Multidimensional Anxiety Scale for Children, Second Edition™ (MASC 2™)
Paulhus Deception Scales™ (PDS™)
Profile of Mood States, Second Edition® (POMS 2®)

## Issues Related to Timing Accuracy

Issues related to timing accuracy of computers existed prior to the introduction of Internet-based assessment. As early as the late 1970s, researchers identified technical deficiencies arising from inaccurate timing procedures (Reed, 1979). Even for the simplest of stimulus-response paradigms, synchronization between the computer's core processor and the display (previously referred to as the "monitor") has some inherent delay/error in timing, which may be further magnified by the use of peripheral devices for input or response. Cernich and colleagues (Cernich, Brennana, Barker, & Bleiberg, 2007) summarized potential sources of systematic error in computer-based testing as coming from the system clock, monitor, and peripherals (see Box 2.2). All told, a single trial on a computer-based measure could contain 28–98 milliseconds (ms) of error. This may seem trivial in the context of documenting response time for more complex decision-making tasks (e.g., 0.5% to 2% error in a task requiring 5,000 ms). However, such timing error may represent a significant percentage of the total time required to complete a simple reaction time task (e.g., 11% to 39% error in a task requiring 250 ms).

Such potential sources of timing error may be magnified when computer-based measures are administered via the Internet. Test measures utilizing technologies like Flash and Java allow for "store and forward," in which the application or task is fully downloaded to the resident computer, stimuli are presented, response times and accuracy information are collected, and data are then uploaded or forwarded to the server (see Table 2.1). These measures are susceptible to the same types of timing error listed above. However, measures utilizing JavaScript or HTML5 perform all stimulus presentation and data collection at the level of the server, creating new potential sources of timing error. To best understand this distinction, consider a layer cake analogy, in which the "mother board" or core processor makes up the base layer. Above this layer is the operating system, such as Windows or Unix. Above this layer is the program, in the form of a Java applet or an installed program from a test manufacturer, assuming the program is running "resident" on the computer. Also at this level is the graphic user interface (GUI), which presents the actual pull-down menus, start button, etc., in the operating system. For tasks using the Internet for data collection, the Internet browser resides at this level, above which is the plug-in for Flash or Shockwave, or specific code interpretations, such as JavaScript or HTML5. Thus, the steps required for the computer to interpret code, display information, collect response data from peripherals, and report the data, may involve passing through several hierarchical layers, all of which may introduce potential timing error. Researchers have shown that timing accuracy for tasks programmed in Java (which runs at a lower "level") was better, relative to tasks programmed in Flash or Javascript (Eichstaedt, 2001; Schmidt, 2001).

Others (Schatz, Gibney, & Leitner, 2009) documented significant differences between Windows laptops versus desktop computers, specific programming languages (e.g., JavaScript versus resident applications), and timing intervals (e.g., 250, 500, 1,000, 10,000, and 29,000 ms; see Box 2.2). All three PCs were running Windows XP, with PC1 a Gateway Desktop, PC2 an IBM Lenova Desktop, and PC3 an HP Laptop. Differences were documented in timing accuracy between the three computers for all types of software, and across timing intervals on two

BOX 2.2 Potential Sources of Timing Error in Computer-Based Testing

**SYSTEM CLOCK (WINDOWS 95, 98, XP)**

Timing delays ranging from 10 to 55 ms

**MONITOR REFRESH RATES**

10 to 18 ms required for one screen refresh (dependent on Hertz, size, display type)

**KEYBOARDS AND PERIPHERAL INPUT DEVICES**

8 to 25 ms potential error (dependent on interface type, such as USB vs. serial port)

(Adapted from Cernich et al., 2007)

TABLE 2.1 Variation in Millisecond Accuracy in Microcomputers by Response Interval, Computer Type, and Software Type

Commercially available software

| Interval | PC1 | PC2 | PC3 |
|----------|-----|-----|-----|
| 250 ms | 49.54 (38.76) | 40.54 (24.75) | 59.11 (26.90) |
| 500 ms | 54.61 (37.11) | 43.64 (36.24) | 50.86 (24.34) |
| 1,000 ms | 48.93 (29.28) | 38.75 (21.50) | 43.32 (5.69) |
| 10,000 ms | 53.31 (33.67) | 53.43 (40.14) | 46.96 (21.61) |
| 29,000 ms | 35.54 (31.22) | 43.39 (35.87) | 42.93 (20.52) |

Computer: $F (2,409) = 1.09$, $p = .34$, partial $\eta^2 = .01$

Time: $F (4,409) = 2.00$, $p = .09$, partial $\eta^2 = .02$

Note: Numbers represent Mean(Standard Deviation)

Experiment-grade software

| Interval | PC1 | PC2 | PC3 |
|----------|-----|-----|-----|
| 250 ms | 39.85 (5.45) | 32.86 (2.73) | 43.21 (2.53) |
| 500 ms | 39.85 (5.45) | 32.86 (2.73) | 43.21 (2.53) |
| 1,000 ms | 40.22 (3.17) | 34.96 (0.84) | 43.14 (2.51) |
| 10,000 ms | 37.22 (2.62) | 29.43 (2.33) | 40.36 (2.42) |
| 29,000 ms | 34.11 (7.83) | 24.79 (2.54) | 33.07 (3.17) |

Computer: $F (2,401) = 314.34$, $p = .001$, partial $\eta^2 = .61$

Time: $F (4,401) = 87.07$, $p = .001$, partial $\eta^2 = .465$; 29k < 250, 500, 1k, 10k

JavaScript

| Interval | PC1 | PC2 | PC3 |
|----------|-----|-----|-----|
| 250 ms | 63.46 (5.66) | 70.18 (7.98) | 89.89 (5.92) |
| 500 ms | 63.68 (6.19) | 68.75 (7.59) | 89.86 (5.67) |
| 1,000 ms | 59.79 (5.07) | 71.07 (8.08) | 84.39 (14.12) |
| 10,000 ms | 60.14 (8.11) | 67.96 (5.92) | 90.18 (11.82) |
| 29,000 ms | 56.96 (7.15) | 62.29 (5.73) | 82.71 (5.17) |

Computer: $F (2,405) = 441.05$, $p = .001$, partial $\eta^2 = .69$

Time: $F (4,405) = 11.61$, $p = .001$, partial $\eta^2 = .10$; 29k < 250, 500, 1k, 10k of the three software types. With respect to software type, while timing error ranged from 25 to 100 ms across all three programs, overall error was lower for commercially available software and experiment-grade software. However, standard deviation was quite low and consistent for the experiment-grade software (3–8 ms) and JavaScript (5–10 ms) as compared to the commercially available software (5–39 ms). While these results apply only to simple reaction time trials, they have potentially significant implications for test results obtained on two different types of computers, as in the case of serial assessments. Clinicians need to use consistent presentation methods (screen sizes, refresh rates), on similar computers, with similar input devices, in order to ensure continuity across assessments.

## Controversies Related to Marketing and Intended End-Users

Using the area of sports concussion as an example, as computer-based assessment has become more common, various position papers and summary statements have addressed assessment-related issues. The first international conference on concussion in sport (Aubry et al., 2002) discussed computer-based testing platforms as having variable testing paradigms that were thought to overcome the practice effects seen in paper-and-pencil measures. By 2013, neuropsychological assessment was considered the "cornerstone" of concussion management, and computer-based neuropsychological screening measures were described as the "mainstay" of these assessments (McCrory et al., 2013). Since the introduction of computer-based neuropsychological screening measures for the purpose of assessment and management of sports-related concussion, their reliability, validity, and clinical utility have been debated in the scholarly literature (Broglio, Ferrara, Macciocchi, Baumgartner, & Elliott, 2007; Broglio, Macciocchi, & Ferrara, 2007; Collie, Maruff, McStephen, & Darby, 2003; Echemendia et al., 2012; Elbin, Schatz, & Covassin, 2011; Iverson, Lovell, & Collins, 2002; Iverson, Gaetz, Lovell, & Collins, 2005; Lau, Collins, & Lovell, 2011; Lovell, 2006; Mayers & Redick, 2012; Nakayama, Covassin, Schatz, Nogle, & Kovan, 2014; Randolph, 2011; Randolph, McCrea, & Barr, 2005, 2006; Resch et al., 2013; Schatz, 2009; Schatz, Kontos, & Elbin, 2012; Schatz, Pardini, Lovell, Collins, & Podell, 2006; Schatz & Sandel, 2012). Despite the relatively superior sensitivity of computer-based measures to concussion at 24 to 48 hours—79% according to Broglio, Macciocchi, et al. (2007), 82% according to Schatz et al. (2006), and 91% according to Schatz & Sandel (2012)—versus the sensitivity of traditional pencil and paper-based measures—23% according to McCrea et al. (2005) and 44% according to Broglio, Macciocchi, et al. (2007)—significant critical attention continues to be directed at the developers and users of computer-based neuropsychological assessment devices.

The American Academy of Clinical Neuropsychology and the National Academy of Neuropsychology issued a joint position paper regarding the accurate and appropriate use of computerized neuropsychological assessment devices (Bauer et al., 2012). They addressed issues related to: marketing and performance claims, who should appropriately administer tests and interpret results, technological factors, privacy of the individual and data security, psychometric reliability and validity, factors affecting examinee interaction (e.g., cultural, experiential, and disability), automated testing and reporting services, and assessment of response validity and effort. While each of these issues is worthy of detailed discussion, for a complete discussion, the reader is directed to the original manuscript. However, two of the issues are unique to computer-based assessment, remain current, and are widely discussed at conferences and on neuropsychology-related LISTSERVs, mainly: marketing and performance claims, and who should administer tests and interpret results.

An example a test marketed to be used by untrained, nonclinician end-users is the King-Devick test. This measure has been available since the 1980s (Oride, Marutani, Rouse, & DeLand, 1986), but has only recently been marketed and researched with respect to sports-related concussion (Galetta et al., 2011; Heitger, Jones, & Anderson, 2008; Leong et al., 2015). Cited among the research articles on the test's website (King & Devick, 2015) is a study promoting the test as being "effectively administered by non-medically trained laypersons," in this case the parents of amateur boxers who assessed participants (Leong, Balcer, Galetta, Liu, & Master, 2014). While all neuropsychological screening measures and sideline batteries are not intended to be administered solely by neuropsychologists, return-to-play decisions are medical in nature and must be made in consultation with neuropsychologists when using neuropsychological test data (McCrory et al., 2013). Even when athletic trainers (ATCs) are responsible for administering sideline assessments, it is recommended that a combination of screening tools be utilized, and test administrators obtain appropriate training with respect to standardized administration and scoring (Guskiewicz et al., 2004). Even though baseline neuropsychological testing/screening is considered to be a technical procedure that can be conducted or administered by technicians, it should take place under the supervision or guidance of a neuropsychologist (Echemendia, Herring, & Bailes, 2009), and interpretation of results should always be under the purview of a neuropsychologist.

An example of potentially inappropriate administration of test measures is the documented instructions provided by CNS Vital Signs (Gualtieri & Johnson, 2006), which was introduced within the last decade, and has been documented as a means of assessing mild cognitive impairment (Brooks, Iverson, Sherman, & Roberge, 2010; Gualtieri & Johnson, 2005; Iverson, Brooks, & Young, 2009) as well as mild traumatic brain injury (Brooks, Khan, Daya, Mikrogianakis, & Barlow, 2014). On their web page (CNSVitalSigns, 2015) the test's developers claim that the test was designed for "self-administration" and that test subjects can be left alone during testing. While they recommend that the test be "ideally administered in a quiet environment with minimal interruptions," a separate room is not required.

The test is described as appropriate for use with individuals 8 to 80 years old, with the caveat that "younger children and older adults . . . often need a family member with them to ensure that they understand the instructions." Research has shown that individualized test administration is preferable over group administration (Moser, Schatz, Neidzwski, & Ott, 2011), especially in younger youth populations (Lichtenstein, Moser, & Schatz, 2013). However, absence of a test administrator and "at home" assessment have the potential to introduce significant confounds and sources of measurement error. Further, assistance with test instructions does not ensure that the test is administered properly. The presence of a "third party" in neuropsychological test administration has been thought to create distractions and interruptions (Axelrod et al., 2000), and parental presence during testing has been shown to negatively affect the validity of neuropsychological test results (Yantz & McCaffrey, 2009). While discussions of "third persons" typically involve the presence of *another* individual, in addition to the test administrator and test taker, in this case, the presence of a parent may be counterproductive. In addition, in their discussion of "identity verification" of test takers, Bauer and colleagues (2012) specifically recognize the challenges posed by remote, web-based administration that may not be present during in-person administration. In this regard, the promotion of "self-assessment" as a marketing feature appears to be out of register with the best practices of the discipline.

## The Introduction of Tablet-Based Assessment Systems

As cited above, ownership of tablet computing devices is on the rise. Commensurate with this trend is the current availability of numerous cognitive assessment "apps" for download and use. Widely used psychological tests have recently been modified for the touchscreen, including the Wechsler adult and child scales, and tablet-based versions have been developed for computer-based neurocognitive measures commonly used for assessment of attention-deficit hyperactivity disorder (the CANTAB battery), memory dysfunction (the Memory Orientation Screening Test; MOST), mild cognitive impairment (the Computer Assessment of Mild Cognitive Impairment; CAMCI), dementia (the Cognitive Assessment for Dementia, iPad version; CADi), and sports-related concussion (the C3 Logix Comprehensive Concussion Care test, and the Immediate Post-Concussion Assessment and Cognitive Testing instrument). Pearson has introduced the Q-Interactive system (Pearson, 2013b), which allows the clinician to create client profiles, to plan and administer test batteries, and to review scores and archive results using two interconnected tablet devices connected by Bluetooth technology. The rationale behind the development of the Q-Interactive system appears to be to allow the clinician to access unique, client-centric batteries and to choose from available test instruments and subtests, as well as to use automated or facilitated scoring. In addition, whereas clinicians have traditionally been required to purchase, store, transport, and set up test kits and batteries, most of this burden is alleviated by the use of a tablet device. That said, it is not clear that transitioning from "arranging blocks" in a physical, three-dimentional space to tapping on, and dragging, three-dimensional representations of blocks on a tablet device represents and measures the same construct.

Unfortunately, describing the perceived limitations of tablet-based assessments after they have been developed, marketed, and implemented may amount to "closing the barn door after the horse has left the barn." A list of apps currently available from major test developers is provided in Box 2.3. Widely used neuropsychological and psychological tests and batteries, including the Wechsler scales (i.e., the WAIS, WISC, WMS, WPPSI), Mini-Mental Status Exam, Peabody Picture Vocabulary Test, and California Verbal Learning Test, provide significant components of a comprehensive test battery, which can be administered on a tablet device.

---

BOX 2.3 Available Psychological Assessment Apps

---

**PEARSON Q-INTERACTIVE**

CELF®-5 (Clinical Evaluation of Language Fundamentals®–Fifth Edition)
CMS (Children's Memory Scale™)
CVLT-C (The California Verbal Learning Test–Children's Version)
CVLT-II (The California Verbal Learning Test–Second Edition)
D-KEFS (Delis-Kaplan Executive Function System)
GFTA-3 (Goldman-Fristoe Test of Articulation–3) and the KLPA-3 (Khan-Lewis Phonological Analysis, Third Edition)
GFTA™-2 (Goldman-Fristoe Test of Articulation 2)
KTEA-3 (Kaufman Test of Educational Achievement, Third Edition)
NEPSY®-II (NEPSY-Second Edition)
PPVT™-4 (Peabody Picture Vocabulary Test, Fourth Edition)
WAIS-IV (Wechsler Adult Intelligence Scale–Fourth Edition)
WIAT®-III (Wechsler Individual Achievement Test®–Third Edition)
WISC®-V (Wechsler Intelligence Scale for Children®–Fifth Edition)
WISC®-IV (Wechsler Intelligence Scale for Children®–Fourth Edition)
WMS-IV (Wechsler Memory Scale®–Fourth Edition)
WPPSI™-IV (Wechsler Preschool and Primary Scale of Intelligence™–Fourth Edition)

**PAR APPS**

MMSE® (Mini Mental Status Exam)
MMSE®-2 (Mini Mental Status Exam, Second Edition)

Tablet devices offer advantages over traditional computers in use for neuro-cognitive assessment, including decreased costs, increased portability, and longer battery life. The joint position paper on computerized neuropsychological assessment devices (Bauer et al., 2012) called for standardization in administering computerized neuropsychological assessments. While considerable research efforts have focused on the administration of computerized assessment measures, tablet-based measures have only just begun to receive the same level of attention. The size of a tablet screen has been shown to have no effect on time to complete common tasks, such as identifying objects on the screen, moving from one object to another, and typing words (Lai & Wu, 2012). Psychometric equivalencies (with respect to response accuracy) have been established between iPad and paper-based versions of batteries used to screen for dementia (Onoda et al., 2013), memory dysfunction (Clionsky & Clionsky, 2014), and multiple sclerosis (Rudick et al., 2014). The study by Rudick and colleagues was exemplary in documenting considerable detail regarding test validation and psychometric equivalence between subscales and external measures of shared constructs.

Despite preliminary research establishing the utility of tablet devices, the timing accuracy of these devices for measuring human performance has not been established. Recently, greater timing error was documented in Android-based tablet devices than in Apple-based tablet devices (Schatz, Ybarra, & Leitner, 2015), raising implications for developers with respect to targeted delivery platforms. In addition, the different input method (e.g., touchscreen) and greater portability/mobility inherent in tablets, as compared to traditional computers (e.g., able to be held in hands), as well as unforeseen "human-tablet interaction" variables, could possibly affect the results obtained from tablet-based assessments, such as reaction time. Computer-based assessment typically utilizes a mouse or keyboard input, which maintain very close contact with the test taker, whereas the tablet-based device may be held in one hand or placed on a table or lap, allowing for a much wider range of movement by the test-taker (Wagner, Hout, & Mackay, 2012). In this context, significantly faster reaction times were documented for simple- and choice-reaction time trials in which the respondents' hands were held close to the center of the tablet screen, as compared to several inches from the center (Kelley & Schatz, 2014).

## The Need for Ongoing Validation and Updated Norming for Technology-Based Assessment Devices

As stated above, the position statement authored by Bauer and colleagues (2012) called for standardization in administering computerized neuropsychological assessments. Based on their foundational premise that "when a traditional examiner-administered test is programmed for computer administration, it becomes a new and different test" (p. 363), when a computer-based or paper-based test is programmed for tablet-based administration, it becomes a new and different test. Within the same position statement is the requirement that "test developers ... provide psychometric data relevant to the claimed purpose or application of the test" (p. 367), including sensitivity, specificity, and positive and negative predictive value. Using Pearson's Q-Interactive format for the WAIS-IV as an example, the only available psychometric data are published on the developer's website (Daniel, 2012). Within the WAIS-IV comparison study, the only psychometric data presented represent test-retest reliability and correlations between traditional and tablet-based administration techniques. Test-retest data reflect significant improvement (practice effects), and only six of thirty correlations between traditional and tablet administrations are above .80. However, the same website states that the Q-Interactive system is "built on a solid foundation of research," that each "new type of subtest undergoes an equivalency study to evaluate whether scores from Q-Interactive testing are interchangeable with those scored from paper-and-pencil testing," and that the validity of the practice of the interpretation of raw scores from Q-Interactive using paper-pencil norms is supported by the equivalency studies posted on the site.

Contrast Pearson's standardization approach to that employed for the National Institutes of Health's (NIH) Toolbox. Originally developed in 2012, the NIH Toolbox includes a cognition assessment as one of four domains measured by the more comprehensive NIH Toolbox for the Assessment of Neurological and Behavioral Function (NIH-TB), complementing the other modules testing motor function, sensation, and emotion. The NIH Toolbox was widely validated in a nine-part series of publications, ranging from pediatric samples (Weintraub et al., 2013), validation of working memory (Tulsky et al., 2013) and processing speed (Carlozzi, Tulsky, Kail, & Beaumont, 2013) trials, to development of age-based composite scores (Akshoomoff et al., 2013). More recently, in August 2015, an iPad version was made available. There are no specific validation studies comparing the web-based versus the iPad-based versions, and a query to NIH Toolbox Support regarding validation returned the response:

> The NIH Toolbox cognition measures were originally validated using a touch screen, so there is effectively little difference between the iPad version and original version. However, in order to clearly demonstrate the independent validity of the iPad version, and to further compare normative data, we are in process of a new NIH-sponsored validation study, which should be concluded in early 2016. This study employs the same methodology used to validate the iPad versions of the WISC and the WAIS. (NIH, 2015)

While use of the iPad application is restricted to Apple iPad devices running iOS 8.4 or later, and publication of upcoming validation is encouraging, the lack of research documenting consistency across platforms appears out of register with the comprehensive validation of the online version of the NIH Toolbox. While there is no reason to suspect accuracy of responses in the form of "yes/no" or item recall would or should be affected by input or platform differences, timing issues related to the accuracy of reaction time assessment (Schatz et al., 2015) warrant more comprehensive validation research.

## Summary and Conclusion

Assessment of human cognitive performance has clearly moved from paper-based to computer-based platforms, and we are currently in a paradigm shift to tablet-based devices. Just as the introduction of computer-based assessment brought forth research on timing issues (Cernich et al., 2007) and recommendations for validation of the new measures (Bauer et al., 2012), there is a commensurate need for similar research as we move to the new frontier of tablet-based assessment.

## References

Akshoomoff, N., Beaumont, J. L., Bauer, P. J., Dikmen, S. S., Gershon, R. C., Mungas, D., . . . Heaton, R. K. (2013). VIII. NIH Toolbox Cognition Battery (CB): Composite scores of crystallized, fluid, and overall cognition. *Monographs of the Society for Research in Child Development, 78*(4), 119–132. doi:10.1111/mono.12038

American Psychological Association. (1986). *Guidelines for computer-based tests and interpretations.* Washington, DC: American Psychological Association.

American Psychological Association. (2009). *2009 Presidential Task Force on the Future of Psychology Practice final report.* Washington, DC: American Psychological Association.

American Psychological Association. (2010). *Ethical principles of psychologists and code of conduct.* Washington, DC: American Psychological Association.

Aubry, M., Cantu, R., Dvorak, J., Graf-Baumann, T., Johnson, K., Kelly, J., . . . Schamasch, P. (2002). Summary and agreement statement of the first international conference on concussion in sport, Vienna 2001. *Sports Medicine Alert, 8*(3), 17–19.

Axelrod, B., Barth, J., Faust, D., Fisher, J., Heilbronner, R., Larrabee, G., . . . Silver, C. (2000). Presence of third party observers during neuropsychological testing: Official statement of the National Academy of Neuropsychology. Approved 5/15/99. *Archives of Clinical Neuropsychology, 15*(5), 379–380.

Bauer, R. M., Iverson, G. L., Cernich, A. N., Binder, L. M., Ruff, R. M., & Naugle, R. I. (2012). Computerized neuropsychological assessment devices: Joint position paper of the American Academy of Clinical Neuropsychology and the National Academy of Neuropsychology. *Archives of Clinical Neuropsychology, 27*(3), 362–373.

Broglio, S. P., Ferrara, M. S., Macciocchi, S. N., Baumgartner, T. A., & Elliott, R. (2007). Test-retest reliability of computerized concussion assessment programs. *Journal of Athletic Training, 42*(4), 509–514.

Broglio, S. P., Macciocchi, S. N., & Ferrara, M. S. (2007). Sensitivity of the concussion assessment battery. *Neurosurgery, 60*(6), 1050–1057; discussion 1057–1058. doi:10.1227/01.NEU.0000255479.90999.Co

Brooks, B. L., Iverson, G. L., Sherman, E. M., & Roberge, M. C. (2010). Identifying cognitive problems in children and adolescents with depression using computerized neuropsychological testing. *Applied Neuropsychology, 17*(1), 37–43. doi:10.1080/09084280903526083

Brooks, B. L., Khan, S., Daya, H., Mikrogianakis, A., & Barlow, K. M. (2014). Neurocognition in the emergency department after a mild traumatic brain injury in youth. *Journal of Neurotrauma, 31*(20), 1744–1749. doi:10.1089/neu.2014.3356

Camara, W. J., Nathan, J. S., & Puente, A. E. (2000). Psychological test usage: Implication in professional psychology. *Professional Psychology: Research and Practice, 31*(2), 141–154.

Carlozzi, N. E., Tulsky, D. S., Kail, R. V., & Beaumont, J. L. (2013). VI. NIH Toolbox Cognition Battery (CB): Measuring processing speed. *Monographs of the Society for Research in Child Development, 78*(4), 88–102. doi:10.1111/mono.12036

Cernich, A. N., Brennana, D. M., Barker, L. M., & Bleiberg, J. (2007). Sources of error in computerized neuropsychological assessment. *Archives of Clinical Neuropsychology, 22*(Suppl 1), S39–48.

Clionsky, M., & Clionsky, E. (2014). Psychometric equivalence of a paper-based and computerized (iPad) version of the Memory Orientation Screening Test (MOST®). *The Clinical Neuropsychologist, 28*(5), 747–755. doi:10.1080/13854046.2014.913686

CNSVitalSigns. (2015). Retrieved June 18, 2015, from http://www.cnsvitalsigns.com/FAQs.html

Collie, A., Maruff, P., McStephen, M., & Darby, D. G. (2003). Psychometric issues associated with computerised neuropsychological assessment of concussed athletes. *British Journal of Sports Medicine, 37*(6), 556–559.

Daniel, M. H. (2012). Equivalence of Q-Interactive administered cognitive tasks: WAIS-IV®. NCS Pearson, Inc. Retrieved June 18, 2015, from http://www.helloq.nl/wp-content/uploads/2014/01/QinteractiveTechnical-Report-1_WAIS-IV.pdf

Echemendia, R. J., Bruce, J. M., Bailey, C. M., Sanders, J. F., Arnett, P., & Vargas, G. (2012). The utility of post-concussion neuropsychological data in identifying cognitive change following sports-related MTBI in the absence of baseline data. *The Clinical Neuropsychologist, 26*(7), 1077–1091. doi:10.1080/13854046.2012.721006

Echemendia, R. J., Herring, S., & Bailes, J. (2009). Who should conduct and interpret the neuropsychological assessment in sports-related concussion? *British Journal of Sports Medicine, 43*(Suppl 1), i32–35.

Eichstaedt, J. (2001). An inaccurate-timing filter for reaction time measurement by JAVA applets implementing Internet-based experiments. *Behavior Research Methods, Instruments, & Computers, 33*(2), 179–186.

Elbin, R. J., Schatz, P., & Covassin, T. (2011). One-year test-retest reliability of the online version of ImPACT in high school athletes. *The American Journal of Sports Medicine.* doi:10.1177/0363546511417173

File, T., & Ryan, C. (2014). *Computer and Internet use in the United States: 2013.* Washington, DC: U.S. Census Bureau.

Galetta, K. M., Brandes, L. E., Maki, K., Dziemianowicz, M. S., Laudano, E., Allen, M., . . . Balcer, L. J. (2011). The King-Devick test and sports-related concussion: Study of a rapid visual screening tool in a collegiate cohort. *Journal of the Neurological Sciences, 309*(1–2), 34–39. doi:10.1016/j.jns.2011.07.039

Gualtieri, C. T., & Johnson, L. G. (2005). Neurocognitive testing supports a broader concept of mild cognitive impairment. *American Journal of Alzheimer's Disease and Other Dementias, 20*(6), 359–366.

Gualtieri, C. T., & Johnson, L. G. (2006). Reliability and validity of a computerized neurocognitive test battery, CNS Vital Signs. *Archives of Clinical Neuropsychology, 21*(7), 623–643. doi:10.1016/j.acn.2006.05.007

Gur, R. C., Ragland, J. D., Moberg, P. J., Turner, T. H., Bilker, W. B., Kohler, C., . . . Gur, R. E. (2001). Computerized neurocognitive scanning: I. Methodology and validation in healthy people. *Neuropsychopharmacology, 25*(5), 766–776.

Guskiewicz, K. M., Bruce, S. L., Cantu, R. C., Ferrara, M. S., Kelly, J. P., McCrea, M., . . . Valovich McLeod, T. C. (2004). National Athletic Trainers' Association position statement: Management of sport-related concussion. *Journal of Athletic Training, 39*(3), 280–297.

Heitger, M. H., Jones, R. D., & Anderson, T. J. (2008). A new approach to predicting postconcussion syndrome after mild traumatic brain injury based upon eye movement function. *Conference Proceedings: Annual International Conference of the IEEE Engineering in Medicine and Biology Society, 2008*, 3570–3573. doi:10.1109/IEMBS.2008.4649977

Iverson, G., Lovell, M., & Collins, M. (2002). Validity of ImPACT for measuring the effects of sports-related concussion. *Archives of Clinical Neuropsychology, 17*(8), 769.

Iverson, G. L., Brooks, B. L., & Young, A. H. (2009). Identifying neurocognitive impairment in depression using computerized testing. *Applied Neuropsychology, 16*(4), 254–261. doi:10.1080/09084280903297594

Iverson, G. L., Gaetz, M., Lovell, M., & Collins, M. (2005). Validity of ImPACT for measuring processing speed following sports-related concussion. *Journal of Clinical & Experimental Neuropsychology, 27*, 683–689.

Kelley, T., & Schatz, P. (2014). *Evaluation of different administration methods of a tablet-based reaction time test.* Paper presented at the Second Annual Meeting of the Sports Neuropsychology Society, Dallas TX.

King, A., & Devick, S. (2015). King-Devick Test. Retrieved June 18, 2015, from http://king-devicktest.com/for-concussions/research-and-publications/

Lai, C. C., & Wu, C. F. (2012). Size effects on the touchpad, touchscreen, and keyboard tasks of netbooks. *Perceptual and Motor Skills, 115*(2), 481–501. doi:10.2466/24.31.PMS.115.5.481–501

Lau, B. C., Collins, M. W., & Lovell, M. R. (2011). Sensitivity and specificity of subacute computerized neurocognitive testing and symptom evaluation in predicting outcomes after sports-related concussion. *The American Journal of Sports Medicine, 39*(6), 1209–1216. doi:10.1177/0363546510392016

Leong, D. F., Balcer, L. J., Galetta, S. L., Evans, G., Gimre, M., & Watt, D. (2015). The King-Devick test for sideline concussion screening in collegiate football. *Journal of Optometry, 8*(2), 131–139. doi:10.1016/j.optom.2014.12.005

Leong, D. F., Balcer, L. J., Galetta, S. L., Liu, Z., & Master, C. L. (2014). The King-Devick test as a concussion screening tool administered by sports parents. *The Journal of Sports Medicine and Physical Fitness, 54*(1), 70–77.

Lichtenstein, J. D., Moser, R. S., & Schatz, P. (2013). Age and test setting affect the prevalence of invalid baseline scores on neurocognitive tests. *The American Journal of Sports Medicine, 42*(2), 479–484. doi:10.1177/0363546513509225

Lovell, M. R. (2006). Letters to the editor. *Journal of Athletic Training, 41*(2), 137–140.

Mayers, L. B., & Redick, T. S. (2012). Clinical utility of ImPACT assessment for post-concussion return-to-play counseling: Psychometric issues. *Journal of Clinical and Experimental Neuropsychology, 34*(3), 235–242. doi:10.1080/13803395.2011.630655

McCrea, M., Barr, W. B., Guskiewicz, K., Randolph, C., Marshall, S. W., Cantu, R., . . . Kelly, J. P. (2005). Standard regression-based methods for measuring recovery after sport-related concussion. *Journal of the International Neuropsychological Society, 11*(1), 58–69.

McCrory, P., Meeuwisse, W. H., Aubry, M., Cantu, B., Dvorak, J., Echemendia, R. J., . . . Turner, M. (2013). Consensus statement on concussion in sport: The 4th International Conference on Concussion in Sport held in Zurich, November 2012. *British Journal of Sports Medicine, 47*(5), 250–258. doi:10.1136/bjsports-2013-092313

McMinn, M. R., Bearse, J., Heyne, L. K., Smithberg, A., & Erb, A. L. (2011). Technology and independent practice: Survey findings and implications. *Professional Psychology: Research and Practice, 42*(2), 176–184.

MHS. (2015). MHS Online Assessment Center. Retrieved June 19, 2015, from http://www.mhs.com/infocenter.aspx

Moser, R. S., Schatz, P., Neidzwski, K., & Ott, S. D. (2011). Group versus individual administration affects baseline neurocognitive test performance. *The American Journal of Sports Medicine, 39*(11), 2325–2330. doi:10.1177/0363546511417114

Naglieri, J. A., Drasgow, F., Schmit, M., Handler, L., Prifitera, A., Margolis, A., & Velasquez, R. (2004). Psychological testing on the Internet: New problems, old issues. *The American Psychologist, 59*(3), 150–162. doi:10.1037/0003-066X.59.3.150

Nakayama, Y., Covassin, T., Schatz, P., Nogle, S., & Kovan, J. (2014). Examination of the test-retest reliability of a computerized neurocognitive test battery. *The American Journal of Sports Medicine, 42*(8), 2000–2005. doi:10.1177/0363546514535901

Newburger, E. C. (2001). *Current population reports: Home computers and Internet use in the United States, August 2000.* Washington, DC: U.S. Department of Commerce, U.S. Census Bureau.

Onoda, K., Hamano, T., Nabika, Y., Aoyama, A., Takayoshi, H., Nakagawa, T., . . . Yamaguchi, S. (2013). Validation of a new mass screening tool for cognitive impairment: Cognitive Assessment for Dementia, iPad version. *Clinical Interventions in Aging, 8*, 353–360. doi:10.2147/CIA.S42342

Oride, M. K., Marutani, J. K., Rouse, M. W., & DeLand, P. N. (1986). Reliability study of the Pierce and King-Devick saccade tests. *American Journal of Optometry and Physiological Optics, 63*(6), 419–424.

PAR. (2012). PAR iConnect. Retrieved June 19, 2015, from https://www.pariconnect.com/

Pearson. (2013a). Q-Global™ web-based administration, scoring, and reporting. Retrieved June 19, 2015, from http://www.pearsonclinical.com/psychology/products/100000680/q-global-usages.html

Pearson. (2013b). Q-Interactive. Retrieved November 5, 2014, from http://www.helloq.com/home.html

Randolph, C. (2011). Baseline neuropsychological testing in managing sport-related concussion: Does it modify risk? *Current Sports Medicine Reports, 10*(1), 21–26. doi:10.1249/JSR.obo13e318207831d 00149619-201101000-00009 [pii]

Randolph, C., McCrea, M., & Barr, W. (2006). Letters to the editor. *Journal of Athletic Training, 41*(2), 137–140.

Randolph, C., McCrea, M., & Barr, W. B. (2005). Is neuropsychological testing useful in the management of sport-related concussion? *Journal of Athletic Training, 40*(3), 139–152.

Reed, A. V. (1979). Microcomputer display timing: Problems and solutions. *Behavior Research Methods Instruments and Computers, 11*, 572–576.

Resch, J., Driscoll, A., McCaffrey, N., Brown, C., Ferrara, M. S., Macciocchi, S., . . . Walpert, K. (2013). ImPACT test-retest reliability: Reliably unreliable? *Journal of Athletic Training, 48*(4), 506–511. doi:10.4085/1062-6050-48.3.09

Rudick, R. A., Miller, D., Bethoux, F., Rao, S. M., Lee, J. C., Stough, D., . . . Alberts, J. (2014). The Multiple Sclerosis Performance Test (MSPT): An iPad-based disability assessment tool. *Journal of Visualized Experiments* (88), e51318. doi:10.3791/51318

Schatz, P. (2009). Long-term test-retest reliability of baseline cognitive assessments using ImPACT. *The American Journal of Sports Medicine, 38*(1), 47–53. doi:0363546509343805 [pii] 10.1177/0363546509343805

Schatz, P., & Browndyke, J. N. (2002). Applications of computer-based neuropsychological assessment. *Journal of Head Trauma Rehabilitation, 17*(5), 395–410.

Schatz, P., Gibney, B., & Leitner, D. (2009). Validation of millisecond timing accuracy in microcomputers. *Archives of Clinical Neuropsychology, 24*, 538.

Schatz, P., Kontos, A., & Elbin, R. (2012). Response to Mayers and Redick: "Clinical utility of ImPACT assessment for postconcussion return-to-play counseling: Psychometric issues." *Journal of Clinical and Experimental Neuropsychology, 34*(4), 428–434; discussion 435–442. doi:10.1080/13803395.2012.667789

Schatz, P., Pardini, J. E., Lovell, M. R., Collins, M. W., & Podell, K. (2006). Sensitivity and specificity of the ImPACT test battery for concussion in athletes. *Archives of Clinical Neuropsychology, 21*(1), 91–99.

Schatz, P., & Sandel, N. (2012). Sensitivity and specificity of the online version of ImPACT in high school and collegiate athletes. *The American Journal of Sports Medicine, 41*(2), 321–326. doi:10.1177/0363546512466038

Schatz, P., Ybarra, V., & Leitner, D. (2015). Validating the accuracy of reaction time assessment on computer-based tablet devices. *Assessment, 22*(4), 405–410. doi:10.1177/1073191114566622

Schatz, P., & Zillmer, E. A. (2003). Computer-based assessment of sports-related concussion. *Applied Neuropsychology, 10*(1), 42–47.

Schmidt, W. C. (2001). Presentation accuracy of web animation methods. *Behavior Research Methods Instruments and Computers, 33*(2), 187–200.

Space, L. G. (1975). A console for the interactive on-line administration of psychological tests. *Behavior Research Methods and Instrumentation, 7*, 191–193.

Tulsky, D. S., Carlozzi, N. E., Chevalier, N., Espy, K. A., Beaumont, J. L., & Mungas, D. (2013). V. NIH Toolbox Cognition Battery (CB): Measuring working memory. *Monographs of the Society for Research in Child Development, 78*(4), 70–87. doi:10.1111/mono.12035

Wagner, J., Hout, S., & Mackay, W. (2012). *BiTouch and BiPad: Designing bimanual interaction for hand-held tablets*. Paper presented at the Proceedings of the SIGCHI Conference on Human Factors in Computing Systems, Austin, Texas, USA.

Waterfall, R. C. (1979). Automating standard intelligence tests. *Journal of Audiovisual Media in Medicine, 2*, 21–24.

Weintraub, S., Bauer, P. J., Zelazo, P. D., Wallner-Allen, K., Dikmen, S. S., Heaton, R. K., . . . Gershon, R. C. (2013). I. NIH Toolbox Cognition Battery (CB): Introduction and pediatric data. *Monographs of the Society for Research in Child Development, 78*(4), 1–15. doi:10.1111/mono.12031

Yantz, C. L., & McCaffrey, R. J. (2009). Effects of parental presence and child characteristics on children's neuropsychological test performance: Third party observer effect confirmed. *The Clinical Neuropsychologist, 23*(1), 118–132. doi:10.1080/13854040801894722

Zickuhr, K., & Rainie, L. (2014). E-reading rises as device ownership jumps. Retrieved October 1, 2014, from http://www.pewinternet.org/2014/01/16/e-reading-rises-as-device-ownership-jumps/

# 3

# Technologies for Functionally Relevant Neuropsychological Assessment

## Maria T. Schultheis and Matthew Doiron

Over the course of its history, the field of neuropsychology has shifted its focus to meet the demands of the medical landscape. Before the advent of neuroimaging, neuropsychologists were relied on to determine brain lesion location and to diagnose brain-behavior pathologies. As time progressed, neuroimaging was able to provide faster and more consistent lesion identification and neuropsychology began to adapt its skills and services for other related fields, such as education, law, and rehabilitation. As a result, some neuropsychological methods were adapted to assess broader cognitive functions in a variety of populations and the general public; however, these assessments have been heavily rooted in the field's diagnostically focused past, which creates limitations in the ecological validity of this approach.

Ecological validity can be generally defined as a measure's ability to predict functional performance or mimic activities of everyday living (i.e., performance at work, driving). For example, batteries of neuropsychological tests and questionnaires have been used to infer level of function and general performance at work or school. These batteries were developed due their statistical associations with different populations, concordance with neurological theories and constructs, and general face validity. However, very few assessments resembled any activity a person would perform in daily life. For many measures, ecological validity was defined by correlating performance with everyday functioning (verdicality; Franzen & Wilhelm, 1996). In contrast, another approach to ecological validity involved designing measures to resemble or mimic an everyday function (verisimilitude; Franzen & Wilhelm, 1996). The major difference between the two approaches determines the primary goal of designing the measure at the onset. It must be decided if the measure will prioritize construct validity at the onset and subsequently infer a link to everyday function, or vice versa. Many researchers interested in predicting functional outcome have relied on verisimilitude, as it more closely resembles "real-world" performance; however, it often comes at a

TABLE 3.1  Comparison of Traditional and Technological Neuropsychological Measures

| Category | Traditional Neuropsychological Measures | Technological Neuropsychological Measures | Example |
|---|---|---|---|
| Engagement | Abstract and not engaging | Engaging and motivating | Gaming mechanics |
| Verisimilitude | Measure cognition and simple behaviors in an isolated way | Measure real-world behavior and complex cognitive constructs | Driving simulator |
| Context | Sterile environment; ignore environmental and situational context | Can take place in everyday life or simulated environment | Smart homes |
| Objectivity | Self-report of real-world behaviors | Objective measurement of real-world behavior | Pedometers and other measures of physical behavior |
| Precision | Low temporal resolution (e.g., <4 observations per year) | High temporal resolution (e.g., possibly real-time data) | Parkinsonian tremor measurement |
| Adaptability | Static stimuli, tasks, and administration | Dynamic and adaptive stimuli, tasks, and administration | Patient-Reported Outcomes Measurement Information System (PROMIS®) |

cost of interpretability within the context of current neuropsychological frameworks and models.

In recent years, a growing body of literature has examined both approaches to ecological validity in existing neuropsychological methods and is leading the way for development of new neuropsychological methodologies to enhance our ability to define and predict the cognitive contributions of functionally relevant everyday activities. It is within this context that the advancement in technologies can offer neuropsychological assessment multiple advantages (see Table 3.1). Not unlike other clinical fields that have capitalized on technological advancement, neuropsychology is well positioned to be a leader in advancing our knowledge of brain-behavior interactions, by defining the interaction between cognition and other constructs (i.e., physical, environmental) that result in complex real-world behaviors.

This chapter outlines how technology can improve current methods of measuring functionally relevant neuropsychological behaviors, and it highlights how novel technologies could measure cognitive processes and behaviors in ways not previously possible.

## Promising Neuropsychological Technologies

### VIRTUAL REALITY—A NEW APPROACH IN BEHAVIORAL METRICS

Virtual reality (VR) systems have become an increasingly valuable tool for achieving ecological validity (see Box 3.1). With a high degree of verisimilitude, VR systems often attempt to replicate real-world activities in a controlled and

BOX 3.1 Technology Highlight: Virtual Reality

---

- *Engagement—People often report enjoying interactive virtual tasks*
- *Verisimilitude—Systems can simulate a range of real world tasks*
- *Context—People can be safely placed in any virtual environment*
- *Objectivity—Behaviors are already defined and represented digitally*
- *Precision—Systems measure phenomena at speeds not otherwise possible*
- *Adaptability*—Digital tasks can be preprogrammed to adapt to performance

---

objectively measured way. VR systems can utilize varying types of technology (i.e., head-mounted screens, motion detecting, and interactive interfaces) and offer different levels of immersion. The benefit of VR systems is that the tests are conducted within a digital space where complex activities and behaviors must be broken down into smaller components in order to be rendered and interacted with. In essence, all computer programs operate on a myriad of if-then statements and stored values. Assessments using VR systems simply capture some of the variables that are calculated by the program as a participant interacts with the virtual environment. In this way, participants often don't know what they are and are not being assessed on, which may lead to participants' feeling more relaxed and comfortable during the assessment. One study comparing the Wisconsin Card Sorting Task (WCST) and Look for a Match (LFAM) test, a virtual executive function measure modeled on the WCST, showed that participants found the LFAM to be more enjoyable and interesting, yet also more difficult (Elkind, Rubin, Rosenthal, Skoff, & Prather, 2004).

## FUNCTIONAL NEAR-INFRARED SPECTROSCOPY—A NEW APPROACH IN NEUROIMAGING

In conjunction with the drive to make cognitive assessment and treatment more ecologically valid, there has also been a demand for more ecologically valid neuroimaging techniques. Functional near-infrared spectroscopy (fNIRS) is one such technology: it uses an array of light-emitting diodes and receptor sensors to measure blood-oxygen-level dependent (BOLD) activation on the surface of the cortex. Like EEG arrays, fNIRS arrays have portable qualities. Rather than presenting a participant with a stimulus in a small enclosed scanner, fNIRS allows the assessment to take place in an open environment in a much more ecological way. Activities are not limited to button presses and small movements, but instead can incorporate gross motor performance tasks with simultaneous BOLD signal data acquisition.

While fNIRS is a relatively new imaging technique, fNIRS systems and techniques have advanced substantially in the past 20 years from limited single-channel systems to portable multichannel systems. fNIRS systems operate on the well-known notion that brain function is associated with specific physiological changes. By projecting near-infrared light into the cortex, optical sensors are able to detect the light reflecting off oxygenated ($HbO_2$) and deoxygenated hemoglobin (HbR) with a temporal resolution in the millisecond range. Infrared light is able to penetrate only 3 to 4 cm into the brain, which limits the accessible brain structures to the surface of the cortex. The spatial resolution of fNIRS has also increased over time, as systems are now able to monitor activity across the entire cortex instead of just a single region of interest.

Often, due to the scanners' tight enclosures, sensitivity to movement, and uncomfortable scanner noise, neuroimaging is severely limited in monitoring brain activity during functionally relevant tasks in any ecologically valid way. Motor tasks are extremely difficult, and sometimes impossible, to assess using large scanners, and often involve mental imagery rather than actual motor movement. In contrast, fNIRS has been used to monitor cortical activity and cognition during multiple physical activities, including balance assessments (Fujimoto et al., 2014; Mihara, Miyai, Hatakenaka, Kubota, & Sakoda, 2008; Mihara et al., 2012), maximal exertion tasks (Rupp, Thomas, Perrey, & Stephane, 2008; Subudhi & Miramon, 2009), and gait assessments (Harada, Miyai, Suzuki, & Kubota, 2009; Suzuki, Miyai, Ono, & Kubota, 2008). These types of physically intensive tasks simply cannot be studied in an ecological way using stationary neuroimaging.

While fNIRS has been used in multiple settings, there are still limitations to its portability (see Box 3.2). Data collection for fNIRS allows free range of motion for the participants, but studies often limit the person to sitting, standing, or moving in a restricted area (e.g., a treadmill). Advancements in wireless systems (Muehlemann, Haensse, & Wolf, 2008) and signal-correction techniques (Solovey et al., 2009) have greatly helped to improve the real-world portability of fNIRS systems to the point that they can be worn while participants perform tasks in a real-world situation. A recent study by Piper et al. (2014) set out to validate fNIRS signal accuracy across multiple settings, including an unrestrained environment. Researchers used a wearable multichannel fNIRS imaging system to measure cortical activity during outdoor bicycle riding, pedaling on a stationary bicycle, and sitting on a stationary bicycle. In all three conditions, a focal HbR decrease over the contralateral motor cortex was seen in left-hand gripping tasks. An event-related increase in $HbO_2$, which is considered to be more susceptible to physiological changes than HbR (Gregg, 2010), was seen only in the stationary condition; however, the lack of significance in the other conditions was attributed to the increased variability associated with movement and cardiovascular phenomena during pedaling.

BOX 3.2  Technology Highlight: fNIRS

- *Engagement—People can feel more relaxed out of scanner enclosure*
- *Verisimilitude—Physical tasks can be performed and not just imagined*
- *Context—Systems are portable and can be brought to actual activity sites*

## WEARABLE SENSORS AND ENVIRONMENTAL
## SYSTEMS—NEW METHODS OF OBSERVATION

With the dawn of the Information Age, we have witnessed computers shrink from the size of a room to the size of a home appliance to as small as a deck of cards. With the rise in popularity of smartphones, tiny microprocessors and associated sensors (i.e., cameras, microphones, accelerometers, motion detectors, etc.) are becoming increasingly affordable, easier to use, and small enough that they can be worn on the body or placed in household objects. The proliferation of ubiquitous computing and digital sensing offers an ocean of data and valuable clinical insight if harnessed correctly. Technology now allows us to objectively observe behavioral patterns of our clients outside of the clinic and in everyday life.

Precise data in mass volume, however, is not a silver bullet for researchers trying to understand complex behavioral patterns. A review of current psychological constructs related to physical activity (Bussmann, 2013) urges readers to distinguish between *physical activity* and *physical behaviors*, and to consider the inferential pitfalls within this burgeoning method of data collection. *Physical activity* has previously been defined as "bodily movement produced by skeletal muscles that requires energy expenditure" (Caspersen, Powell, & Christenson, 1985), whereas *physical behavior* was defined more broadly as "behavior of a person in terms of body postures, movements, and/or daily activities in his/her own environment." The distinction between physical activity and behavior is critical for neuropsychologists, for whom the amount of bodily activity is often not of interest but rather the presence of specific cognitively relevant behaviors. Researchers must remain mindful of the fact that data collected from these systems are measurements of very specific movements and only approximations of more complex constructs (e.g., daily steps taken versus level of fitness). When considering the alternative of self-report questionnaires, neuropsychologists may find value in definitive behavioral measurements in their client's daily routine, even if they are approximations needing clinical judgment to interpret.

One method of objectively observing daily behaviors is to collect data from sensors that are comfortably worn directly on the body, as the sensors remain with the person throughout the day (see Box 3.3). Body sensors that measure acceleration and rotational forces (e.g., accelerometers, gyroscopes, and pizoelectric sensors) can be valuable tools to gain insight into functional activities and specific motor patterns associated with neuropsychological conditions. One of

---

BOX 3.3 Technology Highlight: Wearable Motion Sensors

---

- *Context—Data gathered in the day-to-day environment*
- *Objectivity—Unbiased data collected based on concrete parameters*
- *Precision—Speed and volume of data gathering are impossible for humans*

---

the greatest benefits of sensor technology is that it can objectively measure physical behaviors that are often subjectively rated via clinicians or self-report.

Currently, one of the leading fields using wearable sensors to understand patterns of physical behavior is Parkinson's disease (PD) research. In many PD studies, people with PD perform their daily activities as they are monitored using wearable motion sensors to detect overall movement, posture, and movement dynamics. Patterns of physical activity derived from the sensors have been correlated with widely accepted clinical measures (e.g., the Unified Parkinson's Disease Rating Scale; Garcia Ruiz & Sanchez Bernardos, 2008) and levels of specific symptom severity (e.g., degree of bradykinesia; Salarian et al., n.d.).

Besides enhancing and modernizing widely used clinical tools, wearable motion sensors can also provide new diagnostic techniques for populations that have historically been heavily reliant on self-report and subjective clinical judgment. The diagnosis of attention deficit hyperactivity disorder (ADHD) has been controversial recently due to public perception of subjective diagnostic criteria based on clinical interviewing and self-report questionnaires. In contrast, wearable technology may offer a new diagnostic method entirely. ADHD's unique behavioral symptoms, including fidgeting and other excessive movements, are often rated using imprecise Likert scales, but some researchers are now targeting these behaviors for objective measurement. In ADHD clinical studies, diagnostic accuracy of greater than 90% has been reported solely using accelerometer data and classification algorithms (Martín-Martínez et al., 2012; O'Mahony, Florentino-Liano, Carballo, Baca-García, & Rodríguez, 2014). These contemporary assessments are conducted passively as the children are free to play and behave normally in real-world scenarios, while the machine-learning algorithms are able to classify subtle differences in the motion data. As with all clinical tools, a level of clinical judgment will always be needed, but the modern additions of wearable technology and statistical techniques could provide a more impartial and evidence-based basis for several diagnoses.

Similar to wearable sensors, the rise of mobile computing has also ushered in the opportunity to augment our environments. Advances in low-energy wireless connectivity, battery capacity, and low-cost sensors have now made it feasible to plant multiple sensors in our environment and to connect household objects (e.g., light bulbs, appliances, etc.) into a larger digital network. Clinically, these systems have been primarily implemented in the home (i.e., "smart homes"), but similar systems and principles have been demonstrated in shopping environments (Schneider, 2003), public spaces (Filipponi et al., 2010), parking systems (Idris, Leng, Tamil, & Noor, 2009), and automobiles (Sun, Wu, & Pan, 2009).

A majority of the current smart-home research has focused on rehabilitation and on geriatric populations to assist people in living safely and independently. Due to an aging population and increasing healthcare costs, there has been an ever-increasing interest in allowing individuals to safely live in their homes without direct supervision of clinical professionals or family members. While some

BOX 3.4  Technology Highlight: Smart Homes

---

- *Immersion—Behavioral data are collected passively and in the moment*
- *Context—Data gathered in the day-to-day environment*
- *Objectivity—Unbiased data collected based on concrete parameters*
- *Precision*—Computerized data collection saves hours of direct observation

---

systems have focused on increasing resident safety in emergency situations, such as falls and fires (K. C. Lee & Lee, 2004), other studies have attempted to objectively measure more complex behaviors (e.g., activities of daily living) and cognitive function (e.g., presence of mild cognitive impairment). Systems may include motion detectors (i.e., infrared sensors or optical cameras), microphones, and radio frequency identification (RFID) chips, as well as several other types of sensors, as data inputs.

Research related to smart homes has shown three major hurdles that need to be overcome when implementing smart-home systems (see Box 3.4): detecting and classifying functionally relevant behaviors within the home (Rashidi, Cook, Holder, & Schmitter-Edgecombe, 2011), linking the behaviors to known cognitive processes and diagnoses (Dawadi, Cook, Schmitter-Edgecombe, & Parsey, 2013), and using the systems to assess and intervene to improve functioning (Seelye, Schmitter-Edgecombe, Cook, & Crandall, 2013). Collectively, the studies suggest we can detect changes in behaviors associated with activities of daily living for people with mild cognitive impairment, dementia, and Alzheimer's disease, and even intervene and prompt someone when they have forgotten a step within a specific procedure (i.e., turn off the stove when cooking).

## New Directions for Technology and Neuropsychology

### A CHANGING LANDSCAPE

Neuropsychology is defined as the study of the relationship between behavior and brain function; however, it is important to recognize that the types of behaviors neuropsychologists target are subject to change as day-to-day demands vary. For example, as the storage capacity of cell phones for phone numbers increased, the need to memorize phone numbers for different people dramatically decreased. This example highlights a broader societal change in which several everyday functions and behaviors are now being performed in a digital space or via a form of technology. More recently, the advent of the mainstream smartphones has allowed the majority of Americans to stay connected 24/7 while carrying around a multitude of informative sensors and sources of data in their pocket. As these technologies have become ubiquitous, several daily behaviors (e.g., communication, navigation, scheduling, shopping, and personal entertainment) are now conducted either solely through, or in conjunction with, technology.

The growing universal integration of technology into everyday activities may offer neuropsychologists a novel approach to understanding brain-behavior relationships in the "real world." For example, massive amounts of digital information/data are being created as a byproduct of our daily activities, with some data existing for fleeting moments and never being fully utilized. It is estimated that the amount of digital information worldwide will grow from 130 exabytes to 40,000 exabytes (i.e., 40 trillion gigabytes) between 2005 and 2020 (Gantz & Reinsel, 2012). While it may be challenging to find the appropriate datasets and extract meaningful information from this digital "noise," clinicians and researchers can look at it as an opportunity to detect and to study functional and cognitive status in an ecologically valid manner. Rather than relying on self-report measures or a single administration of a clinical assessment, clinicians and researchers can use patterns in digital behaviors and sensor data to obtain objectively identified, individually contextualized information and to provide a proxy metric for real-life behavioral and cognitive phenomena.

The idea of using digital patterns to infer real-world behaviors and cognitive processes is a growing topic in several scientific fields, gathering labels like "reality mining," "social sensing," and "social network analysis" (Eagle & Sandy Pentland, 2005; Madan, Cebrian, Lazer, & Pentland, 2010). While these methods have become routine in the field of marketing and intelligence gathering, few medical fields have fully embraced the possibilities of the new methodologies; however, some research in the computer science literature has shown how the methods might be applied to medical and psychological studies. In a longitudinal study of 70 undergraduates living in a single dormitory, data collected via smartphones were correlated with daily questionnaires in order to determine if patterns of behavior were associated with mental health and epidemiological symptoms (Madan et al., 2010). For the study, students were given a smartphone to use throughout the semester that passively sampled data regarding their communication, proximity to other participants and nonparticipants, and approximate location on campus (see Table 3.2). Software in the phone anonymized all unique identifiers and uploaded the data to a remote server. It should be noted that researchers were not able to read or to listen to any personal communication of any of the participants; the majority of data were simple timestamps of when specific communication and movement events took place.

The passively collected data were then correlated with the subjects' responses to brief daily electronic questionnaires regarding their current mood, anxiety level, and the presence of low-intensity and high-intensity medical symptoms. Results suggested that participants who often reported feeling anxious had less overall communication diversity (i.e., less unique phone numbers communicated with), while participants who often reported feeling depressed had decreased overall communication during late night and early morning hours. In addition, both groups

TABLE 3.2  Cell Phone Data and Related Behaviors

| Source | Data Collected | Behaviors Inferred |
|---|---|---|
| Phone call metadata | Phone call start timestamp<br>Phone call end timestamp | • Call time<br>• Call length |
| | Remote caller phone number | • Participants contacted<br>• Nonparticipants contacted |
| | Phone call incoming or outgoing flag (binary) | Communication initiation |
| Text messaging metadata | Text message timestamp | Message time |
| | Remote text phone number | • Participants contacted<br>• Nonparticipants contacted |
| Bluetooth logs | Detection timestamp | When physical interaction occurred |
| | Detected phone identifier | • Number of participants physically interacted with<br>• Number of nonparticipants physically interacted with |
| Wi-Fi logs | Detection timestamp | • General location on campus |
| | Detected Wi-Fi transmitter identifier | |
| | Signal strength | |

showed more physical proximity predictability with other people during the late night and early morning. Besides associations with mental health, patterns in the passively collected data were also associated with different intensities of common illnesses (i.e., common cold and influenza). While this study has numerous clinical limitations, it exemplifies the idea of using commonly available technology to passively detect behaviors associated with clinically relevant states and symptoms. The direct observations of anxiety and depression behavior patterns represent a new stream of clinical data previously never feasible or even available to clinicians, as these types of behaviors are often quantified only via self-report.

While studies like the one described above require a high degree of technical expertise for both data collection and security, they could allow psychologists to understand people's functional abilities in ways not otherwise possible. Any data collected through these methods are from the person's natural environment, avoiding any biases due to artificial assessment environments, and can represent a clearer picture of the person's functioning because the data are collected over days or weeks, instead of during a limited number of assessments with the clinician. As more and more aspects of our daily lives leave a digital footprint behind (e.g., email, Internet browsing, digital calendars, etc.), new areas of research are possible, including how socializability affects our cognition and functioning, how we process and take in digital information, and how we manage or solve problems. A plethora of data related to these areas already exist, it is just a matter of how to capture the data technically and ethically.

While there are many opportunities for ecologically valid cognitive assessment, there are also several limitations to shifting cognitive assessment in the clinic to indirectly monitoring behaviors in the community. By drawing inferences from real-world observations, we run the risk of trading ecological validity for construct validity (i.e., we are not truly measuring what we claim to be). Bussman et al. (2013) illustrate this by pointing out that, in several medical fields, our ability to collect real-world behavioral data can easily be overstated and oversimplified. The case is made that physical activity is not synonymous with physical behavior and that a technology like a pedometer cannot solely define a complex concept like "fitness."

Another limitation of the method is that extracting signal from the noise within vast datasets will continue to become increasingly difficult. A common research fallacy is that more data will make predictions easier and more accurate. In order to avoid construct-validity problems, greater care in understanding where and how data originate will be paramount in understanding how the data can be used appropriately, if at all.

## Future Directions

As the history of neuropsychology has been marked with adaptation to meet the needs of the times, the field is adopting new technologies and methods to provide more accurate and empirically based care. Using new technology to objectively identify and assess behaviors harkens back to the pioneers in psychology and their interests in directly observing human behavior. Observational research has historically been a time-consuming and labor-intensive undertaking; however, the combination of advancing technology and increasing digital footprints is beginning to usher in a new era of behavioral observation.

While some digital measurements may be simple or limited, the value of this next-wave technology will be seen in the integration of multiple technologies and sources of data. Individual differences in research will no longer have to be simplified into basic demographics and other nominal data, as influences like daily habits, diet, and physical activity could be incorporated into a larger analysis. Medical conditions could be understood in a social context using data from social media. Perceived social support is one of the most well-documented psychosocial predictors of outcome in multiple medical and psychological conditions (Uchino, Bowen, Carlisle, & Birmingham, 2012), yet its integration into individual case conceptualizations is often based on limited self-report. Pending more ubiquitous adoption of social media by the general public, a combination of neuropsychological data and social data could help neuropsychologists come to understand cognitive function in a more holistic and social context.

As we move toward a future where everything is connected and the line between the digital world and real world begins to blend, some technological leaders have labeled the next wave of technology the "Internet of things." Looking far into the future, even our own bodies could become connected for improved treatment or assessment. Embedded sensors and neuroprostheses that restore or alter neurocognitive processes represent the cutting edge of our technical understanding. Systems like chronically implanted closed-loop neuromodulation (Stanslaski et al., 2012) could revolutionize targeted treatment of multiple psychological disorders and neurological conditions. With everything from implantable biosensors to home appliances emerging as possible sources of information, there is no certainty in what data or systems may be the most useful for neuropsychologists.

In closing, modern technologies are being developed to be small, unintrusive, and preferably offering a seamless and ubiquitous interaction with people's everyday life. The new technologies offer novel and unique data about an individual's functioning in the world, and therefore may represent a new opportunity for improving ecological validity of neuropsychological assessment. Integrating novel technologies can offer an alternate approach that can supplement the traditional single test administration or self-reporting approach currently used for clinical assessments of everyday functioning. The wealth of information offered by patterns in digital behaviors and sensor data may be able to provide objectively identified, individually contextualized information and to provide a proxy metric for real-life behavioral and cognitive phenomena. The challenge and opportunity lie in future research defining how to best integrate the traditional methods with evolving technologies and successfully transition neuropsychology into the digital age.

## References

Bussmann, J. B. J. (2013). To total amount of activity and beyond: Perspectives on measuring physical behavior, 1–6. http://doi.org/10.3389/fpsyg.2013.00463/abstract

Caspersen, C. J., Powell, K. E., & Christenson, G. M. (1985). Physical activity, exercise, and physical fitness: Definitions and distinctions for health-related research. *Public Health Reports (Washington, D.C.: 1974)*, 100(2), 126–131.

Dawadi, P. N., Cook, D. J., Schmitter-Edgecombe, M., & Parsey, C. (2013). Automated assessment of cognitive health using smart home technologies. *Technology and Health Care: Official Journal of the European Society for Engineering and Medicine*, 21(4), 323–343. http://doi.org/10.3233/THC-130734

Eagle, N., & Sandy Pentland, A. (2005). Reality mining: Sensing complex social systems. *Personal and Ubiquitous Computing*, 10(4), 255–268. http://doi.org/10.1007/s00779-005-0046-3

Elkind, J. S., Rubin, E., Rosenthal, S., Skoff, B., & Prather, P. (2004). A simulated reality scenario compared with the computerized Wisconsin Card Sorting Test: An analysis of preliminary results. *Dx.Doi.org*, 4(4), 489–496. http://doi.org/10.1089/109493101750527042

Filipponi, L., Vitaletti, A., Landi, G., Memeo, V., Laura, G., & Pucci, P. (2010). Smart city: An event driven architecture for monitoring public spaces with heterogeneous sensors. *Fourth International Conference On Sensor Device Technologies and Applications*, Barcelona, Spain. August 25–31 (pp. 281–286). IEEE. http://doi.org/ 10.1109/SENSORCOMM.2010.50

Franzen, M. D., & Wilhelm, K. L. (1996). Conceptual foundations of ecological validity in neuropsychological assessment. In R. J. Sbordone & C. J. Long (Eds.), *Ecological validity of neuropsychological testing*. Delray Beach, FL, St. Lucie Press.

Fujimoto, H., Mihara, M., Hattori, N., Hatakenaka, M., Kawano, T., Yagura, H., Miyai, I., & Mochizuki, H. (2014). Cortical changes underlying balance recovery in patients with hemiplegic stroke. *NeuroImage, 85*(Pt 1), 547–554. http://doi.org/10.1016/ j.neuroimage.2013.05.014

Gantz, J., & Reinsel, D. (2012). The digital universe in 2020: Big data, bigger digital shadows, and biggest growth in the Far East. *IDC iView: IDC Analyze the Future, 2007*, 1–16.

Garcia Ruiz, P. J., & Sanchez Bernardos, V. (2008). Evaluation of ActiTrac® (ambulatory activity monitor) in Parkinson's disease. *Journal of the Neurological Sciences, 270*(1-2), 67–69. http://doi.org/10.1016/j.jns.2008.02.002

Gregg, N. M., White, B. R., Zeff, B. W., Berger, A. J., & Culver, J. P. (2010). Brain specificity of diffuse optical imaging: Improvements from superficial signal regression and tomography. *Frontiers in Neuroenergetics, 2*, 161–168. http://doi.org/10.3389/ fnene.2010.00014

Harada, T., Miyai, I., Suzuki, M., & Kubota, K. (2009). Gait capacity affects cortical activation patterns related to speed control in the elderly. *Experimental Brain Research, 193*(3), 445–454. http://doi.org/10.1007/s00221-008-1643-y

Idris, M., Leng, Y. Y., Tamil, E. M., & Noor, N. M. (2009). Car park system: A review of smart parking system and its technology. *Information Technology Journal, 8*(2), 101–113.

Lee, K. C., & Lee, H.-H. (2004). Network-based fire-detection system via controller area network for smart home automation. *Consumer Electronics, IEEE Transactions on, 50*(4), 1093–1100. http://doi.org/10.1109/TCE.2004.1362504

Madan, A., Cebrian, M., Lazer, D., & Pentland, A. (2010). Social sensing for epidemiological behavior change (p. 291). Presented at the the 12th ACM International Conference, New York, New York. New York: ACM Press. http://doi.org/10.1145/ 1864349.1864394

Martín-Martínez, D., Casaseca-de-la-Higuera, P., Alberola-López, S., Andrés-de-Llano, J., López-Villalobos, J. A., Ardura-Fernández, J., & Alberola-López, C. (2012). Nonlinear analysis of actigraphic signals for the assessment of the attention-deficit/ hyperactivity disorder (ADHD). *Medical Engineering & Physics, 34*(9), 1317–1329. http://doi.org/10.1016/j.medengphy.2011.12.023

Mihara, M., Miyai, I., Hatakenaka, M., Kubota, K., & Sakoda, S. (2008). Role of the prefrontal cortex in human balance control. *NeuroImage, 43*(2), 329–336. http://doi.org/ 10.1016/j.neuroimage.2008.07.029

Mihara, M., Miyai, I., Hattori, N., Hatakenaka, M., Yagura, H., Kawano, T., . . . Kubota, K. (2012). Neurofeedback using real-time near-infrared spectroscopy enhances motor imagery related cortical activation. *PLoS ONE, 7*(3), e32234. http://doi.org/ 10.1371/journal.pone.0032234

Muehlemann, T., Haensse, D., & Wolf, M. (2008). Wireless miniaturized in-vivo near infrared imaging. *Optics Express, 16*(14), 10323–10330.

O'Mahony, N., Florentino-Liano, B., Carballo, J. J., Baca-García, E., & Rodríguez, A. A. (2014). Objective diagnosis of ADHD using IMUs. *Medical Engineering & Physics, 36*(7), 922–926. http://doi.org/10.1016/j.medengphy.2014.02.023

Piper, S. K., Krueger, A., Koch, S. P., Mehnert, J., Habermehl, C., Steinbrink, J., Obrig, H., & Schmitz, C. H. (2014). A wearable multi-channel fNIRS system for brain imaging in freely moving subjects. *NeuroImage, 85*(0), 64–71. http://doi.org/10.1016/j.neuroimage.2013.06.062

Rashidi, P., Cook, D. J., Holder, L. B., & Schmitter-Edgecombe, M. (2011). Discovering activities to recognize and track in a smart environment. *IEEE Transactions on Knowledge and Data Engineering, 23*(4), 527–539. http://doi.org/10.1109/TKDE.2010.148

Rupp, T., Thomas, R., Perrey, S., & Stephane, P. (2008). Prefrontal cortex oxygenation and neuromuscular responses to exhaustive exercise. *European Journal of Applied Physiology, 102*(2), 153–163. http://doi.org/10.1007/s00421-007-0568-7

Salarian, A., Russmann, H., Wider, C., Burkhard, P. R., Vingerhoets, F. J. G., & Aminian, K. (n.d.). Quantification of tremor and bradykinesia in Parkinson's disease using a novel ambulatory monitoring system. *IEEE Transactions on Biomedical Engineering, 54*(2), 313–322. http://doi.org/10.1109/TBME.2006.886670

Schneider, M. (2003). A smart shopping assistant utilizing adaptive plan recognition. In A. Hoto & G. Stumme (Eds.), *Lehren - Lernen - Wissen - Adaptivitat¨ (LLWA04)* (pp. 331–334). Karlsruhe, Germany:

Seelye, A. M., Schmitter-Edgecombe, M., Cook, D. J., & Crandall, A. (2013). Naturalistic assessment of everyday activities and prompting technologies in mild cognitive impairment. *Journal of the International Neuropsychological Society: JINS, 19*(4), 442–452. http://doi.org/10.1017/S135561771200149X

Solovey, E. T., Girouard, A., Chauncey, K., Hirshfield, L. M., Sassaroli, A., Zheng, F., Fantini, S., & Jacob, R. J. K. (2009). Using fNIRS brain sensing in realistic HCI settings: Experiments and guidelines. *The 22nd annual ACM symposium* (pp. 157–166). New York: ACM. http://doi.org/10.1145/1622176.1622207

Stanslaski, S., Afshar, P., Cong, P., Giftakis, J., Stypulkowski, P., Carlson, D., . . . Denison, T. (2012). Design and validation of a fully implantable, chronic, closed-loop neuromodulation device with concurrent sensing and stimulation. *IEEE Transactions on Neural Systems and Rehabilitation Engineering, 20*(4), 410–421. http://doi.org/10.1109/TNSRE.2012.2183617

Subudhi, A. W., Miramon, B. R., Granger, M. E., & Roach, R. C. (2009). Frontal and motor cortex oxygenation during maximal exercise in normoxia and hypoxia. *Journal of Applied Physiology, 106*(4), 1153–1158.

Sun, J., Wu, Z.-H., & Pan, G. (2009). Context-aware smart car: From model to prototype. *Journal of Zhejiang University SCIENCE A, 10*(7), 1049–1059. http://doi.org/10.1631/jzus.A0820154

Suzuki, M., Miyai, I., Ono, T., & Kubota, K. (2008). Activities in the frontal cortex and gait performance are modulated by preparation. An fNIRS study. *NeuroImage, 39*(2), 600–607. http://doi.org/10.1016/j.neuroimage.2007.08.044

Uchino, B. N., Bowen, K., Carlisle, M., & Birmingham, W. (2012). Psychological pathways linking social support to health outcomes: A visit with the "ghosts" of research past, present, and future. *Social Science & Medicine, 74*(7), 949–957. http://doi.org/10.1016/j.socscimed.2011.11.023

# 4

# On the Use of Virtual Reality as an Outcome Measure in Neuropsychological Rehabilitation

Diana Jovanovski and Konstantine K. Zakzanis

## Introduction

Despite the prevalence of executive dysfunction across multiple neurological and psychiatric conditions, there have been few validated rehabilitative interventions targeting it. One intervention holding promise for patients with executive dysfunction is Robertson's Goal Management Training (GMT; Robertson, 1996). GMT is based on Duncan's (1986) theory of goal neglect (or failure to execute intentions), in which disorganized behavior is attributed to impaired construction and use of "goal lists," considered to direct behavior by controlling actions that promote or oppose task completion. GMT attempts to ameliorate goal neglect through verbally mediated, metacognitive strategies that systematically target planning abilities by teaching individuals to structure their intentions. Through presentations, discussions, exercises, and homework assignments, GMT trains participants to use strategies like stopping and orienting to relevant information, partitioning goals into more easily managed subgoals, encoding and retaining goals, and monitoring performance.

Investigations into the efficacy of GMT have been promising in both normal older adults and in patients with acquired brain injury (ABI). In order to investigate the efficacy of GMT for older adults with cognitive complaints, van Hooren and colleagues (2007) randomly assigned 69 normal, community-dwelling adults age 55 years or older to a six-week GMT program or to a waitlist control group. After the intervention, participants from the GMT group reported significantly fewer anxiety symptoms, were significantly less annoyed by their cognitive failures, and reported improved ability to manage their executive failures as compared to control participants. Though this study reported positive results for subjective outcome measures, the intervention showed no effect on the Stroop Colour Word Test (Houx, Jolles, & Vreeling, 1993; Stroop, 1935).

Levine and colleagues (2000) reported on 30 traumatic brain injury (TBI) patients who were randomly assigned to receive a brief trial (1-hour session) of GMT or motor skills training. Upon completion of the intervention, the GMT group, but not the motor skills group, showed significant improvement on paper-and-pencil tasks designed to mimic everyday executive tasks that are problematic for patients with goal neglect. In the same report, Levine and colleagues described a case study of a postencephalitic patient seeking to improve her meal-preparation abilities. For this patient, GMT was expanded over two sessions and was supplemented with exercises requiring the implementation of GMT stages while following recipes, some of which were performed as homework assignments. Both naturalistic observation and self-report measures demonstrated improved meal-preparation performance after the intervention. Other studies also support the efficacy of GMT in the rehabilitation of executive dysfunction in patients with brain disease (Levine et al., 2011; Schweizer et al., 2008). Taken together, results of investigations into the efficacy of GMT in brain-injured individuals have been very promising.

In addition to evaluating the efficacy of cognitive interventions, another figural concern in neuropsychological rehabilitation is demonstrating generalization. In order to determine the true effectiveness and clinical value of an intervention, it is imperative to demonstrate that abilities or strategies learned during treatment will be utilized in the real world so that they lead to sustained improvement in everyday functioning. In studies by Levine and colleagues (2000, 2007), tasks were devised that mimicked everyday activities presenting problems for individuals with brain dysfunction. Both studies (Levine et al., 2000, 2007) provided evidence that the effects of GMT are generalizable by way of improvements on the everyday tasks devised. Other studies have also noted generalizable effects of GMT in everyday task performance (Bertens, Kessels, Fiorenzato, Boelen, & Fasotti, 2015) or in self-report evidence from participants (Levine et al., 2007; McPherson, Kayes, & Weatherall, 2009; Schweizer et al., 2008), although Levine and colleagues (2011) did not find significant effects of GMT on self-report questionnaires.

## MULTITASKING IN THE CITY TEST

Virtual reality (VR) technology is increasingly being used in the assessment and rehabilitation of cognitive functions. In particular, researchers are devising VR systems for detailed response measurement and analysis to examine specific behaviors characteristic of patients with executive dysfunction. VR-based versions of more naturalistic, ecologically valid tools for assessing executive functions have been developed. For example, VR tasks have been modeled on the Multiple Errands Test (MET; Shallice & Burgess, 1991). The MET is a test of multitasking and planning ability that is carried out at a real-life shopping center and involves the completion of a variety of tasks (e.g., purchasing various merchandise, being at a certain place by a specified time, and obtaining specific information, such as the exchange rate for a specific foreign currency). VR-based versions of the MET, called the Virtual Multiple Errands Test (VMET), take place in a virtual supermarket; a number of studies have demonstrated the test's ecological validity in the assessment and rehabilitation of executive functions and its sensitivity to aging and brain injury (e.g., stroke, Parkinson's disease; see Cipresso et al., 2014; Rand, Basha-Abu, Weiss, & Katz, 2009; Rand, Weiss, & Katz, 2009; Raspelli et al., 2011).

We have developed a variation of the MET using VR technology in our laboratory. It is called the Multitasking in the City Test (MCT) and has been described in detail elsewhere (Jovanovski, Zakzanis, Campbell, Erb, & Nussbaum, 2012; see also Methods section below). The setting and task requirements distinguish the MCT from the VMET. Briefly, MCT is a test of multitasking and planning ability that takes place in a virtual city and requires participants to complete everyday errands that consist of shopping tasks, attending a doctor's appointment, and withdrawing money from the bank. A previous study of patients with ABI found that the MCT had good ecological validity (Jovanovski et al., 2012).

The main objective of our work was to explore whether the MCT is an appropriate measure to evaluate the effectiveness and generalization of GMT in patients experiencing everyday executive dysfunction. We also sought to compare the MCT with other methods of evaluating the effects of GMT. Thus, patients' pre- and post-GMT performance was compared on the following: the MCT; a brief battery of standardized neuropsychological tests, including both executive (i.e., verbal fluency) and non-executive measures; and a behavioral rating scale assessing behavioral manifestations of executive impairment in everyday functioning (DEX). Data from the DEX scale were included to provide subjective information about how the effects of GMT may generalize to everyday behaviors. Given the focus of GMT on training everyday executive functions, it was hypothesized that the most substantial gains in test performance would be observed on the MCT when compared to the other neuropsychological tests in the battery. It was also of interest to explore whether performance on the standardized executive function tests would show more substantial gains in postintervention performance than the non-executive tests. These findings would address the clinical utility of traditional executive tests in evaluating the effects of executive function rehabilitation.

A second objective of our work was to evaluate the ecological validity of the two types of executive measures in the battery. Given that the MCT and a verbal (semantic) fluency measure were already found to be predictive of everyday behavior in a previous study using the Frontal Systems Behavior Scale (FrSBe; Grace & Malloy, 2001; see Jovanovski et al., 2012), a different informant questionnaire (i.e., DEX) was used in the current study in an attempt to obtain confirmatory evidence of ecological validity.

In short, our work was undertaken to address the following questions:

1. Which executive function task (MCT or verbal fluency) is most appropriate as an outcome measure for the evaluation of the effectiveness and generalization of GMT-trained strategies?
2. Do the two executive measures have ecological validity? Which of the measures is most predictive of real world behavior?

# Method

## PARTICIPANTS AND DESIGN

Patients were recruited for the study after being referred for GMT from either the Brain Health Clinic at Baycrest Centre or the Neuropsychology Consultation Service at Sunnybrook Health Sciences Centre. Both institutions are teaching hospitals fully affiliated with the University of Toronto. For inclusion in the GMT program and this research study, patients were required to have subjective complaints of executive impairment in their everyday activities as a result of acquired damage to the brain or psychiatric disorder. The inclusion criterion was based on the suggestion by Levine and colleagues (2000) that individuals selected for real-life disorganized behavior, as opposed to simply those with brain damage, would be most likely to benefit from GMT. Exclusion criteria consisted of uncorrected hearing loss, uncorrected visual impairment, current or past history of substance abuse, or poor English language comprehension and communication. The study involved a pre–post design in which patients underwent baseline testing one to two weeks before commencement of the GMT program and underwent posttesting within one week of completion of the program. All testing was conducted by an undergraduate or graduate psychology student under the supervision of a clinical neuropsychologist. The study was approved by the ethics review boards at both Baycrest and the University of Toronto at Scarborough and all patients provided informed consent.

## GOAL MANAGEMENT TRAINING

Patients met as a group with three trainers (a registered clinical psychologist, a postdoctoral psychology graduate student, and an undergraduate psychology student) for two hours per week for seven consecutive weeks. The GMT protocol involves an interactive format, including presentations, discussions, exercises, and homework assignments. The main goal of training was to assist patients in developing awareness of attentional control lapses in everyday life and strategies to overcome them. In the first few sessions, patients and trainers discuss the idea of "absent-minded slips" and the internal and external contextual factors that may contribute to their occurrence. The main training focus is the acquisition of a simple self-command (e.g., "stop") to interrupt ongoing automatic behaviors that occur during the attentional lapses in order to resume executive control. Once the opportunity for more controlled processing has been established, patients are encouraged to remain present-minded, to refocus on the goal of the task at hand, to divide the task into manageable steps, and to check continuously on their progress toward the goal. Briefly, the topics covered in each session are: Session 1—Definition of absent-minded slips and discussion of contexts that make them more likely and methods of preventing them;

Session 2—Discussion of what it means to be on automatic pilot and methods to stop this from happening, and introduction of personalized STOP phrases; Session 3—Introduction to the concept of short-term memory as a mental blackboard and demonstration of present-mindedness breathing technique; Session 4—Training in defining the main goal of a task, discussion of methods for remembering goals, and descriptions of different memory systems; Session 5—Description of how to partition main goals into subgoals and application of STOP phrases to goal execution; Session 6—Discussion of problem-solving techniques and description of techniques for monitoring performance and goal execution; and Session 7—Discussion and review. Throughout the intervention, discussion of patients' real-life executive problems was encouraged and application of the GMT strategies to the difficulties was reviewed. For instance, one patient required assistance with disorganization and poor time management that resulted in reduced productivity in job-related tasks. Another patient felt overwhelmed by managing finances and asked for help in this area to avoid making careless errors.

OUTCOME MEASURES

### Neuropsychological Test Battery

A brief battery of standardized neuropsychological tests, along with the MCT (described below) and DEX, were administered pre- and postintervention in order to provide a means of objectively evaluating any cognitive changes following GMT. In addition to executive-function tests, non-executive cognitive measures of verbal memory, visual memory, and confrontation naming were also included. A brief measure of IQ, the National Adult Reading Test (NART; Nelson, 1991), was administered at baseline only. At postintervention testing, alternate versions of tests or the split-half method (i.e., odd items at pretesting, even items at post-testing) was employed for all tests, except the MCT, in order to minimize practice effects. In regard to the MCT, there is no alternate form and the test is not amenable to administration using the split-half method. Thus, the same form of the MCT was administered at baseline and postintervention. The battery included the California Verbal Learning Test-II (CVLT-II; Delis, Kramer, Kaplan, & Ober, 2000; Pre-GMT: Standard Form; Post-GMT: Alternate Form); Brief Visuospatial Memory Test-Revised (BVMT-R; Benedict, 1997; Pre-GMT: Form A; Post-GMT: Form B); Boston Naming Test (BNT; Kaplan, Goodglass, & Weintraub, 1983; split-half method used); and the Delis-Kaplan Executive Function System (D-KEFS) Verbal Fluency Test (Spreen & Benton, 1977; Delis, Kaplan, & Kramer, 2001; Pre-GMT: Standard Form; Post-GMT: Alternate Form).

### Administration of the Multitasking in the City Test (MCT)

A detailed description of the MCT is provided elsewhere (Jovanovski, Zakzanis, Campbell, Erb, & Nussbaum, 2012). In brief, the virtual environment is displayed on a 17-inch color monitor and is viewed from a first-person perspective (i.e., without a graphical representation of the user in the environment). Participants navigate the environment through the use of a standard joystick and make action decisions by pressing the number keys on the keyboard. For observation and coding purposes, each participant's trial is recorded by way of a program that creates video files of computer screen activity (Screen Recorder Gold Version 2.1). The virtual environment of the MCT consists of a post office, drug store, stationary store, coffee shop, grocery store, optometrist's office, doctor's office, restaurant and pub, bank, dry cleaners, pet store, and the participant's home.

(a)

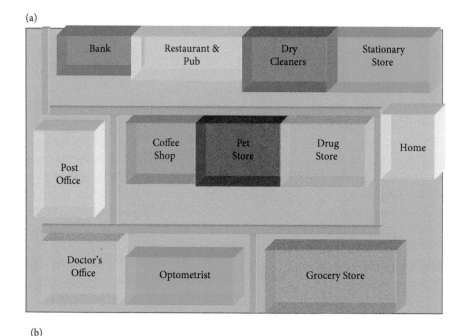

(b)

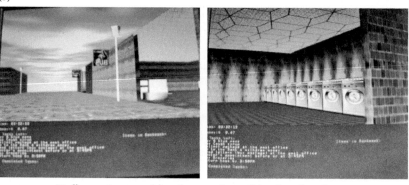

FIGURE 4.1 *Bird's eye view map (a) and screen shots of the virtual environment (b) for the Multitasking in the City Test.*

Participants are required to purchase several items, to obtain money from the bank, and to attend a doctor's appointment within a period of 15 minutes. At the bottom of the computer monitor, participants can view a list of the errands they are to perform, as well as the errands they have already successfully completed, the amount of money in their wallet, the items in their backpack, and a clock displaying the time (i.e., in hours, minutes, and seconds).

Participants initially underwent a training/learning session for three minutes in which they were instructed to familiarize themselves with the joystick and navigate through the city prior to completing the task. A map of the city was placed beside them so they could refer to it at all times (see Figure 4.1 for map and screen shots of task). After the training session, the instructions were read to them and they were then required to construct a plan for how they would go about completing the task prior to task initiation (see Appendix for task instructions). A sequence score out of six was assigned to each participant's plan of how to complete the task. Plan scores were based on the logic of the sequence, whereby higher scores were reflective of plans that were logical from both a spatial perspective (i.e., completing errands sequentially according to shortest distance between previous location and current location visited) in addition to judicious decision making (e.g., plans to go to the bank before any stores). In cases where the most spatially practical sequence was discordant with the more judicious sequence, points were always allocated for more judicious plans even if they were spatially inefficient.

The following scores were obtained from the data files of each patient: *Completion Time* (in seconds); number of *Tasks Completed* (maximal score of 8); and *Task Repetitions*, defined as performing the same task more than once and on two separate occasions (i.e., the participant must have left the building after performing the task and then re-entered and performed the same task, usually after completing other tasks in the interim). Each patient's video file of task performance was used to determine qualitative errors made by the sample, which included *Insufficient Funds* errors, defined as the number of times participants tried to make a purchase for which they had insufficient money in their wallet to buy. Other qualitative errors were categorized as *Inefficiencies,* which included entering a "task" building but not performing a task that was still incomplete; performing the post office task in two separate visits instead of one visit; entering a building in which there was no task to perform; and notable wandering behavior (defined as walking around the city for more than 30 seconds without performing a task and not necessarily involving visits to any buildings). Number of incomplete tasks and insufficient funds errors were categorized as *Task Failures.* Other possible task failures involved purchasing a more expensive item over the more economical option (in the case of the pens that must be purchased) and not meeting the scheduled time deadlines (i.e., not attending the doctor's appointment on time and/or not returning home on time). Thus, all qualitative errors were categorized as *Task Failures, Task Repetitions,* or *Inefficiencies.*

## Dysexecutive Questionnaire (DEX)

The DEX (Burgess, Alderman, Wilson, Evans, & Emslie, 1996) is a behavioral rating scale designed to assess difficulties commonly associated with executive dysfunction in emotion or personality, motivation, behavior, and cognition. The DEX has two forms, one to be completed by the patient (DEX-S) and the other, the DEX-I, to be completed by someone who interacts with the patient on a regular basis (i.e., an informant), such as a spouse. The items in the DEX-S and DEX-I are direct parallels. Additionally, certain items were selected from the DEX that were felt to be most reflective of the types of functions evaluated on executive-function measures, and the total scores from only these items were calculated to derive an "Executive Function" (EF) scale. Items included on the EF scale evaluated abstract thinking, planning, temporal sequencing, lack of insight, perseveration, inhibition, knowledge-response dissociation, distractibility, and decision making. An index of "insight" was also computed by totaling the difference between patient (self) and informant ratings (informant scores were subtracted from patient scores; S-I) on each of the 20 questions to create a composite S-I discrepancy score. Positive S-I scores reflect overestimation of deficits by patients, while negative scores are reflective of underestimation of dysexecutive problems.

## Data Analysis

Descriptive analyses (qualitative and quantitative) were conducted for all MCT measures. Qualitative analysis of MCT performance involved pre- and postintervention comparisons. All statistical analyses were performed using Statistical Package for the Social Sciences (SPSS) for Windows, version 17.0. Statistical analyses were limited to nonparametric statistics due to the small sample size. Corrections to significance levels were not made (i.e., $p$ values of .05 or less were considered significant) due to the exploratory nature of the research. Only the plan time, completion time, and tasks completed scores from the MCT were entered into the analyses, as the other variables (plan score and total errors) lacked sufficient variability pre- and/or postintervention for statistical analyses. To evaluate whether GMT had a significant effect on test scores and questionnaire results, the nonparametric Wilcoxon Signed Ranks Test for paired samples was computed. In addition, the magnitude of the difference between pre- and postintervention scores was computed via effect sizes (Cohen's raw $d$ in addition to corrected $d$). Finally, scatter plots of the postintervention relationship between DEX-I EF scores and both the MCT and verbal fluency tasks were assembled to explore whether informant ratings of everyday executive functioning were related to the executive-function test measures.

# Results

At baseline, the sample consisted of five adults, with one (a 35-year-old male) patient withdrawing from the study after baseline testing and before commencement of treatment because he was "too busy with other commitments." Thus, four patients (three females) were included in the study. The mean age of the sample was approximately 50 years (mean ± *SD* = 48.5 ± 9.3 years, range: 38–60), with above-average education levels (mean ± *SD* = 19.5 ± 1.9 years; range: 18–22) and mean IQ (as estimated by the NART) in the average range (mean ± *SD* = 100.4 ± 2.8; range: 97.39–104.01). The sample was composed of patients with various neurological or psychiatric conditions, including stroke, meningitis and septicemia, multiple sclerosis (MS), and bipolar II disorder comorbid with posttraumatic stress disorder. According to their self-report and clinical records, all patients had been experiencing executive dysfunction, such as difficulty multitasking, distractibility, and disorganization for at least 2 years at the time of baseline testing.

### TEST PERFORMANCE

Test performance scores are summarized in Table 4.1. One patient performed within normal limits on all neuropsychological tests administered. The second patient performed in the borderline range on a visual memory task (BVMT-R Delayed Recall) preintervention but within normal limits across all measures postintervention. The third patient had scores in the impaired range on all three fluency tasks (D-KEFS Letter, Category, and Switching) both pre- and postintervention. This patient also performed in the borderline or impaired range on measures of learning and memory and confrontation naming both preintervention (i.e., BVMT-R Total Recall and Delayed Recall and BNT) and postintervention (i.e., CVLT-II Learning and BNT). Finally, the fourth patient's test scores were in the impaired range on a verbal memory measure (CVLT-II Recognition) prior to treatment and were borderline or impaired on visual and verbal memory tests and confrontation naming (i.e., BVMT-R Total Recall and Delayed Recall, CVLT-II Long Delay and Recognition, and BNT) after treatment. For the latter two patients, all other scores were within normal limits.

Table 4.1 also shows DEX-S and DEX-I scores. All scores, both pre- and postintervention, were below the mean scores of self and informant ratings in the validation sample from the BADS manual (Wilson, Alderman, Burgess, Emslie, & Evans, 1996), indicating that the current sample's executive dysfunction symptoms were less severe than the sample of 78 mixed neurological patients (mainly patients with closed head injury) who were included in validation of the DEX. Indeed, in the current study, all patients and their informants rated their executive impairments in the 50th percentile or below when compared to the ratings

TABLE 4.1 Neuropsychological Test Performance and Questionnaire Results of Sample Before and After Intervention ($N = 4$)

| | Pretreatment | | | Posttreatment | | |
|---|---|---|---|---|---|---|
| | Mean | SD | Range | Mean | SD | Range |
| **MCT** | | | | | | |
| Plan Time (seconds) | 183.50 | 72.95 | 120–287 | 233.25 | 75.33 | 175–340 |
| Plan Score (/6) | 4.75 | 2.50 | 1–6 | 6 | 0 | N/A |
| Budget (/1) | 0.25 | 0.50 | 0–1 | 0 | 0 | 0 |
| Completion Time (seconds) | 624.75 | 199.08 | 494–920 | 338.75 | 127.18 | 211–455 |
| Tasks Completed (/8) | 7.25 | 0.96 | 6–8 | 7.75 | 0.50 | 7–8 |
| Insufficient Funds | 1.00 | 1.15 | 0–2 | 0 | 0 | 0 |
| Time Deadlines Met (/2) | 1.75 | 0.50 | 1–2 | 2 | 0 | N/A |
| Task Repetitions | 0.50 | 0.58 | 0–1 | 0 | 0 | 0 |
| Total Inefficiencies | 1.00 | 0.82 | 0–2 | 0 | 0 | 0 |
| Total Errors | 2.75 | 1.50 | 1–4 | 0 | 0 | 0 |
| **EXECUTIVE FUNCTION TESTS** | | | | | | |
| D-KEFS Letter Fluency (# of words) | 33.25 | 21.42 | 5–57 | 34.50 | 17.18 | 13–55 |
| D-KEFS Category Fluency (# of words) | 31.00 | 12.19 | 14–42 | 29.25 | 11.24 | 16–40 |
| D-KEFS Category Switching (# of words) | 11.50 | 6.46 | 2–16 | 12.50 | 5.80 | 4–17 |
| **NON-EXECUTIVE COGNITIVE TESTS** | | | | | | |
| BVMT-R Total Recall | 21.00 | 4.97 | 15–27 | 20.00 | 7.07 | 11–27 |
| BVMT-R Delayed Recall | 6.50 | 2.89 | 3–10 | 9.00 | 3.16 | 5–12 |
| CVLT-II Learning (Trial 1-5 words) | 54.25 | 14.20 | 36–66 | 52.25 | 21.88 | 24–71 |
| CVLT-II Long-Delay Free Recall | 11.25 | 4.03 | 7–16 | 10.75 | 5.50 | 6–16 |
| BNT (# of words) | 26.00 | 5.23 | 19–30 | 26.50 | 4.04 | 23–30 |
| **QUESTIONNAIRE SCORES** | | | | | | |
| DEX-S | 19.50 | 4.65 | 13–24 | 23.00 | 1.15 | 22–24 |
| DEX-S EF | 11.50 | 1.91 | 9–13 | 12.25 | 1.26 | 11–14 |
| DEX-I | 14.50 | 6.25 | 8–23 | 15.50 | 5.51 | 9–21 |
| DEX-I EF | 9.25 | 4.35 | 5–15 | 8.75 | 3.59 | 4–12 |
| Insight | 5.00 | 8.76 | –3–16 | 7.50 | 5.74 | 3–15 |

Abbreviations: MCT, Multitasking in the City Test; D-KEFS, Delis-Kaplan Executive Function System; BVMT-R, Brief Visuospatial Memory Test-Revised; CVLT-II, California Verbal Learning Test-II; BNT, Boston Naming Test; DEX-S, Dysexecutive Questionnaire-Self; EF, Executive Function scale; DEX-I, Dysexecutive Questionnaire-Other provided in the manual, suggesting relatively mild executive problems both pre- and post-GMT. Mean DEX-S and DEX-I scores increased from pre- to post-GMT, suggesting that patients' dysexecutive symptoms worsened after treatment, contrary to the expectation that executive functioning would improve postintervention. Upon closer inspection, however, the increase in DEX-I scores was minimal and only two patients endorsed more dysexecutive symptoms postintervention, while the other two patients endorsed fewer such symptoms. Moreover, mean DEX-I EF scores decreased postintervention (see Table 4.1), albeit a similar pattern was found here wherein the first two patients' scores increased while the latter two patients' scores decreased. The increase in DEX-S scores postintervention may reflect increased insight. Indeed, two of the patients obtained negative scores on the insight index at baseline, reflecting underestimation of deficits by these individuals (the other two scores were positive and suggested intact insight). All patients obtained scores indicative of good insight post-GMT, endorsing more severe dysexecutive symptoms than their informants. Moreover, in all but one patient, insight scores improved postintervention (as indicated by more positive scores when compared to baseline scores).

### MCT PLAN ANALYSIS: PRE- AND POSTTREATMENT

An unexpected finding observed when comparing pre- and postintervention plans was the increase in planning time after GMT. In the current sample, preintervention planning times were in line with those observed in a previous normal sample (approximately 3 minutes; see Jovanovski, Zakzanis, Campbell, Erb, & Nussbaum, 2012) whereas average planning times postintervention were almost a whole minute longer (i.e., approximately 4 minutes). Indeed, in all four patients, planning time increased. Qualitatively, the comparison of plans produced pre- and postintervention initially appeared to be a fruitless task. Other than the stark contrast in one patient's plan score (baseline = 1/6; post-GMT = 6/6), the other three patients obtained perfect scores both pre- and postintervention. This finding was indicative of ceiling effects and thus little room for, or need for, improvement via GMT training. Closer inspection of the plans constructed, however, revealed some interesting findings. With the exception of one patient who produced essentially the same plan pre- and postintervention, the plans produced were more detailed postintervention, such that patients constructed sentences detailing *what they were going to do* (e.g., go to bank—withdraw money) as opposed to simply listing *where* they were going to go (e.g., bank → post office → doctor, etc.). Another notable difference was the improved spatial efficiency of plans after treatment. Again, with the one exception noted above (i.e., identical pre- and postintervention plans), postintervention plans appeared better thought-out from a spatial perspective and involved less back-and-forth travel when compared to preintervention plans. For instance, the preintervention plan of one patient involved traveling from the bank backward to the stationary store, drug store, and grocery store, and then forward again to the doctor's office and post office (both in the vicinity of the bank). Postintervention, this patient was more strategic in navigating through the city and planned to complete errands at the bank, post office, and doctor's office prior to completing the grocery store, drug store, and stationary store errands on the way back home. It is important to note here that patients can obtain a perfect plan score with a variety of location sequences, some of which are not the most spatially efficient. This explains why patients' scores were (for the most part) "perfect" from a quantitative perspective both pre- and postintervention yet a qualitative improvement after GMT was still observed.

A more detailed analysis of the plan that improved (and substantially so) from pre- to postintervention is warranted here. It is noteworthy that the patient who devised the plan obtained a neuropsychological profile that was within normal limits across all standardized tests administered, with the exception of one borderline score. The main reason for the poor plan score preintervention was that the bank was indicated as the last location visited in the plan sequence. The plan appears to have been constructed with only spatial efficiency in mind, as the planned route indicates that the first location visited would be the one closest to home (stationary store) followed by the location that was closest to the stationary store (drug store) and so forth around the city. In addition to planning to visit the bank last, visiting the doctor's office was also planned according to the point in the sequence when it would be most practical from a spatial perspective, with no apparent regard for appointment time. These mistakes were not repeated postintervention, yet the plan was still spatially efficient in addition to being judicious. A final note about this plan comparison is the increase in planning time, which was observed to be the largest increase from pre- to postintervention across the sample (i.e., the postintervention plan took 66 seconds longer to complete).

## MCT PERFORMANCE: PRE- AND POSTTREATMENT

In contrast with plan times, completion times pre- to postintervention decreased from over 10 minutes to less than 6 minutes (see Table 4.1). Preintervention completion times were in line with those of a previous sample of patients with ABI (see Jovanovski et al., 2012) while postintervention completion times were in the same range as a previous normal sample (see Jovanovski, Zakzanis, Campbell, Erb, & Nussbaum, 2012).

Qualitative comparison of errors is presented in Table 4.2. Most noteworthy here is the ceiling effects obtained postintervention, where a total of one error across the sample was made. This is contrasted with the comparatively high frequency of errors made preintervention. The most common errors were those that were categorized as task failures, including incomplete tasks and insufficient

TABLE 4.2 Qualitative Comparison of Errors Made by the Sample on the MCT Before and After Intervention (*N* = 4)

| | Pretreatment | | Posttreatment | |
|---|---|---|---|---|
| | Number of participants who made error | Total error frequency | Number of participants who made error | Total error frequency |
| **TASK FAILURES** | | | | |
| Incomplete Task | 2 | 3 | 1 | 1 |
| Tried to make purchase before bank (Insufficient Funds error) | 2 | 4 | 0 | 0 |
| Did not meet scheduled time deadline | 1 | 1 | 0 | 0 |
| | | Total: 8 | | Total: 1 |
| **TASK REPETITIONS** | | | | |
| Attended doctor's appointment two times | 1 | 1 | 0 | 0 |
| Purchased the same item more than once | 1 | 1 | 0 | 0 |
| | | Total: 2 | | Total: 0 |
| **INEFFICIENCIES** | | | | |
| Entered a task building but did not perform a task | 1 | 2 | 0 | 0 |
| Performed two tasks in two separate visits to post office instead of one visit | 1 | 1 | 0 | 0 |
| Notable wandering behavior (not necessarily involving visits to buildings) | 1 | 1 | 0 | 0 |
| | | Total: 4 | | Total: 0 |

Abbreviations: MCT, Multitasking in the City Test

funds errors. Only two patients made task repetition errors (one each) and three of the four patients made one inefficiency error. None of the patients in the present study entered any building in which there was no task to perform. The only error made postintervention was that one task was not completed by one patient. In total, 14 errors were made preintervention compared to one error made postintervention.

## CONCORDANCE BETWEEN MCT PLANS AND
## PERFORMANCE: PRE- AND POSTINTERVENTION

As would be expected given the high plan scores obtained, plan–performance concordance was generally very good. The patient who obtained the poor preintervention plan score performed the task in a very different sequence from the one planned, undoubtedly because of the error message that appeared upon attempting to make a purchase prior to going to the bank. Obviously, this necessitated revising the plan on an impromptu basis and would explain the poor plan–performance concordance. Preintervention, concordance between plan and performance was "almost" the same in two patients (defined as visiting three or more, but not all, places in the planned sequence) and was perfect in one patient. Postintervention, all four patients obtained perfect plan–performance concordance.

### INTERRATER RELIABILITY

Errors were scored separately by two independent raters (D. J. and Z. C.). The Intraclass Correlation Coefficients (ICCs) were computed for each category of error (number of tasks completed, insufficient funds errors, task repetitions, time deadlines met, and inefficiency errors) for both pre- and postintervention MCT performance. All ICCs were perfect (1.00) and indicative of excellent interrater reliability.

### TREATMENT EFFECTS

The nonparametric Wilcoxon Signed Ranks Test revealed that there were no significant differences between pre- and postintervention scores for any of the neuropsychological test measures or DEX scores. Interestingly, the only variables to even approach significance were from the MCT (i.e., plan time and completion time; $Z = -1.83$, $p = .07$ for both variables). The effect-size analysis revealed that the differences between pre- and postintervention scores were of variable magnitudes across the different test measures. The interpretation of the magnitude of effect sizes obtained followed Cohen's (1988) conventional criteria for a small, medium, or large effect to provide a frame of reference, although it is recognized that these heuristic criteria are also dependent on context (for example, see Zakzanis, 2001). As shown in Table 4.3, medium to large differences in scores were observed on the MCT, while differences on the other neuropsychological test measures were mostly small or negligible. The one exception was a medium to large effect size obtained on the BVMT-R Delayed Recall score. The DEX scores were more variable, with a medium to large effect found for the DEX-S

TABLE 4.3  Effect Sizes of Neuropsychological Test and Questionnaire Scores from Before to After Intervention ($N = 4$)

| | Effect size[a]: raw $d$ | Interpretation[b] | Effect size: corrected $d$ | Interpretation |
|---|---|---|---|---|
| **MCT** | | | | |
| Plan Time (seconds) | −0.67 | medium | −0.49 | medium |
| Completion Time (seconds) | 1.71 | large | 1.25 | large |
| Tasks Completed (/8) | 0.65 | medium | 0.48 | medium |
| Total Errors | 1.89 | large | 1.37 | large |
| **EXECUTIVE FUNCTION TESTS** | | | | |
| D-KEFS Letter Fluency (# of words) | 0.06 | nil | 0.05 | nil |
| D-KEFS Category Fluency (# of words) | −0.15 | nil | −0.11 | nil |
| D-KEFS Category Switching (# of words) | 0.16 | nil | 0.12 | nil |
| **NON-EXECUTIVE COGNITIVE TESTS** | | | | |
| BVMT-R Total Recall | −0.16 | nil | −0.12 | nil |
| BVMT-R Delayed Recall | 0.83 | large | 0.60 | medium |
| CVLT-II Learning (Trial 1-5 words) | −0.11 | nil | −0.08 | nil |
| CVLT-II Long-Delay Free Recall | −0.10 | nil | −0.08 | nil |
| BNT (# of words) | 0.11 | nil | 0.08 | nil |
| **QUESTIONNAIRE SCORES** | | | | |
| DEX-S Total | −1.03 | large | −0.75 | medium |
| DEX-I Total | −0.17 | nil | −0.12 | nil |
| DEX-S EF | −0.46 | medium | −0.34 | small |
| DEX-I EF | 0.13 | nil | 0.09 | nil |
| Insight | 0.34 | small | 0.25 | small |

Abbreviations: MCT, Multitasking in the City Test; D-KEFS, Delis-Kaplan Executive Function System; BVMT-R, Brief Visuospatial Memory Test-Revised; CVLT-II, California Verbal Learning Test-II; BNT, Boston Naming Test; DEX-S, Dysexecutive Questionnaire-Self; EF, Executive Function scale; DEX-I, Dysexecutive Questionnaire-Other

[a]Raw $d$ computation is equivalent to formula for Hedge's $g$. The corrected $d$ statistic is also reported, as it does not overestimate the population effect size, especially in the case of a small sample size (Hedges & Olkin, 1985).

[b]As outlined in Cohen (1988), conventional criteria for a "small," "medium," and "large" effect size were used to provide a frame of reference for obtained effect sizes.

score and a small to medium effect for DEX-S EF score (both opposite to the expected direction, suggesting worsening of symptoms), while negligible effects were obtained for the DEX-I and DEX-I EF ratings. The insight index increased post-GMT, indicating better insight by patients, although the magnitude of the effect size was considered small.

ECOLOGICAL VALIDITY: RELATIONSHIP BETWEEN DEX-I EF
RATINGS AND EXECUTIVE-FUNCTION TESTS

In order to explore the ecological validity of the executive-function measures
included in the battery (i.e., MCT and D-KEFS Verbal Fluency), scatter plots
of their relationship with DEX-I EF scores were assembled (see Figure 4.2). The
graphs show a positive linear relationship between MCT completion time and
DEX-I EF score (perfect rank order correlation using Spearman's $\rho$). D-KEFS
Category and Switching Fluency scores were negatively related to DEX-I EF

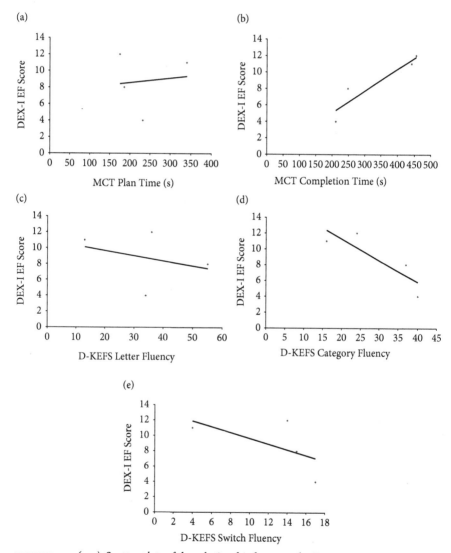

FIGURE 4.2  (a–e). Scatter plots of the relationship between the Dysexecutive
Questionnaire-Other Executive Function scale and executive function measures.

ratings (i.e., in the expected direction), with the scatter plots and trend lines demonstrating a good linear relationship (Spearman's $\rho$ = -.80 for both). The scatter plots for MCT plan time and D-KEFS Letter Fluency demonstrate a poor linear relationship with DEX-I EF, as patients' scores are relatively distant from the trend lines.

## Discussion

Our work has sought to determine whether the MCT and verbal fluency tasks were appropriate outcome measures for the evaluation of a treatment program (GMT) in a small sample of patients with everyday executive dysfunction. A second objective of the study was to explore the ecological validity of the MCT and verbal fluency task performance. The findings with regard to the generalizability of training-induced benefits suggest that they may extend to performance on the MCT but not necessarily to verbal fluency performance. The study also provided evidence of the ecological validity of the MCT and semantic fluency tasks.

### NEUROPSYCHOLOGICAL TEST MEASURES AND TREATMENT OUTCOME

The generalizability and effectiveness of GMT was evaluated using neuropsychological test measures and subjective ratings of executive impairments (the former measures are discussed here, while the latter are discussed in a later section). Inclusion of the verbal fluency tests in the outcome measures allowed for the evaluation of abilities not directly targeted for rehabilitation, but instead executive language functions in this instance. All three measures of verbal fluency (i.e., letter, category, and switching), however, had negligible to small effects when pre- and postintervention performance were compared. This contrasts with a previous study that found improved scores on phonetic fluency of medium to large effects after a GMT intervention (Winocur et al., 2007). In the current study, however, it appears that strategies trained during GMT did not generalize to those required on fluency tasks. Thus, GMT showed poor generalization and effectiveness when evaluated using standardized measures of verbal fluency.

Similar findings were observed on the other neuropsychological test measures utilized in this battery. The effect-size analysis revealed negligible effects of GMT across measures of verbal and visual memory and confrontation naming, with the exception of medium to large effects on a delayed visual memory task. A possible explanation for the relatively large effects on this measure include differences in the level of difficulty across alternate forms of the BVMT-R (i.e., the form used post-GMT may have been less challenging than the one used pre-GMT). Another possibility is the greater potential for large improvements post-GMT due to relatively poor scores at baseline. Indeed, two of the four patients obtained borderline or impaired scores during baseline testing, thus increasing the likelihood for more substantial improvements during postintervention testing. Finally, there is the possibility that the improvements on delayed visual memory were in fact due to GMT. The gains may be attributable to training of encoding and retrieval strategies during Stage 4 of the program. Overall, the findings of mainly negligible effects across neuropsychological test measures suggest that standardized executive function tests are not superior to non-executive tests for indexing treatment efficacy or demonstrating generalization of strategies learned in GMT. The results are consistent with some previous studies that demonstrated no effect or only modest improvements on standardized executive-function measures after GMT (Schweizer et al., 2008; van Hooren et al., 2007) although significant improvements on a standardized executive test (Tower Test) after GMT were found by Levine and colleagues (2011). In sum, the findings in the literature are inconsistent in regard to whether standardized executive measures have adequate clinical utility in the assessment of GMT effects. A possible explanation is that many of the tests are not measuring the constructs specifically targeted by GMT.

A different account emerges, however, when MCT performance is analyzed. The findings from this measure suggest that the training effects associated with GMT were generalizable, at least within the constraints of behavior assessed in the laboratory, as the MCT was not included in the training protocol. Strategies trained in GMT do indeed appear more applicable to those required on the MCT than on fluency tasks. For instance, it is conceivable that GMT instruction on the partitioning of a goal into subgoals and the prioritization of tasks would be more relevant to performance on the MCT than on a verbal fluency test. Indeed, there was a notable improvement in MCT performance, both qualitatively and quantitatively, from baseline to postintervention. Although nonparametric statistical analyses did not reveal any significant differences from pre-GMT to post-GMT on any of the neuropsychological test measures administered, this was likely due to low power. Accordingly, the findings from the effect-size analysis, which is not moderated by the small sample size, were taken to be a more accurate estimate of the effectiveness of treatment. The analysis revealed that overall the largest effects were found on the MCT variables, all of which showed medium to large effect sizes (when compared to negligible effects on the fluency tasks).

The potential influence of practice effects on the MCT must be addressed. It was not possible to use different forms of the test for the pre- and post-GMT evaluations, as only one version of the test exists at present. Thus, there is the obvious possibility that postintervention performance was more reflective of the benefits of practice than the application of goal-management strategies learned during rehabilitation. Some evidence, however, refutes the notion that practice effects alone were responsible for improvements in performance. One such piece of evidence is the substantial increase in plan time that was noted post-GMT across all four patients. If the results obtained were simply a practice effect, one would expect plan time to decrease, rather than increase, due to the benefits of familiarity with the task. The largest increase in plan time and plan score was found in the one patient who obtained a very poor plan score pre-GMT, suggesting that the extra time taken to carefully plan the route, rather than just the effect of practice, contributed to the improved performance. Finally, plans were noted to be more detailed and accurate post-GMT. One might expect that patients would require less detail in plans to accomplish the required tasks if practice effects were solely responsible for the change in their performance. Instead, the increased detail in plans appears more reflective of the effects of GMT, and perhaps more specifically training, on the partitioning of a goal into clearly defined subgoals.

The slower plan times postintervention are consistent with the findings from the study by Levine and colleagues (2000), in which they found that the portion of their sample that received GMT (when compared to the group receiving motor skills training) performed slower on post-GMT tasks. They suggested that GMT increased participants' care and attention to the tasks, in turn reducing errors. This was also found here, where patients reduced errors to virtually zero on the MCT during postintervention testing (i.e., one error was made across the entire sample). It should be noted, however, that while reductions in specific types of errors were found, in some cases the errors occurred so infrequently preintervention that they were already at ceiling, thus limiting the extent of any gains attributable to GMT. Nevertheless, improvements in performance were evident. There was a slight reduction in task repetitions, possibly as a result of improved checking and monitoring skills taught in GMT. It was expected that training in planning and maintaining goals and subgoals would result in completing more tasks within the time limit, fewer missed time deadlines, and faster completion times. Improvements in all of these aspects of performance were indeed found, although only modestly so, in part due to better than expected pre-GMT performance. A main focus of GMT is the acquisition of a simple self-command ("stop") to interrupt ongoing automatic behaviors that occur during attentional lapses in order to resume executive control (Schweizer et al., 2008). Such training may have helped prevent patients from making "automatic pilot errors," defined as absent-minded slips due to inappropriate habitual responding (Levine et al., 2000). In particular, training of the stop command, along with instruction on the prioritization of subgoals, may have helped patients avoid making insufficient funds errors (i.e., attempting to make purchases without money), as this was the error type with the most notable decrease postintervention.

The increased planning times post-GMT coincided with decreased completion times. While faster completion times may be reflective of a practice effect, it could also be argued that the extra care and attention devoted to devising more detailed and accurate plans aided patients in completing the task more efficiently. Indeed, only one patient had perfect plan–performance concordance prior to the intervention, while perfect plan–performance concordance was obtained for all patients post-GMT. The perfect concordance between plans and performance post-GMT was undoubtedly due to the fact that all patients produced "perfect" plans. Although patients produced good plans preintervention, their postintervention plans showed improved detail, logic, and spatial efficiency. Moreover, actual performance on the MCT also improved post-GMT. In line with van Hooren and colleagues' (2007) GMT study, the current results demonstrate that, postintervention, patients were better able to perform activities according to a plan and better able to structure activities in daily life (or in this case, activities resembling those one would perform in daily life).

Some preliminary data exploring practice effects on the MCT have been collected in a sample of four normal participants (age: mean ± $SD$ = 31.0 ± 1.6 years; education: mean ± $SD$ = 20.5 ± 5.8 years), who performed the task on two occasions 4 weeks apart. In contrast to the patient sample, the plan time of the normal sample decreased during the second administration of the task (mean ± $SD$ = 165.3 ± 157.8 seconds to mean ± $SD$ = 86.0 ± 84.7 seconds), with an obtained effect size in the medium range ($d$ = 0.63). Additionally, completion times and total errors decreased, as they did in the patient sample, with a very large effect size obtained for the completion time variable (mean ± $SD$ = 321.5 ± 59.6 seconds to mean ± $SD$ = 217.8 ± 8.8 seconds; $d$ = 2.44) but only small to medium effects on the total errors variable (mean ± $SD$ = 1 ± 1.2 to mean ± $SD$ = 0.5 ± 1.0; $d$ = 0.46). The number of tasks completed was perfect across all four participants on both trials. The results are consistent with the presence of practice effects on the MCT. The plan score, however, decreased during the second testing period (mean ± $SD$ = 3.8 ± 2.6 to mean ± $SD$ = 3.0 ± 3.5), although the effect size obtained on this measure was small to negligible ($d$ = −0.24). Plan score would be expected to improve due to practice effects alone, yet it did not in the normal sample. Moreover, from a spatial perspective, the efficiency of the route taken improved for only one participant; while two of the participants' paths were spatially inefficient on both trials, and the other participant's route was spatially efficient on both occasions. These findings contrast with those from the patient sample, who appeared to put forth more effort in their plans (as evidenced by an increase in plan time and plan detail) and took more spatially efficient routes during the second, postintervention administration of the task. Thus, practice effects may not be responsible for the particular improvements in the patient sample given that the normal sample did not demonstrate the same improvements in performance. From the preliminary data, it can be deduced that while certain MCT variables, such as completion time and total errors, may be subject to practice effects, other MCT scores (i.e., plan time, plan score) likely improved in the patient sample for reasons other than practice, such as benefits gained during GMT.

FURTHER EVIDENCE OF ECOLOGICAL VALIDITY

The DEX-I EF score was utilized to explore relationships with the executive-function variables to evaluate ecological validity. The score was shown to have the best linear relationship with MCT completion time. Findings in support of the ecological validity of the completion-time measure were not unexpected, given that this score probably reflects aspects of task performance like duration engaged in completing tasks, efficiency and accuracy of the sequence of errands performed, and presence or absence of errors made, such as task repetitions and inefficiencies. These aspects of MCT performance indeed appear very relevant to everyday behaviors and seem particularly reflective of an individual's productivity and efficiency in real life.

The DEX-I EF scores were also linearly related, albeit to a lesser extent, to the two semantic fluency measures (D-KEFS Category Fluency and Category Switching Fluency) administered. It is interesting to note that the MCT and a semantic fluency task (Animal Naming) were the only tests associated with subjective ratings of real-world executive functioning in a previous study of patients with ABI (Jovanovski et al., 2012). Thus, the results provide further evidence of the ecological validity of the MCT and semantic fluency tasks. The seemingly more direct relationship between MCT task requirements and daily activities, when compared to semantic fluency, suggests that performance on the MCT may be better suited for the prediction of real-life executive functions. It is also worth noting that several MCT variables (i.e., plan score and total errors) did not have sufficient variability across the small sample to allow for the computation of correlations with the DEX. Accordingly, future studies with larger sample sizes, a matched control group, and perhaps more severely impaired patients, are required to evaluate whether the MCT scores are also predictive of real-world behavior.

## DEX AND TREATMENT OUTCOME

Overall, patients and their informants reported fairly mild executive-function impairments on the DEX. Contrary to what would be expected, dysexecutive symptoms as rated by patients worsened immediately postintervention. Taken together with the findings of improved scores on the insight index, there is some evidence that GMT may improve awareness of executive difficulties. This makes sense intuitively, as the executive deficits experienced by the sample were undoubtedly more salient to them immediately after undergoing the seven-week GMT program, in which these deficits were the primary focus. An increased awareness and appreciation of their dysexecutive problems may have been an immediate effect of GMT, thus explaining the increase in reported symptoms and the reporting of more severe symptoms than their informants reported. The increase in symptom severity reported by patients postintervention may have been a product of the timing of the evaluation, as it is likely that patients did not have enough time to fully implement GMT strategies in their daily lives to even notice improvements in executive function at the time of the evaluations (see below for further discussion).

Subjective behavioral ratings from informants showed an overall decrease in symptom severity on the derived DEX EF scale. Informant ratings are generally regarded as more accurate than patient ratings and are therefore preferred for estimating actual executive dysfunction on the DEX. The items from the DEX that were used to derive the EF scale were specifically chosen because they were thought to reflect the particular functions targeted by GMT. The fact that informant ratings on this scale decreased postintervention suggests that specific executive functions targeted by GMT improved even in this sample of relatively mildly impaired patients. This conclusion must be made cautiously and tentatively, however, as two of the informant ratings on the EF scale actually increased slightly (suggestive of worsening of symptoms) and the overall effect size from baseline to post-GMT was considered small.

A possible explanation for the increase in DEX-I total score may be that expectations for immediate improvements postintervention were high and unrealistic and that the postintervention evaluations were more reflective of the discrepancy between the expectations and reality, as opposed to actual observed changes from baseline. Another possibility is the timing of the completion of the DEX questionnaire. The administration of the DEX immediately after GMT was perhaps not the ideal time, as informants may not have had sufficient opportunity to observe any changes in executive functioning. Alternatively, patients may not yet have fully implemented the strategies learned in training. In the case study report by Schweizer and others (2008), the informant did not rate the patient until long-term follow-up four months post-GMT. Indeed, in this earlier study, ratings provided by the patient on another scale (Cognitive Failures Questionnaire; Broadbent, Cooper, Fitzgerald, & Parkes, 1982) indicated the presence of more difficulties immediately postintervention when compared to baseline, similar to the findings of the current study. Levine and colleagues (2007) found nonsignificant improvements on the DEX immediately post-GMT but significantly lower DEX scores at long-term follow-up. They suggested that the real-life effects measured on the DEX needed time to consolidate and that the postintervention assessment may have been too early to detect effects. In the present study, long-term follow-up evaluations using the DEX may have allowed for consolidation of real-life effects in the patient sample.

LONG-TERM BENEFITS OF GMT

The evidence suggests that the effects of GMT extend beyond the immediate postintervention period (Levine et al., 2000, 2007, 2011; McPherson, Kayes, & Weatherall, 2009; Schweizer et al., 2008; van Hooren et al., 2007). Moreover, even in high-functioning samples like the present one, it is often observed that subtle changes like those observed here on neuropsychological test performance and behavioral ratings can result in a substantial change in daily functioning when compared to preintervention abilities. Test performance in particular has been noted to underestimate the degree of therapeutic benefit derived from GMT (Schweizer et al., 2008). Evidence of the long-term beneficial effects of GMT in terms of the positive impact it had on patients' daily lives was provided by reports from the study sample approximately two months post-GMT. At that time, patients were asked to evaluate the training program and their use of the learned strategies in their daily lives with free-form comments. Three of the four patients provided their reviews, all of which were positive and suggested that the techniques taught during GMT were being utilized regularly in their everyday activities. For instance, one patient described GMT as an "excellent program." In particular, this patient noted, "The 'stop' technique is fantastic! Whenever I feel flustered because I don't know what I'm looking for, for example, I 'stop' and get oriented or more focused." Another patient stated, "The GMT program was very helpful. Particularly the emphasis on paying attention to avoid memory slips. That seems so simple when stated, however it is more difficult to put into practice. Taking a moment or two to focus on what I'm doing has improved my effectiveness." These evaluations are indicative of the potential for long-term benefits and the generalizability of GMT techniques to everyday life.

## LIMITATIONS

In addition to the aforementioned limitations of the study (e.g., small sample size, lack of alternate form for MCT and potential practice effects, lack of long-term follow-up evaluations), a design limitation potentially undermining the study findings is the lack of inclusion of a matched control group not receiving treatment or receiving non-executive-function treatment. Without a control group to provide a comparison base for the evaluation of post-GMT effects, it is acknowledged that positive results could be attributed to a variety of factors other than the intervention's effect. In addition to practice effects, patients may show a placebo effect, in which they expect the intervention to help, resulting in improved postintervention performance. Alternatively, patients may be motivated to show improved performance in order to please the experimenter or play the "good subject role" (Weber & Cook, 1972). Furthermore, improved performance at postintervention assessment could reflect nonspecific effects of the GMT intervention, such as an increase in social interaction or therapeutic gain from meeting individuals with similar cognitive difficulties. These potential confounds involving nonspecific effects of GMT can be partially refuted by the fact that patients evaluated themselves as having worsened executive impairments after treatment. Nonetheless, future studies of the efficacy and generalization of GMT would be strengthened by implementing randomized controlled trials in order to control for the confounding variables.

## Conclusion

In conclusion, our work indicates that GMT is an effective therapeutic program for the amelioration of executive deficits in patients with long-standing complaints of dysexecutive symptoms. The strategies learned in GMT appear to be generalizable to activities not specifically trained during intervention, as demonstrated by improvements in MCT performance. Trained strategies do not appear to generalize to a traditional executive-function measure assessing verbal fluency. Further evidence of the ecological validity of the MCT, and to a lesser extent semantic fluency tasks, was suggested by the current results. The potential for long-term beneficial effects of GMT was evinced by subjective reports from patients of continued everyday use of techniques and improvements in daily activities two months after intervention. Several study limitations were noted and further studies, using randomized controlled trials, alternate forms for all neuropsychological tests, and larger sample sizes, are warranted.

## Appendix:  Multitasking in the City Test (MCT) Instructions

### Learning Session Instructions for the MCT

I want you to imagine that you have recently moved to a new city and that you will spend the next 3 minutes becoming familiar with your new city of residence as well as getting used to using the joystick to navigate through the city. The joystick will allow you to move forward by pushing it forward, to the left by pushing it to the left, etc. During this learning session, you should pay close attention to where various stores and other buildings are located in the city. As you want to focus on getting to know places within the city, you will not be able to do anything other than walk around. For example, you will not be able to make any purchases or withdraw money from the bank.

### MCT Instructions

It is now 4:30 p.m. and you are at home. You are planning to spend the next 15 minutes or so running errands within your city of residence. The following errands are on your list of things to do:

  1) You must go to various stores to purchase the following items:
    • 6 blue pens, which cost various prices
    • Cough syrup, which will cost $4.00
    • Groceries, which will cost a total of $12.50

All of these items can be picked up directly at the cashier—the pens are normally found there and the other items have been pre-ordered and have therefore been placed at the cashier's area for you to pick up.

2) You must go to the doctor's office, as you have an appointment for 4:40 p.m. You may arrive early but you cannot be late.
3) You must pick up your mail from the post office.
4) At the post office, you have to drop off a letter for which you must buy postage, which will cost 75 cents.
5) You must go to the bank to withdraw money as you only have 67 cents in your wallet. You must try not to go over your budget of $20.00 for all the items you need to buy today.
6) You should be back at home no later than 4:45 p.m.

You should attempt to complete as many of the errands as possible within a period of 15 minutes. It is up to you to decide the best order in which to complete these errands. There will be a clock on the screen at all times to assist you with this. In addition, the list of errands will also be on the screen at all times. To perform a task, you must simply walk up close to a desired location using your joystick, such as the cashier, and another screen will immediately appear that will prompt you to choose what you would like to do from a list of options. Each option corresponds to a particular number, so you will have to enter the appropriate number from the number keys on the keyboard. When a task is completed, it will appear under the "Tasks Completed" section of the screen and all of the items you acquire will appear in the "Items in Backpack" section of the screen. You will have a map of the city beside you at all times to help you plan and navigate through your route.

Please take as long you need to construct a plan for the task using the map and paper and pen to record your plan on paper. Please let me know as soon as you have finished constructing your plan and are ready to begin the task.

# References

Benedict, R. H. B. (1997). *Brief Visuospatial Memory Test–Revised: Professional manual.* Odessa, FL: Psychological Assessment Resources, Inc.

Bertens, D., Kessels, R.P., Fiorenzato, E., Boelen, D.H., & Fasotti, L. (2015). Do old errors always lead to new truths? A randomized controlled trial of errorless goal management training in brain-injured patients. *Journal of the International Neuropsychological Society, 21,* 639–649.

Broadbent, D. E., Cooper, P. F., Fitzgerald, P. & Parkes, K. R. (1982). The Cognitive Failures Questionnaire (CFQ) and its correlates. *British Journal of Clinical Psychology, 21,* 1–16.

Burgess, P. W., Alderman, N., Wilson, B. A., Evans, J. J., & Emslie, H. (1996). The Dysexecutive Questionnaire. In B. A. Wilson, N. Alderman, P. W. Burgess, H. Emslie, & J. J. Evans, *Behavioural assessment of the dysexecutive syndrome.* Bury St. Edmunds: Thames Valley Test Company.

Cipresso, P., Albani, G., Serino, S., Pedroli, E., Pallavicini, F., Mauro, A., & Riva, G. (2014). Virtual multiple errands test (VMET): A virtual reality-based tool to detect early executive functions deficit in Parkinson's disease. *Frontiers in Behavioral Neuroscience, 8,* 405. doi:10.3389/fnbeh.2014.00405.

Cohen, J. (1988). *Statistical power analysis for the behavioral sciences* (2nd ed.). Hillsdale, NJ: Lawrence Erlbaum Associates.

Delis, D., Kaplan, E., & Kramer, J. (2001). *Delis-Kaplan Executive Function Scale*. San Antonio, TX: The Psychological Corporation.

Delis, D. C., Kramer, J. H., Kaplan, E., & Ober, B. A. (2000). *California Verbal Learning Test-Second Edition (CVLT-II)*. San Antonio, TX: The Psychological Corporation.

Duncan, J. (1986). Disorganization of behavior after frontal lobe damage. *Cognitive Neuropsychology, 3*, 271–290.

Grace, J., & Malloy, P. F. (2001). *Frontal Systems Behavior Scale professional manual*. Lutz, FL: Psychological Assessment Resources, Inc.

Houx, P. J., Jolles, J., & Vreeling, F. W. (1993). Stroop interference: Aging effects assessed with the Stroop Color-Word Test. *Experimental Aging Research, 19*, 209–224.

Jovanovski, D., Zakzanis, K., Campbell, Z., Erb, S., & Nussbaum, D. (2012). Development of a novel, ecologically oriented virtual reality measure of executive function: The Multitasking in the City Test. *Applied Neuropsychology, 19*, 171–182.

Jovanovski, D., Zakzanis, K., Ruttan, L., Campbell, Z., Erb, S., & Nussbaum, D. (2012). Ecologically valid assessment of executive dysfunction using a novel virtual reality task in patients with acquired brain injury. *Applied Neuropsychology, 19*, 207–220.

Kaplan, E. F., Goodglass, H., & Weintraub, S. (1983). *The Boston Naming Test*. Philadelphia: Lea & Febiger.

Levine, B., Robertson, I. H., Clare, L., Carter, G., Hong, J., Wilson, B. A., et al. (2000). Rehabilitation of executive functioning: An experimental-clinical validation of Goal Management Training. *Journal of the International Neuropsychological Society, 6*, 299–312.

Levine, B., Schweizer, T.A., O'Connor, C., Turner, G., Gillingham, S., Stuss, D.T., Manly, T., & Robertson, I.H. (2011). Rehabilitation of executive functioning in patients with frontal lobe brain damage with Goal Management Training. *Frontiers in Human Neuroscience, 5*, 9. doi:10.3389/fnhum.2011.00009.

Levine, B., Stuss, D. T., Winocur, G., Binns, M. A., Fahy, L., Mandic, M., et al. (2007). Cognitive rehabilitation in the elderly: Effects on strategic behaviour in relation to goal management. *Journal of the International Neuropsychological Society, 13*, 143–152.

McPherson, K. M., Kayes, N., & Weatherall, M. (2009). A pilot study of self-regulation informed goal setting in people with traumatic brain injury. *Clinical Rehabilitation, 23*, 296–309.

Nelson, H. E. (1991). *National Adult Reading Test* (2nd ed.). London: NFER-Nelson Publishing Co., Ltd.

Rand, D., Basha-Abu Rukan, S., Weiss, P. L., & Katz, N. (2009). Validation of the virtual MET as an assessment tool for executive functions. *Neuropsychological Rehabilitation, 19*, 583–602.

Rand, D., Weiss, P. L., & Katz, N. (2009). Training multitasking in a virtual supermarket: A novel intervention after stroke. *The American Journal of Occupational Therapy, 63*, 535–542.

Raspelli, S., Pallavicini, F., Carelli, L., Morganti, F., Poletti, B., Corra, B., Silani, V., & Riva, G. (2011). Validation of a neuro virtual reality-based version of the multiple errands test for the assessment of executive functions. In B.K. Wiederhold, S. Bouchard, &

G. Riva (Eds.), *Annual review of cybertherapy and telemedicine 2011: Evidence-based clinical applications of information technology.* San Diego: Interactive Media Institute.

Robertson, I. H. (1996). *Goal management training: A clinical manual.* Cambridge, UK: PsyConsult.

Schweizer, T. A., Levine, B., Rewilak, D., O'Connor, C., Turner, G., Alexander, M. P., et al. (2008). Rehabilitation of executive functioning after focal damage to the cerebellum. *Neurorehabilitation and Neural Repair, 22,* 72–77.

Screen Recorder Studio Corp. (1999). Screen Recorder Gold (Version 2.1). [Computer software]. Retrieved from www.capture-screen.com.

Shallice, T., & Burgess, P. (1991). Deficits in strategy application following frontal lobe damage in man. *Brain, 114,* 727–741.

Spreen, O., & Benton, A. L. (1977). *Neurosensory Center Comprehensive Examination for Aphasia.* Victoria, BC: Neuropsychology Laboratory, University of Victoria.

Stroop, J. R. (1935). Studies of interference in serial-verbal reaction. *Journal of Experimental Psychology, 18,* 643–662.

van Hooren, S. A. H., Valentijn, S. A. M., Bosma, H., Ponds, R. W. H. M., van Boxtel, M. P. J., Levine, B., Robertson, I., & Jolles, J. (2007). Effect of a structured course involving goal management training in older adults: A randomised controlled trial. *Patient Education and Counseling, 65,* 205–213.

Weber, S. J., & Cook, T. D. (1972). Subject effects in laboratory research: An examination of subject roles, demand characteristics, and valid inferences. *Psychological Bulletin, 77,* 273–295.

Wilson, B. A., Alderman, N., Burgess, P. W., Emslie, H., & Evans, J. J. (1996). *Behavioural assessment of the dysexecutive syndrome.* Bury St. Edmunds: Thames Valley Test Company.

Winocur, G., Craik, F. I. M., Levine, B., Robertson, I. H., Binns, M. A., Alexander, M., et al. (2007). Cognitive rehabilitation in the elderly: Overview and future directions. *Journal of the International Neuropsychological Society, 13,* 166–171.

Zakzanis, K. K. (2001). Statistics to tell the truth, the whole truth, and nothing but the truth: Formulae, illustrative numerical examples, and heuristic interpretation of effect size analyses for neuropsychological researchers. *Archives of Clinical Neuropsychology, 16,* 653–667.

# 5

# Teleneuropsychology

Robert L. Kane and C. Munro Cullum

## Introduction

The growth of telemedicine has been rapid. Initially, telemedicine was seen as a way to bring services to remote areas that lacked access to aspects of health-care delivered through traditional means. This view of telemedicine has changed. Current views toward telemedicine have broadened, with telemedicine now viewed as an effective way to deliver various health services and to bring together patients and providers to increase access to care in various locations and communities. Reimbursement has been a challenge for some aspects of telemedicine development. Initially, Medicare limited reimbursement for telehealth to designated underserved areas. This approach to telehealth reimbursement has lagged behind developments in the field and has been challenged by various groups and legislative initiatives. In April 2016, the Centers for Medicare and Medicaid Services (CMS) released its Managed Care Final Rule (Federal Register, 2016) with wording that potentially will permit reimbursement for expanded telemedicine-based services. The revised standards, in attempting to ensure that Medicaid beneficiaries have reasonable access to care, acknowledge a role for technology and telemedicine. The impact the new standards will have on the development of telemedicine throughout the United States will become evident with time.

Tele-mental health has grown along with other aspects of remote healthcare delivery. Extant literature supports the use of remotely delivered telehealth for a variety of conditions and services, including remote psychiatric consultation, diagnosis, and various therapies (Myers & Turvey, 2012; Shore, 2013). However, the idea that one can provide an adequate neuropsychological evaluation remotely is newer and less intuitive, and would appear to have obvious challenges. Neuropsychological examinations frequently require the use of test stimuli that the examinee has to handle and manage, such as blocks, pencils, or other manipulatives. Some tests, such as the Wisconsin Card Sorting Test (Heaton, 2003), have been adapted for computer but not for Internet-based or remote administration. In some approaches to neuropsychological assessment, the examiner takes careful note of the specific strategies examinees employ when attempting to perform tasks. Hence, performing an examination when the examiner and the patient are in different locations can seem daunting. In this respect, while Medicare reimburses for tele-mental health, at the time of this writing, they do not reimburse for remotely conducted psychological or neuropsychological testing.

Despite the challenges, there are compelling reasons to develop and validate approaches for remote neurocognitive assessment. The two principal drivers for telemedicine, reducing cost and increasing access, are also the main forces driving the development of teleneuropsychology. While neuropsychology has experienced significant growth over the past few decades, not all patients in need of its services have ready access to providers, and the challenge of reaching providers can be exacerbated by limitations brought on by neurological conditions. Implementing telemedicine for remote cognitive assessment has the potential to expand the reach of neuropsychologists, permitting them to serve more locations while reducing the burden of travel for patients. Remote cognitive assessment can also facilitate patient follow-up for both clinical and research applications. From a clinical perspective, tracking a patient's neurocognitive status at intervals can provide critical information to practitioners about how a patient is recovering from an injury or whether there are indications that a patient's cognitive status is worsening or remaining stable. More detailed assessment can reveal patterns of neuropsychological performance over time that might help inform diagnosis or prognosis.

From a research standpoint, having the ability to evaluate and monitor subjects remotely can potentially improve compliance in clinical trials and reduce dropout rates in longitudinal studies. Remote assessment can also reduce interexaminer variability by using the same examiners to remotely perform evaluations, rather than training and monitoring different examiners across multiple sites.

The challenge for neuropsychologists is to develop models for remote neurocognitive assessment and to demonstrate that they can obtain valid results using the models and achieve test scores that are comparable to those obtained from a traditional in-person examination where the examiner and patient are co-located. To date, four models have emerged for remote neuropsychological assessment. Each model is discussed below, along with data supporting its use.

## MODEL 1

Neuropsychologists frequently make use of technicians to administer and score tests in the same way that medical practitioners rely on trained technologists to administer procedures like medical tests and brain imaging studies, among others. Typically, the neuropsychologist reviews the available medical record, interviews the patient, and then works with the technician to plan the examination based on the patient's presentation and the referral question. A model that has been implemented in some health systems modifies slightly the technician-based approach to assessment by having the technician administer tests in the usual face-to-face manner but with the neuropsychologist remotely conducting the interview and providing guidance to the individual administering the tests. This model is enhanced by the use of the electronic medical record, which permits clinicians to access patient records at different locations. This method of implementing remote cognitive assessment hasn't been formally studied, likely due to the fact that the actual tests are given in the traditional manner and there is extant literature supporting using video links to accomplish patient interviews (Myers & Turvey, 2012). This model represents the easiest, most intuitive, and least disruptive method of implementing the neuropsychological examination when the responsible clinician is at a different location than the patient. The strength of the model is that it permits testing to take place in the usual manner and consistent with how tests were normed, while at the same time expanding the reach of the . neuropsychologist. The weakness of the model is that it requires a trained technician to be available at a remote clinic location, or in some cases that the technician be able to travel to the patient. While the model offers an approach to teleneuropsychology that is a logical extension of traditional practice, its success rests on the availability of a trained tester at the site where the patient is. In a number of situations, having a technician co-located with the patient is an obtainable objective. In other situations, having a technician available at the same location as the patient may not be possible, and requiring the presence of a trained tester could prevent the patient from being examined neuropsychologically.

## MODEL 2

In the second model, both the clinical interview and neuropsychological tests are administered to the patient via video teleconference (VTC). Instructions are given by the remote examiner, who also records responses and presents stimuli using an audiovisual connection. An assistant may be available at the same site as the patient to help initiate the process and to establish the video link. However, the assistant does not have to be a trained tester, and once the patient is in place and the connection is established, the remote clinician and/or technician administers all examination procedures. Since Model 2 is a departure from the typical method of in-person test administration, the acceptance of this approach is dependent on research demonstrating the equivalency of results, along with patient acceptance.

Research support for Model 2 has grown since the early days when very brief omnibus screening tools were deployed in healthy and/or minimally impaired populations. In the beginning, the challenges included limited bandwidth and blurred or jerky images during movement, sound-video time delays, limited scope of camera vision, and occasional loss of connectivity. Modern videoteleconferencing allows for near-real-time interactions, high-definition video and sound, and moveable, remotely controlled cameras at the far end to monitor patient behaviors during testing.

Many neuropsychological measures are orally administered and require oral responses, thereby making for an easy transition to the VTC environment. Patient satisfaction with general VTC interactions has been high across studies in various contexts, including psychiatric interviewing and psychotherapy (Myers & Turvey, 2012). Patient satisfaction with teleneuropsychological assessment has only recently been demonstrated, but evidence was supportive among older individuals with and without cognitive impairment (Parikh et al., 2013). As noted above, some tests lend themselves much better to the VTC environment than others, as some traditional measures require manipulable stimuli. Some difficulties can be addressed by having stimuli at the remote end and by giving careful instruction to, and monitoring of, the patient during motor tasks, while some tests are not suitable to the remote testing model or might require re-norming under VTC conditions if procedural adaptations might affect test instructions or response recording/scoring.

Test norms are one of the cornerstones of neuropsychological assessment, and the ability for neuropsychologists to use standard normative reference data derived from large healthy samples for tests administered in the VTC environment is important, lest alternate norms be needed. Therefore, most teleneuropsychological studies have used verbally oriented assessment tools and have examined the reliability of traditional face-to-face administration compared to VTC-based administration. Early studies generally did not counterbalance test conditions or test forms, but showed good promise in terms of overall reliability (Loh et al., 2004).

One of the largest teleneuropsychology investigations to date (Cullum, Hynan, Grosch, Parikh, & Weiner, 2014) included over 200 participants and used counterbalanced test conditions (face-to-face vs VTC) and counterbalanced alternate test forms for most measures studied. Subjects included 119 healthy individuals and 83 patients diagnosed with mild cognitive impairment or Alzheimer's disease. The focus of the investigation was to examine the feasibility and reliability of VTC versus face-to-face administration of a brief yet reasonably broad array of neuropsychological measures commonly used in the evaluation of older patients with and without cognitive impairment (see Table 5.1 for list of tests).

All participants completed all tests, reflecting good feasibility, and no significant problems occurred during VTC test sessions to disrupt the assessment process. Results revealed highly similar test scores across face-to-face and VTC test conditions, with no significant differences in means. Likewise, good to strong intraclass correlations were obtained (all $p$'s < .0001), with most values in the .7 to .9 range ($M = .74$) with only Digit Span forward and backward showing intraclass correlation coefficients (ICCs) of .59 and .55, respectively. The results were consistent with the findings from previous small studies in the literature and also consistent with general test–retest results using the measures under traditional administration conditions.

TABLE 5.1 Neuropsychological Measures Examined

| Measure | Domain Assessed |
| --- | --- |
| MMSE | Global cognitive function |
| Hopkins Verbal Learning Test-Revised (Forms 1 & 4) | Verbal learning and memory |
| Digit Span: Forward and Backward | Attention/working memory |
| 30-Item Boston Naming Test | Confrontation naming |
| Letter & Category Fluency Tests | Verbal fluency |
| Clock Drawing Test | Visuospatial skills |

Given the generally verbally oriented nature of most of the tests, the findings were not surprising, although it remained to be seen whether similar results would be found using other tests and in other populations. Cullum and colleagues expanded the initial findings by examining the Repeatable Battery for Neuropsychological Status (RBANS; Randolf, (2012) administered in face-to-face and VTC conditions using Forms A and B of the RBANS in counterbalanced fashion. The results revealed very similar scores in both testing conditions, thereby further attesting to the utility and reliability of VTC-based neuropsychological test administration (Galusha, Horton, Weiner, & Cullum, 2016). In terms of applicability to remote and underserved populations, Cullum's group found similar results among members of the Choctaw Nation in Oklahoma, with ICCs on these same tests ranging from .65 to .93 ($M = .82$) in individuals with and without cognitive impairment (Wadsworth et al., 2016). In addition to supporting the feasibility and reliability of VTC-based neuropsychological assessment with the tools examined, these results proved reliable for subjects with or without cognitive impairment.

While individuals with severe cognitive impairment may not be able to undergo unassisted remote assessment, in over 200 VTC-based testing sessions, Cullum and colleagues encountered only one subject with dementia who became confused and left the test session. This sample included individuals with MMSE scores as low as 15, even though the majority of subjects with dementia were only mildly impaired. Interestingly, while all participants found the VTC testing condition acceptable (Parikh et al., 2013), patients with cognitive impairment expressed a slight preference to be tested in-person compared with healthy controls.

Thus, a growing literature suggests the feasibility, reliability, and validity of remote VTC-based neuropsychological assessment, although still only a handful of tests have been examined in the VTC environment. More work using additional visuospatial tasks and executive-function measures in particular is needed, and modifications to existing test procedures must be carefully documented and studied. Along these lines, Cullum and his colleagues have experimented with the remote administration of WAIS-IV Block Design, but this requires the subject at the remote end to access, arrange, and manipulate the blocks while viewing the target stimulus via TV monitor and obviously requires some procedural modifications. Since alterations to test instructions or modified testing procedures could potentially affect test results, more systematic research in this area is needed.

MODEL 3

Tests and test batteries that are computer administered have become increasingly available in neuropsychology. A number of these tests present the patient with on-screen instructions and practice items and may require the patient to attain a certain score during the practice samples before proceeding to the actual test. This approach to presenting instructions enhances the ability of tests to be administered with minimum examiner input. The structure of the tests, and the fact that they are computer administered, make them adaptable for remote testing. The cognitive measures can reside, or be downloaded temporarily, on the computer being used by a patient who is in video communication with the examiner or they can be given over the web. Test data can be sent to the remote examiner or can be directly retrieved by the remote examiner over the Internet.

A number of issues have to be addressed when developing or adapting computerized tests for remote administration. The issues involve the usability of the system for the patient, the impact of the test administration method on test performance and response timing, test security, and the protection of health information. Usability is important and the ability of patients to take tests remotely on a computer is a function of the test design, user interface, and the way in which the remote examiner remains part of the process. It also depends on the cognitive resources of the patient; not all patients are suitable for all assessment approaches. Whether computerized tests run locally on the system the patient is using or are accessed via a web browser has implications for test measures that attempt to precisely capture response time. Capturing response times over the Internet is complicated by the type and reliability of the connection and its bandwidth, program and browser characteristics, and data management methods. It is incumbent for publishers of a test running over the Internet to demonstrate how they have approached the timing challenges and to provide data demonstrating the precision and possible variance in their response-time scores. To circumvent the challenges of obtaining reliable Internet-based timing, store-and-forward approaches can be implemented. It is possible to run a test on the computer being used by the patient while transferring the data to the remote examiner's location. Likewise, when using computerized tests remotely, it is important to verify that programs running in conjunction with the cognitive tests that attempt to add functionality—such as monitoring the patient along with his or her responses—do not conflict with the ability of the test software to accurately control the display of test stimuli or to record response times at the level required by the cognitive task.

A recent study by Settle and colleagues (Settle, Robinson, Kane, Maloni, & Wallin, 2015) demonstrated the ability to employ this model for both remote clinic and home-based evaluations. In the study, the investigators reported results from 20 patients with multiple sclerosis (MS). Patients were assessed under three conditions using a set of tests from the Automated Neuropsychological Assessment Metrics (ANAM) test system (Reeves, Winter, Bleiberg, & Kane, 2007). ANAM is a library of computer-administered neurocognitive tests that permits the configuration of batteries for specific uses. For this study, a number of tests were selected that had proven efficacious in previous studies of patients with MS (Kane, Roebuck-Spenser, Kabat, & Wilken, 2007; Pellicano et al., 2013; Wilken et al., 2003, 2013). Initially, subjects were randomized into one of two conditions: 1) test administration with the examiner in the room with the patient; and 2) the examiner in a different room but in contact with the patient through video and audio links. Approximately one month later, patients assessed under condition 1 were assessed under condition 2, and vice versa. ANAM throughput scores for each test were used in the analysis and a summary throughput score was computed as a general indicator of how well a patient performed. There was no statistical difference between individual test scores or the summary score as a function of method of administration. Approximately eight months later (median = 252.5 days), patients underwent the same battery remotely from their homes. Scores from three ANAM tests were significantly different when taken at home compared to the in-person or adjacent remote office administration. When differences occurred, subjects scored slightly better when taking the test at home, likely a result of practice effects, since the home remote administration was the third time patients had been tested using the same battery. Test forms were held constant so as to reduce any form differences as a source of variance. While the study had only 20 subjects taking the test battery under all three conditions, and while all subjects had the same neurological diagnosis, findings gave support to the feasibility of using tests from the ANAM system for remote administration. Findings also supported the utility of this model of using automated tests to assess patients in a different location than the examiner.

A variation of this model currently in use is the store-and-forward computer-based testing that has been implemented in the Department of Defense (DoD) and in the athletic arena for the assessment of concussion at all levels of sport. The implementation is based on a risk-for-injury paradigm and involves obtaining cognitive baseline data that can be used later for postinjury comparison, in addition to the use of norms. Baseline computerized testing can be administered to individuals or to groups of individuals making use of a pretest instructional brief and proctors, and there are a number of popular testing platforms (see Resch, McCrea, & Cullum, 2013). Data are then stored and can be used later to assess potential postinjury changes. In some implementations of this model, comparing pre- and postinjury data can be accomplished independently of the patient's location.

## Hybrid Models

While the three models described above were presented as distinct, they can be combined in implementing a remote cognitive assessment program. For example, it is possible to implement remote testing combining traditional with computerized measures, although this approach has not been studied extensively to date. In Model 2, the remote examiner can make use of a helper to arrange blocks to administer the Wechsler Block Design Test or to place a tapping device or pegboard in front of the patient. Patients can also be instructed to access certain test stimuli at different times during the examination (e.g., "take out the piece of paper from the blue folder on the table labeled Folder #1") previously set up by a remote assistant. Drawings can be done remotely and either observed and scored via video, can be done on a digitizing bitpad that transmits the image electronically, or can be done on paper and sent via fax by an assistant. Whether such modifications significantly affect test results or scoring remains unknown but should be carefully considered.

While additional data are needed to fully support the implementation of remote neurocognitive assessment, the largest obstacles to this approach to care delivery are likely to be regulatory and involve licensing and reimbursement. Studies validating remote neurocognitive assessment as an effective method for care delivery are in their early stages but have been consistently supportive of the concept that valid patient assessments can obtained remotely. It is highly likely that future studies will also confirm that valid assessments can be obtained remotely, even if additional norms are required along with some modifications of procedures. Little if any additional data should be required to support the first model discussed above where the actual testing is done by a technician co-located with the patient. However, once the science is established, licensing and reimbursement are likely to remain a challenge. Currently, a neuropsychologist providing remote assessment across state lines is required to be licensed in both the state from which the neuropsychologist is operating and the state where the patient is located. Psychologists can be licensed in more than one state, but the process of maintaining licenses in more than one state can be expensive and time consuming, depending on state requirements. There are current efforts to make the process easier for a psychologist licensed in one state to obtain licenses in other states. However, the process of obtaining multiple licenses is still involved and efforts to institute a national licensing process remain aspirational and unlikely to bring about changes in state licensing in the foreseeable future. For remote neurocognitive assessment to become an option for patients, third-party payers will have to acknowledge that this approach to assessment is valid and that it constitutes a reasonable standard of care. If healthcare continues to move in the direction of outcome-based payments, studies of remote neuropsychological assessment will need to demonstrate the utility of the information gained, patient satisfaction, improved patient access, and cost savings associated with remote assessment. These goals appear achievable in light of studies accomplished to date, but additional research with larger and more diverse samples is needed to definitely establish remote cognitive assessment as a standard of practice.

## Remote Cognitive Rehabilitation

The models discussed so far focus primarily on assessment. Neuropsychologists are also involved in the provision of therapy services and cognitive rehabilitation. Implementing rehabilitation remotely has received insufficient attention despite the cognitive enhancement programs available commercially through the Internet. The development of remote cognitive interventions also needs to follow a programmatic and sequential process. First, the method employed has to be shown to be effective when delivered in a traditional manner, and this is best done through randomized clinical trials. Treatment effect sizes in the arena of cognitive rehabilitation tend to vary with study design and are often smaller in studies that employ control groups (Rohling, Faust, Beverly, & Demakis, 2009). Once an intervention is demonstrated as efficacious, it should be evaluated for adaptability for remote implementation. The next step is to conduct a clinical trial to demonstrate that the method retains effectiveness when implemented remotely, that the technology runs smoothly, and that patients respond positively when engaging in an intervention provided through telehealth. Based on the growing body of literature pertaining to telehealth in general, there is little reason to believe that therapies cannot be delivered effectively and won't meet with substantial patient satisfaction. Nevertheless, telemedicine-based cognitive rehabilitation needs to be evidence based from the standpoint of both patient care and obtaining reimbursement. Chapter 12 in this volume by Anthony Chen and his colleagues gives an example of a theoretically driven and evidence-based research program that makes use of a computer-game interface that can be implemented either in person or remotely.

## Conclusion

A driving force behind telemedicine is access to care. Access can be narrowly viewed as referring to whether care is available within an individual's broad geographic area. However, access is better viewed by factoring in issues of cost, travel, and the likelihood that obstacles to care will result in an evaluation or treatment's not taking place. Despite the growth of neuropsychology as a field, locating nearby services can be a problem for many patients. For other individuals, travel can be a financial or physical burden. Bringing services to the home or to a more convenient location can result in both improved care and reduced costs. Teleneuropsychology is in its early stages of development from both an assessment and treatment perspective. However, studies to date support the viability of this approach to patient assessment. As telehealth continues to grow and to become an important part of the healthcare system both in the United States and in other countries, it will be important for neuropsychology to continue to develop evidence-based capabilities relating to remote assessment and treatment.

## References

Cullum, C. M., Hynan, L. S., Grosch, M., Parikh, M., & Weiner, M. F. (2014). Teleneuropsychology: Evidence for video conference-based neuropsychological assessment. *Journal of the International Neuropsychological Society, 20*, 1–6.

Galusha, J. M., Horton, D. K., Weiner, M. F., & Cullum, C. M. (2016). Video teleconference administration of the Repeatable Battery for the Assessment of Neuropsychological Status. *Archives of Clinical Neuropsychology, 31*, 8–11.

Heaton, R. K. (2003). *Wisconsin Card Sorting Test computer version 4.0.* Odessa, FL: Psychological Assessment Resources.

Kane, R. L., Roebuck-Spenser, T. M., Kabat, M. H., & Wilken, J. A. (2007). Identifying and monitoring cognitive deficits in a clinical population using Automated Neuropsychological Assessment Metrics (ANAM) tests. *Archives of Clinical Neuropsychology, 22*(S1), s115–s126.

Loh, P. K., Ramesh, P., Maher, S., Saligari, J., Flicker, L., & Goldswain, P. (2004). Can patients with demenita be assessed at a distance? The use of telehealth and standardized assessments. *Internal Medicine Journal, 34*, 239–242.

Myers, K., & Turvey, C. (Eds.). (2012). *Telemental health: Clinical, technical and administrative foundations for evidence-based practice.* Amsterdam: Elsevier.

Federal Register (2016). *Federal Register: Managed care and revisions related to third party liability; Final Rule.* Washington, DC: Centers for Medicare & Medicaid Services.

Parikh, M., Grosch, M. C., Graham, L. L., Hynan, L. S., Weiner, M., Shore, J. H., & Cullum, C. M. (2013). Consumer acceptability of brief videoconference-based neuropsychological assessment in older individuals with and without cognitive impairment. *The Clinical Neuropsychologist, 27*(5), 808–817.

Pellicano, C., Kane, R. L., Gallo, A., Xiaobai, L., Stern, S. K., Ikonomidou, V. E., … Bagnato, F. (2013). Cognitive impairment and its relation to imaging measures in multiple sclerosis: A study using a computerized battery. *Journal of Neuroimaging, 23*(3), 445–452.

Randolf, C. (2012). *RBANS update: Repeatable Battery for the Assessment of Neuropsychological Status.* Bloomington, NCSPearson: PsychCorp.

Reeves D. L., Winter, K., Bleiberg, J., Kane R. L. (2007). ANAM genogram: Historical perspectives, description, and current endeavors. *Archives of Clinical Neuropsychology, 22S*, S15–S37.

Resch, J. E., McCrea, M. A., & Cullum, C. M. (2013). Computerized neurocognitive testing in the management of sport-related concussion: An update. *Neuropsychology Review, 23,* 335–349.

Rohling, M. L., Faust, M. E., Beverly, B., & Demakis, G. (2009). Effectiveness of cognitive rehabilitation following acquired brain injury: A meta-analytic re-examination of Cicerone et al.'s (2000, 2005) systematic reviews. *Neuropsychology, 23*(1), 20–39.

Settle, J. R., Robinson, S. A., Kane, R., Maloni, H. W., & Wallin, M. T. (2015). Remote cognitive assessments for patients with multiple sclerosis: A feasibility study. *Multiple Sclerosis Journal, 21*(8), 1072–1079. doi:10.1177/1352458514559296

Shore, J. H. (2013). Telepsychiatry: videoconferencing in the delivery of psychiatric care. *American Journal of Psychiatry, 170,* 256–262.

Wadsworth, H. E., Galusha-Glasscock, J. M., Womack, K. B., Quiceno, M., Weiner, M. F., Hynan, L. S., Shore, J., & Cullum, C.M. (2016). Remote neuropsychological assessment in rural American Indians with and without cognitive impairment. *Archives of Clinical Neuropsychology, 31*(5), 420–425.

Wilken, J. A., Kane, R. L., Sullivan, C. L., Gudesblatt, M., Lucas, S., Fallis, R., . . . Foulds, P. (2013). Changes in fatigue and cognition in patients with relapsing forms of multiple sclerosis treated with natalizumab: The ENER-G Study. *International Journal of MA Care, 15,* 120–128.

Wilken, J. A., Kane, R. L., Sullivan, C. L., Wallin, M. T., Usiskin, J. B., Quig, M. E., . . . Reeves, D. L. (2003). The utility of computerized neuropsychological assessment of cogntive dysfunction in patients with relapsing-remitting multiple sclerosis. *MS, 9,* 119–127.

# PART III

# Domain and Scenario-Based Assessment

# 6

# Advances in Neuropsychological Assessment of Attention

## FROM INITIAL COMPUTERIZED CONTINUOUS PERFORMANCE TESTS TO AULA

### Unai Díaz-Orueta

## What Is a Continuous Performance Test?

Attention is one of the most basic cognitive processes and is a prerequisite for the use of more complex functions, since it is not possible to evaluate perception or memory processes without keeping in mind attention issues (Amador, Forns, & Kirchner, 2006). The ability to maintain an appropriate level of attention is basic for education and learning, especially during childhood and school age. With the aim of studying attention separately from other cognitive functions, the so-called continuous performance tests (CPT) were created. The first series of CPTs were developed by Rosvold, Mirsky, Sarason, Bransome, and Beck (1956) to study vigilance in adults with acquired brain injury (Riccio, Reynolds, & Lowe, 2001), more specifically, persons with seizures (Amador, Forns, & Kirchner, 2006). Nowadays, CPTs are still one of the most widely used measures for the assessment of attention and processing speed. Briefly, it can be said that a CPT is a group of paradigms to evaluate attention, inhibitory response or disinhibition (a component of executive control that provides information about the subject's impulsivity), and processing speed. Basically, CPTs rely on the rapid, random presentation of a series of stimuli to which the subject must respond following instructions given at the beginning of the test. The main value of CPTs is their empirical support. Diverse CPT paradigms have consistently demonstrated their sensitivity for a great variety of both neurological and psychiatric disorders, in adults and in children.

Frequently, CPTs also use a continuous vigilance task, in order to obtain quantitative information about the individual's ability to sustain attention in time. From its creation, the CPT paradigm has been used with many variants of its task component. Greenberg and Walkman (1993) found up to 100 different

versions of CPT in use. Historically, when Rosvold and his collaborators introduced the test, they had the goal of measuring correct answers provided by the
subject as an indicator of selective attention. With subsequent experimentation,
other measures, such as processing speed, impulsivity, inattention, and sustained
attention, divided or alternate, have been included. Among the variations, we
found changes or variants in the shape of the target stimulus, while in more traditional CPTs, the subject is asked to press the button when he sees the letter
X on the screen. Nowadays, target stimuli include letters, numbers, geometric
shapes, sentences, objects, and faces, and there are variations in the way items are
presented (visual, auditory, or mixed presentations).

Use of a CPT is an excellent option for obtaining objective, quantifiable, and
carefully calibrated data about the course of an attention or executive control
problem, according to Riccio et al. (2001). Losier, McGrath, and Klein (1996) performed a meta-analysis of 26 studies that tested children with attention deficit/
hyperactivity disorder (ADHD) using different versions of CPT and confirmed
the children's poorer performance on CPTs, especially with regard to scores
obtained for commission and omission errors (which were significantly higher
in children with ADHD than in healthy children). After an extensive review of
neuropsychological measures, Barkley (1994) concluded that CPTs are the best
and most objective measures for the diagnosis of ADHD.

Usefulness of CPTs in ADHD is based on their ability to differentiate children with a clinical diagnosis from healthy children. As Fernández-Jaén, Martín
Fernández-Mayoralas, Calleja-Pérez, Moreno-Acero, and Muñoz-Jareño (2008)
state, CPTs have numerous advantages in evaluating patients with ADHD, such
as validity in measuring sustained attention, objectivity, ease of administration,
and lack of conditioning by visual perceptive or motor problems or learning or
mood difficulties. In the specific case of ADHD, CPTs have shown a greater sensitivity and specificity in diagnosis. Undoubtedly, no psychometric test can diagnose ADHD by itself, but CPTs have shown a sensitivity of 90% and a specificity
of 70% in many cases, values that have improved with the latest developments in
virtual reality (VR), as described below.

Some studies have focused their efforts on investigating which parameters
of CPTs correlate with already defined features of ADHD. Epstein, Erkanli,
Conners, Kleric, Castello, and Angold (2003), using Conners' CPT, found that
omission errors correlate with inattention symptoms described in ADHD,
and commission errors correlate with impulsivity symptoms. Moreover, some
variables also showed significant relationships with many hyperactivity and
impulsivity symptoms. In addition, the Conners group found that reaction time
acted as a predictor of ADHD symptomatology, showing overall a slower reaction when pressing the button in front of the target stimuli, and showing that
children with ADHD have more difficulty differentiating between target and
nontarget stimuli. Miranda, Barbosa, Muszkalt et al. (2008) confirmed some of

these findings and demonstrated that children with ADHD made more omission and commission errors, showed a more variable response time, had more perseverative responses, and were less able to discriminate between target and nontarget stimuli, but they did not find any differences from controls in terms of reaction time.

Many studies (reviewed by Silvana and Nada, 2009) have compared different variations of the CPT presentation format. For example, Baker, Taylor and Leyva (1995), cited by Silvana and Nada (2009), administered the Gordon Diagnostic System (Gordon, 1983) and the Comprehensive Auditory Visual Attention Assessment System (Becker, 1993) to 82 university students between 17 and 45 years old. Students completed four tasks: auditory vigilance, visual vigilance, and auditory and visual distraction. Based on the comparison of omission and commission errors, the investigators found that university students performed better on visual, rather than auditory, tasks. Sandford and Turner (1995) found similar results, that is, more commission errors when stimuli are presented on an auditory basis, especially in children with ADHD. These findings suggest that tasks of auditory attention can be more sensitive, and hence more useful, for the identification of sustained attention and executive control problems.

Currently, new developments in virtual reality (VR) offer interesting alternatives for the neuropsychological evaluation of cognitive processes. Recently, VR has been considered a reliable method for testing ADHD children's ability to sustain performance over time, especially as a consequence of the research produced by Rizzo et al. (Bioulac, Lallemand, Rizzo, Philip, Fabrigoule, & Bouvard, 2012; Rizzo, Bowerly, Buckwalter, Limchuk, Mitura, & Parsons, 2006), with the development of the Virtual Classroom. In the Virtual Classroom VR test (described in detail in Rizzo et al., 2006), participants are instructed to view a series of letters presented on the blackboard and to hit the response button only after viewing the letter X preceded by the letter A (i.e., a successive discrimination task) and to withhold their response to any other sequence of letters. Stimuli are presented for 150 milliseconds each, with a fixed interstimulus interval of 1,350 milliseconds. There are two 10-min testing conditions, one without distractors and one with distractors (pure auditory, pure visual, and mixed audiovisual distractors). In addition to the results reported in this study (with a sample of 18 participants, comparing eight physician-referred 6- to 12-year-old males with ADHD and ten nondiagnosed males), the Virtual Classroom is currently undergoing wider administration in a larger study currently in progress at the National Institute of Health, which may help in its standardization (http://clinicaltrials.gov/ct2/show/ NC-T01721720).

The AULA test was developed with the aim of taking advantage of VR as an increasingly useful resource for multiple health-related applications and also to overcome the absence of ecological validity for computerized tests of attention

(Climent & Banterla, 2010). The AULA ("classroom," in Spanish) is based on the CPT paradigm but it is performed in a VR environment that employs a set of three-dimensional VR glasses with movement sensors.

The next sections of this chapter review the existing computerized environments based on the CPT paradigm that have been used for the evaluation of attention processes, and ultimately focus on the AULA test, because AULA is the only VR test that has undergone an extensive normative study with a clinical population, and therefore AULA can be used in a standardized and systematic way to evaluate attention processes in ADHD and other conditions. Hence, the features of the AULA test are discussed in detail and a compendium of the most significant AULA test results (in terms of reliability, validity, sensitivity, and specificity, among others) is presented, with the aim that it may serve as a model for future developments of VR-based tests for neuropsychological assessment and their validation as standardized tools.

## Overview of Computerized CPTs for Evaluating Attention

### GORDON DIAGNOSTIC SYSTEM

The Gordon Diagnostic System (GDS; Gordon, 1983) is a CPT that measures impulsivity, inattention, and distractibility. It is specifically designed to support diagnosis of attention disorders, especially ADHD. According to its author, it provides reliable and objective information about a subject's sustained attention and self-control (impulsivity). The GDS is a portable unit based on a microprocessor that administers a series of game-like tasks. The vigilance task assesses an individual's ability to focus and sustain attention throughout time and in absence of feedback. A series of digits are shown, one by one, on an electronic screen. The child is ask to press a button whenever the number 1 is followed by a 9 (an AX paradigm, which has been considered by some authors as a measure of working memory rather than an attention measure; Climent & Banterla, 2010; Rizzo et al., 2006). The GDS registers correct and incorrect responses, as well as errors in responding to a 1–9 combination. A more complex version of this paradigm, known as the Distractibility Test, is designed for older children and adults and shows irrelevant digits on each side of a column that shows target stimuli. For the youngest children, GDS has a variant that requires the child to press the button only when the number 1 appears. The GDS also offers parallel forms for each task and an impulse-control test (delayed task) that requires a child to inhibit the answer to obtain points. Each task can be administered in less than 9 min. The microprocessor generates the tasks and registers quantitative features of the child's performance. The GDS is recognized as a medical device by the Food & Drug Administration and has been widely standardized.

Mayes, Calhoun, Chase, Mink, and Stagg (2009) examined common features of distractibility and processing speed indexes from WISC and the GDS in 587 children with ADHD, combined and inattentive subtypes. They found that results for attention were low in all the groups, with the group with the combined subtype showing more impulsivity in the GDS delayed task and inattentive children showing lower processing speed than children with the combined subtype.

## CONNERS' CONTINUOUS PERFORMANCE TEST

Conners' Continuous Performance Test (Conners & MHS Staff, 2004) is considered the gold standard of attention evaluation worldwide, so that everyone refers to it as "the CPT," as if there were no other tasks that follow the CPT paradigm. In this computerized test, patients are required to press the space bar or to click the mouse at the appearance of any letter that is not the letter X. Interstimulus intervals range from 1 or 2 to 4 s, with a stimulus presentation time of 250 milliseconds. The order in which different interstimulus intervals are used varies between the presented stimuli blocks. The Conners' CPT is conceived to be applicable to anyone more than 6 years old. One of its advantages is its database of results from 2,686 clinical and nonclinical subjects, with large subsamples of individuals with neurological damage. It allows comparing subjects' answers with normative data from the general population, ADHD norms, and brain injury norms. It can be used to monitor the efficiency of pharmacological or any other kind of treatment, with high sensitivity (low false-positive rate) and specificity (low false-negative rate). Conners' CPT captures and registers response times in milliseconds. The program classifies reaction times lower than 100 milliseconds as perseverations, since it considers that it is virtually impossible for a test taker to answer so fast, being more likely that such rapid answering is perseverative or anticipatory rather than a response to the processed signal. Errors are divided into omission and commission errors. An omission error takes place when the subject does not provide an answer when he should (with any letter that is not an X), and a commission error takes place when the subject answers when he should not (when the letter X appears). Other measures are reaction time for correct answers (as a measure of processing speed); variability in reaction time (as a measure of sustained attention or vigilance); d' or attentiveness (a kind of quality of attention), which indicates to what extent the person discriminates between target and nontarget stimuli; perseverations (as already described, anticipatory answering indicative of impulsivity, as well as random answers indicative of decline), and very low responses to the previous stimulus that may indicate inattention. Normative data are obtained from the U.S. population. The sample groups described in the test manual are 1,259 children between 6 and 16 years old and an ADHD clinical sample of 271 children in the same age range.

## TEST OF VARIABLES OF ATTENTION

Test of Variables of Attention (TOVA) was developed in the 1960s and its latest version, version 7, was published in 1997. TOVA is a computerized test for the evaluation of inattention, with normative data by age and gender and with an approximate administration time of 21.5 min. Its length allows efficient measurement of attention deficits. The subject is placed in front of a computer screen, where shiny squares appear for 0.1 s in 2-s intervals. Each square shines in the upper part of another, bigger square, or else in the bottom part. If it appears in the upper part, it is considered a target stimulus, and if it appears in the bottom part, it is a nontarget stimulus. Each time the target square appears, the person must press a small switch as soon as he sees the target. Each time the nontarget appears, the person must avoid pressing the switch. Omission errors are the number of times the subject does not press the switch when he should, and commission errors the number of times he presses the switch in response to a nontarget stimulus. Response time is the amount of time taken to press after the target stimulus is presented, and variability refers to the subject's response consistency.

TOVA has been used successfully for the diagnosis of ADHD and its subtypes (Forbes, 1998; Llorente, Voigt, Jensen, Fraley, Heird, & Rennie, 2007; Riccio, Garland, & Cohen, 2007; Wada, Yamashita, Matsuishi, Ohtani, & Kato, 2000; Weyandt, Mitzlaff, & Thomas, 2002). In this sense, pure inattention would correlate with omission errors, impulsivity with commission errors, psychomotor delay with a slow reaction time, and inconsistency with a high variability in TOVA reaction time. However, a recent study by Zelnik, Bennett-Back, Miari, Goez, & Fattal-Valevski (2012) states that one of the biggest problems with TOVA and other CPTs is the discrepancy between satisfactory sensitivity with a high predictive value and poor specificity. In other words, TOVA's ability to establish that children without ADHD are actually non-ADHD is poor (for example, in children who have learning difficulties or behavioral disorders). In this sense, relying only on tests like TOVA can lead to overdiagnosis and misuse of the term ADHD for many conditions that may contribute to poor school performance.

## CHILDREN SUSTAINED ATTENTION TASK

Children Sustained Attention Task (CSAT) is a computerized test that can be administered to children from 6 to 11 years old, with a length of 7.5 min. Its goal is to assess sustained attention by means of a vigilance task. The child must press the space bar whenever he is shown the sequence 6–3 (the number 6 followed by a 3). According to CSAT's authors (Servera & Llabrés, 2004), raw scores of correct answers, reaction times, and commission errors are obtained, while several combined indexes based on signal detection theory are interpreted in terms of a neurocognitive response to attention (Servera & Llabrés, 2004, p. 20). The indexes include the subject's ability to sustain attention (d'), the response criterion or bias (C), and the sustained attention ability as a function of the discrimination level shown (A'). The raw value of A' ranges between 0 and 1, and values close to 0.5 indicate that there has been a similar percentage of correct and incorrect answers; values close to 0 (many more errors than correct answers) indicate low attentional capacity and values close to 1 (many more correct answers than errors) indicate that discrimination takes place (due to a high attentional capacity). The CSAT's main problem is the narrow interstimulus interval (only 500 ms), which may misclassify children with low processing speed as ADHD (either inattentive or impulsive) since these children may require a larger interval (up to 1,500 ms) to provide an answer. For example, a child who is slow to respond to the target stimulus A might erroneously provide an answer to stimulus B due to the narrow interstimulus interval. In this example, the child may obtain an omission error with stimulus A and a commission error with B, when he was neither inattentive nor impulsive, just slow.

## Virtual Classrooms in Neuropsychology: An Overview

Since virtual environments (VEs) were implemented to be used in the neuropsychological evaluation of children, the most logical environment to be used as an emulator of the environment children are most frequently exposed to is the classroom. Probably one of the most well-known versions of the Virtual Classroom is the one developed by Rizzo et al. (2001, 2006). In the Virtual Classroom VR test (described in detail in Rizzo et al., 2006), participants are instructed to view a series of letters presented on the blackboard and to hit the response button only after viewing the letter X preceded by the letter A (i.e., a successive discrimination task) and to withhold their response to any other sequence of letters. Stimuli are presented for 150 milliseconds each, with a fixed interstimulus interval of 1,350 milliseconds. There are two 10-min testing conditions, one without distractors and one with distractors (pure auditory, pure visual, and mixed audiovisual distractors). The Virtual Classroom is currently undergoing wider administration in a larger study currently in progress at the National Institutes of Health, which may help with its standardization (http://clinicaltrials.gov/ct2/show/NCT01721720).

To help with discussion of the various versions of the Virtual Classroom, Table 6.1 collects different studies and versions that have been used so far, providing details about the sample used, research design followed, and results obtained.

As can be seen, despite the studies focusing on normally developing children and adolescents and those with ADHD, very few studies have extended their focus to other populations likely to suffer attention problems and whose proper assessment may have benefits in establishing the relevant neuropsychological rehabilitation program. The study by Nolin et al. (2009) was the first one documented that focused on children with traumatic brain injury (TBI) in

TABLE 6.1 Overview of Neuropsychological Studies Using a Virtual Classroom Environment

| Authors/study | VR class version | Sample | Research design | Tests used | Results |
|---|---|---|---|---|---|
| Lee et al. (2001) | Their own developed version, used as an environment for training, not evaluation. | $N = 20$ (10 undergoing VR training and 10 controls). | Intergroup comparison of experimental versus control group. | A continuous performance test (CPT), not specified which. | Decrease of omissions and commissions in VR, significant when compared to control group. |
| Cho et al. (2002) | Their own developed version, used as an environment for training, not evaluation. | $N = 50$, ages 14–18, with learning difficulties, inattentiveness, impulsivity, hyperactivity, and distractibility. 30% of subjects most likely had ADHD. | Randomly assigned to one of five 10-subject groups: a control group, two placebo groups (desktop VR EEG biofeedback training, and desktop VR cognitive training), and two experimental groups (Group 1: VR EEG biofeedback training; Group 2: VR cognitive training). | A continuous performance test (CPT), not specified which. | Experimental groups showed significant improvement with regard to inattentiveness ($p < .01$), while control group indicated no significant change. The experimental groups showed no significant difference between them. |
| Parsons, Bowerly, Buckwalter, & Rizzo (2007) | Three 10-min conditions followed the 1-min hit command phase.<br>• Condition 1 (AX task without distraction).<br>• Condition 2 (AX task with distraction).<br>• Condition 3 (Boston Naming Test Match). | $N = 20$ (10 boys diagnosed with ADHD and 10 normal control boys). | Intergroup comparison of participants with ADHD and normal controls. | The SWAN Behavior Checklist (Swanson et al., 2009); Conners' CPT II (Conners, 2000); Stroop (Golden, 1978); Trail Making tests (Reitan, 1971; Reitan & Wolfson, 2004); NEPSY (visual attention, design fluency, verbal fluency); WISC-III (Digit Span, Coding B, Arithmetic, Vocabulary); Judgement of Line Orientation (Benton et al., 1983) | Participants with ADHD exhibited more omission errors, commission errors, and overall body movement than normal control children in the Virtual Classroom; participants with ADHD were more affected by distraction than normal control children in the Virtual Classroom; Virtual Classroom measures were correlated with traditional ADHD assessment tools, the Behavior Checklist, and flatscreen CPT. No negative side effects were associated with use of the Virtual Classroom. |

| Study | Sample | Design | Measures | Results |
|---|---|---|---|---|
| Adams et al. (2009) | The version by Rizzo et al., (2000) | $N = 35$ (19 boys ages 8 to 14 with a diagnosis of ADHD and 16 age-matched controls). | Both versions of the CPT (with and without the Virtual Classroom) were presented to the participants on a 3D virtual reality dome by Elumens. This provides a field of view (horizontal and vertical) of 140°. | Behavior Assessment System for Children (BASC); Vigil Continuous Performance Test (Cegalis, 1991) | While differences between the two groups did not attain statistical significance, there was a strong trend toward a significant difference in percent of targets correctly identified and in number of commission errors. Furthermore, compared to a standard CPT (Vigil), specificity was improved. |
| Gutiérrez-Maldonado et al. (2009) | A virtual CPT developed by the authors, similar to the Virtual Classroom, with four different tasks: two auditory tasks (with and without distractors) and two visual tasks (with and without distractors). | $N = 20$, ages 6 to 11, divided into two groups. | Group comparison after administration of the virtual CPT: 10 diagnosed with ADHD (experimental group), medicated with methylphenidate, and 10 in the non-ADHD group. | EDAH test (Farré & Narbona, 1998) | Differences between groups were expressed in both auditory and visual tasks and became more evident with the presence of distractors. |
| Nolin et al. (2009) | Version revised by the Digital MediaWorks team (http://www.dmw.ca/) under the name ClinicaVR: Classroom-CPT. | Eight children from 8 to 12 years old with a TBI. | Mean comparison tests with repeated measures. | Vigil Continuous Performance Test (Cegalis, 1991) | No difference between the two kinds of CPT on the total of omissions. Children made significantly more commissions and had longer reaction times in the Virtual Classroom than in the traditional CPT. |
| Pollak et al. (2009) | Modified version for Israel by Rizzo and colleagues and Digital MediaWorks (2006). The alterations included digits used instead of letters and instructions in Hebrew. | Thirty-seven boys, 9 to 17 years old, with ADHD ($n = 20$) and without ADHD ($n = 17$). | Crossover design. | Virtual Classroom on regular computer screen; Test of Variables of Attention (TOVA; Greenberg & Waldman, 1993); Short Feedback Questionnaire. | Children with ADHD performed worse on all CPTs. The VR-CPT showed similar effect sizes to the TOVA. Subjective feelings of enjoyment were most positive for VR-CPT. |

TABLE 6.1 Continued

| Authors/study | VR class version | Sample | Research design | Tests used | Results |
|---|---|---|---|---|---|
| Pollak et al. (2010) | Modified version for Israel by Rizzo and colleagues and Digital MediaWorks (2006). The alterations included digits used instead of letters and instructions in Hebrew. | $N = 27$ (16 boys and 11 girls with clinical diagnosis of ADHD). | Double-blind, placebo-controlled, crossover design. | Virtual Classroom on regular computer screen (Rizzo et al., 2000). Test of Variables of Attention—TOVA (Greenberg & Waldman, 1993). | Methylphenidate (MPH) reduced omission errors to a greater extent on the VR-CPT compared to the no VR-CPT and the TOVA, and decreased other CPT measures on all types of CPT to a similar degree. Children rated the VR-CPT as more enjoyable than the other types of CPT. |
| Gilboa et al. (2011) | Modified version for Israel by Rizzo and colleagues and Digital MediaWorks (2006). The alterations included digits used instead of letters and instructions in Hebrew. | $N = 54$ (29 children diagnosed with neurofibromatosis type 1 according to the NIH criteria [9 males, 20 females; mean age 12.2] and 25 controls [7 males, 18 females; mean age = 12.2]). | Cross-sectional design. Mean comparison tests. | The Conners' Parent Rating Scales–Revised: Long (CPRS-R:L) (Conners, 1997) | Significant differences were found between the NF1 and the control groups on the number of targets correctly identified (omission errors) and the number of commissions (commission errors) in the VC, with poorer performance by the children with NF1 ($p < .005$). Significant correlations were obtained between the number of targets correctly identified, the number of commission errors, and the reaction time. |

| Study | Test/Version | N | Design | Measures | Results |
|---|---|---|---|---|---|
| Bioulac et al. (2012) | Version by Rizzo and colleagues and Digital MediaWorks (2006), adapted to French by the research team. | $N = 36$ (boys 7 to 10 years old). | Children with ADHD and controls were tested at the beginning in the afternoon to try to minimize potential testing effects due to different times of the day. The same physician assessed the children with first the CPT and, after 10 min, the test of the VC. | Continuous Performance Test (CPT II); Conners' Parent Rating Scale; Child Behavior Checklist; State-Trait Anxiety Inventory (STAI) (State form). | Boys with ADHD had a different evolution of performances on this task than control children. Controls sustained performances over time in the VR task, but patients with ADHD showed a significant performance decrement, with a decrease of correct hits and an increase of reaction time. Worse performance in children with ADHD than in controls was then observed both in the VC task and in the CPT. |
| Iriarte et al. (2012) | AULA Nesplora VR test (Climent & Banterla, 2010) | $N = 1,282$ (children ages 6 to 16). | Normative study to obtain normative data. Single application and processing of data obtained. Descriptive design. | None | Variables provided by AULA were clustered in different categories for their posterior analysis. Differences by age and gender were analyzed, resulting in 14 groups, seven per sex. Differences between visual and auditory attention were also obtained. |

(*Continued*)

TABLE 6.1 Continued

| Authors/study | VR class version | Sample | Research design | Tests used | Results |
|---|---|---|---|---|---|
| Nolin et al. (2012) | Version revised by the Digital MediaWorks team (http://www.dmw.ca/) under the name ClinicaVR: Classroom-CPT. | N = 50 (25 sports-concussed and 25 non-sports-concussed adolescents enrolled in a sport and education program). | Students participated individually in testing sessions during regular class hours. The order of the traditional and virtual tests was counterbalanced across participants to prevent skewing of the results due to practice or fatigue effects. The data were collected over a period of 5 weeks. | Vigil Continuous Performance Test (Cegalis, 1991) | Neuropsychological assessment using VR showed greater sensitivity to the subtle effects of sports concussion than the traditional test, which showed no difference between groups. The results also demonstrated that the sports concussion group reported more symptoms of cybersickness and more intense cybersickness than the control group. |
| Lalonde et al. (2013) | Version revised by the Digital MediaWorks team (http://www.dmw.ca/) under the name ClinicaVR: Classroom-Stroop test. See Henry et al. (2012) for a task description and initial validation results. | N = 38 (adolescents 13 to 17 years old). | Descriptive/correlational study. Convergence validity study | Subjects: Delis–Kaplan Executive Function System (D-KEFS, Delis et al., 2001). 5 subtests (Trail Making, Tower, Twenty Questions, Verbal Fluency and Color-Word Interference). Parents: Behavior Rating Inventory of Executive Function (BRIEF; Gioia et al., 2000); Child Behavior Checklist (CBCL, Achenbach and Rescoria, 2001) | Performance on the VR-Stroop task correlates with both traditional forms of EF assessment (D-KEFS, BRIEF). In particular, performance on the VR-Stroop task was closely associated with performance on a paper–pencil inhibition task. Furthermore, VR-Stroop performance more accurately reflected everyday behavioral EF than paper–pencil tasks. |

| | | | | | |
|---|---|---|---|---|---|
| Diaz-Orueta et al. (2014) | AULA Nesplora VR test (Climent & Banterla, 2010) | $N = 57$ children ages 6 to 16 years (26.3% female) with average cognitive ability (IQ mean = 100.56, $SD = 10.38$) with diagnosis of ADHD according to DSM-IV-TR criteria. | One single measure with AULA and Conners' CPT. Convergent validity study between both tests. Comparison of children with ADHD undergoing medical treatment versus those not medicated. Comparison of capacity of AULA and Conners' CPT to differentiate between both groups. | Conners' Continuous Performance Test (Conners, 2000); WISC-III (Wechsler, 1991) | Both tests showed significant correlations in the measures that were comparable between them. In addition, AULA (but not Conners' CPT) was able to differentiate between ADHD patients with and without pharmacological treatment over a wide range of measures related to inattention, impulsivity, processing speed, motor activity, and quality of attention focus. |
| Rohani et al. (2014) | Their own VC version. The VR classroom environment was created with the game engine UNITY, the 3D modeling software Blender, and the Kinect (an infrared camera developed by Microsoft). | Five healthy young subjects participated in the preliminary experiment to test the developed prototype system. | Descriptive study | None | P300 potentially can be used as a measure of attention in a gaming environment. |

(Continued)

TABLE 6.1 Continued

| Authors/study | VR class version | Sample | Research design | Tests used | Results |
|---|---|---|---|---|---|
| Gilboa et al. (2015) | French version of the virtual classroom— .digits are used instead of letters and the test instructions are in French. | $N = 76$ (41 children with acquired brain injury and 35 age- and gender-matched controls, ages 8 to 16). | Cross-sectional design. The patients underwent the WASI subtests, the TEA-Ch, and the VC assessment and parents answered the CPRS-R:S questionnaire while their child was being tested. In order to reduce the assessment-related burden for the control children, the controls did not perform the TEA-Ch. Parents answered a demographic questionnaire and the CPRS-R:S scale. | The Test of Everyday Attention for Children (TEA-Ch) (Manly et al., 1999); Wechsler Abbreviated Scale of Intelligence (WASI): Matrix Reasoning and Vocabulary (Wechsler, 1999); Conners Parent Rating Scales–Revised: Short Form (CPRS-R:S) (Conners, 1997) | Significant differences were found between the groups regarding the number of targets correctly identified in the VC. Based on the VC results, 45% of the children with ABI suffered marked deficits in sustained attention (lower rates of total correct hits). The concurrent validity of the VC in comparison with neuropsychological tests and a parental questionnaire was sufficient. Attentional performance was found to be related to age, age at injury/ diagnosis, and treatment (radiotherapy dose). The VC appears to be a sensitive, playful, and ecologically valid assessment tool for use in the diagnosis of attention deficits among children with ABI. |

| Parsons & Carlew, 2016) | Virtual Classroom Bimodal Stroop task (Clinica VR: Lalonde et al., 2013; Parsons, 2014) | Study #1: Fifty undergraduate students (mean age = 20.37; range = 18–30; 78% female) Study #2: Eight adults diagnosed with high-functioning autism (mean age = 22.88; range = 18–34) and ten neurotypical adults (mean age = 18.8; range = 18–20). | Study #1: Descriptive study. Study #2: Cross-sectional design. Mean comparison tests. | Study #1: Wechsler Test of Adult Reading (WTAR) (Holdnack, 2001); Delis-Kaplan Executive Functioning System (D-KEFS; Delis et al., 2001); Color Word Interference Test; Automated Neuropsychological Assessment Metrics (ANAM; Stroop task (Johnson et al., 2007) Study #2: Wechsler Abbreviated Scale of Intelligence– Second Edition (WASI-II) | Study #1: Virtual Classroom Bimodal Stroop task may be validly used to examine interference control in a typically developing population. The task elicited an interference effect similar to those found in classic Stroop tasks. Study #2: When under conditions of distraction, individuals with ASD are compromised in their ability to activate external distractor inhibition, though their response time may not suffer. |

order to determine whether VEs increase the accuracy and sensitivity of evaluation beyond that obtained with traditional computerized flatscreen CPTs. The Nolin group's subsequent study with sports-concussed adolescents, the study by Gilboa et al. (2011) of patients with neurofibromatosis type 1 (NF1), and most recently, the study by Gilboa et al. (2015) that compares children with acquired brain injury and controls, are studies that extend the VR classroom environment as a useful neuropsychological tool for clinical conditions beyond ADHD. The latest study by Parsons and Carlew (2015) is also promising, because it includes autism spectrum disorders (ASD) as a target for VR-based neuropsychological assessment.

With the exception of AULA, which is discussed in depth in the next section, the majority of studies lack sufficient sample size to establish the most appropriate standardized administration of the Virtual Classroom to characterize the attention profile with sensitivity and specificity. One of the main challenges of getting a level of accuracy is to precisely identify clinical cases and, with the same precision, to correctly discard those who are not clinical cases at all. Both false-positive and false-negative findings incur, respectively, the administration of an unnecessary treatment (with potential physical, psychological, and social side effects) or overlooking a patient who could potentially benefit from early diagnosis and appropriate early treatment. From the procedural point of view, the main difference between ClinicaVR and Aula Nesplora, for example, is that the latter deliberately omits the AX paradigm (i.e., press whenever the X stimulus appears right after the stimulus A), because the authors (Climent & Banterla, 2010) considered that the AX paradigm was more related to working memory, a fact that could have distorted the goals for which the AULA test was developed. As the next section describes, the AULA Nesplora test is so far the only VR-based test with a standardized administration procedure as a result of a normative study.

## AULA NESPLORA: VR TEST FOR NEUROPSYCHOLOGICAL EVALUATION OF ATTENTION

### Description

AULA Nesplora (Climent & Banterla, 2010) is a computerized CPT developed for a VE that is visualized by means of a special set of VR glasses with movement sensors. AULA was developed for the purpose of providing the clinician an accurate and comprehensive evaluation of attention processes, and it has been mainly been used to assess the cognitive domain in the diagnostic decision about ADHD. The AULA scenario resembles a primary or secondary school classroom, and the first-person view provides the subject with the opportunity to be a student sitting at his desk, looking at the blackboard. AULA targets attention processes in children between 6 and 16 years old, and its goal is to analyze the behavior deployed by the child inside the virtual classroom, as shown by means of three-dimensional vision glasses that integrate earphones and movement sensors. The software updates the user's perspective according to head movements, giving the person the impression of actually being inside the classroom. The virtual blackboard and the earphones present a series of visual and auditory stimuli to which the user must respond.

Previous to the test administration, and before their first contact with the VE, the children are asked about their experience with computers and how familiar they are with VR and video games. Clues about the test content are avoided (to prevent test administration biases) and once the child is wearing the equipment (e.g., head-mounted display), the test begins with a series of basic auditory instructions ("Hello, you are in AULA, with the glasses you are wearing you can see the whole classroom, to your left, to your right, up and down . . . you can see everything.") followed by a description of the classroom and the type of stimuli and tasks that may be presented. In order to promote a habituation to the initial impact of being inside a video-game environment, children are presented with a task in which they have to use their head as the mouse to search for, and the 1-button switch as a way to explode a series of red balloons that appear throughout the classroom (see Figure 6.1). This task is expected to lower the activation related to the novelty and to harmonize the performance of all children before the actual attention test begins; that is, all children undergo a pretest phase in which they get familiar with the virtual classroom environment, regardless of their previous experience with computers or video games.

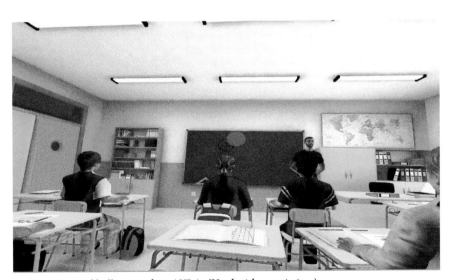

FIGURE 6.1 *Red balloons task in AULA. (Used with permission.)*

Once the habituation/usability task is performed, AULA comprises two main tasks:

- A No-X (No-go paradigm) task: The child must press the button whenever the presented stimulus is different from the target stimulus. More specifically, the child is required to press the button whenever he does not see or hear "apple."
- An X (Go paradigm) task: The child must press the button whenever he sees or hears the target stimulus. More specifically, the child is required to press the button when he sees or hears "seven."

In AULA, both visual and auditory stimuli are presented (see Table 6.2), and, simultaneously, ecological distractors appear progressively, similar to those that may be found in a real-life school classroom.

The combination of visual and auditory stimuli provides more diagnostic information than unimodal CPTs (Doyle, Biederman, & Seidman, 2000), but combined stimuli are rare in computerized CPTs (Cornblatt, Risch Neil, Faris, Friedman & Erlenmeyer-Kimling, 1988; Xu, Zhou, & Wang, 2004). Distractors in AULA, both visual and auditory, are:

- Paper ball: A child throws a paper ball from his desk. The flight lasts about 3 s, then the ball hits the floor and rolls.

TABLE 6.2  Visual and Auditory Stimuli in AULA

|   | Auditory | Visual | Auditory | Visual |
|---|----------|--------|----------|--------|
| 1 | Árbol (Tree) | | Cinco (Five) | 5 |
| 2 | Botella (Bottle) | | Seis (Six) | 6 |
| 3 | Libro (Book) | | Siete (Seven) | 7 |
| 4 | Manzana (Apple) | | Ocho (Eight) | 8 |
| 5 | Tarta (Cake) | | Nueve (Nine) | 9 |
|   |  |  | Siervo* | – |
|   |  |  | Siembro* | – |

*Distractor in Spanish for the word *siete* (seven).

- Teacher's walk: The teacher walks smoothly across the classroom. While he walks by, his steps are heard by the user. From time to time, the teacher observes the work performed by the children (see Figure 6.2).
- Whispers on the right side: Whispers heard to the right of the user include "pss, pss, hey, you, pss, pss, hey. . . ."
- The teacher's pen drops: A ballpoint pen drops from teacher's desk. The pen rolls across the teacher's table and falls to the floor, making a dry and localized noise. The teacher retrieves it and takes it back to the table.
- A child passes a note to another student: Children in front of the user pass each other a note while they look straight at the blackboard, stretching out one arm each. The boy on the left stretches his hand with the paper and the girl on the right reaches tworad the paper in order to take it.
- Cough on the left: The user can hear a loud cough on the left.
- One child gives a paper to the teacher: A student stands up from a desk behind the user, approaches the teacher's desk (see Figure 6.3), leaves a paper, and goes back and sits down at his desk again. When he stands up and sits down, his chair makes considerable noise.
- An ambulance passes by: On the right side of the classroom there is a large window. At a certain time, an ambulance passes very fast across the street (see Figure 6.4), very close to the window, and the sound of its siren is heard clearly, moving from behind the user to in front of him.
- The bell rings: The bell indicating the change to the next lesson rings.
- A car passes by: Moving from in front of the child to behind him, as can be seen through the window on the right, a red car passes by. When

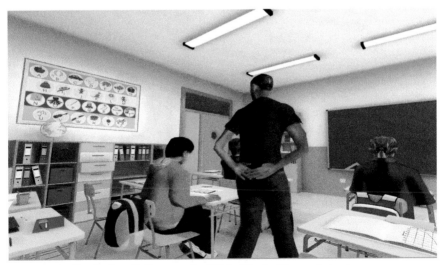

FIGURE 6.2 *Teacher's walk distractor in AULA. (Used with permission.)*

it passes by the window, its horn sounds, as if to greet somebody, it decreases its speed a little bit, and then it continues on its way.

- Voice on the left: A voice is heard to the left of the user: "pss, pss, hey, you, pss, pss, hey. . . ."
- Cough on the right: Someone suffers a coughing attack on the right side of the user.
- Step noise in the corridor: In the corridor to the left of the classroom, steps can be heard approaching the classroom door from the back.

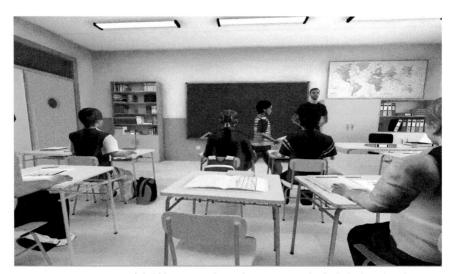

FIGURE 6.3 *Distractor of child leaving a sheet of paper on teacher's desk. (Used with permission.)*

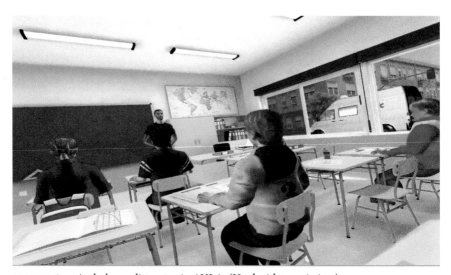

FIGURE 6.4 *Ambulance distractor in AULA. (Used with permission.)*

TABLE 6.3  Variables and Corresponding Measures in AULA Test

| Variable | Measure |
| --- | --- |
| Inattention | Omission errors |
| Impulsivity | Commission errors |
| Processing speed | Mean reaction time |
| Sustained attention | Deviation of reaction time |
| Hyperactivity | Motor activity |
| Quality of attention | Number of total visual errors while watching the blackboard. |

A turmoil of children speaking is heard, noise and steps progressively go in the opposite direction, and a door closing is heard.

- A child on the left raises his hand: A child at a desk on the left raises his hand as if he were about to ask something.
- Laughter: On the right side of the user someone laughs, and immediately after the laugh somebody demands silence: "sssh!"
- Somebody knocks on the door: The sound of someone knocking on the door is heard; the teacher approaches the door, opens it, pops his head out of the room (it looks like he is talking to the person outside), closes the door again, and goes back to his place.
- A child on the right raises his hand: A child at a desk on the right raises his hand as if he were about to ask something.

AULA's complete administration, including the initial training or habituation task, takes around 20 min. As a result of its administration, AULA provides information about sustained attention, divided attention (visual and auditory), impulsivity, excessive motor activity, tendency to distraction, and processing speed. Table 6.3 provides a list of measures obtained with AULA and related variables.

## Theoretical Foundations of AULA

The reason for the sequence of presentation of tasks in AULA (first NO-X and then X) is that the NO-X task generates an overstimulation that results in fast, inaccurate, and inadequate responses, while the X task leads to a hypoactivation, and, thus, to slow, variable, and inefficient responses (Artigas-Pallarés, 2009). It is assumed that this sequence of presentation reproduces more accurately the problem that a child with self-regulation problems (such as a child with attention problems) must face to adapt to new requirements of the environment, once he has developed an overstimulating activity, as described in the State Regulation Model by Sergeant, Oosterlaan, and Van der Meer (1999). The model proposes that, in order to achieve a goal, it is necessary to activate and to mobilize mental energy in order to adapt cognitive resources to external demands and consequently to optimize the response. This concept is similar to mental effort or motivation. State regulation can be considered an executive function, dependent on the frontal lobe and on its connection with the limbic system. This hypothesis, as well as Barkley's Unique Deficit Model, conceptualizes executive dysfunction as a nuclear aspect of ADHD (Iriarte, Díaz-Orueta, Cueto, Irazustabarrena, Banterla, & Climent, 2016).

In computerized neuropsychological tools, state-regulation deficit can be observed as a disruption of reaction time, either slowness or lack of regularity, and the basic deficit is elicited by go/no-go tasks like the ones used in AULA. In other words, the child with self-regulation problems shows a reduced ability to generate the necessary energy adjustment to respond to environmental demands. The relationship between ADHD symptoms and reaction time variability has been reported in both clinical samples (Johnson, Kelly, Bellgrove, et al., 2007) and general population studies (Berwid, Curko Kera, Marks, Santra, & Bender, 2005).

## Comparison of AULA with Other Established CPTs

The stimuli used in AULA differ from those used in Conners' CPT, since the more complex nature of the stimuli presented in AULA (visual images and words instead of letters) require longer presentation times than the letters presented in Conners' CPT. Time of exposure to visual stimuli is 250 milliseconds in both tests. However, in the original development of the AULA tool (described in Climent & Banterla, 2010), it was established that auditory stimuli would have a mean duration of presentation of 650 milliseconds, depending on the concrete word, in a range from 470 milliseconds for the word *tarta* ("cake") up to a maximum of 891 milliseconds for *manzana* ("apple"). In addition, in the pilot part of the AULA normative study, developed with 200 children, it was seen that children with slow reaction times required a mean of 1,200 to 1,500 milliseconds to provide an answer (Climent & Banterla, 2010). Therefore, in that study it was decided to leave a maximum interstimulus interval of 2,500 milliseconds, in order to obtain a more accurate measure of the extension of inattention and processing speed, and thus avoid having the slowest responses fall within the frame of the subsequent stimulus (in other words, to avoid counting the answer as a commission error if the next stimulus is not a target stimulus, or as a correct answer by chance). In summary, the interstimulus interval is a key feature in AULA that differentiates between inattention and processing-speed slowness, with each child having a maximum of 2,500 milliseconds to press the button and thus register the answer in the correct interval (i.e., the interval that corresponds to the presented stimulus).

In relation to total items, the total of items in AULA is 360, as in Conners' CPT, 180 per task (No-X and X). Moreover, 180 items are target stimuli and 180 are nontarget. With regard to distractors (used in AULA but not in Conners' CPT), they were initially programmed as visual, auditory, and mixed, and then were adapted to the ecological environment of the classroom (to avoid having a stimulus appear on the blackboard at the same time that the teacher or another student is walking in front of it). Because the presence of distractors does not interfere with the items' presentation, it is possible to distinguish which part of the results correspond to the child's performance and which were affected for other reasons. In addition, the distribution of distractors differs in AULA tasks, being greater in the No-X task than in the X task (with the aim of generating overstimulation and hypoactivation, respectively).

## Results from Studies Performed with AULA

### NORMATIVE STUDY

The normative study, performed on approximately 1,300 children (boys and girls) with an age range between 6 and 16 years (Iriarte, Díaz-Orueta, Cueto, Irazustabarrena, Banterla y Climent, 2016), showed a general pattern of differences by sex, with a tendency for boys to provide faster responses (both correct responses as well as commission errors) across all age groups, for boys to have greater motor activity (thus worsening their test performance), and for boys to have higher deviation from the attention focus (which implies that the child is not looking where he should, that is, at the blackboard). In other words, girls appear to be slower in providing answers but exhibit better performance across all tasks (both No-X and X) and in all testing conditions (with and without distractors).

Age differences are more clear in the younger age groups (children between 6 and 8 years old), and they are no longer statistically significant in children more than 12 years old, which led to two composite age groups of 12- to 16-year-old boys and girls. In this sense, all participants between 12 and 16 years old showed stable attention parameters regardless of age. It is possible that this stability is a consequence of normal development of cognitive processes in this age interval.

### SENSITIVITY STUDY

Rufo-Campos and colleagues (Rufo-Campos, Cueto, Iriarte & Rufo-Muñoz, 2012) studied the ability of AULA to discriminate between children with a clinical diagnosis of ADHD and a control group. AULA was administered to 124 children, 62 with a clinical diagnosis of ADHD and 62 without any diagnosis. Results showed that, using all the variables included in the test, 93.5% of cases were correctly classified, with a sensitivity of 95.2% and a specificity of 91.8%. Based on these results, it was concluded that both the sensitivity and the diagnostic power of AULA were excellent. With respect to the small percentage of children not correctly identified by AULA, a study by Fernández-Fernández, Morillo-Rojas, and Alonso-Romero (2012) relates this issue to children with high intellectual abilities, which may to some extent mask the presence of ADHD by allowing a test performance significantly higher than what would be expected in other children with similar sociodemographic features and a clinical diagnosis.

## TEST–RETEST STUDY

A study developed by Férnandez-Fernández and Morillo-Rojas (2012) administered AULA twice, at a 1-week interval, to a clinical sample of children with ADHD. Based on the lack of statistically significant differences between the first and second test data, obtained in the same clinical conditions and just a week apart, they concluded that AULA administered at a 1-week interval does not have a learning effect, and thus a 1-week period is long enough to detect variations in the clinical course of the patients studied, a fact that appears to be very useful for short-term evaluation of clinical progress with any particular treatment (either pharmacological or of another type).

## STUDY OF DISTRACTORS

An in-depth study about the influence of distractors in the normative group (Díaz-Orueta, Iriarte, Climent & Banterla, 2012) showed a general pattern of slower processing speed and a higher deviation from the attention focus in the presence of distractors, confirming the disruptive effect of distractors on performance in both boys and girls of the general population.

With regard to the qualitative effect of distractors, anecdotes were gathered, especially about children between 6 and 8 years old, who reacted to AULA avatars as if they were dealing with real people, raising their hands, standing up from their chairs, talking to the teacher and asking him where he was going, etc. In the presence of the auditory distractor that is a voice talking or whispering to the user, one girl turned around completely without removing her VR glasses and told her virtual peer to shut up. In the sensitivity study described above, a boy stood up wearing the VR glasses and said he wanted to take a walk to visit the rest of the school facilities.

In administration of AULA to clinical populations, it has been seen that children and adolescents react to the VE the way they would react in real life. For example, a 10-year-old boy with ADHD, hyperactive-impulsive type, raised his hand continuously to formulate questions for the teacher, and also to complain about the whispers behind him: "Hey, teacher, somebody is annoying me!" Another boy, 9 years old, with ADHD and behavior problems, started to tell his virtual peers "Hey, guys, why do you all stare at the blackboard? Don't you want to go outside? Are you deaf or what? I want to see the playground!" He started to insult a virtual peer while he was trying to beat him. Later, he turned around and shouted at the teacher, "Hey, teacher, why can't we go out to the playground?" This moment was coincidental with the distractor of the teacher approaching the classroom door, and the child reacted: "You do not even listen to me, and now you go away!" In some circumstances, childrens' natural and spontaneous reactions showed a great level of concentration. For example, a 12-year-old adolescent said "Shut up!" to his whispering virtual peer and continued performing the test, while another 9-year-old child replied "OK" to some of the virtual teacher's instructions.

### FACTORIAL VALIDITY STUDY

The goal of the study by Díaz-Orueta et al. (2014) was to study the factorial validity of AULA. Two exploratory factorial analyses of the 18 main variables of AULA were performed with 2,074 children from different Spanish schools and clinical centers. Both a one-dimensional structure and a three-dimensional structure (accounting for aspects of inattention, impulsivity, and hyperactivity) were explored, by means of the Unweighted Least Squares (ULS) extraction method. The 18 studied variables tended to saturate a single factor ($F$ values from .527 to .946), with two factors appearing as residual dimensions. The adequacy of the variables' correlation matrix was analyzed in order to perform the factorial analysis (Bartlett = 55505.0, $p < .00001$; Kaiser-Meyer-Olkin = 0.89), indicating good data adjustment (RMSEA = 0.071; Goodness of Fit index (GFI) = .98; α = .98), with a total explained variance of 66% for the single dimension. These results support the structure of AULA comprising one single factor that includes all the cognitive variables that correlate with ADHD in any of its subtypes.

## Convergent Validity Studies

### COMPARISON OF AULA WITH D2: CONVERGENT VALIDITY AND PRELIMINARY RESULTS OF AULA IN THE ASSESSMENT OF READING DIFFICULTIES

In the study developed recently by Diaz-Orueta, Alonso-Sanchez, and Climent (2014), the goal was to analyze the convergent validity between AULA and the d2 Attention Test (BrickenKamp, 1962), a paper-and-pencil visual cancellation test, and to show AULA's preliminary results in detecting attention problems and information-processing patterns in children with reading disorders.

The d2 test, developed in Germany by BrickenKamp (1962), and validated with a Spanish population by Seisdedos (2002), is an attention test that evaluates different aspects of selective attention and concentration. It takes a maximum of 10 min, including explanation of instructions, although there is a time limit of 20 s for the performance of each of the 14 lines in the test. The test comprises 14 lines with 47 letters in each line. The symbols or characters are the letters d and p, for a total of 658 letters, which may be accompanied by one or two little lines that may go in the upper or lower side of each letter. The test task is to closely review the content of each line and to mark all the d letters that have two little lines attached (either two lines in the upper side, two lines in the lower side, or one line above and one below).

Convergent validity analysis of AULA and the d2 test needs to consider that the measures that can be compared between the tests are limited, since the d2 test has only visual stimuli, lacks distractors, and has a number of total stimuli dependent on the number of items the user can mark in a given time (which may therefore vary from one test taker to another). These conditions reduce the amount of comparable data to the following: total correct answers (in AULA, visual correct answers); total errors (sum of visual omissions and commissions); commission errors (visual only in both tests); omission errors (visual only in both tests); and concentration index (an original measure of the d2 test obtained from the total correct answers minus commissions; the same index was calculated for AULA using total visual answers minus total visual commission errors).

The sample for this study was 60 children (42% female) from 6 to 17 years old (mean age = 10.20, $SD$ = 2.68), and 68% of the sample had some type of learning disorder. Table 6.4 shows the proximities analyses for total correct answers, total errors, commission errors, omission errors, and concentration index.

As can be seen in Table 6.4, relationships between the results obtained in the d2 test and in AULA offer a significant guarantee of an adequate convergent validity for correct answers and concentration indexes. For errors, visual errors as a whole show a good relationship, but the relationship becomes weaker in detailed analysis of the convergence between commissions and errors from both tests, with values lower than 0.50, as if both tests were giving the same name ("omissions" and "commissions") to different measures.

Due to the small sample size, the purpose of the preliminary analysis was also to check whether either of the tests could add value in differentiating between

TABLE 6.4  AULA–d2 Convergent Validity Analysis Results

|  | d2 Test | | | | |
|---|---|---|---|---|---|
|  | Total correct answers | Total errors | Commissions | Omissions | Concentration Index |
| AULA—Total visual correct answers | .944 |  |  |  |  |
| AULA—Total visual errors |  | .566 |  |  |  |
| AULA—Visual commission errors |  |  | .460 |  |  |
| AULA—Visual omission errors |  |  |  | .332 |  |
| AULA—Concentration Index |  |  |  |  | .929 |

the two subgroups with higher frequencies in the studied sample: children with reading-writing difficulties ($n = 29$) and children with no difficulties ($n = 18$).

Mann-Whitney $U$ test analysis was performed in order to check whether there were gender differences in performance on d2 and AULA by children with reading-writing difficulties versus those who presented no difficulties. Table 6.5 shows an overview of obtained differences.

As can be seen from the data above, no significant differences were found on the d2 test between the subgroups with and without literacy problems. However, in AULA, children without reading difficulties produced significantly more visual correct answers ($M = 29.28$) than children with literacy problems ($M = 20.72$; $U = 166, p < .05$), as well as fewer visual errors ($M_{no\ diff} = 18.72$; $M_{diff} = 27.28$; $U = 166$, $p < .05$). The AULA omission error rate and concentration index are also better for children without difficulties, but do not reach statistical significance.

One additional analysis based on the previous results was to take advantage of AULA's multisensory evaluation to study the possibility of differentiating information-processing patterns among children with reading-writing diffi-culties. A Wilcoxon test showed that the children with difficulties ($n = 29$) per-formed significantly better in response to auditory stimuli than to visual stimuli, showing a significantly higher amount of auditory correct answers ($z = -2.142$, $p < .05$) than visual correct answers, fewer auditory errors ($z = -4.444, p < .001$) and, among those, significantly fewer auditory omissions ($z = -3.774, p < .001$) than visual omissions. No statistically significant differences appeared for com-mission errors; the rate was similar in both visual and auditory modalities.

In summary, the present study examined the convergent validity of two differ-ent attention tests, with only a subset of measures from both tests that could actu-ally be compared. This led to a significantly high convergence in concentration indexes, total visual correct answers, and total visual errors, while "omissions" and "commissions" seem to have a different meaning in each test, as their prox-imity values seem to be somewhat weaker. A possible explanation for this is that, in AULA, scores for visual commissions and omissions are total scores for visual errors performed in the presence of distractors and in both No-X and X tasks.

TABLE 6.5 Differences Between Group with Reading-Writing Problems and Group with No Problems

| | d2 CON | d2 TA | d2 O | d2 C | d2 Errors | AULA CON | AULA Correct visual answers | AULA visual errors | AULA visual comissions | AULA visual commissions |
|---|---|---|---|---|---|---|---|---|---|---|
| U | 261.5 | 268 | 222.5 | 227 | 224 | 180.5 | 166 | 166 | 179 | 209.5 |
| Z | −.181 | −.043 | −1.013 | −.926 | −.981 | −1.762 | −2.080 | −2.080 | −1.795 | −1.130 |
| p | .856 | .966 | .311 | .354 | .327 | .078 | .038* | .038* | .073 | .258 |

*p<.05, Abbreviations: C = commissions; CON = Concentration Index; O = omissions; TA = Total Correct Answers.

Moreover, AULA's administration is longer and the sequence No-X followed by X (overstimulation followed by hypoactivation) does not have any homologous condition in the d2 test. The configuration of the AULA task sequence may mean that omissions and commissions in AULA are measuring information that is more precise but quite different from what they measure in the d2 test, a pure visual cancellation test.

Finally, the ability of both tests to differentiate between children with and without reading-writing difficulties was studied. The d2 test did not show any differences, which in treatment planning would not allow the clinician to know whether the child shows better auditory or visual processing abilities. With AULA, the pattern is more clear: children with reading-writing problems seem to show a worse response to visual stimuli than children who do not have those difficulties, and when studied separately, results show a general pattern of better performance with auditory stimuli (more correct answers, fewer errors, and fewer omissions) than with visual stimuli.

## COMPARISON OF AULA WITH FACES–DIFFERENCES PERCEPTION TEST

In their study analyzing the convergent validity between AULA and Faces–Differences Perceptions Test (F-DFT), Zulueta, Iriarte, Díaz-Orueta, and Climent (2013) used an incidental sample of 62 children between the ages of 6 and 16. The F-DPT test (Thurstone & Yela, 1985) requires the patient to visually search, within a series of schematic triads of faces that are essentially equal, for the face in each triad that has a differentiating detail. This paper-and-pencil test was initially used as a visual discrimination task, but performance is affected when the administration time is lengthened, due to the amount of sustained attention and the control of impulsive answers that are required for a correct performance, especially if the administration time is increased from its original 3 min to 6 min, as was done by the team of Crespo-Eguílaz, Narbona, Peralta, & Repáraz (2006). Taking into account correct answers and errors, an Impulsivity Control Index (ICI) was calculated for each age group between 6 and 10 years old. The convergent validity analysis for F-DPT and AULA is shown in Table 6.6.

TABLE 6.6  Convergent Validity Analysis for AULA and F-DPT

| | F-DPT | | | | | |
|---|---|---|---|---|---|---|
| | Correct answers 3′ | Correct answers 6′ | Errors 3′ | Errors 6′ | ICI 3′ | ICI 6′ |
| AULA correct answers | .938 | .953 | −.635 | −.677 | .990 | .991 |
| AULA errors | −.674 | −.682 | .552 | .606 | −.812 | −.809 |
| AULA ICI | .938 | .953 | −.615 | −.652 | .969 | .971 |

*Source*: Zulueta et al. (2013); Abbreviations: ICI = Impulsivity Control Index

As can be seen, all the correlations are very high, especially those for correct answers and for ICIs from both tests (which were extracted from the comparison between correct answers and errors). Correlations for commission and omission errors are moderate, but most of them are higher than 0.6. These results show an excellent convergent validity for AULA and F-DPT (extended version).

## COMPARISON OF AULA WITH CONNERS' CPT: AULA SHOWS BETTER DIFFERENTIATION OF ADHD PATIENTS WITH AND WITHOUT PHARMACOLOGICAL TREATMENT

This study (Díaz-Orueta, García-López, Crespo-Eguílaz, Sánchez-Carpintero, Climent, & Narbona, 2014) included 57 children (42 males and 15 females) ranging in age from 6 to 16 years, with an average cognitive ability as measured by the Spanish version of the Wechsler Intelligence Scale for Children-Fourth Edition (WISC-IV; Wechsler, 2003). Participants were diagnosed by a qualified neuropediatrician according to diagnostic criteria from the *Diagnostic and Statistical Manual of Mental Disorders*, Revised (DSM-IV-TR; American Psychiatric Association, 2000). The majority of the children met the criteria for ADHD combined subtype (56.1%). The other participants met the criteria for ADHD inattentive subtype (40.4%) and hyperactive/impulsive (3.5%). Table 6.7 provides an overview of the convergent validity analysis between AULA and Conners' CPT for the variables for which it was possible to establish a comparison.

TABLE 6.7 Convergent Validity Analyses for Conners' CPT and AULA

| AULA | Conners' CPT | | | |
| --- | --- | --- | --- | --- |
| | Omissions | Commissions | Reaction time | Variability |
| Visual (O, C, RT, VRT) | .596** | .495** | .672** | .786** |
| Auditory (O, C, RT, VRT) | .492** | .358* | .520** | .671** |
| With distractors (O, C, RT, VRT) | .546** | .414** | .600** | .641** |
| Without distractors (O, C, RT, VRT) | .630** | .416** | .699** | .704** |
| No-X task (visual) (O, C) | .569** | .471** | N/A | N/A |
| X task (visual) (O, C) | .562** | .311* | N/A | N/A |
| No-X task (auditory) (O, C) | .497** | .362** | N/A | N/A |
| X task (auditory) (O, C) | .451** | .303* | N/A | N/A |

$**p < .01$, $*p < .05$, N/A = not available.

Abbreviations: C = commissions; O = omissions; RT = reaction time; VRT = Variability in reaction time.

*Source*: Diaz-Orueta et al. (2014)

From the total sample of 57 participants, 29 were receiving pharmacological treatment at the time they were evaluated, while the other 28 were not under treatment. The capacity of both Conners' CPT and AULA to discriminate between the two conditions was analyzed using Mann-Whitney $U$ test. For Conners' CPT, statistically significant differences were found in variability of reaction time for correct answers, which was significantly lower in patients under pharmacological treatment ($M = 24.31$) than in children without treatment ($M = 33.86$; $U = 270$, $p < .05$). In the case of the AULA test, some of the measures were particularly sensitive to the condition of receiving treatment. Specifically, it was shown that AULA could differentiate between children with and without pharmacological treatment on variables such as inattention, impulsivity, processing speed, motor activity, and quality of attention focus, as seen in Table 6.8.

Moreover, AULA contains additional measures (not included in Conners' CPT) that may support more accurate ADHD diagnosis, such as:

- Auditory attention (and therefore divided visual and auditory attention);
- Measures of resistance to distractors (Conners' CPT lacks these) that provide information about ADHD subtypes, which some studies gather (Xu et al., 2004; Parsons, Bowerly, Buckwalter, & Rizzo, 2007);
- Measures of head motor activity and deviation from attentional focus. In the study by Diaz-Orueta et al. (2014) these measures differentiated between ADHD children with and without pharmacological treatment;
- Quality of attention focus, which allows ecologic transferral of results to child's daily life functioning (by evaluating how the child attends the blackboard stimuli and the types of stimuli that can be put in place to affect his performance).

In summary, the results of this study show that the AULA is a valid test for measuring attention and impulsivity and complements the diagnosis of ADHD and the progress of its treatment (either pharmacological or other) with information on cognitive performance in an ecologically relevant simulation of a real-world context (i.e., a classroom).

### CONVERGENT VALIDITY WITH DSM SCALES

The goal of a recent study by Diaz-Orueta et al. (2014) was to study the convergent validity of AULA with DSM-IV-TR criteria. For that purpose, a sample of 360 children with ADHD was analyzed, using cosine similarity analyses. Results showed low-to-moderate correlations between AULA and DSM-IV-TR, with the highest correlation values, from .379 to .473, for inattention. It is very likely that differences between AULA, an objective measure, and DSM-IV-TR, an observational scale, mean they target different aspects or dimensions of patients' behavior and hence may complement each other by increasing the accuracy of

TABLE 6.8 Differences in AULA Performance Based on Treatment Condition

| | Under treatment ($n = 29$)[a] | Without treatment ($n = 28$)[a] | $U$ | $z$ | $p$ |
|---|---|---|---|---|---|
| **TOTAL** | | | | | |
| Reaction time (RT)—correct answers | 768.18 (136.11) | 864.00 (168.48) | 262 | −2.299 | .022 |
| Variability in RT—correct answers | 348.29 (121.01) | 410.50 (80.73) | 260 | −2.331 | .020 |
| Motor activity | 0.82 (0.82) | 1.52 (1.19) | 216.5 | −3.026 | .002 |
| Deviation of the focus | 21417.17 (37823.90) | 56200.71 (77346.63) | 247 | −2.572 | .010 |
| **VISUAL** | | | | | |
| Reaction time (RT)—correct answers | 623.29 (119.62) | 724.55 (192.79) | 272 | −2.139 | .032 |
| Variability in RT—correct answers | 267.04 (135.01) | 347.27 (133.73) | 260 | −2.331 | .020 |
| Variability in RT—commissions | 284.75 (221.52) | 464.71 (260.28) | 246.5 | −2.546 | .011 |
| **AUDITORY** | | | | | |
| Omissions | 7.24 (13.30) | 10.79 (10.84) | 234.5 | −2.747 | .006 |
| Reaction time (RT)—correct answers | 899.92 (164.74) | 990.51 (142.69) | 263 | −2.283 | .022 |
| Variability in RT—correct answers | 341.70 (133.56) | 408.50 (74.65) | 250 | −2.490 | .013 |
| **WITH DISTRACTORS** | | | | | |
| Reaction time (RT)—correct answers | 773.63 (140.40) | 857.57 (155.06) | 270 | −2.171 | .030 |
| Variability in RT—correct answers | 351.35 (170.80) | 394.69 (92.59) | 275 | −2.091 | .037 |
| Motor activity | 0.87 (0.90) | 1.49 (1.22) | 244 | −2.586 | .010 |
| Deviation of the focus | 31767.24 (58687.28) | 58003.14 (90625.13) | 268 | −2.260 | .024 |
| **WITHOUT DISTRACTORS** | | | | | |
| Omissions | 15.72 (19.02) | 22.96 (18.96) | 279 | −2.029 | .042 |
| Reaction time (RT)—correct answers | 766.92 (140.02) | 868.50 (183.57) | 269 | −2.187 | .029 |
| Variability in RT—correct answers | 351.50 (117.45) | 416.77 (83.70) | 275 | −2.091 | .037 |

(*Continued*)

TABLE 6.8  Continued

| | Under treatment (n = 29)[a] | Without treatment (n = 28)[a] | U | z | p |
|---|---|---|---|---|---|
| Reaction time (RT)—commissions | 667.87 (240.43) | 795.31 (292.80) | 282.5 | −1.971 | .049 |
| Motor activity | 0.86 (0.86) | 1.63 (1.26) | 209.5 | −3.137 | .002 |
| Deviation of the focus | 19500.97 (35678.31) | 51953.18 (76501.39) | 257 | −2.450 | .014 |
| **NO-X TASK** | | | | | |
| Reaction time (RT)—correct answers | 743.32 (129.31) | 839.92 (164.69) | 260 | −2.331 | .020 |
| Variability in RT—correct answers | 346.21 (131.05) | 413.27 (84.86) | 254 | −2.426 | .015 |
| Motor activity | 0.78 (0.86) | 1.28 (1.09) | 248 | −2.522 | .012 |
| Deviation of the focus | 10874.45 (21397.55) | 24805.11 (41834.05) | 265 | −2.352 | .019 |
| Omissions (auditory) | 5.93 (12.90) | 7.61 (8.91) | 257.5 | −2.393 | .017 |
| **X TASK** | | | | | |
| Omissions (total) | 3.24 (3.81) | 7.21 (6.05) | 206 | −3.224 | .001 |
| Reaction time (RT)—correct answers | 839.71 (181.25) | 959.39 (229.77) | 265 | −2.251 | .024 |
| Variability in RT—commissions | 793.66 (303.36) | 934.02 (476.13) | 278.5 | −2.050 | .040 |
| Motor activity | 0.86 (0.84) | 1.70 (1.36) | 203.5 | −3.233 | .001 |
| Deviation of the focus | 10542.72 (19768.99) | 31395.61 (49802.20) | 250 | −2.555 | .011 |
| Omissions (visual) | 1.93 (2.85) | 4.04 (3.54) | 211 | −3.164 | .002 |

[a]Expressed as mean (SD).

ADHD diagnosis. In future research, this convergent validity analysis will be repeated on a item-by-item basis (i.e., convergence between individual items of DSM scales and AULA scores), in order to focus on only those DSM criteria that cover the cognitive domain, and therefore on using AULA to add objectivity to the observations made by parents, teachers, and/or clinicians.

## STUDIES ON COGNITIVE PROFILES OF EXECUTIVE DYSFUNCTION

Sánchez-Carpintero, Crespo-Eguílaz, Banterla, & Climent (2013) developed a study to analyze the neuropsychological processes of executive function underlying performance in AULA (e.g., selective and sustained visual and auditory attention; processing speed; inhibitory control of distractors, of impulsive responses, and of motor activity) in order to precisely determine the cognitive profile that complements the behavioral diagnosis in ADHD. The study participants were 130 patients with ADHD (mean age = 10.61, *SD* = 2.62; 36.2% female; WISC-IV = 82–102, with a mean of 102.8 and *SD* of 9.8) from the Pediatric Neurology Unit of the Clínica Universidad de Navarra (Spain). The researchers show that, according to their performance in AULA, subjects with ADHD could be classified into six groups that predominantly showed the following neuropsychological features:

- inattention
- inattention and cognitive impulsivity
- inattention and hyperactivity
- inattention, impulsivity, and hyperactivity
- moderate inattention and severe impulsivity-hyperactivity
- normal performance with an impulsive although efficient
  cognitive style

The researchers concluded that the exhaustive analysis of neuropsychological variables measured by the test allows further precision and accuracy when describing the cognitive functioning in children with an ADHD diagnosis, and that the detailed cognitive profiles of executive dysfunction obtained would help in planning relevant intervention strategies.

## Future Directions

Results of the studies described above show that AULA is a valid test to measure attention and impulsivity, and is very useful to complete the diagnosis of ADHD with information about cognitive performance in an ecologically relevant simulation. This does not mean that AULA is ecologically valid per se (which it is not, since it is based on a CPT paradigm), but AULA's creation of a virtual classroom with all its components, monitoring of motor activity and attention focus, and introduction of distractors typical of those found in a real school setting and that may interfere with performance, are all in all components that add value to the evaluation of attention processes that is required to substantially support the diagnosis of ADHD. In the short term, it is expected that current and future research with larger clinical samples will provide more accurate information about the utility of the AULA test in the differentiation of ADHD subtypes and cognitive performance profiles in children with ADHD, as well as in the study of the correlations between neuropsychological features and behavioral symptoms of children with ADHD. In addition, because AULA is available in different variants of Spanish (from Spain, Mexico, Colombia, Argentina, Colombia, Peru, and Chile), in Brazilian Portuguese, and American English (with some independent research groups already devoted to performing research with AULA worldwide, including Latin America, the United States, and Australia), it is expected that the growing body of research on AULA will serve as a model for development of additional VR tools that will enhance the quality and reputation of neuropsychological assessment in clinical diagnosis of neurological and neurodegenerative conditions.

# References

Achenbach, T. M., & Rescorla, L. A. (2001). *Manual for the ASEBA School-Age Forms and Profiles*. Burlington, VT: University of Vermont, Research Center for Children, Youth, and Families.

Adams, R., Finn, P., Moes, E., Flannery, K., & Rizzo, A. A. (2009). Distractibility in attention deficit hyperactivity disorder (ADHD): The virtual reality classroom. *Child Neuropsychology, 15*, 120–135.

Amador, J. A., Forns, M., & Kirchner, T. (2006). Cognitive repertoires of attention, perception and memory. Department of Personality, Assessment and Psychological Treatment. Faculty of Psychology, University of Barcelona. [Document in Spanish] (online). http://diposit.ub.edu/dspace/bitstream/2445/345/1/144.pdf

Artigas-Pallarés, J. (2009). Cognitive models in attention deficit hyperactivity disorder. [Article in Spanish]. *Revista de Neurología, 49*, 587–593.

Baker, D. B., Taylor, C. J., & Leyva, C. (1995). Continuous Performance Tests: A Comparison of Modalities. *Journal of Clinical Psychology, 51*, 548–551.

Barkley, R. A. (1994). Can neuropsychological tests help diagnose ADD/ADHD? *The ADHD Report, 2*, 1–3.

Becker, L. E. (1993). *Comprehensive auditory visual attention assessment system*. Fort Wayne, IN: Becker & Associate.

Benton, A. L., Hamsher, K., Varney, N. R., & Spreen, O. (1983). *Contributions to Neuropsychological Assessment: A Clinical Manual*. New York: Oxford University Press.

Berwid, O. G., Curko Kera, E. A., Marks, D. J., Santra, A., & Bender, H. A. (2005). Sustained attention and response inhibition in young children at risk for attention deficit/hyperactivity disorder. *Journal of Child Psychology and Psychiatry, 46*, 1219–1229.

Bioulac, S., Lallemand, S., Rizzo, A., Philip, P., Fabrigoule, C., & Bouvard, M. P. (2012). Impact of time on task on ADHD patients' performances in a virtual classroom. *European Journal of Paediatric Neurology, 16*(5), 514–521. doi:10.1016/j.ejpn.2012.01.006

Brickenkamp, R. (1962). *Aufmerksamkeits-Belastungs-Test* [Attention Stress Test] *(Test d2)*. Göttingen, Germany: Hogrefe.

Cegalis, J. A. (1991). *Vigil: Software for Testing Concentration and Attention, Manual*. Nashua, NH: Forthought Ltd.

Cho, B. H., Lee, J. M., Ku, J. H., Jang, D. P., Kim, J. S., et al. (2002). Attention enhancement system using virtual reality and EEG biofeedback. *Virtual Reality, Proceedings IEEE* (pp. 156–163). Orlando, FL: March 24–28. Los Alamitos, CA: IEEE Computer Society.

Climent, G., & Banterla, F. (2010). *AULA Nesplora. Ecological evaluation of attention processes*. [Book in Spanish]. San Sebastián: Nesplora.

Conners, C. K. (1997). *The Conners Rating Scales - Revised Manual*. North Towanda, NY: Multi-health Systems.

Conners, C. K. (2000). *Conners' Continuous Performance Test: User's Manual*. Toronto, Canada: Multi-Health Systems.

Conners, C.K., & MHS Staff (2004). *Conners' CPT II: Continuous Performance Test II*. New York: MHS.

Cornblatt, B., Risch Neil, J., Faris, G., Friedman, D., & Erlenmeyer-Kimling, L. (1988). The Continuous Performance Test, Identical Pairs version (CPT-IP): I. New findings about sustained attention in normal families. *Psychiatry Research, 26*(2), 223–228.

Crespo-Eguílaz, N., Narbona, J., Peralta, F., & Repáraz, R. (2006). Measure of sustained attention and impulsivity control in children: A new administration modality for the "Faces" Differences Perception Test. [Article in Spanish]. *Infancia y aprendizaje, 29*(2), 219–232.

Delis, D. C., Kaplan, E., & Kramer, J. H. (2001). *Delis-Kaplan Executive Function System (D-KEFS)*. San Antonio, TX: The Psychological Corporation.

Díaz-Orueta, U., Alonso-Sánchez, B., & Climent, G. (2014, February). *AULA versus d2 test of attention: Convergent validity and applicability of virtual reality in the study of reading disorders. Preliminary results*. Poster presented at the 42nd Annual Meeting of the International Neuropsychological Society, Seattle, WA.

Diaz-Orueta, U., Cueto, E., Alonso-Sánchez, B., Crespo-Eguílaz, N., Fernández, M., Otaduy, C., Pérez-Lozano, C., & Zulueta, A. (2014, July). *AULA VR based attention test: Factorial validity and convergent validity with commonly used ADHD diagnostic tools*. Poster presented at the 9th Conference of the International Test Commission, San Sebastian, Spain.

Díaz-Orueta, U., Garcia-López, C., Crespo-Eguílaz, N., Sánchez-Carpintero, R., Climent, G., & Narbona, J. (2014). AULA virtual reality test as an attention measure: Convergent validity with Conners' Continuous Performance Test. *Child Neuropsychology, 20*(3), 328–342.

Díaz-Orueta, U., Iriarte, Y., Climent, G., & Banterla, F. (2012). AULA: An ecological virtual reality test with distractors for evaluating attention in children and adolescents. *Journal of Virtual Reality, 5*, 1–20.

Doyle, A. E., Biederman, J., & Seidman, L. J. (2000). Diagnostic efficiency of neuropsychological test scores for discriminating boys with and without attention deficit-hyperactivity disorder. *Journal of Consulting and Clinical Psychology, 68*(3), 477–488.

Epstein, J. N., Erkanli, A., Conners, C. K., Kleric, J., Castello, J. E., & Angold, A. (2003). Relations between continuous performance test performance measures and ADHD behaviors. *Journal of Abnormal Child Psychology, 31*(5), 543–554.

Farré, A., & Narbona, J. (1998). *EDAH, Escalas Para la Evaluación del Trastorno por Déficit de Atención con Hiperactividad*. Madrid: TEA Ediciones.

Fernández-Fernández, M., & Morillo-Rojas, M. (2012, May). *Test–retest validation of AULA Nesplora (virtual reality continuous performance test) for ADHD*. Poster presented at the 2nd International ADHD Conference, Barcelona, Spain.

Fernández-Fernández, M., Morillo-Rojas, M., & Alonso-Romero, L. (2012, May–June). *Utility of AULA Nesplora in the assessment of ADHD*. Paper presented at the XXXVI Annual Meeting of the Spanish Society of Pediatric Neurology, Santander, Spain.

Fernández-Jaén, A., Martín Fernández-Mayoralas, D., Calleja-Pérez, B., Moreno-Acero, N., & Muñoz-Jareño, N. (2008). Effects of methylphenidate in cognitive-attentional processes. Use of continuous performance tests. [Article in Spanish]. *Revista de Neurología, 46*(Suppl. 1), S47–49.

Forbes, G. B. (1998). Clinical utility of the Test of Variables of Attention (TOVA) in the diagnosis of attention-deficit/hyperactivity disorder. *Journal of Clinical Psychology, 54*, 461–476.

Gilboa, Y., Kerrouche, B., Longaud-Vales, A., Kieffer, V., Tiberghien, A., Aligon, D., ... Paule Chevignard, M. (2015). Describing the attention profile of children and adolescents with acquired brain injury using the virtual classroom. *Brain Injury, 29*(13–14), 1691–1700. doi:10.3109/02699052.2015.1075148

Gilboa,Y., Rosenblum, S., Fattal-Valevski, A., Toledano-Alhadef, H., Rizzo, A. A., & Josman, N. (2011). Using a virtual classroom environment to describe the attention deficits profile of children with neurofibromatosis type 1. *Research in Developmental Disabilities, 32*(6), 2608–2613. doi:10.1016/j.ridd.2011.06.014

Gioia, G. A., Isquith, P. K., Guy, S. C., & Kenworthy, L. (2000). *Behavior Rating Inventory of Executive Function (BRIEF): Professional manual*. Lutz, FL: Psychological Assessment Resources.

Golden, C. (1978). *Stroop Color and Word Test*. Illinois: Stoelting Company.

Gordon, M. (1983). The Gordon Diagnostic System (GDS): The standard in computerized assessment of attention and self control. (online). http://www.devdis.com/gds.html

Greenberg, L. M., & Walkman, I. D. (1993). Developmental normative data on the Test of Variables of Attention (TOVA). *Journal of Child Psychology and Psychiatry, 34*, 1019–1030.

Gutiérrez-Maldonado, J., Letosa-Porta, A., Rus-Calafell, M., & Peñaloza-Salazar, C. (2009). The assessment of attention deficit hyperactivity disorder in children using continuous performance tasks in virtual environments. *Anuario de Psicología, 40*(2), 211–222.

Henry, M., Joyal, C. C., & Nolin, P. (2012). Development and Initial Assessment of a New Paradigmfor Assessing Cognitive and Motor Inhibition: the Bimodal Virtual-Reality Stroop. *Journal of Neuroscience Methods, 210*, 125–131.

Holdnack, H. A. (2001). *Wechsler Test of Adult Reading: WTAR*. San Antonio. The Psychological Corporation.

Iriarte, Y., Díaz-Orueta, U., Cueto, E., Irazustabarrena, P., Banterla, F., & Climent, G. (2016). AULA—Advanced virtual reality tool for the assessment of attention: Normative study in Spain. *Journal of Attention Disorders, 20*(6), 542–568. doi:10.1177/1087054712465335

Johnson, K. A., Kelly, S. P., Bellgrove, M. A., Barry, E., Cox, M., Gill, M., & Robertson, I. H. (2007). Response variability in attention deficit hyperactivity disorder: Evidence for neuropsychological heterogeneity. *Neuropsychologia, 45*, 630–638.

Lalonde, G., Henry, M., Drouin-Germain, A., Nolin, P., & Beauchamp, M. H. (2013). Assessment of executive function in adolescence: A comparison of traditional and virtual reality tools. *Journal of Neuroscience Methods, 219*(1), 76–82. http://dx.doi.org/10.1016/j.jneumeth.2013.07.005

Lee, J. M., Cho, B. H., Ku, J. H., Kim, J. S., Lee, J. H., Kim, I. Y, & Kim, I. S. (2001). A study on the system for treatment of ADHD using virtual reality. *Engineering in Medicine* and Biology Society, 2001. *Proceedings of the 23rd Annual International Conference of the IEEE, 4,* 3754–3757.

Llorente, A. M., Voigt, R., Jensen, C. L., Fraley, J. K., Heird, W. C., & Rennie, K. M. (2007). The Test of Variables of Attention (TOVA): Internal consistency (Q(1) vs Q(2) and Q(3) vs Q(4)) in children with attention deficit/hyperactivity disorder (ADHD). *Child Neuropsychology, 3,* 1–9.

Losier, B. J., McGrath, P. J., & Klein, R. M. (1996). Error patterns on the continuous performance test in non-medicated and medicated samples of children with and without ADHD: A meta-analytic review. *Journal of Child Psychology and Psychiatry, 37,* 971–987.

Manly, T., Robertson, I. H., Anderson, V., & Nimmo-smith, I. (1999). *TEA-Ch: The Test of Everyday Attention for Children Manual.* Bury St. Edmunds, UK: Thames Valley Test Company Limited.

Mayes, S. D., Calhoun, S. L., Chase, G. A., Mink, D. M., & Stagg, R. E. (2009). ADHD subtypes and co-occurring anxiety, depression, and oppositional-defiant disorder: Differences in Gordon Diagnostic System and Wechsler Working Memory and Processing Speed index scores. *Journal of Attention Disorders, 12*(6), 540–550.

Miranda, M. C., Barbosa, T., Muszkalt, M., Rodrigues, C., Sinnes, E., Coelho, L., Rizzuti, S., . . . Bueno, O. (2008). Patterns of performance on the Conners' CPT in children with ADHD and learning disabilities. *Journal of Attention Disorders, 11*(5), 588–598.

Nolin, P., Martin, C., & Bouchard, S. (2009). Assessment of inhibition deficits with the virtual classroom in children with traumatic brain injury: A pilot study. *Studies in Health Technology and Informatics, 144,* 240–242.

Nolin, P., Stipanicic, A., Henry, M., Joyal, C. C., & Allain, P. (2012). Virtual reality as a screening tool for sports concussion in adolescents. *Brain Injury, 26*(13–14), 1564–1573.

Parsons, T. D. (2014). Virtual Teacher and Classroom for Assessment of Neurodevelopmental Disorders. In *Technologies of inclusive well-being* (pp. 121–137). Berlin & Heidelberg: Springer.

Parsons, T. D., Bowerly, T., Buckwalter, J. G., & Rizzo, A. A. (2007). A controlled clinical comparison of attention performance in children with ADHD in a virtual reality classroom compared to standard neuropsychological methods. *Child Neuropsychology, 13* (4), 363–381.

Parsons, T. D., & Carlew, A. R. (2016). Bimodal virtual reality Stroop for assessing distractor inhibition in autism spectrum disorders. *Journal of Autism and Developmental Disorders, 46*(4), 1255–1267. doi:10.1007/s10803-015-2663-7

Pollak, Y., Shomaly, H. B., Weiss, P. L., Rizzo, A. A., & Gross-Tsur, V. (2010). Methylphenidate effect in children with ADHD can be measured by an ecologically valid continuous performance test embedded in virtual reality. *CNS Spectrums, 15*(2), 125–130.

Pollak, Y., Weiss, P. L., Rizzo, A. A., Weizer, M., Shriki, L., Shalev, R. S., & Gross-Tsur, V. (2009). The utility of a continuous performance test embedded in virtual reality in measuring ADHD-related deficits. *Journal of Developmental and Behavioral Pediatrics, 30,* 2–6.

Reitan, R. M. (1971). Trail Making Test Rresults for Normal and Brain-Damaged Children. *Perceptual and Motor Skills, 33,* 575–581.

Reitan, R. M., & Wolfson, D. (2004). The Trail Making Test as an Initial Screening Procedure for Neuropsychological Impairment in Older Children. *Archives of Clinical Neuropsychology, 19*(2), 281–288.

Riccio, C. A., Garland, B. H., & Cohen, M. J. (2007). Relations between the Test of Variables of Attention (TOVA) and the Children's Memory Scale (CMS). *Journal of Attention Disorders, 11,* 167–171.

Riccio, C. A., Reynolds, C. R., & Lowe, P. (2001). *Clinical applications of continuous performance tests.* New York: John Wiley & Sons.

Rizzo, A. A., Bowerly, T., Buckwalter, J. G., Limchuk, D., Mitura, R., & Parsons, T. D. (2006). A virtual reality scenario for all seasons: The virtual classroom. *CNS Spectrums, 11,* 35–44.

Rizzo, A. A., Buckwalter, J. G., Bowerly, T., Van der Zaag, C., Humphrey, L., Neumann, U., . . . Sisemore, D. (2000). The Virtual Classroom: A Virtual Reality Environment for the Assessment and Rehabilitation of Attention Deficits. *Cyberpsychology & Behavior, 3*(3), 483–499.

Rohani, D. A., Sorensen, H. B., & Puthusserypady, S. (2014). Brain-computer interface using P300 and virtual reality: A gaming approach for treating ADHD. *Conference Proceedings. Annual International Conference of the IEEE Engineering in Medicine and Biology Society,* 3606–3609. doi: 10.1109/EMBC.2014.6944403.

Rosvold, H. E., Mirsky, A. F., Sarason, I., Bransome, E. D., Jr., & Beck, L. H. (1956). A continuous performance test of brain damage. *Journal of Consulting Psychology, 20,* 343–350.

Rufo-Campos, M., Cueto, E., Iriarte, Y., & Rufo-Muñoz, M. (2012, May–June). *Sensitivity study of a new diagnostic method for ADHD: Aula Nesplora.* Paper presented at the XXXVI Annual Meeting of the Spanish Society of Pediatric Neurology, Santander, Spain.

Sánchez-Carpintero, R., Crespo-Eguílaz, N., Banterla, F., & Climent, G. (2013, February–March). *Cognitive profiles of executive dysfunction in ADHD according to performance in AULA virtual reality test.* Poster presented at the XV International Course of Updates in Neuropediatrics and Child Neuropsychology, Valencia, Spain.

Sandford, J.A., & Turner, A. (1995). *Manual for the Integrated Visual and Auditory (IVA) continuous performance test.* Richmond, VA: BrainTrain.

Seisdedos, N. (2002). *d2 attention test.* [Spanish version]. Madrid: TEA.

Sergeant, J., Oosterlaan, J., & Van der Meere, J. (1999). Information processing and energetic factors in attention-deficit/hyperactivity disorder. In C. Herbert & A. E. Hogan (Eds.), *Handbook of disruptive behavior disorders* (pp. 75–104). Dordrecht, Netherlands: Kluwer.

Servera, M., & Llabrés, J. (2004). *CSAT: Children Sustained Attention Task.* [Book in Spanish]. Madrid: TEA.

Silvana, M. S., & Nada, P. J. (2009). Comparison of visual and emotional continuous performance test related to sequence of presentation, gender and age. *Contributions, Section of Biological and Medical Sciences, 1,* 167–178.

Swanson, J. M., Wigal, T., & Lakes, K. (2009). DSM-V and the Future Diagnosis of Attention-Deficit/Hyperactivity Disorder. *Current Psychiatry Reports, 11,* 399–406.

Thurstone, L., & Yela, M. (1985). *Faces –Differences Perception Test.* [Book in Spanish]. Madrid: TEA.

Wada, N., Yamashita, Y., Matsuishi, T., Ohtani, Y., & Kato, H. (2000). The Test of Variables of Attention (TOVA) is useful in the diagnosis of Japanese male children with attention deficit hyperactivity disorder. *Brain Development, 22,* 378–382.

Wechsler, D. (1991). *The Wechsler Intelligence Scale for Children—Third Edition*. San Antonio, TX: The Psychological Corporation.

Wechsler, D. (1999). *Wechsler Abbreviated Scale of Intelligence. Manual.* San Antonio, TX: The Psychological Corporation.

Wechsler, D. (2003). *Wechsler Intelligence Scale for Children–Fourth Edition*. San Antonio, TX: The Psychological Corporation.

Weyandt, L. L., Mitzlaff, L., & Thomas, L. (2002). The relationship between intelligence and performance on the Test of Variables of Attention (TOVA). *Journal of Learning Disabilities, 35*, 114–120.

Xu, Y., Zhou, X. L., & Wang, Y. F. (2004). Effects of distractors on sustained attention in children with attention-deficit hyperactivity disorder. *Chinese Journal of Pediatrics, 42*, 44–48.

Zelnik, N., Bennett-Back, O., Miari, W., Goez, H. R., & Fattal-Valevski, A. (2012). Is the Test of Variables of Attention reliable for the diagnosis of attention-deficit hyperactivity disorder (ADHD)? *Journal of Child Neurology, 27*: 703. doi:10.1177/0883073811423821

Zulueta, A., Iriarte, Y., Díaz-Orueta, U., & Climent, G. (2013). AULA Nesplora: Progress in assessing attention processes—a convergent validity study with the Faces—Perception of Differences Test (extended version). *ISEP Science, 4*, 3–10.

# 7

# Virtual Environment Grocery Store

Thomas D. Parsons, Timothy McMahan, Patrick Melugin,
and Michael Barnett

Neuropsychologists are increasingly being asked to determine whether a patient can return to work, classroom, or play (e.g., sports). A difficulty for the neuropsychological assessment of cognitive functioning is that patients' performance on a cognitive test may have little or no predictive value for how they may perform in a real-world situation (Burgess, Alderman, Evans, Emslie, & Wilson, 1998; Chaytor, Schmitter-Edgecombe, & Burr, 2006). To address this issue, neuropsychologists are increasingly emphasizing the need for tasks that represent real-world functioning and that tap into a number of executive domains (Chaytor & Schmitter-Edgecombe, 2003; Jurado & Rosselli, 2007). Burgess and colleagues (2006) argue that the majority of neuropsychological assessments currently in use today were developed to assess abstract cognitive "constructs" without regard for their ability to predict "functional" behavior. For example, although the construct-driven Wisconsin Card Sorting Test (WCST) is one of the most widely used measures of executive function, it was not originally developed as a measure of executive functioning. Instead, the WCST was preceded by a number of sorting measures that were developed from observations of the effects of brain damage (e.g., Weigl, 1927). While Milner (1963) found that patients with dorsolateral prefrontal lesions had greater difficulty on the WCST than patients with orbitofrontal or nonfrontal lesions, other studies have shown that patients with frontal lobe pathology do not always differ from control subjects on the WCST (Stuss et al., 1983). Some may argue that while there have been some inconsistencies in the literature, data from the construct-driven WCST do appear to provide information relevant to the constructs of *set shifting* and *working memory*. However, it can also be argued that the data do not necessarily offer information that would allow a neuropsychologist to predict what situations in everyday life require the abilities that the WCST measures.

A number of investigators have argued that performance on traditional tests has little correspondence to everyday activities of daily living. This can leave the neuropsychologist uncertain of the efficacy of the tests for predicting the way in which patients will manage in their everyday lives (Bottari, Dassa, Rainville, & Dutil, 2009; Manchester, Priestly, & Howard, 2004; Sbordone, 2008). Chan and colleagues (2008) have pointed out that most of these traditional measures assess at the impairment level. Moreover, they do not delineate the complexity of responses required in the numerous multistep tasks found in everyday activities. Burgess et al. (2006) suggest that future development of neuropsychological assessments should result in tests that are representative of real-world functions and proffer results that are generalizable for prediction of functional performance across a range of situations. According to Burgess et al. (2006), a "function-led approach" to creating neuropsychological assessments will include neuropsychological models that proceed from directly observable everyday behaviors backward to examine the ways in which a sequence of actions leads to a given behavior in normal functioning; and the ways in which that behavior might become disrupted. Therefore, he calls for a new generation of neuropsychological tests that are function led rather than purely construct driven. The neuropsychological assessments should meet the usual standards of reliability, but discussions of validity should include both sensitivity to brain dysfunction and generalizability to real-world function.

## Multiple Errands Paradigm for Function-Led Assessments

In response to these issues, a number of function-led tests of executive function have been developed to assess real-world planning (e.g., Zoo Map and Six Elements subtests of the Behavioral Assessment of Dysexecutive Syndrome; Wilson et al., 1996) and self-regulation (e.g., the Revised Strategy Application Test, Levine et al., 2000; Sustained Attention to Response Test, Robertson et al., 1997; for review, see Chan et al., 2008). One of the most widely accepted is the Multiple Errands Test (MET). Shallice and Burgess (1991) developed the MET as a function-led assessment of multitasking. The MET requires the patient to perform a number of relatively simple but open-ended tasks in a shopping context. Participants are required to achieve a number of simple tasks without breaking a series of arbitrary rules. The MET has been shown to have increased sensitivity (over traditional neuropsychological measures) to elicit and detect failures in executive function (e.g., distractibility and task implementation deficits). It has also been shown to be better at predicting behavioral difficulties in everyday life (Alderman, Burgess, Knight, & Henman, 2003). Further, the MET has been found to have strong interrater reliability (Dawson et al., 2009; Knight, Alderman, & Burgess, 2002), and performance indices from the MET were able to significantly predict severity of everyday life executive problems in persons with traumatic brain injury (Cuberos-Urbano et al., 2013).

While the MET does overcome some of the limitations of construct-driven neuropsychological assessments, there are some limitations inherent in any naturalistic observation. Potential limitations of the MET are apparent in the obvious drawbacks to experiments conducted in real-life settings (e.g., Bailey, Henry, Rendell, Phillips, & Kliegel, 2010). Logie, Trawley, and Law (2011) point out a number of limitations in the MET:

- It is time consuming
- Transportation is required for participants
- Consent from local businesses is needed
- Experimental control is lacking
- It is difficult to adapt tasks for other clinical or research settings.

Hence, there is need for a function-led approach to neuropsychological assessment that is both function-led and is able to log information in a controlled manner.

This chapter describes attempts to develop a virtual reality-based multiple errands task that is function-led and offers a great deal of experimental control. After a brief discussion of virtual reality-based neuropsychological assessments, attempts to operationalize function-led virtual errands tasks are presented. This is followed by a discussion of the Virtual Environments Grocery Store, which was developed to combine the strengths of the original MET with the various virtual errands tasks. It is believed that this new Virtual Environments Grocery Store reflects an enhanced iteration.

## Virtual Reality-Based Neuropsychological Assessments

Virtual environments (VEs) are increasingly considered potential aids for enhancing the ecological validity of neuropsychological assessments (Campbell et al., 2009; Parsons, 2011; Schultheis, Himelstein, & Rizzo, 2002; Renison, Ponsford, Testa, Richardson, & Brownfield, 2012). VEs are advanced computer interfaces that allow patients to become immersed in a computer-generated simulation of everyday activities. Given that VEs represent a special case of computerized neuropsychological assessment devices (Bauer et al., 2012; Schatz & Browndyke, 2002), they have enhanced computational capacities for administration efficiency, stimulus presentation, automated logging of responses, and data analytic processing. Since VEs allow for precise presentation and control of dynamic perceptual stimuli, they can provide ecologically valid assessments that combine the veridical control and rigor of laboratory measures with a verisimilitude that reflects real-life situations (Parsons, 2011, 2015). Additionally, the enhanced computational power allows for increased accuracy in the recording of neurobehavioral responses in a perceptual environmental that systematically presents complex stimuli. Such simulation technology appears to be distinctively suited for the development of ecologically valid environments, in which three-dimensional objects are presented in a consistent and precise manner (Schultheis et al., 2002). VE-based neuropsy-chological assessments can provide a balance between naturalistic observation and the need for exacting control over key variables (Campbell et al., 2009; Parsons, 2011, 2015). In summary, VE-based neuropsychological assessments allow for real-time measurement of multiple neurocognitive abilities in order to assess complex sets of skills and behaviors that may more closely resemble real-world functional abilities (Matheis et al., 2007; Parsons et al., 2015b).

## Virtual Multiple Errands Tasks

A number of early attempts were made to develop VR versions of the Multiple Errands Test (MET). For example, McGeorge et al. (2001) developed a Virtual Errands Test (VET) that had features similar to the original MET. That said, the VET tasks were more vocationally oriented in format and contained work-related errands instead of the shopping errands found in the MET. Their study included five adult patients with brain injury and five unimpaired matched controls. The participants completed both the real-life MET and the VET. Findings from the study revealed similar performance for real-world and VE tasks. In a larger study that compared 35 patients with prefrontal neurosurgical lesions to 35 controls matched for age and estimated IQ, the virtual reality (VR) scenario was found to successfully differentiate between participants with brain injuries and controls (Morris, Kotitsa, Bramham, Brooks, & Rose, 2002). While the results are interesting, it is important to note that these early VEs had unrealistic graphics, and performance assessment involved video recording test sessions, with subsequent manual scoring.

Recently, a number of VEs with enhanced graphics (and usability) have been developed to model the function-led approach found in the MET. The Multitasking in the City Test (MCT) was developed to reflect the sorts of tasks found in the original MET. The MCT involves an errand-running task that takes place in a virtual city (Jovanovski et al., 2012a, 2012b). The MCT can be distinguished from existing VR and real-life METs in that tasks are performed with less explicit rule constraints. This distinction was intentional in the MCT because the research-ers aimed to investigate behaviors that are clearly not goal-directed. The MCT is made up of a virtual city that includes a post office, drug store, stationary store, coffee shop, grocery store, optometrist's office, doctor's office, restaurant/pub, bank, dry cleaners, pet store, and the participant's home. The MCT has been used to compare poststroke and traumatic brain injury patients to healthy controls.

## Virtual Shopping Tasks for Assessment of Executive Functioning

Virtual shopping scenarios offer an advanced computer interface that allows the clinician to immerse the patient in a computer-generated simulation that reflects activities of daily living. They involve a number of errands that must be completed in a real environment following certain rules that require problem solving. Since they allow for precise presentation and control of dynamic perceptual stimuli, virtual shopping scenarios have the potential to provide ecologically valid assessments that combine the control of laboratory measures with simulations that reflect real-life situations. Due to their resemblance to everyday activities, virtual shopping tasks have quickly become a mainstay in research surrounding function-led assessment tools. In recent years, several iterations of the virtual shopping task have been developed and tested on both clinical and nonclinical samples (see Table 7.1).

## VIRTUAL ACTION PLANNING—SUPERMARKET

The Virtual Action Planning—Supermarket (VAP-S; Klinger, Chemin, Lebreton, & Marié, 2004; Marié, Klinger, Chemin, & Josset, 2003) is a VR assessment tool designed to assess executive functioning. In the VAP-S, participants are introduced to a fully textured virtual supermarket replete with shopping items (e.g., fruits, vegetables, drinks, canned foods, refrigerated goods, flowers, clothes, cleaning equipment), multiple aisles, four check-out counters, a reception point, and a shopping cart. Static customers and employees inhabit the virtual supermarket and obstacles like boxes and cartons obstruct participants' progression through the store aisles. Using a computer, keyboard, and mouse, participants first undergo brief training sessions that teach them how to navigate and interact with the VAP-S. Following the training sessions, participants are given verbal instructions that are also displayed on the screen along with seven products specified by the researcher. Participants stand behind a shopping cart, visualizing the VAP-S from a first-person perspective (i.e., no avatar is visible). They are instructed to navigate the aisles to search for and obtain all seven items. Participants must place the items on a conveyer belt at a check-out line, pay for them, and then place the items back in the shopping cart before walking out the door. In order to complete the shopping task, 12 correct actions (e.g., choosing correct items, leaving supermarket only after acquiring correct items and paying) must be completed. Eight outcome measures can be extracted from the VAP-S, including distance covered, trajectory duration, items purchased, correct/incorrect actions, number of stops, total duration of stops, and the time to pay.

The VAP-S was originally developed by researchers in France to assess cognitive planning (Klinger et al., 2004; Marié et al., 2003). Klinger, Chemin, Lebreton, and Marié (2006) subsequently used the VAP-S to assess cognitive planning in five patients ($M_{age}$ = 74.0, SD = 5.4) with Parkinson's disease (PD) in relation to that of five age-matched healthy controls ($M_{age}$ = 66.6, SD = 7.7). They found that patients with PD walked a significantly longer distance in the VR supermarket relative to the control group, providing preliminary evidence for the feasibility of the VAP-S as an assessment of cognitive planning in individuals with PD.

TABLE 7.1 Virtual Shopping Protocols

| Study | Virtual Environment | | | Outcome Measures | Traditional Tests | Groups | Outcome |
|---|---|---|---|---|---|---|---|
| | Name | Equipment & Software | Setting | | | | |
| Canty et al. (2014) | Virtual Reality Shopping Task (VRST) | Laptop Virtools, 3DVIA-player | Shopping mall | Ongoing task performance, time-based performance, event-based performance, time-checking frequency, total performance | LDPMT, TMT, HVLT-R, COWAT, HSCT, LNS, SPRS | Severe TBI ($n = 30$) vs. healthy controls ($n = 24$) | VRST performance successfully differentiated between TBI patients and the control group. Measures of prospective memory, neurocognitive functioning, and psychosocial functioning were significantly associated with VRST performance among TBI patients. |
| Carelli, Morganti, Weiss, Kizony, & Riva (2008) | n/a | PC, Gamepad NeuroVR, Blender | Supermarket | Execution time, errors, number of trials failed, complexity level reached | n/a | Healthy older adults ($N = 20$) | Results suggest the virtual supermarket may be a useful tool in executive assessment, particularly due to its temporal and accuracy measures. |
| Josman et al. (2006) | Virtual Action Planning Supermarket (VAP-S) | Laptop, 17" LCD monitor, Keyboard, Mouse Virtools Development, Discreet 3D Studio Max 4 | Supermarket | Total trajectory (min), trajectory duration (s), number of items purchased, number of correct/incorrect actions, number of stops, total duration of stops (s), time to pay (s) | BADS | Poststroke ($N = 26$) | VAP-S outcome measures (i.e., number of items purchased, number of correct actions, total duration of stops) were moderately correlated with the Key Search subtest of the BADS, providing preliminary evidence for usefulness of the VAP-S as an assessment tool for cognitive planning in poststroke populations. |

| Study | Instrument | Equipment | Setting | Outcome measures | Assessment | Population | Results |
|---|---|---|---|---|---|---|---|
| Josman et al. (2014) | Virtual Action Planning Supermarket (VAP-S) | 17" LCD monitor, Keyboard, Mouse, 3DVIA Virtools, 3D Studio Max | Supermarket | Total trajectory (min), trajectory duration (s), number of items purchased, number of correct/incorrect actions, number of stops, total duration of stops (s), time to pay (s) | BADS, OTDL-R | Poststroke ($n = 24$) vs. healthy controls ($n = 24$) | Results revealed that poststroke patients purchased significantly fewer items and made significantly fewer correct actions in the VAP-S than the control group. The number of items purchased and the number of correct actions in the VAP-S were also found to be moderately correlated with BADS subtests and highly correlated with the OTDL-R. |
| Josman, Schenirderman, Klinger, & Shevil (2009) | Virtual Action Planning Supermarket (VAP-S) | Laptop, 3DVIA, 3D Studio Max | Supermarket | Total trajectory (min), trajectory duration (s), number of items purchased, number of correct/incorrect actions, number of stops, total duration of stops (s), time to pay (s) | BADS | Schizophrenia ($n = 30$) vs. healthy controls ($n = 30$) | Schizophrenia patients performed significantly worse than the control group on three VAP-S outcome measures (i.e., number of items purchased, number of correct actions, time to pay). Performance in the VAP-S was able to differentiate between patients with differing levels of executive functioning. Two VAP-S outcome measures (i.e., number of items purchased, number of correct actions) displayed moderate to high correlations with all BADS subtests. |

(Continued)

TABLE 7.1 Continued

| Study | Virtual Environment | | | | Traditional Tests | Groups | Outcome |
|---|---|---|---|---|---|---|---|
| | Name | Equipment & Software | Setting | Outcome Measures | | | |
| Kang et al. (2008) | VR Shopping Simulation Program | PC, HMD (Eye-Trek FMD-250W), 3-Degrees of Freedom Position Sensor, Gamepad | Supermarket | Stage 1: Performance score, interaction error<br>Stage 2: Total time (s), immediate recognition memory, delayed recognition memory, auditory memory score, visual memory score, attention index, attention reaction time (s)<br>Stage 3: Total time (s), total distance, executive index | n/a | Poststroke ($n = 20$) vs. healthy controls ($n = 20$) | Significant differences were found between poststroke patients and the control group on the majority of outcome measures, with the patient group performing worse on measures of memory, attention, and executive functioning. |
| Klinger, Chemin, Lebreton, & Marié (2006) | Virtual Action Planning Supermarket (VAP-S) | PC, 21" Screen, Keyboard, Mouse Virtools Dev Education, Discreet 3D Studio Max | Supermarket | Distance (m), duration (min), number of, time of first action (min), time to pay (s), good actions, intrusions, training time (min) | n/a | Parkinson's disease ($n = 5$) vs. healthy controls ($n = 5$) | Patients with Parkinson's disease (PD) walked a significantly longer distance in the VAP-S than the control group, suggesting that the VR supermarket may be a useful tool for assessing cognitive planning in patients with PD. |

| Author | Test | Hardware | Environment | Measures | Cognitive assessments | Population | Results |
|---|---|---|---|---|---|---|---|
| Okahashi et al. (2013) | Virtual Shopping Test (VST) | PC, 19" LCD touch screen Metasequoia, Open GL | Shopping mall | Bag use, list use, cue use, forward movement, reverse movement, correct purchases, total time, time in shops, time on road, mean time per shop | SDMT, SRT, RBMT, BIT (Star and Letter Cancellation task), MMSE, EMC, DEX, BADS (Zoo Map subtest) | Brain damage ($n = 10$) vs. healthy controls ($n = 10$); older adults ($n = 10$) vs. young adults ($n = 10$) | Performance on the VST was significantly associated with conventional cognitive assessments in the patient group, with the exception of the Zoo Map subtest, Star and Letter Cancellation Task, and DEX. The patient group performed significantly worse than the control group on seven of the ten VST outcome measures, while the older adult group performed significantly worse than the young group on four of the VST outcome measures. |
| Rand, Katz, & Weiss (2007) | VMall | GestureTek's GX video-capture VR system | Supermarket | Total time to shop, order of items bought, number of items bought by mistake | n/a | Poststroke ($n = 14$) vs. healthy controls (children $n = 23$; young adults $n = 44$; older adults $n = 26$) | Total time taken to shop in the VMall successfully differentiated between poststroke patients and the control groups, with poststroke patients taking significantly longer to complete the shopping task. |

*(Continued)*

TABLE 7.1 Continued

| Study | Virtual Environment | | | | Traditional Tests | Groups | Outcome |
|---|---|---|---|---|---|---|---|
| | Name | Equipment & Software | Setting | Outcome Measures | | | |
| Rand, Rukan, Weiss, & Katz (2009) | VR version of the Multiple Errands Test (VMET) within VMall | GestureTek's IREX video capture VR system | Supermarket | Total mistakes, mistakes in completing tasks, partial mistakes in completing tasks, non-efficiency mistakes, rule break mistakes, use of strategies mistakes | MET—Hospital version, BADS (Zoo Map subtest), IADL questionnaire | Poststroke (n = 9) vs. older adults (n = 20) vs. young adults (n = 20) | VMET performance successfully differentiated among all three study groups. Moderate to high correlations were found between MET performance and the VMET outcome measures among poststroke patients and healthy older adults. Non-efficiency mistakes and total mistakes committed in the VMET were highly correlated with the Zoo Map subtest and IADL questionnaire, respectively. |
| Raspelli et al. (2012) | VR version of the Multiple Errands Test (VMET) | PC, Gamepad NeuroVR, Blender | Supermarket | Time of execution, total errors, partial task failures, inefficiencies, rule breaks, strategies, interpretation failures | TEA, IGT, Stroop Test | Stroke patients (n = 9) vs. healthy older adults (n = 10) vs. healthy young adults (n = 10) | Significant differences were found among all three study groups on two outcome measures of the VMET (i.e., time of execution, total errors). The TEA (but not the IGT or Stroop) displayed moderate to high correlations with VMET performance in poststroke participants. |

| Ruse et al. (2014) | Virtual Reality Functional Capacity Assessment Tool (VRFCAT) | n/a | Kitchen, bus, supermarket | Completion time, errors made, forced progressions | MCCB, UPSA-B | Schizophrenia ($n = 51$) vs. healthy controls ($n = 54$) | Patients with schizophrenia performed significantly more slowly and with a greater number of errors and forced progressions relative to the control group. Small to moderate correlations were found between VRFCAT performance and the MCCB; however, no relationship was found between VRFCAT performance and the UPSA-B. |
|---|---|---|---|---|---|---|---|
| Werner, Rabinowitz, Klinger, Korczyn, & Josman (2009) | Virtual Action Planning Supermarket (VAP-S) | n/a | Supermarket | Total trajectory (m), trajectory duration (sec), number of items purchased, number of correct/incorrect actions, number of stops, total duration of stops (min), mean time to pay (min) | BADS | MCI ($n = 30$) vs. healthy controls ($n = 30$) | Results indicated that four of the eight VAP-S outcome measures were significantly associated with performance on the BADS. VAP-S performance successfully differentiated between MCI patients and the control group, suggesting the VAP-S is sensitive to deficits in executive functioning. |

(Continued)

TABLE 7.1 Continued

| Study | Virtual Environment | | | Outcome Measures | Traditional Tests | Groups | Outcome |
|-------|------|---------------------------|---------|------------------|-------------------|--------|---------|
| | Name | Equipment & Software | Setting | | | | |
| Zygouris et al. (2015) | Virtual Supermarket (VSM) | n/a | Supermarket | Correct types, correct quantities, correct money, bought unlisted, duration | MMSE, RAVLT, ROCFT, RBMT, TEA, TMT, FRSSD, FUCAS, CDR, "FAS" verbal fluency test, Greek dementia screening scale | MCI (n = 34) vs. healthy controls (n = 21) | VSM performance was moderately correlated with traditional neuropsychological tests. The VSM was able to differentiate between MCI patients and the control group; however, it was unable to differentiate MCI subtypes. |

*Note: MCCB = MATRICS Consensus Cognitive Battery, LDPMT = Lexical Decision Prospective Memory Task, TMT = Trail Making Test, HVLT-R = Hopkins Verbal Learning Test-Revised, COWAT = Controlled Oral Word Association Task, HSCT = Hayling Sentence Completion Test, LNS = Letter Number Sequencing, SPRS = Sydney Psychosocial Reintegration Scale, ROCFT = Rey–Osterrieth Complex Figure Test, RAVLT = Rey Auditory Verbal Learning Test, BADS = Behavioural Assessment of Dysexecutive Syndrome, SDMT = Symbol Digit Modalities Test, SRT = Simple Reaction Time Task, RBMT = Rivermead Behavioural Memory Test, EMC = Everyday Memory Checklist, DEX = Dysexecutive Questionnaire, BIT = Behavioural Inattention Test, MMSE = Mini-Mental State Examination, TEA = Test of Everyday Attention, FRSSD = Functional Rating Scale for Symptoms of Dementia, OTDL-R = Observed Tasks of Daily Living-Revised, FUCAS = Functional Cognitive Assessment Scale, CDR = Clinical Dementia Rating, MET = Multiple Errands Test, IGT = Iowa Gambling Task, UPSA-B = UCSD Performance-Based Skills Assessment-Brief, IADL = Instrumental Activities of Daily Living.

Klinger then adapted the VAP-S for use in an Israeli population (Josman et al., 2006), with the names of aisles, grocery items, and other elements being translated to Hebrew. In the Klinger study, researchers looked at VAP-S performance among 26 poststroke participants ($M_{age}$ = 56.9, SD = 8.9) in relation to performance on the Behavioral Assessment of Dysexecutive Syndrome (BADS; Wilson et al., 1996), a series of tests predicting day-to-day functioning. The study found that VAP-S outcome measures (i.e., number of items purchased, number of correct actions, total duration of stops) were moderately correlated with the Key Search subtest of the BADS, a measure of planning and problem solving, providing evidence for potential of the VAP-S as an assessment of cognitive planning in poststroke patients.

In the wake of research finding significant impairments in executive functioning associated with mild cognitive impairments (MCI), Werner, Rabinowitz, Klinger, Korcyzn, and Josman (2009) further investigated the VAP-S among individuals with MCI. Werner and colleagues (2009) examined 30 patients with MCI ($M_{age}$ = 69.5, SD = 7.3) and 30 age- and gender-matched healthy controls ($M_{age}$ = 69.2, SD = 7.4) and found that four outcome measures of the VAP-S were moderately to highly correlated with the BADS total profile score ($r = -.40$ to $r = -.63$, $p < .001$), with trajectory duration ($r = -.63$) and total duration of stops ($r = -.58$) displaying the strongest associations with the BADS. Three of the VAP-S outcome measures, namely total trajectory, trajectory duration, and total duration of stops, were also found to significantly differentiate between MCI patients and the control group. Used in conjunction with the MMSE, the VAP-S displayed potential at predicting group membership.

The VAP-S has since been validated in several other important clinical populations, including poststroke (Josman et al., 2014) and schizophrenic patients (Josman, Schenirderman, Klinger, & Shevil, 2009). Both of these studies found that the VAP-S outcome measures were able to successfully differentiate between the patient and control groups. Furthermore, the studies found that VAP-S performance was significantly associated with established performance-based measures of everyday functioning.

### VIRTUAL MALL—VIRTUAL MULTIPLE ERRANDS TASK

Another iteration of the virtual shopping paradigm is the Virtual Multiple Errands Task (VMET). The VMET is a virtual shopping task located within a shopping environment called the "VMall." The VMET was designed to serve as a VR adaptation of the MET (Shallice & Burgess, 1991), a measure of executive functioning in everyday life conducted in real-life settings (i.e., shopping malls, hospitals). Although the MET has been shown to be an ecologically valid assessment of executive functioning, the difficulties associated with conducting this type of assessment *in natura* prompted the development of the VMET.

In order to interact with the VMall, participants are placed in front of a video-capture VR system that projects their image onto the VMall and responds to their movements (Rand, Katz, Shahar, Kizony, & Weiss, 2005; Rand, Katz, & Weiss, 2007). The VMall features images of real grocery store items rendered by three-dimensional graphic software that are then inserted into the virtual landscape. Each aisle (nine in total) contains upwards of 60 products that are sorted by category (e.g., baked goods, cleaning products) and features signs displaying the names and images of the products located therein. Users are required to perform gross motor movements with their upper extremities in order to select items and navigate the aisles. In order to prevent inadvertent selections, only actions performed by participants wearing a red glove (or another red accessory) translate to actions within the supermarket. Participants must hover over selections for a minimum of 2 seconds for their decision to register. To help facilitate immersion, background music and intermittent sale announcements were added. Rand et al. (2007) evaluated whether performance on a four-item shopping task within the VMall could differentiate between 14 poststroke patients ($M_{age} = 61$, $SD = 11.2$) and a healthy control group ($n = 93$) comprised of older adults ($M_{age} = 60$, $SD = 5.5$), young adults ($M_{age} = 26$, $SD = 2.6$), and children ($M_{age} = 14.6$, $SD = 2.5$). In this task, participants were given a shopping list containing four items: 1-kg bag of sugar, 1-kg bag of rice, half liter of soda, and half liter of orange juice. Of the VMall outcome measures, total time to shop, order of items bought, and number of items bought by mistake, results indicated that poststroke participants took significantly longer to complete the four-item shopping task than all three healthy control groups. Poststroke participants also reported having to expend significantly greater physical effort than the young control group.

Rand, Rukan, Weiss, and Katz (2009) subsequently implemented a more complex shopping task in the VMall based on the MET, which they named the VMET. This task featured the same instructions as the MET and had participants engage in the same number of tasks; however, products were changed to resemble items that were more appropriate for the VMall. Further, rather than having participants meet with the researcher at a certain time (an additional MET task), participants were instead instructed to check the contents of their shopping cart at a certain time. In total, the VMET (Rand et al., 2009) featured six outcome measures: total mistakes, task mistakes, partial task mistakes, non-efficiency mistakes, rule break mistakes, and strategy use mistakes. Using the VMET, researchers compared the shopping performance of nine poststroke participants ($M_{age} = 64.2$, $SD = 7.7$) to that of 20 healthy young ($M_{age} = 26.3$ $SD = 2.7$) and 20 healthy older controls ($M_{age} = 64.0$, $SD = 9.6$). They also compared outcome measures of the VMET to MET performance in a real-life shopping mall, the Zoo Map subtest of the BADS, and a measure of instrumental activities of daily living. For roughly half of the participants, MET performance was assessed at a small shopping mall located within a medical center, while the remaining participants were assessed at small a university shopping center. Findings indicated that significant differences existed among all three groups on all VMET outcome measures. Further, moderate to high correlations between VMET and MET performance were found among poststroke patients and older adults but not among young adults. The VMET was also shown to be significantly related to cognitive planning (Zoo Map subtest) and a measure of IADL.

A second version of the VMET was later developed by researchers (Raspelli et al., 2010) using a virtual supermarket created with NeuroVR software and a Blender-based application. This same VE was used previously in a pilot study (Carelli, Morganti, Weiss, Kizony, & Riva, 2008), in which researchers illustrated the feasibility of the NeuroVR supermarket as an assessment of executive functioning in a sample of 20 healthy older adults ages 50 to 62. Unlike the VMET conducted in the VMall (Rand et al., 2009), this version of the VMET did not require sophisticated video-capture technology nor did it require participants to engage in active movements in order to interact with the VE. A total of 96 shelves (six identical items per shelf) comprising 12 product sections featured items including frozen goods, beverages, hygiene products, stationary supplies, and animal products. Participants were able to navigate the virtual supermarket via a gamepad. Raspelli et al. (2012) tested their version of the VMET on nine poststroke participants ($M_{age}$ = 62.0, $SD$ = 7.8) and two healthy control groups consisting of young ($M_{age}$ = 26, $SD$ = 1.94) and older adults ($M_{age}$ = 55, $SD$ = 6.03). Their study revealed that two of the seven VMET outcome measures (i.e., time of execution, total errors) successfully differentiated all three study groups. Possibly owing to the absence of conflicting stimuli in the virtual supermarket (e.g., confusing store announcements) as well as the rigid rules and instructions associated with the VMET protocol, no significant correlations were found between the VMET outcome measures, the Stroop Test and the Iowa Gambling Task, in any of the study groups. However, the Test of Everyday Attention (TEA; Zimmerman & Fimm, 1992) was found to be associated with VMET performance among poststroke patients.

### VIRTUAL REALITY SHOPPING SIMULATION PROGRAM

In addition to the VAP-S and the VMET, several other virtual shopping assessment tools have been developed and tested in recent years (see Table 7.1 for a summary of virtual shopping protocols). For example, Kang et al. (2008) developed a VR shopping simulation in which participants sit in a rotating chair and interact with a virtual supermarket using a gamepad and a head-mounted display (HMD). While participants navigate the VR shopping environment, their head movements are tracked by a sensor (3-Degrees of Freedom Position Sensor). When they turn their head, participants' view within the environment changes in a corresponding manner, allowing them to fully visualize the store. In stage 1, participants are tested on their computer interactive ability through a simple task involving them finding three items within an allotted time. Stage 2 tests memory and attention by having participants select items belonging to a specific category and having them react to auditory and visual stimuli in addition to unexpected events (e.g., dropping an item). The final stage (stage 3) evaluates executive functioning by having participants select an item on their own (with some specification) and pay for that item. Kang et al. (2008) tested the shopping simulation on 20 poststroke participants with unilateral brain lesions ($M_{age}$ = 54.8, $SD$ = 8.9) and a healthy control group ($M_{age}$ = 48.7, $SD$ = 10.7) who did not differ significantly with respect to age, education level, or computer experience. The poststroke and control groups were found to differ on a number of shopping outcome measures across all three stages, including the performance index (stage 1), memory scores (i.e., delayed recognition, auditory/visual memory) and attention index (stage 2), and the executive index (stage 3).

## Virtual Shopping Tasks for Assessment of Prospective Memory

While many virtual shopping protocols have been developed to primarily assess executive functioning, several iterations of the virtual shopping paradigm have been developed with the specific aim of studying prospective memory in naturalistic settings (Canty et al., 2014; Kinsella, Ong, & Tucker, 2009). Individuals with traumatic brain injury (TBI) are likely to incur significant deficits in prospective memory that may cause difficulties with day-to-day functioning. Canty et al. (2014) developed the Virtual Reality Shopping Task (VRST) to assess time- and event-based prospective memory in patients with severe TBI. They also sought to examine the ecological validity of the assessment in relation to conventional assessments of prospective memory (i.e., the Lexical Decision Prospective Memory Task; LDPMT). Thirty participants with severe TBI ($M_{age}$ = 54.8, $SD$ = 8.9) and 24 age-, gender-, and education-matched healthy controls ($M_{age}$ = 29.7, $SD$ = 10.4) were assessed using the VRST. From a first-person perspective, participants were required to purchase 12 items from a selection of 20 unique shops in a prespecified order. To assess time-based prospective memory, participants were instructed to send prewritten text messages on a virtual cellphone at 4-min intervals (i.e., 4, 8, and 12 min into the task). To assess event-based prospective memory, participants were instructed to press the T key on the computer keyboard whenever a "sale" announcement was made. Throughout the task, three sale and three non-sale announcements were made. Results from the study revealed that individuals with severe TBI did significantly worse than the control group on the time- and event-based prospective memory tasks in addition to the ongoing component of the study. For the last half of the task, results indicated that TBI patients checked the time significantly less than the healthy control group, which likely explains the differences discovered for time-based prospective memory performance.

Prospective memory performance within the TBI group was also found to be significantly moderately correlated with cognitive measures of mental flexibility, verbal fluency, and verbal memory. Small to moderate correlations were also observed between prospective memory performance in the TBI group and measures of attention, response initiation/suppression, and working memory; however, these associations did not achieve significance. While VRST event-based prospective memory was found to be moderately correlated with event-based prospective memory as measured by the LDPMT, the VRST (but not the LDPMT) was significantly associated with independent living skills and significant others' ratings of patients' occupational activities.

## Virtual Environment Grocery Store

The Virtual Environment Grocery Store (VEGS) was invented by Thomas Parsons. The VEGS is a VR-based neuropsychological assessment that expands upon both VR and real-life MET protocols. The original MET assessed execution of everyday behaviors in an actual shopping center (Shallice & Burgess, 1991). The MET evaluates how patients complete a series of errands that require organization and planning while shopping. Activities in the MET include rule following. Examples of activities include: rules about entering particular shops, making purchases to meet a specified budget, and remembering to meet someone at a predetermined time without additional cues. The VEGS allows broader use of the MET by requiring parallel tasks to be completed in a VE. Shopping-related tasks must be completed in a simulated grocery store according to a particular set of rules.

### NEUROVR VERSION OF THE VIRTUAL ENVIRONMENT GROCERY STORE

Over the years, there have been a number of iterations of the VEGS. The first iteration of the VEGS was developed using NeuroVR (Parsons, Rizzo, Brennan, Silva, & Zelinski, 2008). The open source NeuroVR VE platform includes an Editor and a Player that provide an interactive rendering system based on OpenGL. The NeuroVR Editor makes use of Blender and an integrated suite of three-dimensional creation tools. Users navigate and interact within the VEGS using the NeuroVR Player (see Figure 7.1). This iteration places the subject in an immersive modality, in which the VEGS is displayed using a head-tracked eMagin HMD. The participant interacts bimanually within the VEGS, using keyboard arrows and a mouse to make selections.

A number of limitations in the NeuroVR platform had to be overcome if we were to record a sufficient range of neurobehavioral responses in a perceptual

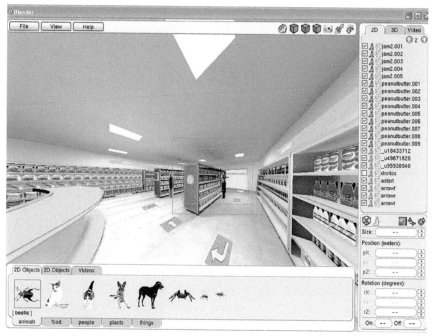

FIGURE 7.1  *NeuroVR Player*

environment that systematically presents complex stimuli. One issue was the difficulty of real-time synchronization of stimulus data from NeuroVR, behavioral responses from users, and psychophysiological assessments of the users. With NeuroVR, it is difficult to match virtual environment stimuli with psychophysiological data from the user. Furthermore, it was difficult to allow third-party applications to tap into the data being generated by the psychophysiological hardware, MATLAB, and NeuroVR during data acquisition. Knowledge of the user state during exposure to the VEGS is imperative for the development and assessment of VE design. Different individuals will invariably have different reactions to the VEGS, and without an assessment tool that can be employed online, the clinician will experience difficulties in identifying the causes of the differences, which may lead to a loss of experimental control of the clinical research paradigms. For example, a user may become increasingly frustrated with some aspect of the VEGS, but without proper measurement techniques to detect the frustration while it occurs, compensatory measures cannot be taken and the user's sense of presence, or feeling of "being there," may be diminished. While the NeuroVR version of the VEGS offers the capability of presenting a realistic simulation of the real world, online assessment of the patient's reactions to that environment is vital to maintaining an understanding of how the environment is affecting the patient in order to preserve experimental control.

## SECOND-GENERATION VIRTUAL ENVIRONMENT GROCERY STORE PLATFORM

To increase the flexibility and usability of patient interaction in the VEGS, we decided to port the VEGS to a new platform that we custom developed using the G3D graphics engine. We imported a variant of the virtual grocery store model from NeuroVR as a set of textured objects in .obj format and redesigned the locomotion and interaction metaphors to be more compatible with an immersive VR experience. We used an nVisorSX HMD to present participants with an immersive view of the VE in stereo over a 60° diagonal field of view on twin SXGA OLED displays with 100% stereo overlap. The VE was rendered in real time on a custom-built PC with an nVidia Quadro FX 5800 graphics card. We attached 19-mm and 14-mm retroreflective tracking markers, respectively, to the HMD and to a fingerless bicycle glove that participants wore on their dominant hand, allowing the head and hand to each be tracked in real time using a collection of 12 Vicon MX40+ cameras focused on a small region in the center of our lab. The hand tracking was used to enable participants to interact with objects in the VE by reaching out and touching them. We used a high-fidelity rigid hand-and-arm model to represent the location of the hand to participants in as realistic a way as our tracking implementation allowed. Participants controlled their viewpoint in the VE using a Logitech Attack 3 joystick that was firmly mounted to a short wooden bar that extended forward beneath the armrest of an Aeron chair. We prepared left- and right-handed versions of the chairs, as well as of the gloves and hand models, so that each participant could both drive and select objects with the dominant hand. Participants were able to use the joystick to translate their viewpoint forward and backward in the VE, but they had to swivel in the chair to turn. We adopted this locomotion model in light of research showing that people are better able to maintain their sense of direction while traveling around in an immersive VE when they are able to physically turn their own bodies within the VE rather than having to virtually turn the VE around themselves while remaining in a fixed physical orientation. While participants were in the VEGS, an audio background consisting of ambient grocery-store sounds was presented via built-in headphones attached to the HMD. We used physiological sensors from Thought Technology along with Biograph Infiniti software to stream time-stamped heart rate and galvanic skin response data to a file. We were able to synchronize this physiological data output stream with an event-logging output stream from our VE software by using a Windows event hook in the Biograph software to time-stamp a key-press event on the single computer that was running both systems. In order to acclimate participants to the experience of using the VE equipment, we began by using the HMD to immerse them in a high-fidelity virtual replica of our lab space (see Figure 7.2). Our goal in doing this was to foster the illusion that VR technology works in a way that is analogous to a magical see-through camera. Previous research has shown that people are able

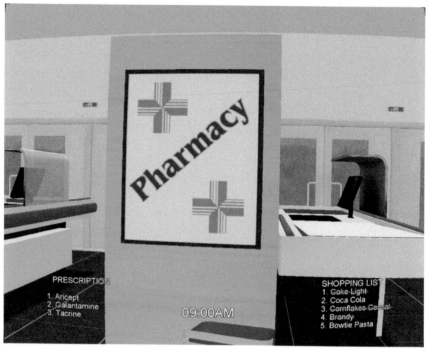

FIGURE 7.2  *Virtual Pharmacy*

to achieve a higher sense of presence and a more accurate spatial understanding
of a remote VE when they are smoothly transitioned into that environment after
first being immersed in a virtual replica room.

Interaction with the VE was done using hand gestures. As a distractor task,
participants were asked to shop for a small set of items specified on a provided
list. When they found one of the items on a shelf in the supermarket, they could
choose it by reaching out to touch it with their hand (see Figure 7.3). When the
hand model intersected the object model, the object disappeared from the shelf
and a red line was drawn through that item on the shopping list. Figure 7.4 shows
what this looked like. We prepared three levels of lists, containing items that were
progressively more difficult to find, to ensure that no participant would run out
of items to search for while at the same time allowing some easy initial successes
to keep people engaged and to avoid frustration.

Although it represented a new platform, the new iteration of the VEGS maintained the neuropsychological characteristics of the original MET-based VEGS.
The neuropsychological assessments included both a time-based and an event-
based prospective memory task. A written list of shopping items was provided
in order to counter the impact of impaired memory in the distractor task. The
scenario was designed to accurately resemble real-world procedure. For the time-
based measure, two points were awarded for turning in the prescription within 2

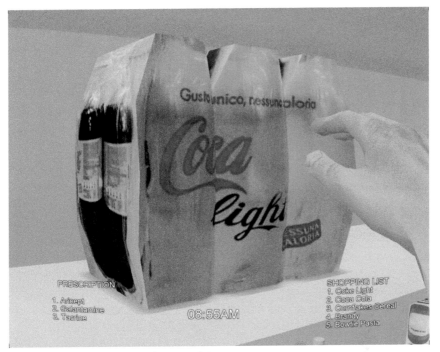

FIGURE 7.3 *Item selection in the Virtual Environment*

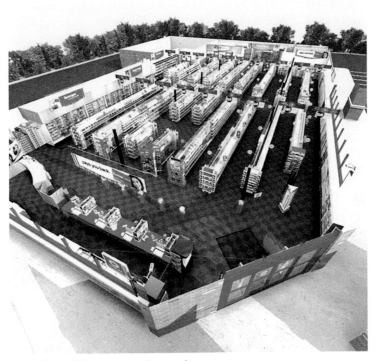

FIGURE 7.4 *Virtual Environment Grocery Store*

min of the time limit, and one point for turning the prescription in after an oral reminder. For the event-based measures, three points were awarded for returning to the pharmacy within 2 min of hearing their number called the first time, two points for retrieving the prescription within 2 min of the second announcement, and one point following an on-screen reminder.

## CURRENT ITERATION OF THE VIRTUAL ENVIRONMENT GROCERY STORE

The current iteration of the VEGS makes use of the Unity simulation engine. This powerful and user-friendly simulation engine integrates a custom rendering engine with the nVidia PhysX engine and Mono, the open source implementation of Microsoft's .NET libraries. There are multiple benefits to using Unity for VEGS when compared to other game engines. First, Unity offers complete documentation with examples for its entire application program interface. This allows for increased productivity when making changes to the VEGS. Furthermore, Unity's editor is very easy to use and VEGS content can be listed in a tree and added to VEGS in a drag-and-drop method. VEGS objects are listed in a separate tree and each can be assigned multiple scripts written in C# as well as physics and rendering properties. We have access to the complete Mono application program interface, and scripts can give VEGS objects interactive behaviors, create the VEGS interface, and manage VEGS information. Through the use of Unity's physics properties (nVidia's PhysX engine), VEGS objects can have collision detection and be assembled using a variety of joints. Unity's custom rendering engine uses a simplified shader language that is compiled into DirectX 9 or OpenGL 2.0 shaders. Multiplatform distribution is possible given the fact that Unity can be compiled for OSX, Windows, or as a web browser via a plugin.

Two monitors were used: one for displaying the Launcher application, which is used by the examiner administering the test, and another for displaying the participant's view of the VE in the HMD (Oculus Rift). To increase the potential for sensory immersion, a tactile transducer was built using a three-foot-square platform with six Bass Shaker speakers (100 W Bass Shaker) attached. The tactile transducer is powered by an amplifier with 100 watts per channel ×2 in stereo mode. Animation software is utilized for development of the VEGS. The environments were rendered in real time using a graphics engine with a fully customizable rendering pipeline, including vertex and pixel shaders, shadows, bumpmaps, and screen space geometric primitives. A MATLAB scoring program and human–computer interface (Computational Neuropsychology and Simulation Interface; CNS-I) is employed for data acquisition. The CNS-I also allows for key events in the environment to be logged and time stamped with millisecond temporal accuracy.

The VEGS has evolved to allow the neuropsychologist a platform for systematic adjustments to a patient's information load (which affects goal maintenance).

This offers an advanced VR version of the MET that includes assessment of learning, memory (including prospective memory), and executive functioning. The VEGS also makes use of several adaptive trials in the assessment procedure. Moreover, the VEGS has a library of "multiple task assignments" for empirically determining a patient's baseline difficulty, and then adding conditions in the environment that affect baseline task difficulty. This includes the ability to adjust the density of items on shelves, the similarity of packaging, and the intensity and types of realistic irrelevant distractions (e.g., loudness/type of music in the background and loudspeaker announcements). The VEGS platform offers a range of difficulties that may be used to make the tasks sufficiently complex that floor or ceiling effects will not be a problem (Parsons, McPherson, & Interrante, 2013). Tasks include:

- navigating through a virtual grocery store by following specified routes through the aisles;
- finding and selecting items needed to prepare simple meals, such as making a peanut butter and jelly sandwich;
- pricing and selecting other items so that no more than a budgeted amount is spent; and
- performing a prospective memory task when a certain individual is encountered.

Further, the difficulty of tasks assigned is increased over trials by adding distractions:

- increasing the number of items on store shelves,
- adding background sounds and music, and
- increasing the loudness and frequency of distractors.

The use of a simulated environment allows patients who may be physically or behaviorally impaired to be safely assessed (see Figure 7.4). This would not be possible with the traditional MET, which requires the tasks to be completed in a real-world shopping environment.

## NEUROCOGNITIVE TASKS AND PROTOCOL

A number of cognitive tasks are found in the VEGS that are involved in multitasking and memory: learning, memory (including prospective memory), and executive functions. Before the patient is immersed in the VE, the neuropsychologist reads a shopping list to the patient. Following the reading of the 16 items on the shopping list, the neuropsychologist requests that the patient repeat the items on the shopping list (immediately) in any order. The interstimulus interval is two seconds. Immediate recall performance is recorded verbatim by a microphone and is logged for each of the immediate recall trials (Trials 1–3). Next the patient is informed that they are going to need to drop off a prescription once the VEGS protocol starts. They are also told that they need to remember to go to the coupon machine after 5 min of shopping. Next, the patient is immersed in the VE and is instructed on how to move about and interact with the environment (5 min). At this point the VEGS protocol begins and the patient must drop off a prescription with the virtual pharmacist (see Figure 7.5). The virtual pharmacist gives the patient a number and instructs the patient to listen for the number while shopping. While the patient shops, the virtual pharmacist announces other prescription numbers at each 1-min interval of the protocol. After 10 min, the virtual pharmacist announces the patient's prescription number. At that time, the patient needs to return to the virtual pharmacist and click on her to end the simulation. At the completion of the VEGS, the patient will be asked to perform delayed recall and recognition trials. Patients are not warned that delayed recall will be tested later.

An important component of the VEGS is its inclusion of prospective memory assessments. There is an event-based prospective memory task, in which patients have to remember to pick up their prescription from the pharmacy when their number is called over the loudspeaker (while also finishing their shopping task). There is also a time-based prospective memory task, in which the client has to remember to pick up the order when the number is called. While waiting for the number to be called, the client shops and after 5 min of shopping must go to the coupon machine (see Figure 7.6).

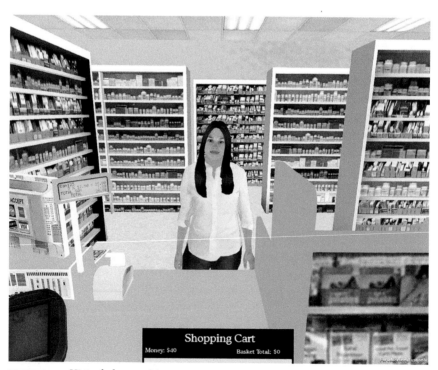

FIGURE 7.5  *Virtual pharmacist*

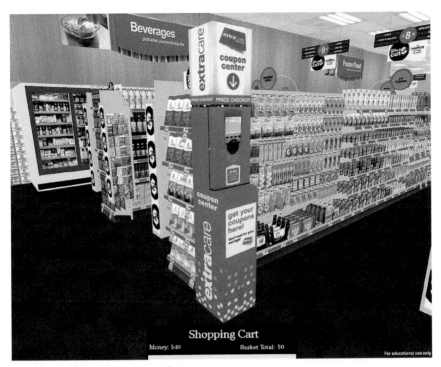

FIGURE 7.6 *Virtual coupon machine*

The VEGS has the advantage of automated logging of behavioral responses. For example, with the VEGS the neuropsychologist has access to the patient's navigation path, response time, accuracy, amount of money spent, activities, items purchased, and a host of others. Perhaps most interesting is the automated logging of the patient's navigation through the store, the strategies used to get from one place to the next, and the amount of time it took (see Figure 7.7). The VEGS records and measures outcomes with the same rigor as is possible in a controlled laboratory environment. Furthermore, it assesses the patient in a simulation of real-world activities that are generalizable to real-world activities of daily living. The use of a simulated environment ensures consistent stimulus presentation and allows the clinician to have better control of the perceptual environment—the number and intensity of distractors is predictable and modifiable. Furthermore, the computerized nature of the VEGS allows for more precise and accurate scoring than is possible with the qualitative scoring method of the traditional MET. The tasks to be completed in the VEGS are directly related to the types of memory, attention, organization, and planning that are required for real-world functioning. The outcomes allow for more precise prediction of similar functional performance across a variety of domains, which means recommendations are based on direct observation and can be customized to the client (Parsons et al., 2013).

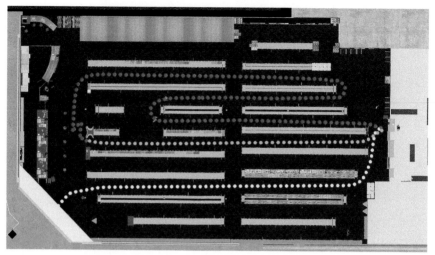

FIGURE 7.7  *Tracking user progress.*

A number of validation studies are currently underway. In a recent study (Parsons et al., 2015a), performance of an older adult cohort was compared with that of college-age students. Participants included 55 undergraduate students ($M_{age}$ = 20.0; $SD$ = 2.89) and 47 older adults ($M_{age}$ = 75.6; $SD$ = 7.4). After completing the virtual shopping task, participants were asked to recall the items shopped for using free recall and cued recall methods. Fifteen minutes after the completion of the short-delay recall, with a distractor task in between, participants were assessed via long-delay free and cued recall. Results of one-way ANOVAs (Bonferroni correction; $p < .0125$) reveal significant differences (favoring younger adults) for short-delay free recall ($F_{(1, 100)}$ = 36.67, $p < 0.001$); short-delay cued recall ($F_{(1, 100)}$ = 21.06, $p < 0.001$); long-delay free recall ($F_{(1, 100)}$ = 31.24, $p < 0.001$); and long-delay cued recall ($F_{(1, 100)}$ = 24.16, $p < 0.001$). The authors concluded that the VR-based shopping task provides a unique opportunity to study memory function within an ecologically valid environment. Results indicate that memory in older individuals may be more vulnerable to external disturbance (e.g., ambient noise and distractors in a VE) than memory in younger controls.

## Conclusion

The aim of the Virtual Environment Grocery Store is to offer the neuropsychologist a function-led neuropsychological assessment that can be used for detailed evaluation of various cognitive domains. It is also believed that the VEGS offers the neuropsychologist the ability to identify particular deficits as areas to work on in rehabilitation and for targeting of real-life activities of daily living. Before the VEGS can be fully implemented by clinical neuropsychologists in rehabilitation settings, it must be fully validated against traditional neuropsychological assessments. Initial pilot studies are underway to validate the VEGS through the use of a standard paper-and-pencil neuropsychological battery for comparisons of older age cohorts and college-age students. Furthermore, there are efforts to assess arousal and engagement using various psychophysiological measures. We believe that this will provide a first step in the development of this tool. Many more steps are necessary to continue the process of test development and to fully establish the VEGS as a measure that contributes to existing assessment procedures for the diagnosis of neurocognitive decline.

The VEGS offers a platform for neuropsychological assessments and builds upon prior developments of VR applications that focus on component cognitive processes. The increased ecological validity of neurocognitive batteries that include assessment using virtual scenarios like the VEGS may aid differential diagnosis and treatment planning. Within the VEGS, it is possible to systematically present cognitive tasks targeting neuropsychological performance beyond what are currently available using traditional methods. Reliability of the planned rehabilitation regimens based on neuropsychological assessment can be enhanced in the VEGS by better control of the perceptual environment, more consistent stimulus presentation, and more precise and accurate scoring. The VEGS may also improve the validity of neurocognitive measurements via the increased quantification of discrete behavioral responses, allowing for the identification of more specific cognitive domains. The VEGS could allow for neurocognition to be tested in situations that are more ecologically valid. Participants can be evaluated in an environment that simulates the real world, not a contrived testing environment.

Through simulation of real-world environments, VR offers promise for increasing the ecological validity of cognitive tasks while maintaining control of manipulations that can affect performance. Even though patients are quite aware that the VEGS is virtual instead of actual reality, they willingly "play along." Moreover, it has been argued that reality is experiential, not based on the external environment, and that tasks performed in a VE may produce subjective engagement that is equivalent to engagement in the real world. For the clinical neuropsychologist focused upon rehabilitation, the VEGS offers the opportunity to immerse the patient in an ecologically valid environment and observe the patient as she or he performs systematically presented and functionally oriented therapeutic activities that are based upon an assessment and understanding of the individual's brain–behavior deficits. From a clinical perspective, neurocognitive rehabilitation using a VE like the VEGS allows for methodical assessment and intervention in activities of daily living that will aid the person affected by cognitive and/or behavioral deficits. As a result, the clinician and patient can work together in a controlled environment that mimics real-world functioning to enable the patient to increase his or her ability to perform activities of daily living.

# References

Alderman, N., Burgess, P. W., Knight, C., & Henman, C. (2003). Ecological validity of a simplified version of the multiple errands shopping test. *Journal of the International Neuropsychological Society, 9*, 31–44. doi:10.1017/s1355617703910046

Bailey, P. E., Henry, J. D., Rendell, P. G., Phillips, L. H., & Kliegel, M. (2010). Dismantling the "age-prospective memory paradox": The classic laboratory paradigm simulated in a naturalistic setting. *The Quarterly Journal of Experimental Psychology, 63*, 646–652. doi:10.1080/17470210903521797

Bauer, R. M., Iverson, G. L., Cernich, A. N., Binder, L. M., Ruff, R. M., & Naugle, R. I. (2012). Computerized neuropsychological assessment devices: Joint position paper of the American Academy of Clinical Neuropsychology and the National Academy of Neuropsychology. *Archives of Clinical Neuropsychology, 27*, 362–373. doi:10.1093/arclin/acs027

Bottari, C., Dassa, C., Rainville, C., & Dutil, É. (2009). The criterion-related validity of the IADL Profile with measures of executive functions, indices of trauma severity and sociodemographic characteristics. *Brain Injury, 23*, 322–335. doi:10.1080/02699050902788436

Burgess, P. W., Alderman, N., Evans, J., Emslie, H., & Wilson, B. A. (1998). The ecological validity of tests of executive function. *Journal of the International Neuropsychological Society, 4*, 547–558. doi:10.1017/s1355617798466037

Burgess, P. W., Alderman, N., Forbes, C., Costello, A., Coates, L. M, Dawson, D. R., . . . Channon, S. (2006). The case for the development and use of "ecologically valid" measures of executive function in experimental and clinical neuropsychology. *Journal of the International Neuropsychological Society, 12*, 194–209. doi:10.1017/S1355617706060310

Campbell, Z., Zakzanis, K. K., Jovanovski, D., Joordens, S., Mraz, R., & Graham, S. J. (2009). Utilizing virtual reality to improve the ecological validity of clinical neuropsychology: An fMRI case study elucidating the neural basis of planning by comparing the Tower of London with a three-dimensional navigation task. *Applied Neuropsychology, 16*, 295–306. doi:10.1080/09084280903297891

Canty, A. L., Fleming, J., Patterson, F., Green, H. J., Man, D., & Shum, D. H. K. (2014). Evaluation of a virtual reality prospective memory task for use with individuals with severe traumatic brain injury. *Neuropsychological Rehabilitation, 24*, 238–265. doi:10.1080/09602011.2014.881746

Carelli, L., Morganti, F., Weiss, P. L., Kizony, R., & Riva, G. (2008). A virtual reality paradigm for the assessment and rehabilitation of executive function deficits post stroke: Feasibility study. *2008 Virtual Rehabilitation* (pp. 99–104). IEEE. doi:10.1109/icvr.2008.4625144

Chan, R., Shum, D., Toulopoulou, T., & Chen, E. (2008). Assessment of executive functions: Review of instruments and identification of critical issues. *Archives of Clinical Neuropsychology, 23*, 201–216. doi:10.1016/j.acn.2007.08.010

Chaytor, N. S., & Schmitter-Edgecombe, M. (2003). The ecological validity of neuropsychological tests: A review of the literature on everyday cognitive skills. *Neuropsychology Review, 13*, 181–197. doi:10.1023/b:nerv.0000009483.91468.fb

Chaytor, N. S., Schmitter-Edgecombe, M., & Burr, R. (2006). Improving the ecological validity of executive functioning tests: Environmental demands and compensatory strategies. *Archives of Clinical Neuropsychology, 21*, 217–227. doi:10.1016/j.acn.2005.12.002

Cuberos-Urbano, G., Caracuel, A., Vilar-Lòpez, R., Valls-Serrano, C., Bateman, A., & Verdejo-García, A. (2013). Ecological validity of the Multiple Errands Test using predictive models of dysexecutive problems in everyday life. *Journal of Clinical and Experimental Neuropsychology, 35*, 329–336. doi:10.1080/13803395.2013.776011

Dawson, D. R., Anderson, N. D., Burgess, P., Cooper, E., Krpan, K. M., & Stuss, D. T. (2009). Further development of the Multiple Errands Test: Standardized scoring, reliability, and ecological validity for the Baycrest version. *Archives of Physical Medicine and Rehabilitation, 90*, S41–S51. doi:10.1016/j.apmr.2009.07.012

Josman, N., Hof, E., Klinger, E., Marie, R. M., Goldenberg, K., Weiss, P. L., & Kizony, R. (2006). Performance within a virtual supermarket and its relationship to executive functions in post-stroke patients. *2006 International Workshop on Virtual Rehabilitation*. doi:10.1109/iwvr.2006.1707536

Josman, N., Kizony, R., Hof, E., Goldenberg, K., Weiss, P. L., & Klinger, E. (2014). Using the Virtual Action Planning-Supermarket for evaluating executive functions in people with stroke. *Journal of Stroke and Cerebrovascular Diseases, 23*, 879–887. doi:10.1016/j.jstrokecerebrovasdis.2013.07.013

Josman, N., Schenirderman, A. E., Klinger, E., & Shevil, E. (2009). Using virtual reality to evaluate executive functioning among persons with schizophrenia: A validity study. *Schizophrenia Research, 115*, 270–277. doi:10.1016/j.schres.2009.09.015

Jovanovski, D., Zakzanis, K., Campbell, Z., Erb, S., & Nussbaum, D. (2012a). Development of a novel, ecologically oriented virtual reality measure of executive function: The Multitasking in the City Test. *Applied Neuropsychology: Adult, 19*, 171–182.

Jovanovski, D., Zakzanis, K., Ruttan, L., Campbell, Z., Erb, S., & Nussbaum, D. (2012b). Ecologically valid assessment of executive dysfunction using a novel virtual reality task in patients with acquired brain injury. *Applied Neuropsychology, 19*, 207–220.

Jurado, M. B., & Rosselli, M. (2007). The elusive nature of executive functions: A review of our current understanding. *Neuropsychology Review, 17*, 213–233. doi:10.1007/s11065-007-9040-z

Kang, Y. J., Ku, J., Han, K., Kim, S. I., Yu, T. W., Lee, J. H., & Park, C. I. (2008). Development and clinical trial of virtual reality-based cognitive assessment in people with stroke: Preliminary study. *CyberPsychology & Behavior, 11*, 329–339. doi:10.1089/cpb.2007.0116

Kinsella, G. J., Ong, B., & Tucker, J. (2009). Traumatic brain injury and prospective memory in a virtual shopping trip task: Does it matter who generates the prospective memory target? *Brain Impairment, 10*, 45–51. doi:10.1375/brim.10.1.45

Klinger, E., Chemin, I., Lebreton S., Marié, R. M. (2004). A virtual supermarket to assess cognitive planning. In: *Proceedings of Cybertherapy 2004, San Diego, California*, Abstract published in: *CyberPsychology and Behavior, 7*, 292–293.

Klinger, E., Chemin, I., Lebreton, S., & Marié, R. M. (2006). Virtual action planning in Parkinson's disease: A control study. *CyberPsychology & Behavior, 9*, 342–347. doi:10.1089/cpb.2006.9.342

Knight, C., Alderman, N., & Burgess, P. (2002). Development of a simplified version of the Multiple Errands Test for use in hospital settings. *Neuropsychological Rehabilitation, 12*, 231–255. doi:10.1080/09602010244000039

Levine, B., Robertson, I. H., Clare, L., Carter, G., Hong, J., Wilson, B. A., . . . Stuss, D. T. (2000). Rehabilitation of executive functioning: An experimental-clinical validation of goal management training. *Journal of the International Neuropsychological Society, 6*, 299–312. doi:10.1017/s1355617700633052

Logie, R. H., Trawley, S., & Law, A. (2011). Multitasking: Multiple, domain-specific cognitive functions in a virtual environment. *Memory & Cognition, 39*, 1561–1574. doi:10.3758/s13421-011-0120-1

Manchester, D., Priestley, N., & Howard, J. (2004). The assessment of executive functions: Coming out of the office. *Brain Injury, 18*, 1067–1081. doi:10.1080/02699050410001672387

Marié, R. M., Klinger, E., Chemin, I., Josset, M. (2003). Cognitive planning assessed by virtual reality. In: *VRIC 2003 Proceedings, Laval Virtual Conference*, Laval, France, pp. 119–125.

Matheis, R. J., Schultheis, M. T., Tiersky, L. A., DeLuca, J., Millis, S. R., & Rizzo, A. (2007). Is learning and memory different in a virtual environment? *Clinical Neuropsychology, 21*, 146–161.

McGeorge, P., Phillips, L. H., Crawford, J. R., Garden, S. E., Sala, S. D., & Milne, A. B., . . . Callender, J. S. (2001). Using virtual environments in the assessment of executive dysfunction. *Presence: Teleoperators and Virtual Environments, 10*, 375–383. doi:10.1162/1054746011470235

Milner, B. (1963). Effects of different brain lesions on card sorting. *Archives of Neurology, 9*, 90–100. doi:10.1001/archneur.1963.00460070100010

Morris, R. G., Kotitsa, M., Bramham, J., Brooks, B. M., & Rose, F. D. (2002). Virtual reality investigation of strategy formation, rule breaking and prospective memory in patients with focal prefrontal neurosurgical lesions. In *Proceedings of the 4th International Conference on Disability, Virtual Reality & Associated Technologies*, Veszprém.

Okahashi, S., Seki, K., Nagano, A., Luo, Z., Kojima, M., & Futaki, T. (2013). A virtual shopping test for realistic assessment of cognitive function. *Journal of NeuroEngineering and Rehabilitation, 10*, 59. doi:10.1186/1743-0003-10-59

Parsons, T. D. (2011). Neuropsychological assessment using virtual environments: Enhanced assessment technology for improved ecological validity. In S. Braham (Ed.), *Advanced computational intelligence paradigms in healthcare: Virtual reality in psychotherapy rehabilitation and assessment* (pp. 271–289). Springer Berlin Heidelberg.

Parsons, T. D. (2015). Virtual reality for enhanced ecological validity and experimental control in the clinical, affective, and social neurosciences. *Frontiers in Human Neuroscience, 9*, 1–19. doi:10.3389/fnhum.2015.00660

Parsons, T. D., Barnett, M., & Dumas, B. (2015a). Virtual Multiple Errands Test for "ecologically valid" assessment of cohort memory effects. *Archives of Clinical Neuropsychology, 30*, 578–578. doi:10.1093/arclin/acv047.244

Parsons, T. D., Carlew, A. R., Magtoto, J., & Stonecipher, K. (2015b). The potential of function-led virtual environments for ecologically valid measures of executive function in experimental and clinical neuropsychology. *Neuropsychological Rehabilitation, 11,* 1–13. doi:10.1080/09602011.2015.1109524

Parsons, T. D., McPherson, S., & Interrante, V. (2013). Enhancing neurocognitive assessment using immersive virtual reality. *IEEE Virtual Reality Workshop on Virtual and Augmented Assistive Technology, pp. 27–34.*

Parsons, T. D., Rizzo, A. A., Brennan, J., Silva, T. M., & Zelinski, E. M. (2008). Assessment of executive functioning using virtual reality: Virtual Environment Grocery Store. *Gerontechnology, 7*(2), 186. doi:10.4017/gt.2008.07.02.123.00

Rand, D., Katz, N., Shahar, M., Kizony, R., & (Tamar) Weiss, P. L. (2005). The virtual mall: A functional virtual environment for stroke rehabilitation. *Annual Review of CyberTherapy Telemedicine: A decade of VR. 2005, 3,* 193–198.

Rand, D., Katz, N., & (Tamar) Weiss, P. L. (2007). Evaluation of virtual shopping in the VMall: Comparison of post-stroke participants to healthy control groups. *Disability and Rehabilitation, 29,* 1710–1719. doi:10.1080/09638280601107450

Rand, D., Rukan, S. B., (Tamar) Weiss, P. L., & Katz, N. (2009). Validation of the Virtual MET as an assessment tool for executive functions. *Neuropsychological Rehabilitation, 19,* 583–602. doi:10.1080/09602010802469074

Raspelli, S., Carelli, L., Morganti, F., Poletti, B., Corra, B., Silani, V., & Riva, G. (2010). Implementation of the Multiple Errands Test in a NeuroVR-supermarket: A possible approach. *Annual Review of CyberTherapy and Telemedicine, 8,* 92–95.

Raspelli, S., Pallavicini, F., Carelli, L., Morganti, F., Pedroli, E., Cipresso, P., . . . Riva, G. (2012). Validating the neuro VR-based virtual version of the Multiple Errands Test: Preliminary results. *Presence: Teleoperators and Virtual Environments, 21,* 31–42. doi:10.1162/pres_a_00077

Renison, B., Ponsford, J., Testa, R., Richardson, B., & Brownfield, K. (2012). The ecological and construct validity of a newly developed measure of executive function: The Virtual Library Task. *Journal of the International Neuropsychological Society, 18,* 440–450. doi:10.1017/S1355617711001883

Robertson, I. H., Manly, T., Andrade, J., Baddeley, B. T., & Yiend, J. (1997). "Oops!": Performance correlates of everyday attentional failures in traumatic brain injured and normal subjects. *Neuropsychologia, 35,* 747–758. doi:10.1016/s0028-3932(97)00015-8

Ruse, S. A., Harvey, P. D., Davis, V. G., Atkins, A. S., Fox, K. H., & Keefe, R. S. E. (2014). Virtual reality functional capacity assessment in schizophrenia: Preliminary data regarding feasibility and correlations with cognitive and functional capacity performance. *Schizophrenia Research: Cognition, 1,* e21–e26. doi:10.1016/j.scog.2014.01.004

Sbordone, R. J. (2008). Ecological validity of neuropsychological testing: Critical issues. In A. M. Horton & D. Wedding (Eds.), *The neuropsychology handbook* (3rd ed., pp. 367–394). New York: Springer.

Schatz, P., & Browndyke, J. (2002). Applications of computer-based neuropsychological assessment. *Journal of Head Trauma Rehabilitation, 17,* 395–410. doi:10.1097/00001199-200210000-00003

Schultheis, M. T., Himelstein, J., & Rizzo, A. A. (2002). Virtual reality and neuropsychology: Upgrading the current tools. *Journal of Head Trauma Rehabilitation, 17,* 378–394. doi:10.1097/00001199-200210000-00002

Shallice, T., & Burgess, P. W. (1991). Deficits in strategy application following frontal lobe damage in man. *Brain, 114*, 727–741. doi:10.1093/brain/114.2.727

Stuss, D. T., Benson, D. F., Kaplan, E. F., Weir, W. S., Naeser, M. A., Leiberman, I., & Ferrill, D. (1983). The involvement of orbitofrontal cerebrum in cognitive tasks. *Neuropsychologia, 21*, 235–248. doi:10.1016/0028-3932(83)90040-4

Weigl, E. (1927). On the psychology of so-called processes of abstraction. *Zeitschrift für Psychologie, 103*, 245–300.

Werner, P., Rabinowitz, S., Klinger, E., Korczyn, A. D., & Josman, N. (2009). Use of the Virtual Action Planning Supermarket for the diagnosis of mild cognitive impairment: A preliminary study. *Dementia and Geriatric Cognitive Disorders, 27*, 301–309. doi:10.1159/000204915

Wilson, B. A., Alderman, N., Burgess, P. W., Emslie, H., & Evans, J. J. (1996). Behavioural Assessment of the Dysexecutive Syndrome (BADS). Bury St Edmunds: Thames Valley.

Zimmerman, P., & Fimm, B. (1992). *Test Batterie zur Auf- merksamkeitsprüfung (TAP)*. Würselen: Psytest.

Zygouris, S., Giakoumis, D., Votis, K., Doumpoulakis, S., Ntovas, K., Segkouli, S., ... Tsolaki, M. (2015). Can a virtual reality cognitive training application fulfill a dual role? Using the virtual supermarket cognitive training application as a screening tool for mild cognitive impairment. *Journal of Alzheimer's Disease, 44*, 1333–1347. doi:10.3233/JAD-141260

{ 8 }

# Virtual Reality Applications for Neuropsychological Assessment in the Military

## HISTORICAL ANTECEDENTS, CURRENT DEVELOPMENTS, AND FUTURE DIRECTIONS

### Joe Edwards and Thomas D. Parsons

Neuropsychological assessment has a long history in the United States military and has played an essential role in ensuring the mental health and operational readiness of service members since World War I (Kennedy, Boake, & Moore, 2010). Over the years, mental health clinicians in the military have developed paper-and-pencil assessment instruments, which have evolved in terms of psychometric rigor and clinical utility, but not in terms of technological sophistication. Since the advent of modern digital computing technology, considerable research has been devoted to the development of computer-automated neuropsychological assessment applications (Kane & Kay, 1992; Reeves, Winter, Bleiberg, & Kane, 2007), a trend that is likely to continue in the future. While many comparatively antiquated paper-and-pencil-based test instruments are still routinely used, it is arguably only a matter of time until they are supplanted by more technologically advanced alternatives.

It is important to note, however, that questions have been raised about the ecological validity of many commonly used traditional neuropsychological tests, whether paper-and-pencil-based or computerized (Alderman, Burgess, Knight, & Henman, 2003; Burgess et al., 2006; Chaytor & Schmitter-Edgecombe, 2003; Chaytor, Schmitter-Edgecombe, & Burr, 2006; Parsons, 2016a; Sbordone, 2008). In the context of neuropsychological testing, *ecological validity* generally refers to the extent to which test performance corresponds to real-world performance in everyday life (Sbordone, 1996). In order to develop neuropsychological test instruments with greater ecological validity, investigators have increasingly turned to virtual reality (VR) technologies as a means to assess real-world performance via true-to-life simulated environments (Campbell et al., 2009; Negut, Matu, Sava, & Davis, 2016; Parsons, 2015a, 2015b, 2016a).

Bilder (2011) described three historical and theoretical formulations of neuropsychology. First, clinical neuropsychologists focused on lesion localization and relied on interpretation without extensive normative data. Next, clinical neuropsychologists were affected by technological advances in neuroimaging and as a result focused on characterizing cognitive strengths and weaknesses rather than on differential diagnosis. Today, clinical neuropsychologists are beginning to leverage advances in neuroimaging, as well as incorporating findings from the Human Genome Project, advances in psychometric theory, and information technologies. Recently, Parsons (2016a) described three technological modalities found in the practice of neuropsychological assessment that refine the three theoretical formulations. Specifically, Parsons presents a discussion of three iterations of neuropsychological assessment technologies: Neuropsychological Assessment 1.0 reflects paper-and-pencil-based testing, Neuropsychological Assessment 2.0 entails computer-based assessment applications, and Neuropsychological Assessment 3.0 represents the potential of VR-based simulation technologies for ecologically valid neuropsychological assessments.

This chapter traces the historical trajectory of neuropsychological assessment technologies in the military, from its roots in the early 1900s through cutting-edge VR-based technologies of today. It is organized according to Parsons' iterative framework, beginning with a discussion of early paper-and-pencil-based procedures. Next, a brief review of computerized assessment technologies is provided. Finally, there is discussion of ecologically oriented VR-based neuropsychological instruments to address real-world outcomes. The discussion includes specific militarily relevant VR-based applications, including their potential advantages and limitations as well as directions for future research.

## Military Neuropsychological Assessment 1.0: Paper-and-Pencil Measures

The historical development of neuropsychological assessment in the U.S. military extends from Alfred Binet's tests of intelligence (Binet & Henri, 1895, 1898; Binet & Simon, 1905, 1908) and was largely cultivated following the United States' entry into World War I in 1917 (Yoakum & Yerkes, 1920). As the military prepared itself for war, there was a clear need for rapid and effective organization of its personnel. In order to assist in that endeavor, presiding members of the American Psychological Association (APA) developed a system for military personnel screening and classification, involving the use of various paper-and-pencil assessment instruments, primarily derived from measures created previously by Binet, but modified and adapted to the needs of the American armed forces. Following a brief provisional period of instrument development and application through preliminary trials, the proposed examination procedures were officially approved by the U.S. Department of War, which sanctioned Army-wide administration of the newly developed tests for all incoming recruits (Yerkes, 1921).

## ARMY ALPHA AND ARMY BETA TEST BATTERIES
## FOR ELIGIBILITY SCREENING

Test development efforts were spearheaded by Robert Yerkes and a panel of many other leading APA psychologists. A partial list of key contributors includes Robert Yerkes, Lewis Terman, Arthur Otis, Henry Goddard, Thomas Haines, Frederic Wells, Walter Bingham, Guy Whipple, Louis Thurstone, and Edward Thorndike (Yerkes, 1921, pp. 299–300). Together they collaborated on the construction and revision of each individual subtest, which eventually culminated in the emergence of the Army Alpha and Army Beta test batteries, which served as the primary group-administered assessment instruments used throughout the war. As reported by Yerkes (1921), the Army tests were given to 1,726,966 service members by the end of the war. The Army Alpha, by far the most frequently administered, was given to well over one million examinees, followed by the Army Beta, which exceeded 400,000 administrations (Yerkes, 1921, pp. 102–103). In addition to the group-administered Alpha and Beta test batteries, several individually administered instruments were also used (pp. 102–103), including the Army Performance Scale (Yoakum & Yerkes, 1920, pp. 100–128), the Stanford-Binet (Terman, 1916), and the Yerkes-Bridges Point Scale (Yerkes, Bridges, & Hardwick, 1915).

As the Army test batteries were being constructed, Yerkes and his colleagues took pains to ensure the scientific and clinical merit of each subtest, as well as their applied practical utility. With the immense influx of new recruits needing to be screened, accompanied by the urgency of war, rapid administration and processing of results were absolute necessities. Therefore, each individual subtest contained in the Alpha and Beta instruments was thoroughly scrutinized to ensure optimal administrative efficiency, in addition to psychometric integrity, and applied practical benefit to the military as a tool for the screening and classification of its personnel. Subtests falling short of their criteria were either revised or discarded, including those deemed to be invalid, unreliable, overly ambiguous, redundant, too easy, too difficult, excessively time-consuming, or too cumbersome to administer and/or score (Yerkes, 1921, pp. 299–311). The finalized Alpha and Beta test materials were logistically streamlined through the use of a multiple-choice format, and quick scoring keys and stencils for use by examiners. In order to expedite program implementation Army-wide, testing facilities were established in 35 Army training camps located throughout the nation (Yerkes, 1921, p. 99); the facilities often accommodated several hundred recruits simultaneously, and examination sessions were completed within an hour (Terman, 1918, p. 178).

While the Army tests were designed to be pragmatic and administratively efficient, they were also constructed to assess a broad range of distinct cognitive abilities (e.g., comprehension, working memory, abstract reasoning, pattern recognition, processing speed, fluid and crystallized intelligence, etc.). Largely based on measures of cognitive ability originally published by Binet and Simon

(1905), and later revised by Terman (1916), most individual subtests were further modified prior to being incorporated into the Army Alpha and Beta test batteries. Upon finalizing their review, selection, and revision of subtests to use for each battery, the Army Alpha included the following examinee tasks: implementing procedural commands, deciphering analogies, sentence rearrangement and comprehension, arithmetical reasoning, numerical sequencing, synonym and antonym discernment, practical judgment, and general knowledge questions. The Army Beta was designed to accommodate examinees unable to take the Alpha due to illiteracy or lack of English language proficiency, so it consisted entirely of nonverbal examinee tasks, including visuospatial pattern analysis, geometric pattern construction, picture completion, maze navigation, numerical sequence matching, symbol series completion, and a digit-symbol coding task. Further details and descriptions, accompanied by administrative instructions, examinee forms, and stimuli used for each individual subtest contained within the original Army Alpha and Beta instruments, may be found in *Army Mental Tests*, compiled and edited by Yoakum and Yerkes (1920).

As noted by Kennedy, Boake, and Moore (2010), the Army tests of World War I have had a lasting and profound influence on the professional practice of neuropsychological assessment, both within the military and for the field of neuropsychology in general. In fact, despite subsequent subtest revisions made throughout the decades following the formation of the original Army test instruments in the early 1900s, echoes of their content may still be found within many of today's neuropsychological assessment batteries (Boake, 2002; Lichtenberger & Kaufman, 2013, pp. 1–10). For instance, variations of the original Army Beta digit-symbol subtest procedure are routinely used today for the assessment of attentional and processing speed abilities, and can be found in several modern neuropsychological test instruments (Ashendorf & Reynolds, 2013, pp. 78–79), such as the Wechsler Adult Intelligence Scale (WAIS-IV; Wechsler, 2008), Symbol Digit Modalities Test (SDMT; Smith, 1991), and the Repeatable Battery for the Assessment of Neuropsychological Status (RBANS; Randolph, 1998, 2012).

From a historical and technological perspective, the success of the Army Alpha and Beta testing initiative is commendable, especially given the enormous volume of tests administered. While most testing procedures performed by Yerkes and colleagues a century ago can now be automated via computers, such technologies had not yet been invented in the year 1917, and Army test examiners had no other option but to rely upon the tools available to them at the time. Therefore, each examination had to be manually administered, using paper-and-pencil-based examinee record forms (Figure 8.1). Moreover, after test administration, examiners were saddled with the laborious task of hand-scoring each individual examinee test booklet, which they ultimately performed no less than 1,726,966 times (Yerkes, 1921, p. 102). Though some efforts were made to expedite statistical analysis of hand-scored Army test data through procurement of punched card tabulator machines, their practical application was significantly

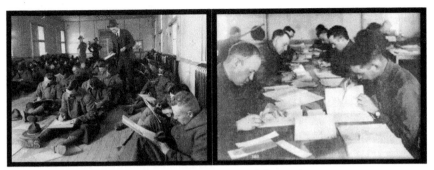

FIGURE 8.1  *Army Alpha group examination (upper left image); Army test examiners scoring examinee record forms (upper right image); October, 1917—Camp Lee, Virginia. Reprinted from Yerkes, R. M. (Ed.). (1921). Psychological examining in the United States Army, p. 90 (plate number 5). Washington, DC: Government Printing Office. Photographs are in the public domain.*

compromised by limited machine availability, shortages of administrative and statistical support staff, clerical errors made during their use, and computational limitations inherent within the machines themselves (Yerkes, 1921, pp. 565–571).

Largely modeled upon the Army tests of World War I, many other screening and classification instruments were developed and implemented in subsequent wars. A few prominent examples include the Army General Classification Test (AGCT; Richardson, 1940) used in World War II, the Armed Forces Qualification Test (AFQT; Uhlaner & Bolanovich, 1952) created in 1950 and used throughout the Korean and Vietnam Wars, and the Armed Services Vocational Aptitude Battery (ASVAB), officially implemented as the primary joint service entrance examination in 1976 (Comptroller General of the United States, 1976) and used to this day.

## CLINICAL APPLICATIONS

While intended to be used primarily for purposes of enlistment eligibility screening, classification, and occupational assignment of military personnel, all of the aforementioned instruments have also been applied for clinical evaluation purposes with war-disabled veterans. For example, while serving as Chief Psychologist at Walter Reed Army Hospital during World War I, Dr. Bird Baldwin used the Army Alpha and Army Performance Scale in his clinical practice with cognitively impaired soldiers as a means to objectively assess their mental capacities, deficiencies, and prospects for rehabilitation (Baldwin, 1919). Military entrance test records have also been a useful means for clinicians to gauge premorbid cognitive capacities during the course of evaluations of service members after the onset of symptoms involving impaired cognition (Grafman, Salazar, Weingartner, Vance, & Amin, 1986; Kennedy, Kupke, & Smith, 2000; Orme, Brehm, & Ree 2001; Orme, Ree, & Rioux, 2001), posttraumatic stress

(Kremen et al., 2007; Macklin et al., 1998), and other forms of psychiatric disturbance (Larson, Booth-Kewley, Highfill-McRoy, & Young, 2009) that may occur
post-deployment.

### BRAIN INJURY ASSESSMENT IN WORLD WAR I

Paper-and-pencil assessment instruments have played an especially vital historical role in shaping our understanding of the neuropsychological aftereffects of
traumatic brain injuries sustained in combat. During World War I, such injuries
were poorly understood, and postconcussive symptoms were often considered
manifestations of "shell shock," a hotly debated and ill-defined phenomenon
(Jones, Fear, & Wessely, 2007). While some clinicians understood the issue in
terms of genuine cognitive disturbance stemming from neurological trauma,
others saw it purely in terms of psychogenic neurosis, weakness of character, or
even malingering (Lumsden, 1916; Shively & Perl, 2012). Unsatisfied by mere theoretical speculation, a few pioneering clinicians took a more empirically driven
approach to the problem through systematic application of cognitive assessment
instruments.

Some of the most innovative and influential developments during World War I
took place in Germany, primarily through the efforts of Kurt Goldstein and his
colleagues, who routinely applied various testing procedures during their clinical encounters with brain-injured soldiers (Gelb & Goldstein, 1920; Goldstein,
1919, 1942; Poppelreuter, 1917). Their novel use of "sorting tasks" for clinical cognitive assessment purposes (Eling, Derckx, & Maes, 2008; Gelb & Goldstein, 1920;
Goldstein & Scheerer, 1941, p. 1) is likely the earliest instance of a practice that
would eventually inspire the development of the Wisconsin Card Sorting Test
(WCST; Grant & Berg, 1948). To this day, the WCST remains one of the most
widely used neuropsychological test instruments for evaluating executive functions (Rabin, Paolillo, & Barr, 2016, p. 216).

Also during World War I, British neurologist Henry Head developed and
applied a battery of paper-and-pencil-based testing procedures in his clinical
practice treating brain-injured soldiers in England (Henderson, 2010, pp. 237–
239). As a specialist in aphasia and related disorders, Head devised several tests
specifically targeting receptive and expressive language functioning, so his
assessment battery primarily consisted of activities involving speech, writing,
reading, object naming, and recognition. However, Head's battery also encom-
passed tasks designed to assess arithmetical reasoning, sensorimotor function,
memory, and visuoconstructive ability (Head, 1926).

### BRAIN INJURY ASSESSMENT IN WORLD WAR II

During World War II, techniques for brain injury assessment continued to evolve
internationally. Oliver Zangwill, a British neuropsychologist, played a significant

role in solidifying the establishment of neuropsychology as a distinct professional discipline (Collins, 2006), and also made significant contributions to neuropsychological assessment theory and methodology through his scholarship and clinical work with brain-injured service members at the Brain Injuries Unit, Royal Infirmary, Edinburg (Benton, 1994a, pp. 36–37; Zangwill, 1945).

Meanwhile, during his tenure serving as director of a rehabilitative facility in the Southern Urals region of Russia (Homskaya, 2001), neuropsychologist Alexander Luria developed flexible, qualitatively oriented, neuropsychological assessment techniques (Sheehy, Chapman, & Conroy, 2002, pp. 365–366), which he applied in his clinical practice with war-disabled soldiers recovering from concussive injuries (Luria, 1948/1963, 1966, 1972). Luria's approach was later adapted and standardized by Charles Golden and colleagues to form the Luria-Nebraska Neuropsychological Battery (LNNB; Golden, Purisch, & Hammeke, 1985).

Several prominent clinicians in the United States treated brain-injured service members throughout the war, while also advancing the field of clinical neuropsychology through their contributions to the professional literature. They include neuropsychologists Ralph Reitan, Hans-Lukas Teuber, and Arthur Benton (Kennedy, Boake, & Moore, 2010, pp. 12–13; Meier, 1992, pp. 552–553), who also each took part in the construction and development of paper-and-pencil-based instruments throughout their careers, including the Halstead-Reitan Neuropsychological Test Battery (HRNB; Reitan & Wolfson, 1993), Personal Orientation Test (Semmes, Weinstein, Ghent, Meyer, & Teuber, 1963), Extrapersonal Orientation Test (Semmes, Weinstein, Ghent, & Teuber, 1955), Benton Visual Retention Test (BVRT; Benton, 1945; Sivan, 1992), and the Judgment of Line Orientation (JLO) test (Benton, 1994b; Benton, Varny, & Hamsher, 1978).

Since the conclusion of World War II until the present, clinical neuropsychology has played a vital role within the military, and it continues to evolve through ongoing theoretical and scientific advancements. However, from a technological point of view, traditional assessment instrumentation and procedures have advanced very little. In fact, many of the instruments routinely implemented today, which are still manually administered and laboriously scored by hand, bear an uncanny resemblance to the paper-and-pencil-based instruments developed by Binet and Simon (1905) over a century ago (Boake, 2002; Castles, 2012, pp. 186–190).

## Military Neuropsychological Assessment 2.0: Emergence of Computerized Assessments

During the past few decades, considerable progress has been made through the advent of computer-based assessment devices, which are in some respects vastly superior to paper-and-pencil alternatives. However, while computerization affords several technological advantages, there are still many challenges and limitations to contend with, as is discussed later in this section.

## PREDIGITAL ELECTRONIC DEVICES

Attempts to automate paper-and-pencil-based assessments through electronic technology first began several decades ago. Prior to the emergence of modern digital computers, various predigital electronic devices were introduced and reached a fairly high level of technological sophistication around the mid 1930s. For instance, an advanced programmable mark-sensing device known as the IBM 805 Test Scoring Machine was invented in 1936 (IBM, 2011; Wood, 1936), and it was used routinely by the U.S. military well into the 1960s (Parker & Auwood, 1966; U.S. Department of the Army, 1962, p. 86). By the 1940s, slightly more efficient analog computing devices were invented to automate the scoring, and data profiling, of psychometric questionnaires (e.g., Campbell, 1971, pp. 359–360; Strong & Hankes, 1947). The U.S. Army Personnel Research Branch relied heavily on such analog computer systems, along with various other tabulation machines, to expedite Army personnel test scoring and analysis procedures (Harman & Harper, 1953). These devices represented an important step forward in the technological progression of assessment methods, but they were soon surpassed by the rise of digital computer devices, which have advanced exponentially from the time of their original emergence in the 1940s (O'Regan, 2012), allowing for increasingly powerful and sophisticated clinical applications ever since.

## U.S. NAVY'S WHIRLWIND I

By the mid 20th century, digital computers were capable of automating highly elaborate statistical algorithms applied to psychological testing data (Tucker, 1953; Wrigley, 1957). One of the most sophisticated systems available at the time was Whirlwind I (Everett, 1952), a high-speed digital computer developed for the U.S. Navy, and used by psychometrician Frederic Lord to automate factor-analytic analysis of test scores he obtained from a broad battery of neuropsychological measures (e.g., measures of verbal fluency, arithmetical reasoning, and processing speed abilities) administered to research participants during the course of his investigations sponsored by the Office of Naval Research (Lord, 1954). Prior to the advent of digital computer systems like Whirlwind I, the factor-analytic calculations performed by Lord were known in theory, but they were not amenable to applied practical use due to the exorbitant degree of mathematical complexity involved (Carroll, 1987, p. 100; Lord, 1955; Nunnally, 1975, pp. 8–12; Tucker & MacCallum, 1997, p. 266). As computer-automated analysis programs continued to advance in terms of computational power and speed, previously unimaginable analytic procedures soon became commonplace throughout the psychological sciences as a means of gleaning novel interpretive insights for applied practical research and clinical assessment use.

## 1960S: COMPUTER SOFTWARE APPLICATIONS

During the 1960s, computer software applications were introduced to automate the scoring and interpretative analysis of well-known psychological measures, such as the Minnesota Multiphasic Personality Inventory (MMPI; Rome et al., 1962), the Rorschach Inkblot Test (RIT; Piotrowski, 1964), and the Sixteen Personality Factor Questionnaire (16PF; Eber, 1964). Computer programs explicitly designed for neuropsychological evaluation purposes began to emerge as well (Knights & Watson, 1968). Also during this period in history, researchers in the military were actively engaged in exploratory research and preliminary prototype development (e.g., Bayroff, 1964), which laid the foundation for fully operational computerized test applications to take shape shortly thereafter.

## 1970S: AUTOMATION OF INTERPRETIVE ANALYSES

In the 1970s, several computer-based applications were developed in order to automate interpretive analysis of neuropsychological test scores (e.g., Adams, 1975; Finkelstein, 1977; Russell, Neuringer, & Goldstein, 1970; Swiercinsky, 1978). Within the military, computerized applications were devised to automate neuropsychological test administration, as well as scoring and analysis of results. One example is the Psychomotor/Perceptual Test Battery, a computer-automated application designed to assess various aspects of memory, attention, associative learning, and processing speed (Hunter, 1975). Early experimental research efforts toward the development of the Computerized Adaptive Testing—Armed Services Vocational Aptitude Battery (CAT-ASVAB) also took place during the late 1970s and early 1980s, but the CAT-ASVAB would not be ready for widespread operational use until much later (Sands, Waters, & McBride, 1997).

## 1980S AND 1990S: COMPUTERIZED NEUROPSYCHOLOGICAL ASSESSMENT BATTERIES

Throughout the 1980s and 1990s, numerous computerized neuropsychological assessment batteries developed through the work of several military-affiliated research and development teams. A few examples include the Criterion Task Set (CTS; Shingledecker, 1984), Automated Portable Test System (APTS; Bittner, Smith, Kennedy, Staley, & Harbeson, 1985), Walter Reed Performance Assessment Battery (WRPAB; Thorne, Genser, Sing, & Hegge, 1985), Unified Tri-Service Cognitive Performance Assessment Battery (UTC-PAB; Reeves & Thorne, 1986), Complex Cognitive Assessment Battery (CCAB; Samet, Gerselman, Zajaczknowski, & Marshall-Mils, 1986), Naval Medical Research Institute Performance Assessment Battery (NMRI-PAB; Thomas & Schrot, 1988), a PC-based series of synthetic work tasks (SYNWORK1; Elsmore, Naitoh, & Linnville,

1992), and the CogScreen–Aeromedical Edition test battery (CogScreen-AE; Kay, 1995), among many others. Thorough reviews of these and similar applications developed through the mid-1990s have been documented by Kane and Kay (1992, 1997), as well as Gilliland and Schlegel (1993).

### CURRENT COMPUTER-AUTOMATED APPLICATIONS

The research efforts behind the earlier test batteries referenced above helped to inform subsequent developments of the many computerized applications used routinely within the Department of Defense (DoD) today. At present, one of the most prominent examples is the Automated Neuropsychological Assessment Metrics (ANAM; Figures 8.2 & 8.3). Originally launched in the early 1990s, the ANAM has since gone through a series of continuous revisions (Friedl et al., 2007; Reeves, Winter, Bleiberg, & Kane, 2007) up until its most current iteration. To this day, the ANAM continues to serve as the DoD-designated predeployment baseline assessment instrument administered to all service members, and it is used to evaluate potential cognitive changes experienced by individuals who subsequently sustain concussive injuries while deployed, or in garrison (Department of Defense, 2015).

Another computerized application currently used DoD-wide is the CAT-ASVAB. Following the early years of its development referenced previously, the CAT-ASVAB became fully operational by the late 1990s (Pommerich,

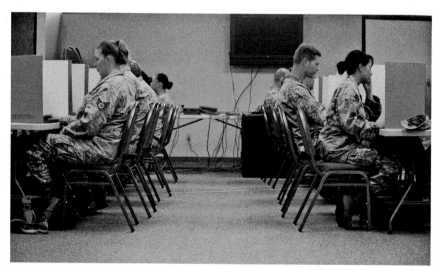

FIGURE 8.2  *ANAM group testing. Photograph taken by Joshua Green, Airman 1st Class, U.S. Air Force (November 5, 2009) at Moody Air Force Base, Georgia. Retrieved from http://media.defense.gov/2009/Nov/09/2000437 066/-1/-1/0/091105-F-8832G-004.JPG. The image is in the public domain.*

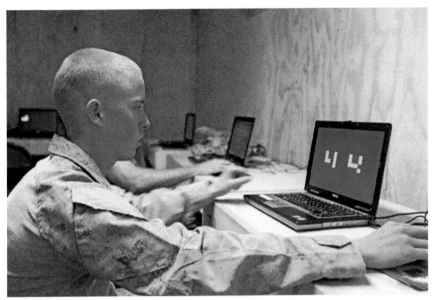

FIGURE 8.3 *Soldier viewing ANAM visuospatial subtest stimuli shown on laptop computer screen. Photograph taken by Corporal Kenneth Jasik, U.S. Marines (2010) at the Concussion Restoration Care Center, Camp Leatherneck, Afghanistan. Retrieved from http://www.usmedicine.com/pageImages/anamstudy1.jpg. The image is in the public domain.*

Segal, & Moreno, 2009), and it is presently utilized by military entrance processing facilities throughout the nation. Though CAT-ASVAB was not expressly designed for neuropsychological assessment purposes, several of its component subtests have been found to be highly correlated with traditional neuropsychological measures (Kennedy, Kupke, & Smith, 2000). Also, review of ASVAB test records is a common practice among military neuropsychologists for evaluating premorbid neuropsychological functioning (French, Anderson-Barnes, Ryan, Zazeckis, & Harvey, 2012, pp. 187–188; Kelly, 2013, p. 51; Kennedy, Kupke, & Smith, 2000; Kratz, Poppen, & Burroughs, 2007). While the range of underlying neuropsychological constructs included in the current version is somewhat lacking, subject-matter experts involved in planning and revision of the ASVAB have recently called for the inclusion of several additional measures specifically targeting neuropsychological capacities (e.g., processing speed, working memory, and visuospatial ability; Held & Carretta, 2013; Held, Carretta, & Rumsey, 2014; National Research Council, 2015, pp. 29–32; Russell, Ford, & Ramsberger, 2014). Though the paper-and-pencil-based version of the ASVAB is still occasionally given, plans are in place for it to be phased out completely, in favor of the CAT-ASVAB (Drasgow, 2014, p. 9), which affords significant advantages in terms of administrative efficiency and cost-effectiveness, as well as enhanced test design flexibility and data-capturing functionality (McCloy & Gibby, 2011; Pommerich, Segall, & Moreno, 2009; Sands, Waters, & McBride, 1997; Segall & Moreno, 1999).

Over the past few decades, a number of reviews appearing in the literature have expressed both optimism and concern about the rise of computer-automated neuropsychological test procedures (e.g., Adams, 1986; Adams & Brown, 1986; Adams & Heaton, 1985; Butcher, Perry, & Hahn, 2004; Crook, Kay, & Larrabee, 2009; Dede, Zalonis, Gatzonis, & Sakas, 2015; Kane & Kay, 1992, 1997; Kane & Reeves, 1997; Moser, Schatz, & Lichtenstein, 2015; Parsey & Schmitter-Edgecombe, 2013; Parsons, 2016a; Rabin et al., 2014; Schlegel & Gilliland, 2007). On the one hand, reviews have highlighted several purported benefits of computerized neuropsychological assessments, including their ability to automate test administration (Parsey & Schmitter-Edgecombe, 2013), scoring (Russell, 2000; Woo, 2008), normative data collection (Bilder, 2011), and interpretive analysis (Ferguson & Iverson, 2011; Horton, Vaeth, & Anilane, 1990; Russell, 1995). Other notable advantages include increased flexibility and complexity of stimulus presentation (Gur et al., 2001a, 2001b; Schatz & Browndyke, 2002), along with automated logging of examinee responses (Crook, Kay, & Larrabee, 2009; Woo, 2008), with millisecond timing accuracy (Schatz & Browndyke, 2002).

On the other hand, a number of concerns have been raised, including the issue of whether the patient's perceptions of computer-generated stimuli, and responses to computerized administration, are significantly different from their perceptions of traditional paper-and-pencil-based procedures (Cernich, Brennana, Barker, & Bleiberg, 2007; Hoskins, Binder, Chaytor, Williamson, & Drane, 2010; Noyes & Garland, 2008; Williams & McCord, 2006). Furthermore, varying levels of patient familiarity and comfort with computer-based assessments could potentially have a confounding effect on their performance (Bush, Naugle, & Johnson-Greene, 2002; Iverson, Brooks, Ashton, Johnson, & Gualtieri 2009). These issues may result in a failure of computer-administered tests to deliver results that are equivalent to paper-and-pencil-based tests administered manually by an examiner (Feldstein et al., 1999; French & Beaumont, 1990; Ozonoff, 1995). For example, there are two commercially available versions of the Wisconsin Card Sorting Test (WCST): a manual version (Heaton, Chelune, Talley, Kay, & Curtis, 1993) and a computer version (Heaton & PAR Staff, 2003). Discrepant patterns of performance observed between the two versions may be due in part to patient cohort issues (e.g., persons with autism; Ozonoff, 1995), but studies suggest that the paper-and-pencil and computerized versions of the WCST are not psychometrically equivalent (Feldstein et al., 1999; Steinmetz, Brunner, Loarer, & Houssemand, 2010). Other concerns raised with respect to computer-automated testing include the potential for hardware or software related technical errors (Cernich, Brennana, Barker, & Bleiberg, 2007), unappealing or unintuitive human–computer interfaces, and lack of ecological validity (Schatz & Browndyke, 2002, p. 406).

## Military Neuropsychological Assessment 3.0: Military-Specific Virtual Environments

All aforementioned concerns regarding traditional computer-automated applications are entirely valid and must be carefully scrutinized so that they may be mitigated through future research and development. But they do not negate the many benefits highlighted. As a special case of computer-based technology, VR-based platforms afford the same advantages, as well as other clinically useful and unique features not found in traditional computerized assessment applications. At the same time, VR-based applications also face a similar range of challenges to contend with.

VR-based technologies have a long-standing track record of use within the military for training and mission rehearsal exercises (Lele, 2013; Seidel & Chatelier, 1997; U.S. Congress, Office of Technology Assessment, 1994, 1995), from pre-digital Link Trainer flight simulators used during the 1930s (De Angelo, 2000; Duchak, 1990, pp. 6–9) to the vast array of high-speed digital-computer-based VR systems in use today (Dando & Tranter, 2016, pp. 197–205; Gourley, 2016; Matthews, 2014). But the military's use of VR-based applications specifically for neuropsychological assessment purposes has only recently emerged within the past few decades. Building upon computer platforms, VR-based neuropsychological assessment applications afford enhanced computational capacities for administration efficiency, stimulus presentation, automated logging of responses, and data analytic processing. Moreover, VR-based technologies offer the potential of increased ecological validity via true-to-life virtual environments (VEs), which may be customized in accordance with specific areas of interest (e.g., virtual battlefield scenarios tailored for dismounted soldier cognitive performance assessments). Specific militarily relevant assessment platforms are summarized below, followed by a brief overview of their advantages and limitations.

### VIRTUAL ENVIRONMENT PERFORMANCE ASSESSMENT BATTERY (VEPAB)

By the early 1990s, researchers in the military were actively exploring the use of VR-based applications specifically for purposes of assessment. One example application developed during this period was the VEPAB. The VEPAB platform was designed to assess various perceptual and psychomotor abilities through a series of examinee tasks performed within immersive three-dimensional VEs, presented visually to examinees via head-mounted display (HMD), with navigational control enabled via joystick or spaceball. Standard desktop computer systems with dual-monitor displays were used by examiners—i.e., primary monitor displaying VEPAB program menu to select, start, and/or terminate tasks, alongside a secondary monitor for examiners to follow the examinee's field of view in real time as tasks were performed (Lampton et al., 1994, 1995).

While the VEPAB project was primarily driven by a desire to more effectively leverage VR for training purposes, it was also largely focused upon ecologically valid measurement of human cognitive performance variables (e.g., visuospatial perception, psychomotor functioning, and processing speed capacity) that are of particular relevance for neuropsychological assessment purposes. As an early exploratory prototype application, VEPAB had stimuli and examinee tasks intentionally designed to be relatively rudimentary and minimalistic. However, the VEPAB effectively demonstrated the practical utility of VE scenarios for human performance assessment, and helped to inspire the development of increasingly sophisticated and contextually nuanced military-themed VR-based assessment interfaces.

## COMPUTER ASSISTED REHABILITATION ENVIRONMENT (CAREN)

One of the most technologically elaborate VR-based assessment platforms available currently is the Computer Assisted Rehabilitation Environment (CAREN; Figure 8.4). Since the time of its inception in the late 1990s (van der Eerden, Otten, May, & Even-Zohar, 1999), interest in the use of CAREN for clinical assessment has continued to build. Presently, within the DoD, CAREN systems are in operation at the following facilities: National Intrepid Center of Excellence (NICoE), Walter Reed National Military Medical Center (WRNMMC), Naval Health Research Center (NHRC), and the Center for the Intrepid (CFI) at Brook Army Medical Center (BAMC; Bartlett, Sessoms, and Reini, 2013). Specific system configurations may vary, but most high-end CAREN systems are arranged to enable fully immersive multisensory VEs via panoramic or dome-display screen enclosures, surround-sound stereo systems, dual-belt treadmill motion platforms, and a customizable suite of VE software applications (van der Meer, 2014). Other components sometimes incorporated into CAREN platforms include synchronized scent systems, motion-capture camera systems, accelerometers, and an assortment of physiological monitoring devices (Bartlett, Sessoms, and Reini, 2013).

CAREN systems have been used to facilitate immersive militarily relevant VE scenarios (Bartlett, Sessoms, and Reini, 2013), which elicit a strong sense of experiential engagement, or *presence*, in rehabilitating service members (Highland, Kreuger, & Roy, 2015). A heightened sense of presence has also proven to be beneficial for neuropsychological assessment purposes (Morganti, 2004, 2016). Numerous studies have been performed to date involving clinical applications of the CAREN platform with service members (Collins et al., 2015), and a few of the studies have specifically referenced neuropsychological assessment applications in particular. For instance, Rabago and Wilken (2011)

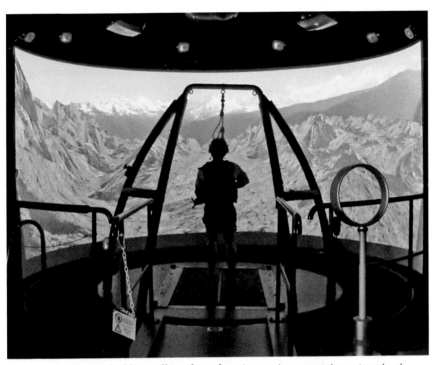

FIGURE 8.4 *Image of soldier walking through an immersive mountainous terrain virtual environment within the CAREN (Computer Assisted Rehabilitation Environment). Reprinted from Collins, J., Markham, A., Service, K., Reini, S., Wolf, E., & Sessoms, P. (2015). A systematic literature review of the use and effectiveness of the Computer Assisted Rehabilitation Environment for research and rehabilitation as it relates to the wounded warrior. Work, 50(1), 122, with permission from IOS Press. doi:10.3233/WOR-141927*

reported a case study involving their use of the CAREN to assess and monitor the vestibular and neuropsychological functioning of a recently concussed service member over a 3-week period of rehabilitation. The specific neuropsychological assessment procedures included a novel VR-based adaptation of the classic Stroop (1935) color-word interference task, along with VR-based symbol recognition and symbol matching tasks. By the end of the 3-week rehabilitative program, the service member demonstrated significant improvements in terms of vestibular function (e.g., static and dynamic postural balance) as well as neuropsychological parameters assessed (e.g., executive function, divided attention, and processing speed). This study lends preliminary empirical support for the potential use of CAREN systems for both assessment and rehabilitation of service members experiencing physical as well as cognitive disturbances, but further research is needed in the form of large-scale clinical trials to further explore and validate potential CAREN-based neuropsychological assessments.

Similar VR-based cognitive tasks have been implemented by other clinician researchers in the context of CAREN-mediated rehabilitation regimes with brain-injured service members (e.g., Gottshall, Sessoms, & Bartlett, 2012; Gottshall & Sessoms, 2015; Sessoms et al., 2015). The CAREN has recently been used to implement a novel VR-based multitasking procedure to evaluate neuropsychological functioning of rehabilitating service member research participants, while attempting to differentiate between diagnoses of mild traumatic brain injury (mTBI) alone and mTBI comorbid with PTSD (Onakomaiya, Kruger, Highland, & Roy, 2016a, 2016b). Initial study findings from pilot clinical trials suggest that the CAREN VR multitasking procedure can be a useful asset for differential diagnostic purposes. Overall, the few preliminary studies performed to date involving the use of the CAREN for neuropsychological assessment purposes are encouraging, but research is required to further evaluate its potential.

## DRIVING SIMULATORS

Driving simulators are another form of VR-based assessment technology that has been researched for use with service members (Amick, Kraft, & McGlinchey, 2013; Classen et al., 2011; Classen, Monahan, Canonizado, & Winter, 2014; Cox et al., 2010; Kraft, Amick, Barth, French, & Lew, 2010; Laferrier et al., 2013, pp. 120–124). As a cohort, service members recovering from mild traumatic brain injury (mTBI) and/or PTSD are considered to be particularly susceptible to developing unsafe driving behaviors (Carlson et al., 2016; Lew et al., 2011; Lew, Amick, Kraft, Stein, & Cifu, 2010). Studies involving the use of driving simulators with veterans affected by mTBI/PTSD suggest the simulators can be useful for facilitating multiple clinical and practical benefits. As reported by Lew et al. (2009), driving simulators afford a safe, therapeutic, and ecologically valid means to assess and rehabilitate impaired driving abilities—mimicking the real-world experience of driving on actual streets, yet removed from the dangers they impose. Moreover, as the act of driving requires engagement of several neuropsychological domains (e.g., attention, processing speed, memory, executive function), driving simulators could theoretically be useful purely in terms of neuropsychological assessment itself (Bedard, Parkkari, Weaver, Riendeau, & Dahlquist, 2010; Schultheis & Chute, 1999; Schultheis & Mourant, 2001; Wald & Liu, 2001). Several preliminary studies have recently documented statistically significant correlations between driving simulator performance and neurocognitive ability (Choi, Yoo, & Lee, 2015; Dumenigo, Scarrino, & Golden, 2015; Guinosso, Johnson, Schultheis, Graefe, & Bishai, 2016; Hayhurst, Babika, Messerly, Williams, & Golden, 2015; Lamargue-Hamel et al., 2015; Lee, Lee, & Choi, 2016; Zusman, & Golden, 2015).

Individual driving simulator interfaces vary in terms of appearance, cost, hardware, and VE scenario presentation (Philips & Morton, 2015), but they often share many of the same essential features of relevance to clinicians for purposes of assessment and rehabilitation. Most driving simulator platforms are fully equipped with an assemblage of external peripheral controls (e.g., vehicle interior mock-up to include steering wheel, brakes, and accelerator pedals), along with built-in driving performance data-capture functionality for clinicians to seamlessly track and monitor multiple behavioral variables simultaneously in real time (e.g., speed regulation, lane deviations, traffic violations, etc.; Classen & Brooks, 2014; Figure 8.5). Also, the immersive, experientially engaging nature of driving simulator VEs can be useful for facilitating service member motivation and adherence to assessment and/or rehabilitation procedures (Lew, Rosen, Thomander, & Poole, 2009). Imhoff, Lavalliere, Teasdale, and Fait (2016) provide a summary of research performed, including descriptions of each driving simulator platform used, in studies exploring their application for assessment and rehabilitation with traumatic brain injury patients.

## WEAPONS TRAINING SIMULATORS

Military-affiliated researchers have begun to explore the potential role of VR-based weapons training platforms to evaluate vestibular functioning and

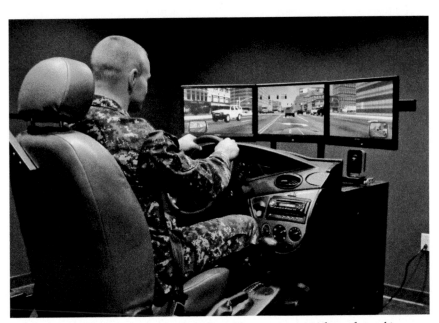

FIGURE 8.5 *Technician demonstration of cognitive assessment tasks performed in a driving simulator. U.S. Air Force courtesy photograph taken at the National Intrepid Center of Excellence (NICoE) in Bethesda, Maryland. Retrieved from http://media. defense.gov/2016/Jul/19/2001577331/-1/-1/0/160718-O-ZZ999-003A.JPG. The image has been officially released by the U.S. Air Force and is in the public domain.*

fitness-for-duty status of military personnel recovering from mTBI (Grandizio et al., 2014). A few studies have been carried out with a more explicitly stated aim of evaluating neuropsychological constructs via VR-based weapons simulators (Biggs, Cain, & Mitroff, 2015; Kelley, Ranes, Estrada, & Grandizio, 2015; Patton & Marusich, 2015; Scribner, 2016). Kelley et al. (2011) have noted significant correlations between objective neuropsychological measures and marksmanship skills using the Engagement Skill Trainer 2000 (EST 2000) weapons training simulator. Patton & Marusich (2015) have described the use of a five-screen 300° VE display unit known as the Immersive Cognitive Readiness Simulator (ICoRS; Figure 8.6) for evaluating militarily relevant tactical decision-making abilities through virtual hostile enemy fire scenarios. Similarly, Scribner (2016) recently reported findings from a study using the Dismounted Infantry Survivability and Lethality Test Bed (DISALT), a VR-based firing range simulator, to examine the cognitive

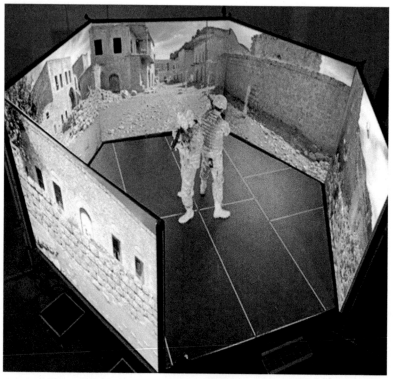

FIGURE 8.6  *Photo of the Immersive Cognitive Readiness Simulator (ICoRS). Reprinted from Patton, D., & Marusich, L. (2015, March). Simulated network effects on tactical operations on decision making. Paper presented at the 2015 IEEE International Inter-Disciplinary Conference on Cognitive Methods in Situation Awareness and Decision Support (CogSIMA), Orlando, FL, with permission from the ICoRS platform developer & manufacturer: VirTra Systems, Inc., www.virtra.com.*
doi:10.1109/COGSIMA.2015.7108190

and affective variables involved in "shoot/don't shoot" decision making. The ICoRS and DISALT platforms are both relatively high-end systems equipped with audio, visual, and tactile sensory inputs, with data-capture functionality, and are capable of facilitating high-fidelity multisensory immersion. As reported by Scribner (2016), and by Patton & Marusich (2015), VR shoot/don't shoot scenario performance does appear to be significantly correlated with various affective and neuropsychological domains (e.g., working memory, processing speed, stress-response/arousal). All of the aforementioned weapons simulator studies have been exploratory and have been limited by small sample sizes. Nevertheless, they represent a promising new avenue of inquiry into VR-based applications for evaluating service member operational readiness and neuropsychological status.

### VIRTUAL CONVOY OPERATIONS TRAINER (VCOT)

Kelley, Ranes, Estrada, and Grandizio (2015) recently published results obtained from an exploratory study involving the newly developed Military Functional Assessment Program (MFAP) that entails a battery of militarily relevant functional assessment tasks, including several VR-based procedures. For instance, one of the MFAP tasks involved the use of a military tactical vehicle simulator (i.e., VCOT), in order to assess neuropsychological and return-to-duty status of brain-injured service members via simulated convoy exercises resembling real-world combat scenarios. Specific examples of soldier tasks performed within the VCOT included identification of environmental threats, such as improvised explosive devices (IEDs) and/or rocket-propelled grenades (RPGs) encountered in a simulated battlefield, as well as the completion of a SALUTE report of enemy information (i.e., Size, Activity, Location, Unit identification, Time, and Equipment). Each task included within the MFAP study battery was primarily based on examples documented in the *Soldier's Manual of Common Tasks* (Department of the Army, 2012), and the tasks were selected on the basis of their relevance to real-world soldier tasks performed in live combat scenarios, as well as their relevance to underlying neuropsychological functions involved while performing such tasks (Kelley, Ranes, Estrada, & Grandizio, 2015, p. E12). For instance, effective performance during the VCOT task requiring identification of IEDs and/or RPGs in a simulated combat scenario would arguably involve multiple neuropsychological variables, such as attention, executive function, processing speed, and visuospatial-perceptual abilities. Correlational analyses performed by the MFAP study team revealed patterns of significant convergence between clinical measures used (e.g., RBANS) and performance on MFAP battery tasks, such as those performed with the VCOT. However, as a preliminary investigation, further research is needed to more fully examine the clinical utility of the VCOT, and related VR-based tactical engagement simulators, as potential tools for augmenting traditional neuropsychological return-to-duty evaluation practices currently performed within the military.

## VIRTUAL REALITY COGNITIVE PERFORMANCE ASSESSMENT TEST (VRCPAT)

Parsons first developed the Virtual Reality Cognitive Performance Assessment Test (VRCPAT) platform at the University of Southern California's Institute for Creative Technologies. The original VRCPAT made use of assets from virtual Iraqi and virtual Afghani scenarios that had been developed for VR exposure therapy (Parsons, Rizzo, Bamattre, & Brennan, 2007; Rizzo et al., 2006). The novel assessment and treatment environments leveraged graphic assets that were initially built for the Army-funded combat tactical simulation scenario and commercially successful X-Box game, Full Spectrum Warrior (Parsons, Silva, Pair, & Rizzo, 2008).

The VRCPAT is different from paper-and-pencil or traditional computerized neuropsychological tests in that it allows soldiers to experience a greater "sense of presence" as they became immersed within militarily relevant VEs (Parsons, Rizzo, Courtney, & Dawson, 2012). Parsons and colleagues made efforts to ensure that the VRCPAT retained the benefits afforded by computer automation (i.e., exacting control over VE task parameters and stimuli, such as number, order, and speed). Furthermore, the VRCPAT allows for automated data capture and scoring of patient task performance (Parsons, Iyer, Cosand, Courtney, & Rizzo, 2009), combined with a capacity to measure complex sets of skills and behaviors in a more ecologically valid fashion. This approach represented a distinctive departure from traditional instruments and procedures whereby clinicians attempt to predict an individuals' real-world performance using stimuli and methods that are inherently contrived and radically dissimilar to a person's actual lived experience and behavior in the real world (see Parsons, 2011).

The VRCPAT included a series of customizable virtual scenarios designed to represent relevant contexts for assessment, including a city and desert road convoy environment. User-centered design feedback needed to iteratively evolve the system was gathered from returning Iraq War veterans in the U.S., and from a system in Iraq tested by an Army Combat Stress Control Team. The VRCPAT evolved into a battery of neuropsychological and psychophysiological measures for diagnostic assessment of soldiers with affective disorders, brain injury, and/ or related neurocognitive deficits (Reger, Parsons, Gahm, & Rizzo, 2010). While soldiers were immersed in the VRCPAT, their neurocognitive and psychophysiological responses were recorded in an attempt to understand how the activation of particular brain areas related to given tasks (Parsons & Rizzo, 2008a). The goal was to better uncover the relationship between the neural correlates of neurocognitive functioning in virtual environments designed to mimic and generalize to real-world functioning. Following the acquisition of the data, Parsons used machine learning and artificial neural networks for nonlinear stochastic approximation and modeling of specific neurocognitive and affective processes of persons immersed in VRCPAT (Iyer, Cosand, Courtney, Rizzo, & Parsons, 2009; Wu &

Parsons, 2011a, 2011b). The VRCPAT includes a battery of neuropsychological measures to assess the ways in which the structure and function of the brain relate to specific psychological processes and overt behaviors: attention-vigilance (Parsons & Rizzo, 2008b), executive functioning (Parsons, Cosand, Courtney, Iyer, & Rizzo, 2009), memory (Parsons & Rizzo, 2008c), and affective responding (Parsons et al., 2009; Parsons, Iyer, Cosand, Courtney, & Rizzo, 2009; Parsons & Courtney, 2011).

### VRCPAT VIRTUAL CITY MEMORY MODULE

In a study aimed at using VRCPAT to assess object learning and memory, Parsons and Rizzo (2008) used the VRCPAT virtual city task that reflected tasks found in the Hopkins Verbal Learning Test–Revised (HVLT-R; Brandt & Benedict, 2001) and the Brief Visuospatial Memory Test–Revised (BVMT-R; Benedict, 1997). Before being immersed in the virtual city, participants took part in a learning task in which they were exposed to language and graphic-based information without any context across three free-learning trials. Next, they were immersed in. the virtual environment and they followed a virtual human guide to five different zones of a virtual city (see Figure 8.7). In each zone, participants searched the area for two target items (i.e., items from the learning phase). Following

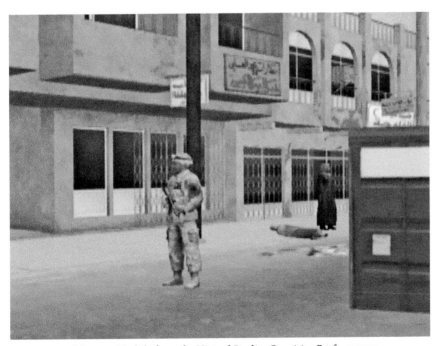

FIGURE 8.7 *Memory Module from the Virtual Reality Cognitive Performance Assessment Test.*

immersion in each of the five zones, participants performed short- and long-delay free and cued recall tasks. Parsons and Rizzo compared results from the virtual city to traditional paper-and-pencil tasks and found the virtual city was significantly related to paper-and-pencil measures (both individual and composite) of both visually and auditorily mediated learning and memory (convergent validity). These results have been replicated in a study with a larger group of participants (Parsons, Iyer, Cosand, Courtney, & Rizzo, 2009).

### VIRTUAL HIGH MOBILITY MULTIPURPOSE WHEELED VEHICLE (HMMWV) ATTENTION MODULE

In another study, Parsons and colleagues (2009) assessed attentional processing using manipulation of stimulus intensity and stimulus complexity while participants took part in a Virtual High Mobility Multipurpose Wheeled Vehicle (HMMWV; Figure 8.8) attention-vigilance scenario. The task involved the presentation of a four-digit number that was superimposed on the virtual windshield (of the HMMWV) as the participants drove the HMMWV. Stimulus complexity was relative to the presentation of stimuli. For simple presentations, the four-digit number always appeared in a fixed central location on the windshield. For the complex presentations, the numbers appeared randomly throughout the

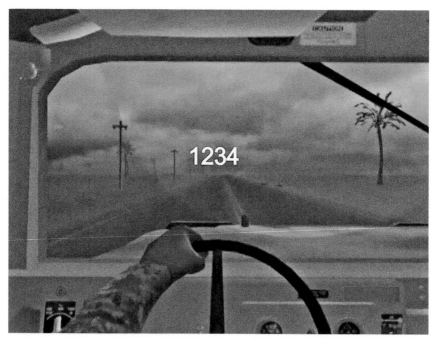

FIGURE 8.8 *Attention Module from the Virtual Reality Cognitive Performance Assessment Test.*

windshield rather than in one fixed central location. Stimulus intensity was modulated by placing the user in "safe" (low intensity) and "ambush" (high intensity) settings: start section, palm ambush, safe zone, city ambush, and bridge ambush. To examine scenario differences, one-way ANOVAs were performed, comparing attentional performance in simple stimulus presentations versus complex stimulus presentations. The results indicated that the increase in stimulus complexity caused a significant decrease in performance on attentional tasks. Participant performance was also found to be significantly diminished by increased stimulus intensity.

### VIRTUAL REALITY STROOP TASK (VRST)

More recently, research and development efforts in Parsons' lab at the University of North Texas have led to the creation of VEs designed to assess both cognitive and affective processes using combat-related scenarios (Parsons, Courtney, & Dawson, 2013; Wu, Lance, & Parsons, 2013), which allow clinicians to assess soldier functioning within high-threat militarily relevant settings, while avoiding the risks posed by live combative exercises. A primary goal of the platforms is to assess the impact of affective arousal upon cognitive processes. For example, Parsons and colleagues (2013) have developed assessment scenarios using the HMMWV, in which participants are immersed in a simulated HMMWV as they drive through zones characterized by low-threat or high-threat conditions. In low-threat zones, participants are exposed to relatively neutral environmental stimuli as they drive down a deserted desert road. Conversely, high-threat zones are characterized by hostile enemy gunfire, explosions, and shouting, among other stressors. In both neutral and high-threat conditions, participants are instructed to perform a VR-based adaptation of the Stroop (1935) color-word interference task, wherein Stroop stimuli are presented on the windshield of the HMMWV (see Figure 8.9). This task is used in order to determine the effect of level of threat upon participant Stroop task performance. The study performed by Parsons et al. (2013) using the HMMWV Stroop task yielded the following findings: As expected, the high-threat zones created a greater level of psychophysiological arousal (heart rate, skin conductance, respiration) than did low-threat zones. Analyses of the effect of threat level on the color–word and interference scores resulted in a main effect of threat level and condition, whereby high-threat conditions were consistently correlated with significantly diminished Stroop-task performance. High-information-load tasks used for cognitive processing appear relatively unaffected by controlled, low-threat zones with little activity. And, last, the total available processing capacities may be decreased by other affective factors, such as arousal (e.g., threat zones with a great deal of activity; Parsons, Courtney, Arizmendi, & Dawson, 2011; Wu et al., 2010). In a replication study, Armstrong et al. (2013) established the preliminary convergent and discriminant validity of the VRST with an active-duty military sample.

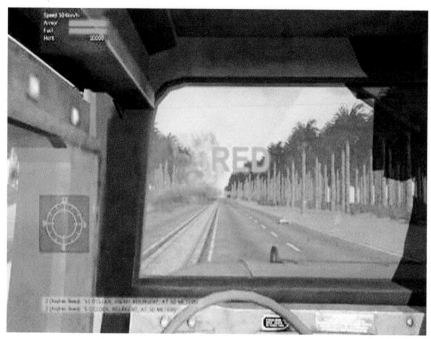

FIGURE 8.9  *Virtual Reality Stroop Task: Virtual High-Mobility Multipurpose Wheeled Vehicle.*

## VIRTUAL REALITY PACED AUDITORY SERIAL ADDITION TEST (VR-PASAT)

In addition to VR-based neuropsychological assessments using HMMWV driving simulators, Parsons has developed other militarily relevant VEs for neuropsychological assessment of cognitive and affective processes. For example, Parsons and colleagues (2012, 2014) used a dismounted soldier VE to immerse participants in a Middle Eastern city context (see Figure 8.10), exposing participants to a cognitive processing task (e.g., paced auditory serial addition test) as they followed a fire team on foot through safe zones and ambush zones (e.g., bombs, gunfire, screams, and other visual and auditory forms of threat). During a route-learning task included as part of the assessment, each zone was preceded by a zone marker, which served as a landmark to assist in remembering the route. The route-learning task was followed immediately by the navigation task, in which the participants were asked to return to the starting point of their tour through the city. Courtney et al. (2013) found that the inclusion of affective stimuli (e.g., high-threat zones) resulted in a greater level of psychophysiological arousal (heart rate, skin conductance, respiration) and predictably decreased performance on cognitive processes. Results from active-duty military (Parsons et al., 2012) and civilian (Parsons & Courtney, 2014) populations offer preliminary support for the construct validity of the virtual PASAT as a measure of

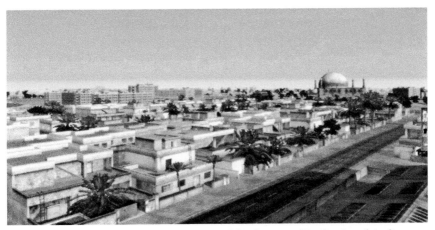

FIGURE 8.10 *Virtual Middle Eastern City used for the Virtual Reality Paced Auditory Serial Addition Test.*

attentional processing. Further, results suggest that the VR-PASAT may provide some unique information related to affective processing not tapped by traditional attentional processing tasks.

## MILITARILY RELEVANT ADAPTIVE VIRTUAL IRAQI/AFGHANI ENVIRONMENTS

A further development in Parsons' lab was the creation of militarily relevant adaptive virtual Iraqi/Afghani environments, in which data gleaned from the assessment module is used for refined analysis, management, and rehabilitation of soldiers suffering from the aftereffects of traumatic brain injury and/or PTSD-related symptoms (Parsons & Courtney, 2011; Parsons & Reinebold, 2012; Wu, Lance, & Parsons, 2013; Wu & Parsons, 2012). This represented a major development that allowed the neuropsychologist to take the neurocognitive and psychophysiological profile information from an assessment module and use that information to create adaptive VEs (see Figure 8.11), which dynamically calibrate in accordance with the unique neurophysiological status of individual soldiers as they progress through rehabilitative treatment protocols. The ultimate goal is to have an adaptive, militarily relevant VE, accompanied by psychophysiological metrics, to assess and profile neurocognitive, affective, and physiological functional status of soldiers recovering from a concussive trauma and/or PTSD. Such adaptive VEs can be used to adjust the presentation of both the difficulty (e.g., simple versus complex) and intensity (safe versus threatening) of stimuli delivered to match the neurocognitive and physiological characteristics of each user (Parsons & Reinebold, 2012), and thereby enhance existing cognitive rehabilitation and/or VR exposure therapy protocols.

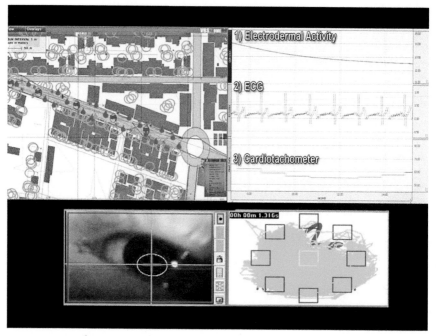

FIGURE 8.11 *Adaptive virtual environment using behavioral metrics and psychophysi-ological responding.*

Although there have been prior attempts to apply adaptive VEs to posttrau-matic stress disorder (Botella et al., 2010; Ćosić, Popović, Kukolja, Horvat, & Dropuljic, 2010; Popović, Horvat, Kukolja, Dropuljic, & Ćosić, 2009;) and neu-rocognitive rehabilitation (Klinger, Cao, Douguet, & Fuchs, 2009; Salva, Alban, Wiederhold, Wiederhold, & Kong 2009), the attempts were made during very early stages of development. Current adaptive VEs represent a shift toward a somewhat more developmentally advanced stage and are novel in that they include both psychophysiological and neurocognitive profiles to enhance adap-tive capabilities. Nevertheless, they are still a work in progress and efforts to further enhance and expand upon their current form are ongoing. Thus far, VR-based assessments have established a well-defined set of neuropsychological tests that have been validated against standard paper-and-pencil, as well as computer-ized, neuropsychological measures.

## Discussion: Advantages and Challenges

### ADVANTAGES

The most attractive aspect of VEs for clinicians working with military service members is the provision of ecologically valid platforms for presenting dynamic and militarily relevant stimuli in a manner that allows for both the veridical control of laboratory measures and the verisimilitude of naturalistic observation of real-life situations. VE-based assessments can provide a balance between nuanced naturalistic observation and the need for exacting measurement of key neuropsychological variables. Other, more traditional approaches to assessment can still be useful, but VR-based assessment applications are arguably among the most promising for facilitating ecological validity (Campbell et al., 2009; Parsons, 2015a, 2015b, 2016a).

Why would a military neuropsychologist be interested in ecological validity? To answer this question, we need to look at common neuropsychological measures and their efficacy for return-to-duty decisions. A difficulty for most assessments is that performance on tests (e.g., WCST, Stroop task) of a given construct (e.g., working memory) may have little or no predictive value for how a person functions in a real-world situation (Burgess et al., 2006; Chaytor, Schmitter-Edgecombe, & Burr, 2006). Neuropsychologists therefore increasingly emphasize the need for tests to represent real-world functioning, while tapping into a number of cognitive domains relevant to an individual's actual behavior in everyday life (Chaytor & Schmitter-Edgecombe, 2003). A next logical question is why would a military neuropsychologist be interested in virtual reality? The most obvious answer is that VE-based assessments allow for real-time evaluation of a service member's neurocognitive, affective, and social functioning, in a manner that more closely resembles real-world militarily relevant functional abilities (Bartlett, Sessoms, & Reini, 2013; Benson, 2016; Cohen, Brinkman, & Neerincx, 2015, p. 517; Edwards, Vess, Reger, & Cernich, 2014; Kennedy, Nesbitt, & Alt, 2014; Moten, 2015; Patton & Gamble, 2016; Reger, Parsons, Gahm, & Rizzo, 2012; Scribner, 2016). Further, virtual reality allows for precise presentation and control of dynamic perceptual stimuli that can be used for assessment of neurocognitive, affective, and social processing while service members are immersed in simulations of contextually familiar military-specific scenarios they would normally encounter in the real world.

VR-based technologies afford many other practical advantages. For instance, as a special type of computer-automated technology, VR-based applications enable increased administrative efficiency through automated data-capture, scoring, and analysis capability (Rizzo, Parsons, Kenny, & Buckwalter, 2012). Also, the underlying software applications used for creating VEs are becoming increasingly more agile, intuitive, and amenable to user-specified customizations in accordance with desired clinical assessment needs and outcomes (Koenig et al., 2014). In the context of the military, VEs can be used by clinicians to assesses service member cognitive performance and operational readiness (Freeman, Nicholson, Squire, & Bolton, 2014) through a wide range of real-world militarily relevant scenarios, including high-threat hostile enemy fire scenarios, in a manner that is safe and controlled (Hildebrandt, McCall, Engen, & Singer, 2016; Parsons & Courtney, 2016; Patton & Gamble, 2016; Patton, Loukota, & Avery,

2013; Patton & Marusich, 2015; Scribner, 2016). Finally, while some of the more elaborate high-end VR platforms, such as the CAREN, can be cost-prohibitive, there are a wide range of VR-based applications that are inexpensive, yet perfectly adequate and effective for clinical use (Cipresso, Serino, & Riva, 2016), requiring little more than a desktop or laptop computer, with a head-mounted display (HMD) unit for increased visual immersion.

## CHALLENGES

Despite the advantages afforded by computerized neuropsychological assessment applications, including VR-based applications, they remain largely underutilized by practicing neuropsychologists (Rabin et al., 2014). With respect to VR-based applications specifically, a relatively new technology, failure to embrace their use may be due in part to simple lack of familiarity, which is likely to fade with time, especially given the continued rise of publications on the topic throughout the professional literature. However, increased familiarity does not necessarily guarantee acceptance. In order for widespread adoption to occur, VR-based applications must be made palatable to clinician end-users in terms of user-friendliness, cost-effectiveness, and applied practical advantages (Gross, 2015; Slater, 2014), as well as theoretical soundness, and strength of supportive empirical evidence with respect to their use for neuropsychological assessment.

In the context of the military, while traditional computerized applications like the ANAM are routinely utilized, use of VR-based platforms for neuropsychological assessment remains a rarity. Integration of VR-based assessment applications into mainstream clinical practice appears likely to occur eventually, but it will require continued concerted efforts to further demonstrate their effectiveness, while raising awareness of their applied practical utility among military affiliated neuropsychologist practitioners.

As previously noted, in terms of equipment costs, while there are many affordable options available, the expense associated with some of the more elaborate high-end VR platforms is a potentially limiting factor. Another possible barrier to increased adoption of VR-based applications for clinical use is the potential for technical difficulties, which may arise from VR hardware and/or software compatibility conflicts (Rizzo & Kim, 2005, pp. 131–132), unintuitive human-computer interfaces, or mechanical failure.

An additional challenge to VR application usability is the occurrence of side-effects, sometimes referred to as "simulator sickness" or "cybersickness," which can involve feelings of general discomfort, headache, dizziness, or nausea (LaViola, 2000). Several attempts have been made to mitigate such effects. Specific mitigation strategies include virtual field-of-view (FOV) modification (Fernandes & Feiner, 2016), galvanic vestibular stimulation (GVS; Cevette et al., 2012), galvanic cutaneous stimulation (GCS; Gálvez-García, Hay, & Gabaude, 2015), tactile stimulation (Gálvez-García, Albayay, Rehbein, & Tornay, 2017), calibrated white noise (Gálvez-García, 2015), hand-eye coordination tasks (Curtis et al., 2015), and other behavioral interventions (Keshavarz, 2016). While most of these strategies have so far proven to be largely effective, there is still a need for continued progress in order for VR-induced side-effects to be further offset or eliminated (Rebenitsch & Owen, 2016; Serge & Moss, 2015).

Though studies involving the use of VR-based applications for neuropsychological assessment continue to produce supportive findings (Cogné et al., 2016; Diaz-Orueta et al., 2016; Negut, Jurma, & David, 2016; Negut, Matu, Sava, & David, 2016; Lopez, Deliens, & Cleeremans, 2016; Parsons & Phillips, 2016; Pedroli et al., 2016), there remains a need for ongoing applied clinical research and development in order to further confirm their validity, reliability, and overall psychometric robustness for all neuropsychological domains they purport to measure. Further research and development are also needed to expand and improve upon VR-based assessment normative properties (Parsey & Schmitter-Edgecombe, 2013), as well as guidelines for standardized administration, scoring, and interpretation of results. To ensure suitability for use with military personnel, military-specific applications will require coordination of large-scale clinical trials, conducted with service member research participants, and led by military-affiliated neuropsychologist researchers.

If VR-based assessment applications are to be introduced for routine clinical use within the military, care must be taken to establish standardized professional guidelines for safe, ethically informed, evidence-based procedures to ensure they are used appropriately. Guidelines presented by Bauer et al. (2012) for the appropriate use of computerized neuropsychological assessment devices are a useful starting point (e.g., guidelines for proper administration, interpretation, and communication of results; examiner qualification standards; privacy and security of patient information; psychometric validity and reliability standards; sensitivity to individual/cultural patient differences, as well as varying levels of comfort with computerized assessment devices, etc.). However, use of VR-based applications in a military clinical setting is a special case (Reger, 2013, pp. 290–292), which will require establishment of guidelines that are specifically tailored for armed forces personnel.

## Future Directions of VR-Based Assessment Applications in the Military

### TECHNOLOGICAL ADVANCEMENTS AND CLINICAL AFFORDANCES

While early VR-based prototypes were often technically unstable, exorbitantly priced, and relatively cumbersome to operate, today's VE systems are far more robust and reliable, cost-effective, and intuitive in terms of patient and clinician user interfaces (Bohil, Alicea, & Biocca, 2011). Also, the degree of high-fidelity immersion afforded by many of today's VEs (Figure 8.12) represents a vast

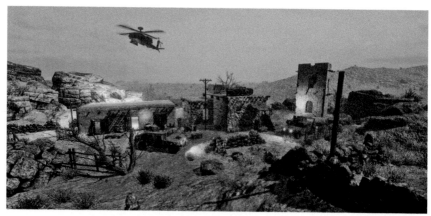

FIGURE 8.12  *High-fidelity military-themed virtual environment. Virtual environment screen capture image taken by Jon Brouchoud (April 4, 2014), Owner/Founder of Arch Virtual, LLC, http://archvirtual.com/. Retrieved from https://www.flickr.com/photos/crescendo/13624601053/in/album-72157645808231107/. Image reproduced with permission of the developer.*

improvement over VEs developed in decades past (Gilson & Glennerster, 2012). The clinical utility of VEs is likely to be further enhanced in years to come as the underlying technology continues to evolve (Parsons, 2015, 2016a; Stanney, Hale, & Zyda, 2015) via increased computational power, improved human-computer interaction design quality, and expanded range of functionalities afforded by future innovations in VR and related immersive user interface platforms and peripherals (LaViola, Bowman, McMahan, Kruijiff, & Poupyrev, 2017).

Continued advancements in VR-based military training platforms are likely to lead to enhanced clinical applications via repurposing for neuropsychological assessment use. Though not designed with clinical affordances in mind, VR-based military training platforms can facilitate multisensory immersion in ecologically oriented VEs that are especially suited for use with service members. Moreover, military training simulators often afford robust human performance monitoring, data-capture, and analysis functionalities via embedded VR software programs (Buxbaum, 2015, pp. 40–42; Kaber et al., 2013; Murphy, Hannigan, Hruska, Medford, & Diaz, 2016; Nicholson, Bartlett, Hoppenfeld, Nolan, & Schatz, 2014; Ross et al., 2016) which may be adapted for assessing neuropsychological constructs (Kelley et al., 2011; Szalma, Schmidt, Teo, & Hancock, 2014; Scribner, 2016), as well as neurophysiological mechanisms (Berka et al., 2011; Ko, Shih, Chikara, Chuang, & Chang, 2016) when paired with functional magnetic resonance imaging (fMRI), electroencephalography (EEG), and related neurophysiological assessment technologies.

Analogous to the trend of ongoing technological advancements, clinical research involving VR-based assessment applications has progressed considerably since the 1990s when it first began to emerge (Andrews, Rose, Leadbetter,

Attree, & Painter, 1995; Pugnetti et al., 1995; Rizzo, 1994), and it appears well primed for continued progress well into the foreseeable future. Several recently published reviews have highlighted current evidence in support of VR-based platforms in terms of their sensitivity (Negut, Matu, Sava, & David, 2016), convergent validity (Negut, Matu, Sava, & David, 2015), ecological validity (Parsons, 2016a, pp. 11–27), and reliability (Negut, 2014). In addition to their use for neuropsychological assessment (Cogné et al., 2016; Diaz-Orueta, Lizarazu, Climent, & Banterla, 2014; Lopez, Deliens, & Cleeremans, 2016; Negut, Jurma, & David, 2016; Parsons, Carlew, Magtoto, & Stonecipher, 2015; Parsons & Phillips, 2016; Pedroli et al., 2016), the utility of VR-based applications for neuropsychological rehabilitation is also well supported (Dores et al., 2016; Dores, Barbosa, Guerreiro, Almeida, & Carvalho, 2016; Lehman, 2015; Negut, 2014; Parsons, 2016a, pp. 113–132; Salisbury, Dahdah, Driver, Parsons, & Richter, 2016; Shin & Kim, 2015).

Military-specific VR-based neuropsychological assessment applications continue to demonstrate their utility for evaluating soldier cognitive abilities via operationally relevant VEs (Armstrong et al., 2013; Chen & Joyner, 2009; Parsons et al., 2012; Parsons & Reinebold, 2012; Parsons et al., 2009; Patton & Marusich, 2015; Scribner, 2016). Exploratory studies continue to accumulate evidence in support of their utility for facilitating fitness-for-duty/return-to-duty evaluations (Grandizio et al., 2014; Kelley, Ranes, Estrada, & Grandizio, 2015; Scherer, Weightman, Radomski, Davidson, & McCulloch, 2013, pp. 1258–1260), traumatic brain injury assessments (Edwards, Vess, Reger, & Cernich, 2014; Onakomaiya, Kruger, Highland, & Roy, 2016a, 2016b; Robitaille et al., 2016; Wright, 2014), and neuropsychological rehabilitation procedures specifically tailored for service members (Hebert et al., 2013; Hoffman, Shesko, & Harrison, 2010, p. 265; Levy et al., 2015; Lew et al., 2009; Parsons & Courtney, 2011; Rabago & Wilken, 2011; Rabago, Pruziner, & Esposito, 2015). However, significant challenges and limitations remain. In order to further validate and build upon the body of evidence accumulated thus far, continued future research and development are needed.

In addition to continued studies involving assessment and rehabilitation for service members whose functioning has become impaired due to neurological injury or psychiatric illness, there is also a need for research involving assessment of cognitive stressors endured by healthy neurologically intact service members. As noted by McNeil and Morgan (2010), operational stressors of war often lead to significant cognitive performance decrements affecting "both normal and elite" (p. 363) individuals, which are distinct from pathognomonic neuropsychological deficits. This observation has important implications for a wide range of research topics involving neuropsychological assessment within the military. Specific examples would include personnel selection, cognitive performance enhancement, and mitigation of performance decrements. Among studies performed thus far, while most have relied upon traditional paper-and-pencil and/or computerized neuropsychological assessment instruments, a significant minority of studies have involved novel VR-based assessment measures. A brief summary of studies performed in the areas of personnel selection, and cognitive enhancement research is provided below.

## PERSONNEL SELECTION

Neuropsychological assessment plays an integral role in military personnel selection procedures, and is an especially important component in the selection process for occupational specialties requiring superior cognitive performance under high-risk, hostile, and often ambiguous circumstances (e.g., aviators; French, Anderson-Barnes, Ryan, Zazeckis, & Harvey, 2012, p. 200). While the idea of using VR-based cognitive assessment measures for personnel selection has been introduced previously (Aguinas, Henle, & Beaty, 2001; Staal, Bolton, Yaroush, & Bourne, 2008, pp. 283–284; Schaub, 2010; Stanney & Cohn, 2012, pp. 656–658), relatively few military-specific examples have been documented in the research literature. However, the use of flight simulators for military aviator candidate selection is one example application of VR, which has been empirically investigated (Darr, 2009; Gress & Willkomm, 1996). Significant correlations between simulated flight performance and test scores from traditional neuropsychological measures have also been identified (Causse, Dehais, & Pastor, 2011; Taylor, O'Hara, Mumenthaler, & Yesavage, 2000; Yesavage et al., 2011). As noted by Carretta and Ree (2003) in their review of military aviator candidate selection methods, "... the validity of simulation-based approaches for pilot selection appears comparable to that for general cognitive ability $(g)$. Further, simulation-based tests may significantly increment the validity of cognitive tests when the two approaches are used together" (p. 375). At present, conventional neuropsychological test instruments remain the most common type of measure administered to military aviator candidates, but VR-based flight simulations continue to be regarded as a useful adjunctive method of assessment (Kozuba & Bondaruk, 2014; Johnston & Catano, 2013; Olson, Walker, & Phillips, 2010, p. 49; Stanney & Cohn, 2012, p. 656).

## VR-BASED ASSESSMENT OF ENHANCED COGNITION

There are several purported methods of enhancing cognitive performance (e.g., psychopharmacological, neurostimulatory) among healthy, neurologically intact individuals, that have been researched for military use. One way of evaluating their efficacy is through the use of VR-based cognitive assessment platforms using operationally relevant VEs (Russo, Fiedler, Thomas, & McGhee, 2005, pp. 14-8–14-11). Some studies have been performed to examine the efficacy of stimulant pharmaceutical cognitive enhancers such as modafinil, in sleep-deprived military pilots performing virtual maneuvering tasks within a flight simulator (e.g., Caldwell et al., 2004; LeDuc et al., 2009), yielding significant results in terms of cognition-enhancing effects (e.g., improved vigilance and decision-making), corresponding to improved simulated flight performance (e.g., better maintenance of target altitudes, headings, velocities, etc.).

Non-pharmacological interventions, such as transcranial direct current stimulation (tDCS), have also been investigated using dismounted soldier VE threat detection scenarios as a means to assess cognitive performance, subsequent to tDCS exposure (Clark et al., 2012; Coffman et al., 2012; Falcone, Coffman, Clark, & Parasuraman, 2012; Parasuraman & Galster, 2013). Other operationally relevant VEs have also been used in some of the more recent tDCS studies. One involved a simulated air-traffic control task, used as a means of evaluating the impact of tDCS on levels of sustained attention, or vigilance (Nelson, McKinley, Golob, Warm, & Parasuraman, 2014). A later study employed a virtual airspace monitoring scenario, wherein participants were tasked with surveilling and identifying each incoming aircraft as either "friend of foe." (McKinley, McIntire, Nelson, Nelson, & Goodyear, 2017, pp. 176–178).

For each of the studies referenced above, significant cognition-enhancing effects were identified—i.e., pharmaceutical stimulants, and tDCS, each appeared to appreciably improve cognitive performance. While not the primary subject matter, study findings also highlight the utility of VR as a platform for assessing enhanced cognitive performance during operationally relevant tasks. As reported by McKinley, McIntire, Nelson, Nelson, & Goodyear (2017), an important objective of their investigation was to examine the effects of tDCS in "complex tasks that are more relevant to real-world activities" (p. 181). For this particular study, that objective was met through the use of VR, which allowed them to simulate a complex operational task (i.e., monitoring of a hostile airspace) relevant to real-world activities performed by their study population (i.e., 32 active duty Air Force service members).

VR continues to serve as a useful platform for assessment among investigators involved in cognitive enhancement research. However, studies that have so far been conducted involving military-specific VR-based assessment are few in number, limited in terms of sample sizes used, and generally exploratory in nature. Preliminary research findings are encouraging, but much remains to be explored through future investigations, with much larger sample sizes and greater methodological rigor.

## EMERGING RESEARCH AND DEVELOPMENT INITIATIVES

As of this writing, there are many innovative developments that are just beginning to emerge. Some of the VR-based applications currently being researched are primarily intended to be used for clinical assessment with patients whose cognitive function has become impaired due to neurological injury or illness. One example is the Avatar-Administered Neuropsychological Test (AVANT) application, a DoD-funded research initiative aiming to develop an advanced form of computer-automated neuropsychological assessment battery, which will guide patients through test administration procedures via an artificially intelligent virtual clinician avatar (Parsons, 2016b).

VR-based platforms are also being researched for purposes of evaluating, and ultimately improving upon, cognitive performance and operational effectiveness of healthy unimpaired soldiers. For instance, researchers from the Center for Applied Brain & Cognitive Sciences (CABSC) at the Natick Soldier Research, Development, and Engineering Center (NSRDEC) are actively engaged in studies evaluating soldier cognitive abilities via operationally relevant VE scenarios, which are presented to soldier research participants within an immersive VR dome enclosure (Benson, 2016;Figure 8.13). While findings have yet to be published, investigators are hopeful that they will obtain novel insights into soldiers' cognitive functioning under conditions which closely approximate their actual experience and behavior in real-world deployed environments. The VR dome enclosure will also serve as a test bed for development and evaluation of new types of soldier equipment and technologies designed to optimize soldier cognitive performance in the field.

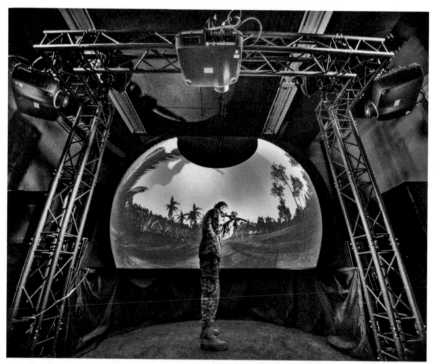

FIGURE 8.13 *Natick Soldier Research, Development, and Engineering Center (NSRDEC) virtual reality dome. Army photograph taken by David Kamm (February 24, 2016), professional photographer, Natick Soldier Research, Development, and Engineering Center (NSRDEC), U.S. Army. Retrieved from http://www.army.mil/media/424525/. The image has been officially released by the Army and is in the public domain.*

The Physiological and Cognitive Operational Research Environment (PhyCORE) VR system located at the Naval Health Research Center (NHRC) is being utilized for a number of ongoing VR-based cognitive assessment research initiatives (Sessoms, 2016). Specific research focus areas include traumatic brain injury assessment and rehabilitation, injury prevention, cognitive readiness, performance optimization and resilience. Similar research is performed at the Sensorimotor Technology Realization in Immersive Virtual Environments (STRIVE) Center at the Massachusetts Institute of Technology (MIT Lincoln Laboratory, 2016). Current STRIVE Center research mission areas include clinical assessment and rehabilitation, technology development, and cognitive performance optimization for improved operational effectiveness of military service members while training or deployed.

## Conclusion

This chapter explores the historical trajectory of neuropsychological assessment technologies within the military, from paper-and-pencil tests developed toward the beginning of the 20th century, to computer-automated neuropsychological assessments, and finally to the cutting-edge VR-based assessment applications of today. Despite 100 years of technological advancements, many neuropsychological assessment instruments in current use bear a striking likeness to paper-and-pencil-based instruments, which predate the Army Alpha and Beta tests of World War I (Boake, 2002).

While limited in some respects, traditional computer-based assessment applications have several demonstrable advantages that have benefited clinicians for over 50 years, but they remain underutilized by many of today's clinical neuropsychologists (Rabin et al., 2014). The military has been somewhat more progressive in its adoption of computer-based instruments, as evidenced by DoD-wide implementation of the Automated Neuropsychological Assessment Metrics (ANAM) application (Department of Defense, 2015), but VR-based neuropsychological assessment applications have yet to become commonplace in any setting, within or outside of the military.

Although there are considerable challenges to be addressed before widespread adoption of VR is to be realized, evidence gathered thus far supports the clinical utility and ecological validity of VR-based applications for neuropsychological assessment (Areces, Rodríguez, García, Cueli, & González-Castro, 2016; Besnard et al., 2016; Cogné et al., 2016; Diaz-Orueta et al., 2016; Diaz-Orueta, Lizarazu, Climent, & Banteria, 2014; Gamito et al., 2016; Lopez, Deliens, & Cleeremans, 2016; Negut, Matu, Sava, & Davis, 2015, 2016; Parsey & Schmitter-Edgecombe, 2013; Parsons, 2016a; Parsons, Carlew, Magtoto, & Stonecipher, 2015; Pedroli et al., 2016; Teel, Gay, Johnson, & Slobounov, 2016). Studies involving military-specific VR-based assessment applications have also yielded positive results in support of their validity and clinical value (Armstrong et al., 2013; Chen & Joyner, 2009; Edwards, Vess, Reger, & Cernich, 2014; Kelley, Ranes, Estrada, & Grandizio, 2015; Onakomaiya, Kruger, Highland, & Roy, 2016a, 2016b; Parsons et al., 2012; Rabago, Pruziner, & Esposito, 2015; Rabago & Wilken, 2011; Robitaille et al., 2016). VR-based neuropsychological assessment applications have not yet actualized their full potential, but they have been steadily evolving. Empirical evidence gathered to date is in aggregate highly supportive and encouraging. Prospects for the continued future progression of VR-based neuropsychological assessment applications within the military appear to be exceptionally favorable.

# References

Adams, K. M. (1975). Automated clinical interpretation of the neuropsychological battery: An ability based approach. *Dissertation Abstracts International: Section B. Sciences and Engineering, 35,* 6085.

Adams, K. M. (1986). Concepts and methods in the design of automata for neuropsychological test interpretation. In S. B. Filskov & T. J. Boll (Eds.), *Handbook of clinical neuropsychology* (Vol. 2, pp. 561–576). New York, NY: Wiley.

Adams, K. M., & Brown, G. C. (1986). The role of the computer in neuropsychological assessment. In I. Grant & K. M. Adams (Eds.), *Neuropsychological assessment of neuropsychiatric disorders* (pp. 87–89). New York, NY: Oxford University Press.

Adams, K. M., & Heaton, R. K. (1985). Automated interpretation of neuropsychological test data. *Journal of Consulting and Clinical Psychology 53*(6), 790–802. doi:10.1037/0022006X.53.6.790

Aguinas, H., Henle, C. A., & Beaty, J. C., Jr. (2001). Virtual reality technology: A new tool for personnel selection. *International Journal of Selection and Assessment, 9*(1/2), 70–83. doi:10.1111/1468-2389.00164

Alderman, N., Burgess, P. W., Knight, C., & Henman, C. (2003). Ecological validity of a simplified version of the multiple errands shopping test. *Journal of the International Neuropsychological Society, 9*(1), 31–44. doi:10.1017/S1355617703910046.

Amick, M. M., Kraft, M., & McGlinchey, R. (2013). Driving simulator performance of veterans from the Iraq and Afghanistan wars. *Journal of Rehabilitation Research and Development, 50*(4), 463–470. doi:10.1682/JRRD.2012.06.0108

Andrews, T. K., Rose, F. D., Leadbetter, A. G., Attree, E. A., & Painter, J. (1995). The use of virtual reality in the assessment of cognitive ability. In I. P. Porrero, & R. Puig de la Bellacasa (Eds.), *The European Context for Assistive Technology: Proceedings of the 2nd TIDE Congress* (pp. 276–279). Amsterdam, Netherlands: IOS Press.

Areces, D., Rodríguez, C., García, T., Cueli, M., & González-Castro, P. (2016). Efficacy of a continuous performance test based on virtual reality in the diagnosis of ADHD and its clinical presentations. *Journal of Attention Disorders.* Advance online publication. doi:10.1177/1087054716629711

Armstrong, C. M., Reger, G. M., Edwards, J., Rizzo, A. A., Courtney, C. G., & Parsons, T. D. (2013). Validity of the Virtual Reality Stroop Task (VRST) in active duty military. *Journal of Clinical and Experimental Neuropsychology, 35*(2), 113–123. doi:10.1080/13803395.2012.740002

Ashendorf, L., & Reynolds, E. (2013). Process analysis of the Digit Symbol task. In L. Ashendorf, R. Swenson, & D. Libon (Eds.), *The Boston process approach to neuropsychological assessment: A practitioner's guide* (pp. 77–87). New York, NY: Oxford University Press.

Baldwin, B. T. (1919). The function of psychology in the rehabilitation of disabled soldiers. *Psychological Bulletin, 16*(8), 267–290. doi:10.1037/h0070987

Bartlett, J. L., Sessoms, P. H., & Reini, S. A. (2013). Strength through science: Using virtual technology to advance the warfighter. *Aviation, Space, and Environmental Medicine, 84*(2), 165–166. doi:10.3357/ASEM.3578.2013

Bauer, R. M., Iverson, G. L., Cernich, A. N., Binder, L. M., Ruff, R. M., & Naugle, R. I. (2012). Computerized neuropsychological assessment devices: Joint position paper of the American Academy of Clinical Neuropsychology and the National Academy of Neuropsychology. *The Clinical Neuropsychologist, 26*(2), 177–196, doi:10.1080/13854046.2012.663001

Bayroff, A. G. (1964). *Feasibility of a programmed testing machine* (Research Study No. 64-63). Washington, DC: U.S. Army Personnel Research Office.

Bedard, M., Parkkari, M., Weaver, B., Riendeau, J., & Dahlquist, M. (2010). Assessment of driving performance using a simulator protocol: Validity and reproducibility. *American Journal of Occupational Therapy, 64*(2), 336–340. doi:10.5014/ajot.64.2.336

Benedict, R. H. B. (1997). *Brief Visuospatial Memory Test—Revised.* Odessa, FL: Psychological Assessment Resources.

Benson, J. (2016, February 24). Virtual reality dome: Impact of real-life scenarios on cognitive abilities. *Natick Soldier Research, Development and Engineering Center (NSRDEC) Public Affairs.* https://www.army.mil/article/162899/virtual_reality _ dome_impact_of_real_life_scenarios_on_cognitive_abilities/

Benton, A. L. (1945). A visual retention test for clinical use. *Archives of Neurology & Psychiatry, 54*(3), 212–216. doi:10.1001/archneurpsyc.1945.02300090051008

Benton, A. L. (1994a). Four neuropsychologists. *Neuropsychology Review, 4*(1), 31–44. doi:10.1007/BF01875020

Benton, A. L. (1994b). Judgement of line orientation. In A. L. Benton, A. B. Sivan, K. Hamsher, N. R. Varney, & O. Spreen (Eds.), *Contributions to neuropsychological assessment: A clinical manual* (2nd ed., pp. 53–64). New York, NY: Oxford University Press.

Benton, A. L., Varney, N. R., & Hamsher, K. D. (1978). Visuospatial judgment: A clinical test. *Archives of Neurology, 35*(6), 364–367. doi:10.1001/archneur.1978.00500300038006

Berka, C., Pojman, N., Trejo, J., Coyne, J., Cole, A., Fidopiastis, C, & Nicholson, D. (2011). NeuroGaming: Merging cognitive neuroscience & virtual simulation in an interactive training platform. In T. Marek, W. Karwowski, & V. Rice (Eds.), *Advances in understanding human performance: Neuroergonomics, human factors design, and special populations* (pp. 313–324). Boca Raton, FL: CRC Press. doi:10.1201/EBK143983 5012-33

Besnard, J., Richard, P., Banville, F., Nolin, P., Aubin, G., Le Gall, D., ... Allain, P. (2016). Virtual reality and neuropsychological assessment: The reliability of a virtual kitchen to assess daily-life activities in victims of traumatic brain injury. *Applied Neuropsychology: Adult, 23*(3), 223–235. doi:10.1080/23279095.2015.1048514

Biggs, A. T., Cain, M. S., & Mitroff, S. R. (2015). Cognitive training can reduce civilian casualties in a simulated shooting environment. *Psychological Science, 26*(8), 1164–1176. doi:10.1177/0956797615579274

Bilder, R. M. (2011). Neuropsychology 3.0: Evidence-based science and practice. *Journal of the International Neuropsychological Society, 17*(1), 7–13. doi:10.1017/S1355617710001396

Binet, A., & Henri, V. (1895). La psychologie individuelle [Individual psychology]. *L'Année Psychologique, 2,* 411–465. doi:10.3406/psy.1895.1541

Binet, A., & Henri, V. (1898). *La fatigue intellectuelle* [Intellectual fatigue]. Retrieved from http://www.archive.org/details/lafatigueintelloobine

Binet, A., & Simon, T. (1905) Méthodes nouvelles pour le diagnostic du niveau intellectuel des anormaux [New methods for the diagnosis of the intellectual level of subnormals]. *L'Année Psychologique, 11,* 191–244. doi:10.3406/psy.1904.3675

Binet, A., & Simon, T. (1908). Le développement de l'intelligence chez les enfants [The development of intelligence in children]. *L'Année Psychologique, 14,* 1–94. doi:10.3406/psy.1907.3737

Bittner, A. C., Smith, M. G., Kennedy, R. S., Staley, C. F., & Harbeson, M. M. (1985). Automated Portable Test (APT) System: Overview and prospects. *Behavior Research Methods, Instruments, & Computers, 17*(2), 217–221. doi:10.3758/BF03214386

Boake, C. (1989). A history of cognitive rehabilitation of head injured patients 1915–1980. *Journal of Head Trauma Rehabilitation, 4*(3), 1–8. doi:10.1097/00001199-198909000-00004

Boake, C. (2002). From the Binet-Simon to the Wechsler-Bellevue: Tracing the history of intelligence testing. *Journal of Clinical and Experimental Neuropsychology, 24*(3), 383–405. doi:10.1076/jcen.24.3.383.981

Bohil, C. J., Alicea, B., & Biocca, F. A. (2011). Virtual reality in neuroscience research and therapy. *Nature Reviews Neuroscience, 12*(12), 752–762. doi:10.1038/nrn3122

Botella, C., García-Palacios, A., Guillen, V., Baños, R. M., Quero, S., & Alcaniz, M. (2010). An adaptive display for the treatment of diverse trauma PTSD victims. *Cyberpsychology, Behavior, and Social Networking, 13*(1), 67–71. doi:10.1089/cyber.2009.0353

Brandt, J., & Benedict, R. H. B. (2001). *The Hopkins Verbal Learning Test–Revised.* Odessa, FL: Psychological Assessment Resources.

Burgess, P. W., Alderman, N., Forbes, C., Costello, A., Coates, L. M., Dawson, D. R., . . . Channon, S. (2006). The case for the development and use of "ecologically valid" measures of executive function in experimental and clinical neuropsychology. *Journal of the International Neuropsychological Society, 12*(2), 194–209. doi:10.1017/S1355617706 060310

Bush, S., Naugle, R., & Johnson-Greene, D. (2002). Interface of information technology and neuropsychology: Ethical issues and recommendations. *The Clinical Neuropsychologist, 16*(4), 536–547. doi:10.1076/clin.16.4.536.13911

Butcher, J. N., Perry, J., & Hahn, J. (2004). Computers in clinical assessment: Historical developments, present status, and future challenges. *Journal of Clinical Psychology, 60*(3), 331–345. doi:10.1002/jclp.10267

Buxbaum, P. (2015, December). Battlespace platform. *Military Training Technology, 20*(7), 38–43.

Caldwell, J., Caldwell, L., Smith, J., Alvarado, L., Heintz, T., Mylar, J., & Brown, D. (2004). *The efficacy of modafinil for sustaining alertness and simulator flight performance in F-117 pilots during 37 hours of continuous wakefulness* (Report No.

AFRL-HE-BR-TR-2004-0003). Brooks City-Base, TX: Human Effectiveness Directorate, Biosciences and Protection Division, Fatigue Countermeasures Branch.

Campbell, D. P. (1971). An informal history of the SVIB. In *Handbook for the Strong Vocational Interest Blank* (pp. 343–365). Stanford, CA: Stanford University Press.

Campbell, Z., Zakzanis, K. K., Jovanovski, D., Joordens, S., Mraz, R., & Graham, S. J. (2009). Utilizing virtual reality to improve the ecological validity of clinical neuropsychology: An fMRI case study elucidating the neural basis of planning by comparing the Tower of London with a three-dimensional navigation task. *Applied Neuropsychology, 16*(4), 295–306. doi:10.1080/09084280903297891

Carlson, K. F., O'Neil, M. E., Forsberg, C. W., McAndrew, L. M., Storzbach, D., Cifu, D. X., & Sayer, N. A. (2016). Risk of hospitalization due to motor vehicle crashes among Iraq and Afghanistan War Veterans diagnosed with traumatic brain injury. *NeuroRehabilitation, 39*(3), 351–361. doi:10.3233/NRE-161367

Carretta, T. R., & Ree, M. J. (2003). Pilot selection methods. In P. S. Tsang & M. A. Vidulich (Eds.), *Principles and practice of aviation psychology* (pp. 357–396). Mahwah, NJ: Lawrence Erlbaum.

Carroll, J. B. (1987). Measurement and educational psychology: Beginnings and repercussions. In J. A. Glover & R. R. Ronning (Eds.), *Historical foundations of educational psychology* (pp. 89–106). New York, NY: Plenum Press.

Castles, E. C. (2012). A century of IQ testing: The more things change the more they stay the same. In D. Carvalko (Ed.), *Inventing intelligence: How America came to worship IQ* (pp. 105–120). Santa Barbara, CA: Praeger/ABC-CLIO.

Causse, M., Dehais, F., & Pastor, J. (2011). Executive functions and pilot characteristics predict flight simulator performance in general aviation pilots. *The International Journal of Aviation Psychology, 21*(3), 217–234. doi:10.1080/10508414.2011.582441

Cernich, A. N., Brennana, D. M., Barker, L. M., & Bleiberg, J. (2007). Sources of error in computerized neuropsychological assessment. *Archives of Clinical Neuropsychology, 22S*, S39–S48. doi:10.1016/j.acn.2006.10.004

Cevette, M. J., Stepanek, J., Cocco, D., Galea, A. M., Pradhan, G. N., Wagner, L. S., ... Brookler, K. H. (2012). Oculo-vestibular recoupling using galvanic vestibular stimulation to mitigate simulator sickness. *Aviation, Space, and Environmental Medicine, 83*(6), 549–555. doi:10.3357/ASEM.3239.2012

Chaytor, N., & Schmitter-Edgecombe, M. (2003). The ecological validity of neuropsychological tests: A review of the literature on everyday cognitive skills. *Neuropsychology Review, 13*(4), 181–197. doi:10.1023/B:NERV.0000009483.91468.fb

Chaytor, N., Schmitter-Edgecombe, M., & Burr, R. (2006). Improving the ecological validity of executive functioning assessment. *Archives of Clinical Neuropsychology, 21*(3), 217–227. doi:10.1016/j.acn.2005.12.002

Chen, J. Y. C., & Joyner, C. T. (2009). Concurrent performance of gunner's and robotics operator's tasks in a multitasking environment. *Military Psychology, 21*(1), 98–113. doi:10.1080/08995600802565785

Choi, S. Y., Yoo, D. H., & Lee, J. S. (2015). Usefulness of the driveABLE cognitive assessment in predicting the driving risk factor of stroke patients. *Journal of Physical Therapy Science, 27*(10), 3133–3135. doi:10.1589/jpts.27.3133

Cipresso, P., Serino, S., & Riva, G. (2016). Psychometric assessment and behavioral experiments using a free virtual reality platform and computational science.

BMC Medical Informatics and Decision Making, 16(37), 1–11. doi:10.1186/s12911-016-0276-5

Clark, V. P., Coffman, B. A., Mayer, A. R., Weisend, M. P., Lane, T. D. R., Calhoun, V. D., … Wassermann, E. M. (2012). TDCS guided using fMRI significantly accelerates learning to identify concealed objects. NeuroImage, 59(1), 117–128. doi:10.1016/j.neuroimage.2010.11.036

Classen, S., & Brooks, J. (2014). Driving simulators for occupational therapy screening, assessment, and intervention. Occupational Therapy in Health Care, 28(2), 154–162. doi:10.3109/07380577.2014.901590

Classen, S., Levy, C., Meyer, D. L., Bewernitz, M., Lanford, D. N., & Mann, W. C. (2011). Simulated driving performance of combat veterans with mild traumatic brain injury and posttraumatic stress disorder: A pilot study. American Journal of Occupational Therapy, 65(4), 419–427. doi:10.5014/ajot.2011.000893

Classen, S., Monahan, M., Canonizado, M., & Winter, S. (2014). Utility of an occupational therapy driving intervention for a combat veteran. The American Journal of Occupational Therapy, 68(4), 405–411. doi:10.5014/ajot.2014.010041

Coffman, B. A., Trumbo, M. C., Flores, R. A., Garcia, C. M., van der Merwe, A. J., Wassermann, E. M., … Clark, V. P. (2012). Impact of tDCS on performance and learning of target detection: Interaction with stimulus characteristics and experimental design. Neuropsychologia, 50(7), 1594–1602. doi:10.1016/j.neuropsychologia.2012.03.012

Cohen, I., Brinkman, W. P., & Neerincx, M. A. (2015). Modelling environmental and cognitive factors to predict performance in a stressful training scenario on a naval ship simulator. Cognition, Technology and Work, 17(4), 503–519. doi:10.1007/s10111-015-0325-3

Collins, A. (2006). An intimate connection: Oliver Zangwill and the emergence of neuropsychology in Britain. History of Psychology, 9(2), 89–112. doi:10.1037/1093-4510.9.2.89

Collins, J., Markham, A., Service, K., Reini, S., Wolf, E., & Sessoms, P. (2015). A systematic literature review of the use and effectiveness of the Computer Assisted Rehabilitation Environment for research and rehabilitation as it relates to the wounded warrior. Work, 50(1), 121–129. doi:10.3233/WOR-141927

Comptroller General of the United States. (1976). An assessment of all-volunteer force recruits: Department of Defense: report to the Congress. Washington, DC: U.S. General Accounting Office.

Cogné, M., Taillade, M., N'Kaoua, B., Tarruella, A., Klinger, E., Larrue, F., … Sorita, E. (2016). The contribution of virtual reality to the diagnosis of spatial navigation disorders and to the study of the role of navigational aids: A systematic literature review. Annals of Physical and Rehabilitation Medicine. Advance online publication. doi:10.1016/j.rehab.2015.12.004

Ćosić, K., Popović, S., Kukolja, D., Horvat, M., & Dropuljic, B. (2010). Physiology-driven adaptive virtual reality stimulation for prevention and treatment of stress related disorders. Cyberpsychology, Behavior, and Social Networking, 13(1), 73–78. doi:10.1089/cyber.2009.0260

Cox, B. D., Edwards, H. M., Service, K. A., Sessoms, P. H., Dominguez, J. A., & Zheng, W., & Reini, S. A. (2015). Toward cognitive two-way interactions in an immersive virtual reality environment (Paper No. 15332). Proceedings of the 2015 Interservice/

*Industry Training, Simulation, and Education Conference (I/ITSEC).* Retrieved from http://www.iitsecdocs.com/volumes/2015

Cox, D. J., Davis, M., Singh, H., Barbour, B., Nidiffer, F. D., Trudel, T., . . . Moncrief, R. (2010). Driving rehabilitation for military personnel recovering from traumatic brain injury using virtual reality driving simulation: A feasibility study. *Military Medicine, 175*(6), 411–416. doi:10.7205/MILMED-D-09-00081

Courtney, C. G., Dawson, M. E., Rizzo, A. A., Arizmendi, B. J., & Parsons, T. D. (2013). Predicting navigation performance with psychophysiological responses to threat in a virtual environment. In R. Schumaker (Ed.), *Virtual augmented and mixed reality: Designing and developing augmented and virtual environments* (pp. 129–138). Berlin: Springer. doi:10.1007/978-3-642-39405-8_16

Crook, T. H., Kay, G. G., & Larrabee, G. J. (2009). Computer-based cognitive testing. In I. Grant, & K. M. Adams (Eds.), *Neuropsychological assessment of neuropsychiatric and neuromedical disorders* (3rd ed., pp. 84–100). New York, NY: Oxford University Press.

Curtis, M. K., Dawson, K., Jackson, K., Litwin, L., Meusel, C., Dorneich, M. C., . . .Winer, E. (2015). Mitigating visually induced motion sickness: A virtual hand-eye coordination task. *Proceedings of the Human Factors and Ergonomics Society Annual Meeting, 59*(1), 1839–1843. doi:10.1177/1541931215591397

Dando, C., & Tranter, C. (2016). Military and defence applications. In A. Attrill & C. Fullwood (Eds.), *Applied cyberpsychology: Practical applications of cyberpsychological theory and research* (pp. 197–215). London, England: Palgrave Macmillan UK. doi:10.1057/9781137517036_12

Darr, W. (2009). *A psychometric examination of the Canadian Automated Pilot Selection System* (CAPSS; Technical Memorandum No. DGMPRA TM 2009-024). Ottawa, Canada: Director General Military Personnel Research & Analysis (DGMPRA). Retrieved from http://cradpdf.drdc-rddc.gc.ca/PDFS/unc126/p532336_A1b.pdf

De Angelo, J. (2000). The Link flight trainer—A historic mechanical engineering landmark, 1-12. *American Society of Mechanical Engineers (ASME) International.* Retrieved from https://www.asme.org/getmedia/d75b81fd-83e8-4458-aba7-166a87d35811/210-Link-C-3-Flight-Trainer.aspx

Dede, E., Zalonis, I., Gatzonis, S., & Sakas, D. (2015). Integration of computers in cognitive assessment and level of comprehensiveness of frequently used computerized batteries. *Neurology, Psychiatry and Brain Research, 21*(3), 128–135. doi:/10.1016/j.npbr.2015.07.003

Department of the Army. (2012). *Soldier's manual of common tasks: Warrior skills level 1* (Publication No. STP 21-1-SMCT). Washington, DC: Department of the Army.

Department of Defense. (2015, September). *Comprehensive policy on traumatic brain injury-related neurocognitive assessments by the military services* (DoD Instruction 6409.13). Retrieved from https://www.hsdl.org/?view&did=787206

Diaz-Orueta, U., Climent, G., Cardas-Ibáñez, J., Alonso, L., Olmo-Osa, J., & Tirapu-Ustarroz, J. (2016). Evaluación de la memoria mediante realidad virtual: Presente y futuro [Memory assessment by means of virtual reality: Its present and future]. *Revista de Neurologia, 62*(2), 75–84.

Diaz-Orueta, U., Lizarazu, B., Climent, G., & Banterla, F. (2014). Virtual reality for neuropsychological assessment. In M. Ma, C. L. Jain, & P. Anderson (Eds.),

*Virtual, augmented reality and serious games for healthcare 1* (pp. 233–255). Berlin, Germany: Springer Science & Business. doi:10.1007/978-3-642-54816-1_13

Dores, A. R., Barbosa, F., Guerreiro, S., Almeida, I., & Carvalho, I. P. (2016). Computer-based neuropsychological rehabilitation: Virtual reality and serious games. In M. M. Cruz-Cunha, I. M. Miranda, R. Martinho, & R. Rijo (Eds.), *Encyclopedia of e-health and telemedicine* (pp. 473–485). Hershey, PA: IGI Global. doi:10.4018/978-1-4666-9978-6.ch037

Dores, A. R., Mendes, L., Carvalho, I. P., Guerreiro, S., Almeida, I., & Barbosa, F. (2016). Significance of virtual reality-based rehabilitation in acquired brain injury. In F. Hu, J. Lu, & T. Zhang (Eds.), *Virtual reality enhanced robotic systems for disability rehabilitation* (pp. 164–179). Hershey, PA: IGI Global. doi:10.4018/978-1-4666-9740-9.ch009

Drasgow, F. (2014). An overview of the ASVAB. In J. D. Held, T. R. Carretta, J. W. Johnson, & R. A. McCloy (Eds.), *Introductory guide to conducting ASVAB validation/standards studies in the U.S. Navy* (Technical Report No. NPRST-TR-15-1, pp. 9–21). Millington, TN: Navy Personnel Research, Studies, and Technology (NPRST), Bureau of Naval Personnel.

Duchak, G. D. (1990). *The conversion of a Singer/Link GAT-1B analog flight simulator into a digital flight simulator* (Accession No. ADA246085). Retrieved from the Defense Technical Information Center (DTIC) website: http://www.dtic.mil/dtic/tr/fulltext/u2/a246085.pdf

Dumenigo, N., Scarrino, N., & Golden, C. (2015). The relationship between WAIS-IV IQ indices and driving simulator performance. *Archives of Clinical Neuropsychology, 30*(6), 580. doi:10.1093/arclin/acv047.250

Eber, H. W. (1964, September). *Automated personality description with 16-PF data.* Paper presented at the meeting of the American Psychological Association, Los Angeles, CA.

Edwards, J., Vess, J., Reger, G., & Cernich, A. (2014). The use of virtual reality in the military's assessment of service members with traumatic brain injury: Recent developments and emerging opportunities. *Applied Neuropsychology: Adult, 21*(3), 220–230. doi:10.1080/09084282.2013.796554

Elkind, J. S., Rubin, E., Rosenthal, S., Skoff, B., & Prather, P. (2001). A simulated reality scenario compared with the computerized Wisconsin Card Sorting Test: An analysis of preliminary results. *CyberPsychology & Behavior, 4*(4), 489–496. doi:10.1089/109493101750527042

Eling, P., Derckx, K., & Maes, R. (2008). On the historical and conceptual background of the Wisconsin Card Sorting Test. *Brain and Cognition, 67*(3), 247–253. doi:10.1016/j.bandc.2008.01.006

Elsmore, T. F., Naitoh, P., & Linnville, S. (1992). *Performance assessment in sustained operations using a computer-based synthetic work task* (Report No. 92-30). San Diego, CA: Naval Health Research Center.

Everett, R. R. (1952). The Whirlwind I computer. *Electrical Engineering, 71*(8), 681–686. doi:10.1109/EE.1952.6437630

Falcone, B., Coffman, B. A., Clark, V. P., & Parasuraman, R. (2012). Transcranial direct current stimulation augments perceptual sensitivity and 24-hour retention in a complex threat detection task. *PLoS ONE, 7*(4), 1–10. doi:10.1371/journal.pone.0034993

Feldstein, S. N., Keller, F. R., Portman, R. E., Durham, R. L., Klebe, K. J., & Davis, H. P. (1999). A comparison of computerized and standard versions of the Wisconsin Card Sorting Test. *The Clinical Neuropsychologist, 13*(3), 303–313. doi:10.1076/clin.13.3.303.1744

Fernandes, A. S., & Feiner, S. K. (2016). Combating VR sickness through subtle dynamic field-of-view modification. In B. H. Thomas, R. Lindeman, & M. Marchal (Eds.), *2016 IEEE Symposium on 3D User Interfaces (3DUI) Proceedings* (pp. 201–210). Piscataway, NJ: Institute of Electrical and Electronics Engineers (IEEE) doi:10.1109/3DUI.2016.7460053

Ferguson, K. E., & Iverson, G. L. (2011). Test interpretations: Computer based. In J. S. Kreutzer, J. DeLuca, & B. Caplan (Eds.), *Encyclopedia of clinical neuropsychology* (pp. 2490–2491). New York, NY: Springer New York. doi:10.1007/978-0-387-79948-3_1259

Finkelstein, J. N. (1977). Brain: A computer program for interpretation of the Halstead-Reitan Neuropsychological Test Battery. *Dissertation Abstracts International: Section B. Sciences and Engineering, 37,* 5349.

Freeman, J., Nicholson, D., Squire, P., & Bolton, A. (2014). Data & analytics tools for agile training & readiness assessment (Paper No. 14064). *Proceedings of the 2014 Interservice/Industry Training, Simulation, and Education Conference (I/ITSEC).* Retrieved from http://www.iitsecdocs.com/volumes/2014

French, C. C., & Beaumont, J. G. (1990). A clinical study of the automated assessment of intelligence by the Mill Hill Vocabulary Test and the Standard Progressive Matrices test. *Journal of Clinical Psychology, 46*(2), 129–140. doi:10.1002/1097-4679(199003)46:2<129::AID-JCLP2270460203>3.0.CO;2-Y

French, L. M., Anderson-Barnes, V., Ryan, L. M., Zazeckis, T. M., & Harvey, S. (2012). Neuropsychological practice in the military. In C. H. Kennedy & E. A. Zilmer (Eds.), *Military psychology: Clinical and operational applications* (2nd ed., pp. 185–210). New York, NY: Guilford Press.

Friedl, K. E., Grate, S. J., Proctor, S. P., Ness, J. W., Lukey, B. J., & Kane, R. L. (2007). Army research needs for automated neuropsychological tests: Monitoring soldier health and performance status. *Archives of Clinical Neuropsychology, 22S,* S7–S14. doi:10.1016/j.acn.2006.10.002

Gálvez-García, G. (2015). A comparison of techniques to mitigate simulator adaptation syndrome. *Ergonomics, 58*(8), 1365–1371. doi:10.1080/00140139.2015.1005168

Gálvez-García, G., Albayay, J., Rehbein, L., & Tornay, F. (2017). Mitigating Simulator Adaptation Syndrome by means of tactile stimulation. *Applied Ergonomics, 58,* 13–17. doi:10.1016/j.apergo.2016.05.004.

Gamito, P., Oliveira, J., Brito, R., Lopes, P., Rodelo, L., Pinto, L., & Morais, D. (2016). Evaluation of cognitive functions through the Systemic Lisbon Battery: Normative data. *Methods of Information in Medicine, 55*(1), 93–97. doi:10.3414/ME14-02-0021

Gelb, A., & Goldstein, K. (1920). *Psychologische analysen hirnpathologischer fälle* [Psychological analysis of cases of brain injury]. Leipzig, Germany: Verlag Von Johann Ambrosius Barth.

Gilliland, K., & Schlegel, R. E. (1993). Review of computer-based performance assessment batteries. Appendix A of *Readiness to perform testing: A critical analysis of the concept and current practices* (Report No. DOT/FAA/AM-93/13, pp. A1–A14). Washington, DC: FAA Office of Aviation Medicine, Federal Aviation Administration.

Gilson, S., & Glennerster, A. (2012). High fidelity immersive virtual reality. In T. Xinxing (Ed.), *Virtual reality—Human computer interaction* (pp. 41–58), InTech. doi:10.5772/ 50655 Available from: http://www.intechopen.com/books/virtual-reality-human-computer-interaction/high-fidelity-immersive-virtual-reality

Golden, C. J., Purisch, A. D., & Hammeke, T. A. (1985). *Luria-Nebraska Neuropsychological Battery: Forms I and II manual.* Los Angeles, CA: Western Psychological Services.

Goldstein, K. (1919). *Die behandlung, fürsorge und begutachtung der hirnverletzten (Zugleich ein beitrag zur verwendung psychologischer methoden in der klinik)* [Treatment, care and evaluation of brain injuries (At the same time a contribution to the use of psychological methods in the clinic)]. Leipzig, Germany: F. C. W. Vogel.

Goldstein, K. (1942). *Aftereffects of brain injuries in war: Their evaluation and treatment.* New York, NY: Grune & Stratton.

Goldstein, K., & Scheerer, M. (1941). Abstract and concrete behavior: An experimental study with special tests. *Psychological Monographs, 53*(2), i–151. doi:10.1037/h0093487

Gottshall, K. R., & Sessoms, P. H. (2015). Improvements in dizziness and imbalance results from using a multidisciplinary and multisensory approach to vestibular physical therapy—A case study. *Frontiers in Systems Neuroscience, 9,* 1–7. doi:10.3389/ fnsys.2015.00106

Gottshall, K. R., Sessoms, P. H., & Bartlett, J. L. (2012, August). Vestibular physical therapy intervention: Utilizing a Computer Assisted Rehabilitation Environment in lieu of traditional physical therapy. *Proceedings of the Engineering in Medicine and Biology Society (EMBS), 34th Annual International Conference of the IEEE,* 6141–6144. doi:10.1109/EMBC.2012.6347395

Gourley, S. (2016). Stimulating simulation: Technology advances and upgrades boost realism in soldier training. *ARMY Magazine, 66*(3). Retrieved from http://www. armymagazine.org/ 2016/02/16/stimulating-simulation-technology-advances-and-upgrades-boost-realism-in-soldier-training/

Grafman, J., Salazar, A., Weingartner, H., Vance, S., & Amin, D. (1986). The relationship of brain-tissue loss volume and lesion location to cognitive deficit. *The Journal of Neuroscience, 6*(2), 301–307. Retrieved from http://www.jneurosci.org/content/6/2/ 301.full.pdf

Grandizio, C., Lawson, B., King, M., Cruz, P., Kelley, A., Erickson, B., . . .Chiaramonte, J. (2014). *Development of a fitness-for-duty assessment battery for recovering dismounted warriors* (USAARL Technical Report No. 2014-18). doi:10.13140/RG.2.1.1982.5688

Grant, D. A., & Berg, E. (1948). A behavioral analysis of degree of reinforcement and ease of shifting to new responses in a Weigl-type card-sorting problem. *Journal of Experimental Psychology, 38*(4), 404–411. doi:10.1037/h0059831

Gress, W., & Willkomm, B. (1996). Simulator based test systems as a measure to improve the prognostic value of aircrew selection. *Selection and Training Advances in Aviation:AGARD Conference Proceedings 588* (AGARD CP-588; pp. 15-1–15-4). Neuilly-sur-Seine, France: Advisory Group for Aerospace Research & Development (AGARD).

Gross, D. (2015). Technology management and user acceptance of virtual environment technology. In K. S. Hale & K. M. Stanney (Eds.), *Handbook of Virtual Environments: Design, Implementation, and Applications* (2nd Edition; pp. 493–504). Boca Raton, FL: CRC Press, Taylor & Francis Group. doi:10.1201/b17360-25

Guinosso, S. A., Johnson, S. B., Schultheis, M. T., Graefe, A. C., & Bishai, D. M. (2016). Neurocognitive correlates of young drivers' performance in a driving simulator. *Journal of Adolescent Health, 58*(4), 467–473. doi:10.1016/j.jadohealth.2015.12.018

Gur, R. C., Ragland, J. D., Moberg, P. J., Bilker, W. B., Kohler, C., Siegel, S. J., & Gur, R. E. (2001a). Computerized neurocognitive scanning: II. The profile of schizophrenia. *Neuropsychopharmacology, 25*(5), 777–788. doi:10.1016/S0893-133X(01)00279-2

Gur, R. C., Ragland, J. D., Moberg, P. J., Turner, T. H., Bilker, W. B., Kohler, C., . . . Gur, R. E. (2001b). Computerized neurocognitive scanning: I. Methodology and validation in healthy people. *Neuropsychopharmacology, 25*(5), 766–776. doi:10.1016/S0893-133X(01)00278-0

Harman, H. H., & Harper, B. P. (1953, October). AGO machines for test analysis. In W. N. Durost (Chair), *Proceedings of the invitational conference on testing problems* (pp. 154–156), New York, NY. Retrieved from http://files.eric.ed.gov/fulltext/ED173434.pdf

Hayhurst, H., Babika, C., Messerly, J., Williams, S., & Golden, C. (2015). Computerized tasks of executive functioning to total number of simulator driving errors. *Archives of Clinical Neuropsychology, 30*(6), 571. doi:10.1093/arclin/acv047.225

Head, H. (1926). *Aphasia and kindred disorders of speech* (Vols. 1–2). Cambridge, England: Macmillan.

Heaton, R. K., Chelune, G. J., Talley, J. L., Kay, G. G., & Curtis, G. (1993). *Wisconsin Card Sorting Test (WCST) manual: Revised and expanded.* Odessa, FL: Psychological Assessment Resources.

Heaton, R. K., & PAR Staff. (2003). *Wisconsin Card Sorting Test: Computer version 4.* Lutz, FL: Psychological Assessment Resources (PAR).

Hébert, L. J., McFadyen, B., Robitaille, N., Larochelle, J., Mercier, C., Jackson, P. L., . . . Richards, C. L. (2013, April). *Interactive virtual reality real-time avatar for military rehabilitation in the Canadian forces.* Paper presented at the NATO Science and Technology Organization Human Factors and Medicine Panel (HFM) Symposium, Milan, Italy. Retrieved from https://www.cso.nato.int/pubs/rdp.asp?RDP=STO-MP-HFM-228

Held, J. D., & Carretta, T. R. (2013). *Evaluation of tests of processing speed, spatial ability, and working memory for use in military occupational classification* (Technical Report No. NPRSTTR-14-1). Millington, TN: Navy Personnel Research, Studies, and Technology (NPRST), Bureau of Naval Personnel.

Held, J. D., Carretta, T. R., & Rumsey, M. G. (2014). Evaluation of tests of perceptual speed/ accuracy and spatial ability for use in military occupational classification. *Military Psychology, 26*(3), 199–220. doi:10.1037/mil0000043

Henderson, V. W. (2010). Cognitive assessment in neurology. In S. Finger, F. Boller, & K. L. Tyler (Eds.), *History of neurology: Handbook of clinical neurology* (Vol. 95, pp. 235–256). doi:10.1016/S0072-9752(08)02117-9

Highland, K. B., Kruger, S. E., & Roy, M. J. (2015). If you build it, they will come, but what will wounded warriors experience?—Presence in the CAREN. In B. Wiederhold, G. Riva, & M. D. Wiederhold (Eds.), *Studies in health technology and informatics: Vol. 219. Annual review of cybertherapy and telemedicine 2015* (pp. 23–27). Amsterdam, Netherlands: IOS Press. doi:10.3233/978-1-61499-595-1-23

Hildebrandt, L. K., McCall, C., Engen, H. G., & Singer, T. (2016). Cognitive flexibility, heart rate variability, and resilience predict fine-grained regulation of arousal during prolonged threat. *Psychophysiology, 53*(6), 880–890. doi:10.1111/psyp.12632

Hoffman, S. W., Shesko, K., & Harrison, C. R. (2010). Enhanced neurorehabilitation techniques in the DVBIC Assisted Living Pilot Project. *NeuroRehabilitation, 26*(3), 257–269. doi:10.3233/NRE-2010-0561

Homskaya, E. D. (2001). The forties: World War II and the rehabilitation hospital—neuropsychology in the making (D. Krotova, Trans.). In D. E. Tupper (Ed.), *Alexander Romanovich Luria: A scientific biography* (pp. 35–40). doi:10.1007/978-1-4615-12073_5

Horton, A. M., Jr., Vaeth, J., & Anilane, J. (1990). Computerized interpretation of the Luria-Nebraska Neuropsychological Battery: A pilot study. *Perceptual and Motor Skills, 71*(1), 83–86. doi:10.2466/pms.1990.71.1.83

Hoskins, L. L., Binder, L. M., Chaytor, N. S., Williamson, D. J., & Drane, D. L. (2010). Comparison of oral and computerized versions of the word memory test. *Archives of Clinical Neuropsychology, 25*(7), 591–600. doi:10.1093/arclin/acq060

Hunter, D. R. (1975). *Development of an enlisted psychomotor/perceptual test battery: Final report* (Report No. AFHRL-TR-75-60). Lackland Air Force Base, TX: Air Force Human Resources Laboratory, Personnel Research Division.

IBM (2011, February 22). *Icons of progress: Automated test scoring.* Retrieved from http://www-03.ibm.com/ibm/history/ibm100/us/en/icons/testscore/

Imhoff, S., Lavalliere, M., Teasdale, N., & Fait, P. (2016). Driving assessment and rehabilitation using a driving simulator in individuals with traumatic brain injury: A scoping review. *NeuroRehabilitation, 39*(2). doi:10.3233/NRE-161354

Iverson, G. L., Brooks, B. L., Ashton, V. L., Johnson, L. G., & Gualtieri, C. T. (2009). Does familiarity with computers affect computerized neuropsychological test performance? *Journal of Clinical and Experimental Neuropsychology, 31*(5), 594–604. doi:10.1080/13803390802372125

Iyer, A. V., Cosand, L. D., Courtney, C. G., Rizzo, A. A., & Parsons, T. D. (2009). Considerations for designing response quantification procedures in non-traditional psychophysiological applications. *Lecture Notes in Computer Science, 5638*, 479–487. doi:10.1007/978-3-642-02812-0_56

Jones, E., Fear, N. T., & Wessely, S. (2007). Shell shock and mild traumatic brain injury: A historical review. *The American Journal of Psychiatry, 164*(11), 1641–1645. doi:10.1176/appi.ajp.2007.07071180

Johnston, J., & Catano, V. M. (2013). Investigating the validity of previous flying experience, both actual and simulated, in predicting initial and advanced military pilot training performance. *The International Journal of Aviation Psychology, 23*(3), 227–244. doi:10.1080/10508414.2013.799352

Kaber, D. B., Riley, J. M., Endsley, M. R., Sheik-Nainar, M., Zhang, T., & Lampton, D. R. (2013). Measuring situation awareness in virtual environment-based training. *Military Psychology, 25*(4), 330–344. doi:10.1037/h0095998

Kane, R. L., & Kay, G. G. (1992). Computerized assessment in neuropsychological assessment: A review of tests and test batteries. *Neuropsychology Review, 3*(1), 1–117. doi:10.1007/ BF01108787

Kane, R. L., & Kay, G. G. (1997). Computer applications in neuropsychological assessment. In G. Goldstein & T. M. Incagnoli (Eds.), *Contemporary approaches in neuropsychological assessment: Critical issues in neuropsychology* (pp. 359–392). New York, NY: Plenum Press.

Kane, R. L., & Reeves, D. (1997). Computerized test batteries. In A. M. Horton, D. Wedding & J. Webster (Eds.), *The neuropsychology handbook* (Vol. 2, pp. 423–467). New York, NY: Springer.

Kay, G. G. (1995). *CogScreen-Aeromedical Edition: Professional manual.* Odessa, FL: Psychological Assessment Resources.

Kelley, A. M., Athy, J. R., King, M., Ericson, B., Chiaramonte, J., Vasbinder, M., & Thompson, A. (2011). *Think before you shoot: The relationship between cognition and marksmanship* (Technical Report No. USAARL 2011-23). Retrieved from the Defense Technical Information Center (DTIC) website: http://www.dtic.mil/dtic/tr/fulltext/u2/a553803.pdf

Kelley, A. M., Ranes, B. M., Estrada, A., & Grandizio, C. M. (2015). Evaluation of the Military Functional Assessment Program: Preliminary assessment of the construct validity using an archived database of clinical data. *Journal of Head Trauma Rehabilitation, 30*(4), E11–E20. doi:10.1097/HTR.0000000000000060

Kelly, M. P. (2013). Military neuropsychology. In B. A. Moore & J. E. Barnett (Eds.), *Military psychologists' desk reference* (pp. 48–52). New York, NY: Oxford University Press. doi:10.1093/med:psych/9780199928262.003.0010

Kennedy, C. H., Boake, C., & Moore, J. L. (2010). A history and introduction to military neuropsychology. In C. H. Kennedy & J. L. Moore (Eds.), *Military neuropsychology* (pp. 1–28). New York, NY: Springer.

Kennedy, C. H., Kupke, T., & Smith, R. (2000). A neuropsychological investigation of the Armed Services Vocational Aptitude Battery (ASVAB). *Archives of Clinical Neuropsychology, 15*(8), 696–697. doi:10.1016/S0887-6177(00)80085-2

Kennedy, Q., Nesbitt, P., & Alt, J. (2014). Assessment of cognitive components of decision making with military versions of the IGT and WCST. *Proceedings of the Human Factors and Ergonomics Society Annual Meeting, 58*(1), 300–304. doi:10.1177/1541931214581062

Keshavarz, B. (2016). Exploring behavioral methods to reduce visually induced motion sickness in virtual environments. In S. Lackey & R. Shumaker (Eds.), *Lecture Notes in Computer Science: Vol. 9740. Virtual, Augmented and Mixed Reality* (pp. 147–155). Cham, Switzerland: Springer International Publishing. doi:10.1007/978-3-319-39907-2_14

Klinger, E., Cao, X., Douguet, A. S., & Fuchs, P. (2009). Designing an ecological and adaptable virtual task in the context of executive functions. *Studies in Health Technology and Informatics, 144*, 248–252. doi:10.3233/978-1-60750-017-9-248

Knights, R. M., & Watson, P. (1968). The use of computerized test profiles in neuropsychological assessment. *Journal of Learning Disabilities, 1*(12), 696–709. doi:10.1177/002221946800101201

Ko, L., Shih, Y., Chikara, R. K., Chuang, Y., & Chang, E. C. (2016). Neural mechanisms of inhibitory response in a battlefield scenario: A simultaneous fMRI-EEG study. *Frontiers in Human Neuroscience, 10*(Article 185), 1–15. doi:10.3389/fnhum.2016.00185

Koenig, S. T., Krch, D., Chiaravalloti, N., Lengenfelder, J., Nikelshpur, O., Lange, B., . . . & Rizzo, A. A. (2014). Agile development of a virtual reality cognitive assessment. *Journal of accessibility and design for all: JACCES*, *4*(2), 53–68.

Kozuba, J., & Bondaruk, A. (2014). Flight simulator as an essential device supporting the process of shaping pilot's situational awareness. *Scientific Research & Education in the Air Force: 2014, Vol. 1* (pp. 41–60). Brasov, Romania: Henri Coanda Air Force Academy.

Kraft, M., Amick, M. M., Barth, J. T., French, L. M., & Lew, H. L. (2010). A review of driving simulator parameters relevant to the Operation Enduring Freedom/Operation Iraqi Freedom veteran population. *American Journal of Physical Medicine & Rehabilitation*, *89*(4), 336–344. doi:10.1097/PHM.0b013e3181d3eb5f

Kratz, K., Poppen, B., & Burroughs, L. (2007). The estimated full-scale intellectual abilities of U.S. Army aviators. *Aviation, Space, and Environmental Medicine*, *78*(5, Suppl. 1), B261–B267.

Kremen, W. S., Koenen, K. C., Boake, C., Purcell, S., Eisen, S. A., Franz, C. E., . . . Lyons, M. J. (2007). Pretrauma cognitive ability and risk for posttraumatic stress disorder: A twin study. *Archives of General Psychiatry*, *64*(3), 361–368. doi:10.1001/archpsyc.64.3.361

Laferrier, J. Z., Rice, I., Beyene, N., Sprunger, N., Simpson, R., Fairman, A., & Collins, D. M. (2013). Assistive technology, accessibility, and universal design. In R. A. Cooper, P. F. Pasquina, & R. Drach (Eds.), *Warrior transition leader: Medical rehabilitation handbook* (pp. 119–158), [Adobe Digital Editions version]. Washington, DC: Government Printing Office. Retrieved from https://www.overdrive.com/media/1311596/warrior-transition-leader

Lamargue-Hamel, D., Deloire, M., Saubusse, A., Ruet, A., Taillard, J., Philip, P., & Brochet, B. (2015). Cognitive evaluation by tasks in a virtual reality environment in multiple sclerosis. *Journal of the Neurological Sciences*, *359*(1-2), 94–99. doi:10.1016/j.jns.2015.10.039

Lampton, D. R., Knerr, B. W., Goldberg, S. L., Bliss, J. P., Moshell, M. J., & Blau, B. S. (1994). The Virtual Environment Performance Assessment Battery (VEPAB): Development and evaluation. *Presence: Teleoperators and Virtual Environments*, *3*(2), 145–157. doi:10.1162/pres.1994.3.2.145

Lampton, D. R., Knerr, B. W., Goldberg, S. L., Bliss, J. P., Moshell, M. J., & Blau, B. S. (1995). *The Virtual Environment Performance Assessment Battery (VEPAB): Development and evaluation* (ARI Technical Report No. 1029). Alexandria, VA: U.S. Army Research Institute for the Behavioral and Social Sciences.

Larson, G. E., Booth-Kewley, S., Highfill-McRoy, R. M., & Young, S. Y. (2009). Prospective analysis of psychiatric risk factors in marines sent to war. *Military Medicine*, *174*(7), 737–744.doi:10.7205/MILMED-D-02-0308

LaViola Jr., J. L. (2000). A discussion of cybersickness in virtual environments. *Special Interest Group on Computer-Human Interaction, SIGCHI Bulletin*, *32*(1), 47–56. doi:10.1145/333329.333344

LaViola Jr., J. L., Bowman, D., Kruijff, E., Pouprev, I., & McMahan, R. P. (2017). *3D user interfaces: Theory and practice* (2nd Edition). Boston, MA: Addison-Wesley Professional.

LeDuc, P., Rowe, T., Martin, C., Curry, I., Wildzunas, R., Schmeisser, E., ... Milam, L. (2009). *Performance sustainment of two man crews during 87 hours of extended wakefulness with stimulants and napping* (Report No. USAARL 2009-04). Fort Rucker, AL: U.S. Army Aeromedical Research Laboratory.

Lee, S., Lee, J. A., & Choi, H. (2016). Driving Trail Making Test part B: A variant of the TMT-B. *Journal of Physical Therapy Science, 28*(1), 148–153. doi:10.1589/jpts.28.148

Lehman, L. A. (2015). The potential value of virtual environments (VEs) in rehabilitation. *Journal of Mobile Technology in Medicine, 4*(3), 26–31. doi:10.7309/jmtm.4.3.5

Lele, A. (2013). Virtual reality and its military utility. *Journal of Ambient Intelligence and Humanized Computing, 4*(1), 17–26. doi:10.1007/s12652-011-0052-4

Letz, R. (2003). Continuing challenges for computer-based neuropsychological tests. *NeuroToxicology, 24*(4–5), 479–489. doi:10.1016/S0161-813X(03)00047-0

Levy, C. E., Halan, S., Silverman, E. P., Marsiske, M., Lehman, L., Omura, D., & Lok, B. C. (2015). Virtual environments and virtual humans for military mild traumatic brain injury and posttraumatic stress disorder: An emerging concept. *American Journal of Physical Medicine & Rehabilitation, 94*(4), e31–e32. doi:10.1097/PHM.0000000000000248

Lew, H. L., Amick, M. M., Kraft, M., Stein, M. B., & Cifu, D. X. (2010). Potential driving issues in combat returnees. *NeuroRehabilitation, 26*(3), 271–278. doi:10.3233/NRE-2010-0562

Lew, H. L., Kraft, M., Pogoda, T. K., Amick, M. M., Woods, P., & Cifu, D. X. (2011). Prevalence and characteristics of driving difficulties in Operation Iraqi Freedom/Operation Enduring Freedom combat returnees. *Journal of Rehabilitation Research and Development, 48*(8), 913–925. doi:10.1682/Jrrd.2010.08.0140

Lew, H. L., Rosen, P. N., Thomander, D., & Poole, J. H. (2009). The potential utility of driving simulators in the cognitive rehabilitation of combat-returnees with traumatic brain injury. *The Journal of Head Trauma Rehabilitation, 24*(1), 51–56. doi:10.1097/HTR.0b013e3181956fe3\r00001199-200901000-00007

Lichtenberger, E. O., & Kaufman, A. S. (Eds.). (2013). Introduction and overview. In *Essentials of WAIS-IV assessment* (2nd ed., pp. 1–53). Hoboken, NJ: John Wiley & Sons, Inc.

Lopez, M. C., Deliens, G., & Cleeremans, A. (2016). Ecological assessment of divided attention: What about the current tools and the relevancy of virtual reality. *Revue Neurologique, 172*(4), 270–280. doi:10.1016/j.neurol.2016.01.399

Lord, F. M. (1954). A study of speed factors in tests and academic grades. *ETS Research Bulletin Series, 1954*(2), 1–28. doi:10.1002/j.2333-8504.1954.tb00251.x

Lord, F. M. (1955). *Use of high-speed digital computers: An introduction to programming*. ETS Research Memorandum (Report No. RM-55-2). Princeton, New Jersey: Educational Testing Services.

Lumsden, T. (1916). The psychology of malingering and functional neuroses in peace and war. *The Lancet, 188*(4864), 860–863. doi:10.1016/S0140-6736(01)19511-5

Luria, A. R. (1948). Vosstanovleniye funkstii mozga posle voennoy travmi [Rehabilitation of brain functions after military wounds]. Moscow, Russia: Akademiia Meditsinskikh Nauk SSSR.

Luria, A. R. (1963). *Restoration of function after brain injury* (B. Haigh, Trans.). New York, NY: Pergamon Press.

Luria, A. R. (1966). *Traumatic aphasia: Its syndromes, psychology and treatment* (D. Bowden, Trans.). The Hague: Mouton.

Luria, A. R. (1972). *The man with a shattered world: The history of a brain wound* (L. Solotaroff, Trans.). Cambridge, MA: Harvard University Press.

Macklin, M., Metzger, L., Litz, B., McNally, R., Lasko, N., Orr, S., & Pitman, R. (1998). Lower precombat intelligence is a risk factor for posttraumatic stress disorder. *Journal of Consulting and Clinical Psychology, 66*(2), 323–326. doi:10.1037/0022-006X.66.2.323

Matthews, W. (2014). Virtual payoff. *National Guard, 68*(1), 24–28.

McCloy, R. A., & Gibby, R. E. (2011). Computerized adaptive testing. In N. T. Tippins & S. Adler (Eds.), *Technology-enhanced assessment of talent* (pp. 153–189). San Francisco, CA: Jossey-Bass. doi:10.1002/9781118256022.ch5

McKinley, R. A., McIntire, L., Nelson, J., Nelson, J., & Goodyear, C. (2017). The effects of transcranial direct current stimulation (tDCS) on training during a complex procedural task. In K. S. Hale & K. M. Stanney (Eds.), *Advances in intelligent systems and computing: Vol. 488. Advances in neuroergonomics and cognitive engineering* (pp. 173–183). doi:10.1007/978-3-319-41691-5_15

McNeil, J. A., & Morgan, C. A. (2010). Cognition and decision making in extreme environments. In C. H. Kennedy & J. L. Moore (Eds.), *Military neuropsychology* (pp. 361–382). New York, NY: Springer.

Meier, M. J. (1992). Modern clinical neuropsychology in historical perspective. *American Psychologist, 47*(4), 550–558. doi:10.1037/0003-066X.47.4.550

MIT Lincoln Laboratory (2016). *MIT Lincoln Laboratory facts 2016-2017* (pp. 20–21). Lexington, MA: Massachusetts Institute of Technology. Retrieved from https://www.ll.mit.edu/publications/MITLL_FactsBook_2016.pdf

Morganti, F. (2004). Virtual interaction in cognitive neuropsychology. In G. Riva, C. Botella, P. Legeron, & G. Optale (Eds.), *Studies in Health Technology and Informatics, 99*, 55–70. doi:10.3233/978-1-60750-943-1-55

Morganti, F. (2016). "Being there" in a virtual world: An enactive perspective on presence and its implications for neuropsychological assessment and rehabilitation. In A. Przepiorka, P. Cipresso, & C. Lau (Eds.), *Human computer confluence: Transforming human experience through symbiotic technologies* (pp. 40–54). Berlin, Germany: De Gruyter Open. doi:10.1515/9783110471137-003

Moser, R. S., Schatz, P., & Lichtenstein, J. D. (2015). The importance of proper administration and interpretation of neuropsychological baseline and postconcussion computerized testing. *Applied Neuropsychology: Child, (4)*1, 41–48, doi:10.1080/21622965.2013.791825

Moten, C. (2015). *Understanding optimal decision-making in war-gaming III* (Technical Report No. TRAC-M-TM-15-030). Monterey, CA: U.S. Army Training and Doctrine Command (TRADOC) Analysis Center.

Murphy, J., Hannigan, F., Hruska, M., Medford, A., & Diaz, G. (2016). Leveraging interoperable data to improve training effectiveness using the Experience API (xAPI). In D. D. Schmorrow & C. M. Fidopiastis (Eds.), *Lecture Notes in Computer Science: Vol. 9744. Foundations of augmented cognition: Neuroergonomics and operational neuroscience* (pp. 46–54). Cham, Switzerland: Springer International Publishing. doi:10.1007/978-3-319-39952-2_5

National Research Council (2015). Fluid intelligence, working memory capacity, executive attention, and inhibitory control. In R. Katt (NRC Consultant Ed.), *Measuring human capabilities: An agenda for basic research on the assessment of individual and group performance potential for military accession* (pp. 29–52). Washington, DC: The National Academies Press. doi:10.17226/19017

Negut, A. (2014). Cognitive assessment and rehabilitation in virtual reality: Theoretical review and practical implications. *Romanian Journal of Applied Psychology, 16*(1), 1–7.

Negut, A., Jurma, A. M., & David, D. (2016). Virtual-reality-based attention assessment of ADHD: ClinicaVR: Classroom-CPT versus a traditional continuous performance test. *Child Neuropsychology.* Advance online publication. doi:10.1080/09297049.2016.1186617

Negut, A., Matu, S. A., Sava, F. A., & David, D. (2015). Convergent validity of virtual reality neurocognitive assessment: A meta-analytic approach. *Transylvanian Journal of Psychology, 16*(1), 31–54.

Negut, A., Matu, S., Sava, F. A., & David, D. (2016). Virtual reality measures in neuropsychological assessment: A meta-analytic review, *The Clinical Neuropsychologist, 30*(2), 165–184. doi:10.1080/13854046.2016.1144793

Nelson, J. T., McKinley, R. A., Golob, E. J., Warm, J. S., & Parasuraman, R. (2014). Enhancing vigilance in operators with prefrontal cortex transcranial direct current stimulation (tDCS). *NeuroImage, 85*(Part 3), 909–917. doi:10.1016/j.neuroimage.2012.11.061

Nicholson, D. M., Bartlett, K., Hoppenfeld, R., Nolan, M., & Schatz, S. (2014, May). *A virtual environment for modeling and testing sensemaking with multisensor information.* Paper presented at the Proceedings of the SPIE Defense and Security Symposium 2014, Baltimore, MD. doi:10.1117/12.2050780

Noyes, J. M., & Garland, K. J. (2008). Computer- vs. paper-based tasks: Are they equivalent? *Ergonomics, 51*(9), 1352–1375. doi:10.1080/00140130802170387

Nunnally, J. C. (1975). Psychometric theory—25 years ago and now. *Educational Researcher, 4*(10), 7–21. doi:10.3102/0013189X004010007

Olson, T. M., Walker, P. B., & Phillips, H. L. (2010). Assessment and selection of aviators in the U.S. military. In P. E. O'Connor & J. V. Cohn (Eds.), *Human performance enhancement in high-risk environments: Insights, developments, and future directions from military research* (pp. 37–57). Santa Barbara, CA: Praeger Security International.

Onakomaiya, M., Kruger, S., Highland, K., & Roy, M. (2016a). Multi-tasking in the Computer Assisted Rehabilitation Environment (CAREN) distinguishes service members with mild traumatic brain injury alone from those with comorbid post-traumatic stress disorder. *Journal of Neurotrauma, 33*(3), A-25. doi:10.1089/neu.2016.29005.abstracts

Onakomaiya, M., Kruger, S., Highland, K., & Roy, M. (2016b). Examining the value of an integrative, sensorimotor, multi-tasking virtual environment in the Computer Assisted Rehabilitation Environment (CAREN) in distinguishing between service members with traumatic brain injury alone and those with comorbid post-traumatic stress disorder. *Brain Injury, 30*(5–6), 675–676. doi:10.3109/02699052.2016.1162060

O'Regan, G. (2012). Early computers. In G. O'Regan (Ed.), *A brief history of computing* (pp. 35–52). London, England: Springer London. doi:10.1007/978-1-4471-2359-0_3

Orme, D. R., Brehm, W., & Ree, M. J. (2001). Armed Forces Qualification Test as a measure of premorbid intelligence. *Military Psychology, 13*(4), 187–197. doi:10.1207/S15327876 MP1304_1

Orme, D. R., Ree, M. J., & Rioux, P. (2001). Premorbid IQ estimates from a multiple aptitude test battery: Regression vs. equating. *Archives of Clinical Neuropsychology, 16*(7), 679–688. doi:10.1016/S0887-6177(00)00091-3

Ozonoff, S. (1995). Reliability and validity of the Wisconsin Card Sorting Test in studies of autism. *Neuropsychology, 9*(4), 491–500. doi:10.1037/0894-4105.9.4.491

Parasuraman, R., & Galster, S. (2013). Sensing, assessing, and augmenting threat detection: Behavioral, neuroimaging, and brain stimulation evidence for the critical role of attention. *Frontiers in Human Neuroscience, 7*(Article 273), 1–10. doi:10.3389/fnhum.2013.00273

Parker, J. W., & Auwood, J. A. (1966). *Ten point weighting with the IBM-805 test scoring machine* (Naval Submarine Medical Research Laboratory, NSMRL Report No. M-66-18). Ft. Belvoir, VA: Defense Technical Information Center.

Parsey, C. M., & Schmitter-Edgecombe, M. (2013). Applications of technology in neuropsychological assessment. *The Clinical Neuropsychologist, 27*(8), 1328–1361. doi:10.1080/13854046.2013.834971

Parsons, T. D. (2011). Neuropsychological assessment using virtual environments: Enhanced assessment technology for improved ecological validity. In S. Brahnam, & L. C. Jain (Eds.), *Advanced computational intelligence paradigms in healthcare 6: Virtual reality in psychotherapy, rehabilitation, and assessment* (pp. 271–289). Berlin, Heidelberg, Germany: Springer-Verlag. doi:10.1007/978-3-642-17824-5_13

Parsons, T. D. (2015a). Virtual reality for enhanced ecological validity and experimental control in the clinical, affective and social neurosciences. *Frontiers in Human Neuroscience, 9*, 1–19. doi:10.3389/fnhum.2015.00660

Parsons, T. D. (2015b). Ecological validity in virtual reality-based neuropsychological assessment. In M. Khosrow-Pour (Ed.), *Encyclopedia of information science and technology* (3rd ed., pp. 214–223). Hershey, PA: IGI Global. doi:10.4018/978-1-4666-5888-2.ch095

Parsons, T. D. (2016a). *Clinical neuropsychology and technology: What's new and how we can use it.* Basel, Switzerland: Springer International Publishing. doi:10.1007/978-3-319-31075-6

Parsons, T. D. (2016b, August). *Avatar Administered Neuropsychological Testing (AVANT).* Paper presented at the 24th annual Military Health System Research Symposium (MHSRS), Kissimmee, Florida.

Parsons, T. D., Carlew, A. R., Magtoto, J., & Stonecipher, K. (2015). The potential of function-led environments for ecologically valid measures of executive function in experimental and clinical neuropsychology. *Neuropsychological Rehabilitation.* Advance online publication. doi:10.1080/09602011.2015.1109524

Parsons, T. D., Cosand, L., Courtney, C., Iyer, A., & Rizzo, A. A. (2009). Neurocognitive workload assessment using the Virtual Reality Cognitive Performance Assessment Test. *Lecture Notes in Computer Science, 5639*, 243–252. doi:10.1007/978-3-642-02728-4_26

Parsons, T. D., & Courtney, C. G. (2011). Neurocognitive and psychophysiological interfaces for adaptive virtual environments. In M. Ziefle, & C. Röcker (Eds.), *Human* centered design of e-health technologies: Concepts, methods and applications (pp. 208–233). Hershey, PA: IGI Global. doi:10.4018/978-1-60960-177-5.ch009

Parsons, T. D., & Courtney, C. G. (2014). An initial validation of the Virtual Reality Paced Auditory Serial Addition Test in a college sample. *Journal of Neuroscience Methods, 222*, 15–23. doi:10.1016/j.jneumeth.2013.10.006

Parsons, T. D., & Courtney, C. G. (2016). Interactions between threat and executive control in a Virtual Reality Stroop Task. *IEEE Transactions on Affective Computing.* Advance online publication. doi:10.1109/TAFFC.2016.2569086

Parsons, T. D., Courtney, C. G., Arizmendi, B., & Dawson, M. (2011). Virtual Reality Stroop Task for neurocognitive assessment. *Studies in Health Technology and Informatics, 163*, 433–439. doi:10.3233/978-1-60750-706-2-433

Parsons, T. D., Courtney, C., Cosand, L., Iyer, A., Rizzo, A. A. & Oie, K. (2009). Assessment of psychophysiological differences of West Point cadets and civilian controls immersed within a virtual environment. *Lecture Notes in Computer Science, 5638*, 514–523. doi:10.1007/978-3-642-02812-0_60

Parsons, T. D., Courtney, C., & Dawson, M. (2013). Virtual Reality Stroop Task for assessment of supervisory attentional processing. *Journal of Clinical and Experimental Neuropsychology, 35*(8), 812–826. doi:10.1080/13803395.2013.824556

Parsons, T. D., Courtney, C., Rizzo, A. A., Edwards, J., & Reger, G. (2012). Virtual Reality Paced Serial Assessment Test for neuropsychological assessment of a military cohort. *Studies in Health Technology and Informatics, 173*, 331–337. doi:10.3233/978-1-61499-022-2-331

Parsons, T. D., Iyer, A., Cosand, L., Courtney, C., & Rizzo, A. A. (2009). Neurocognitive and psychophysiological analysis of human performance within virtual reality environments. *Studies in Health Technology and Informatics, 142*, 247–252. doi:10.3233/978-1-58603-964-6247

Parsons, T. D., & Phillips, A. S. (2016). Virtual reality for psychological assessment in clinical practice. *Practice Innovations, 1*(3), 197–217. doi:10.1037/pri0000028

Parsons, T. D., & Reinebold, J. L. (2012). Adaptive virtual environments for neuropsychological assessment in serious games. *IEEE Transactions on Consumer Electronics, 58*(2), 197–204. doi:10.1109/TCE.2012.6227413

Parsons, T. D., & Rizzo, A. A. (2008a, September). Neuropsychological assessment using the Virtual Reality Cognitive Performance Assessment Test. *Proceedings of the 7th International Conference on Disability, Virtual Reality and Associated Technologies (ICDVRAT 2008)*, Maia, Portugal.

Parsons, T. D., & Rizzo, A. A. (2008b). Neuropsychological assessment of attentional processing using virtual reality. *Annual Review of CyberTherapy and Telemedicine, 6*(1), 23–28.

Parsons, T. D., & Rizzo, A. A. (2008c). Initial validation of a virtual environment for assessment of memory functioning: Virtual Reality Cognitive Performance Assessment Test. *CyberPsychology & Behavior, 11*(1), 17–25. doi:10.1089/cpb.2007.9934

Parsons, T. D., Rizzo, A. A., Bamattre, J., & Brennan, J. (2007). Virtual Reality Cognitive Performance Assessment Test. *Annual Review of CyberTherapy and Telemedicine, 5*, 163–171.

Parsons, T. D., Rizzo, A. A., Courtney, C. G., & Dawson, M. E. (2012). Psychophysiology to assess impact of varying levels of simulation fidelity in a threat environment. *Advances in Human-Computer Interaction, 5*, 1–9. doi:10.1155/2012/831959

Parsons, T. D., Silva, T. M., Pair, J., & Rizzo, A. A. (2008). A virtual environment for assessment of neurocognitive functioning: Virtual Reality Cognitive Performance Assessment Test. *Studies in Health Technology and Informatics, 132*, 351–356.

Patton, D., & Gamble, K. (2016). Physiological measures of arousal during soldier-relevant tasks performed in a simulated environment. In D. D. Schmorrow & C. M. Fidopiastis (Eds.), *Lecture Notes in Computer Science: Vol. 9743. Foundations of augmented cognition: Neuroergonomics and operational neuroscience* (pp. 372–382). Cham, Switzerland: Springer International Publishing. doi:10.1007/978-3-319-39955-3_35

Patton, D., Loukota, P., & Avery, E. (2013, July). *Using the Immersive Cognitive Readiness Simulator to validate the ThreatFire Belt as an operational stressor: A pilot study.* Paper presented at the Proceedings of the 22nd Annual Conference on Behavior Representation in Modeling and Simulation (BRiMS), Ontario, Canada. Retrieved from http://cc.ist.psu.edu/BRIMS/archives/2013/BRIMS2013-140.pdf

Patton, D., & Marusich, L. (2015, March). *Simulated network effects on tactical operations on decision making.* Paper presented at the Proceedings of the 2015 IEEE International Inter-Disciplinary Conference on Cognitive Methods in Situation Awareness and Decision Support (CogSIMA), Orlando, FL. doi:10.1109/COGSIMA.2015.7108190

Pedroli, E., Serino, S., Giglioli, A. C., Pallavicini, F., Cipresso, P., & Riva, G. (2016). The use of virtual reality tools for the assessment of executive functions and unilateral spatial neglect. In F. Hu, J. Lu, & T. Zhang (Eds.), *Virtual reality enhanced robotic systems for disability rehabilitation* (pp. 115–140). Hershey, PA: IGI Global. doi:10.4018/978-1-4666-9740-9.ch007

Philips, B., & Morton, T. (2015). *Making driving simulators more useful for behavioral research—Simulator characteristics comparison and model-based transformation: Summary report* (Report No. FHWA-HRT-15-016). McLean, VA: U.S. Department of Transportation, Federal Highway Administration.

Piotrowski, Z. A. (1964). Digital-computer interpretation of inkblot test data. *The Psychiatric Quarterly, 38*(1), 1–26. doi:10.1007/BF01573364

Pommerich, M., Segall, D.O., & Moreno, K.E. (2009, June). *The nine lives of CAT-ASVAB: Innovations and revelations.* Paper presented at the Proceedings of the 2009 GMAC Conference on Computerized Adaptive Testing, Minneapolis, MN. Retrieved from: http://publicdocs.iacat.org/cat2010/cat09pommerich.pdf

Popović, S., Horvat, M., Kukolja, D., Dropuljic, B., & Ćosić, K. (2009). Stress inoculation training supported by physiology-driven adaptive virtual reality stimulation. *Studies in Health Technology and Informatics, 144*, 50–54. doi:10.3233/978-1-60750-017-9-50

Poppelreuter, W. (1917). *Die psychischen schädigungen durch kopfschuß im Krieg* [Disturbances of lower and higher visual capacities caused by occipital damage]. Leipzig, Germany: Verlag Von Leopold Voss.

Pugnetti, L., Mendozzi, L., Motta, A., Cattaneo, A., Barbieri, E., & Brancotti, A. (1995). Evaluation and retraining of adults' cognitive impairments: Which role for virtual reality technology? *Computers in Biology and Medicine, 25*(2), 213–227. doi:10.1016/0010-4825(94)00040-W

Rabago, C. A., Pruziner, A. L., & Esposito, E. R. (2015). Virtual reality-based assessment and treatment interventions for the combat-injured service member. *Proceedings of the 2015 International Conference on Virtual Rehabilitation (ICVR)*, Valencia, Spain. doi:10.1109/ICVR.2015.7358631

Rabago, C. A., & Wilken, J. M. (2011). Application of a mild traumatic brain injury rehabilitation program in a virtual reality environment: A case study. *Journal of Neurologic Physical Therapy, 35*(4), 185–193. doi:10.1097/NPT.0b013e318235d7e6

Rabin, L. A., Paolillo, E., & Barr, W. B. (2016). Stability in test-usage practices of clinical neuropsychologists in the United States and Canada over a 10-year period: A follow-up survey of INS and NAN members. *Archives of Clinical Neuropsychology, 31*(3), 206–230. doi:10.1093/arclin/acw007

Rabin, L. A., Spadaccini, A. T., Brodale, D. L., Grant, K. S., Elbulok-Charcape, M. M., & Barr, W. B. (2014). Utilization rates of computerized tests and test batteries among clinical neuropsychologists in the United States and Canada. *Professional Psychology: Research and Practice, 45*(5), 368–377. doi:10.1037/a0037987

Randolph. C. (1998). *Repeatable Battery for the Assessment of Neuropsychological Status manual.* San Antonio, TX: The Psychological Corporation.

Randolph. C. (2012). *Repeatable Battery for the Assessment of Neuropsychological Status Update manual.* Bloomington, MN: Pearson.

Rebenitsch, L., & Owen, C. (2016). Review on cybersickness in applications and visual displays. *Virtual Reality, 20*(2), 101–125. doi:10.1007/s10055-016-0285-9

Reeves, D. L., & Thorne, D. R. (1986). *A synopsis of UTC-PAB development* (Technical Report No. NMRI 86-125). Bethesda, MD: Naval Medical Research Institute.

Reeves, D. L., Winter, K. P., Bleiberg, J., & Kane, R. L. (2007). ANAM genogram: Historical perspectives, description, and current endeavors. *Archives of Clinical Neuropsychology, 22S,* S15–S37. doi:10.1016/j.acn.2006.10.013

Reger, G. M. (2013). Technology applications in delivering mental health services. In B. A. Moore & J. E. Barnett (Eds.), *Military psychologists' desk reference* (pp. 288–292). New York, NY: Oxford University Press. doi:10.1093/med:psych/9780199928262.003.0059

Reger, G. M., Parsons, T. D., Gahm, G. A., & Rizzo, A. A. (2010). Virtual reality assessment of cognitive functions: A promising tool to improve ecological validity. *Brain Injury Professional, 7*(3), 24–26.

Reitan, R. M., & Wolfson, D. (1993). *The Halstead-Reitan Neuropsychological Test Battery: Theory and clinical interpretation* (2nd ed.). Tucson, AZ: Neuropsychology Press.

Richardson, M. W. (1940). *Plans for the construction and validation of the Army Classification Test: A report to the Test Committee, National Research Council.* Washington, D.C.: National Research Council.

Rizzo, A. A. (1994, June). Virtual reality applications for the cognitive rehabilitation of persons with traumatic head injuries. In H. J. Murphy (Ed.), *Proceedings of the 2nd International Conference on Virtual Reality and Persons with Disabilities.* Northridge, CA: California State University. Retrieved from http://www.csun.edu/~hfdss006/conf/1994/proceedings/Thi~1.htm

Rizzo, A. A., Graap, K., Pair, J., Reger, G., Treskunov, A., & Parsons, T. D. (2006). User-centered design driven development of a virtual reality therapy application for Iraq war combat-related post traumatic stress disorder. In *Proceedings of the 6th International Conference on Disability, Virtual Reality and Associated Technology (ICDVRAT 2006, pp. 113–122),* Esbjerg, Denmark. doi:10.13140/RG.2.1.2757.9368

Rizzo, A. A., & Kim, G. J. (2005). A SWOT analysis of the field of virtual reality rehabilitation and therapy. *Presence, 14*(2), 119–146. doi:10.1162/1054746053967094

Rizzo, A. A., Parsons, T. D., Kenny, P., & Buckwalter, J. G. (2012). Using virtual reality for clinical assessment and intervention. In L. L'Abate, & D. A. Kasier (Eds.), *Handbook of technology in psychology, psychiatry, and neurology: Theory, research, and practice* (pp. 277–318), Hauppauge, NY: Nova Science Publishers.

Rizzo, A. A., Parsons, T. D., Lange, B., Kenny, P., Buckwalter, J. G., Rothbaum, B. O., . . . Reger, G. (2011). Virtual reality goes to war: A brief review of the future of military behavioral healthcare. *Journal of Clinical Psychology in Medical Settings, 18*(2), 176–187. doi:10.1007/s10880-011-9247-2

Robitaille, N., Jackson, P. L., Hébert, L. J., Mercier, C., Bouyer, L. J., Fecteau, S., . . . McFadyen, B. J. (2016). A Virtual Reality avatar interaction (VRai) platform to assess residual executive dysfunction in active military personnel with previous mild traumatic brain injury: Proof of concept. *Disability and Rehabilitation: Assistive Technology.* Advance online publication. doi:10.1080/17483107.2016.1229048

Rome, H. P., Swenson, W. M., Mataya, P., McCarthy, C. E., Pearson, J. S., Keating, F. R., & Hathaway, S. R. (1962). Symposium on automation techniques in personality assessment. *Proceedings of the Staff Meetings of the Mayo Clinic, 37,* 61–82.

Ross, W. A., Johnston, J. H., Riddle, D., Phillips, H., Townsend, L., & Milham, L. (2016). Making sense of cognitive performance in small unit training. In D. D. Schmorrow & C. M. Fidopiastis (Eds.), *Lecture Notes in Computer Science: Vol. 9744. Foundations of augmented cognition: Neuroergonomics and operational neuroscience* (pp. 67–75). Cham, Switzerland: Springer International Publishing. doi:10.1007/978-3-319-39952-2_7

Russell, E. W. (2000). The application of computerized scoring programs to neuropsychological assessment. In R. D. Vanderploeg (Ed.), *Clinician's guide to neuropsychological assessment* (2nd ed., pp. 483–515). New York, NY: Routledge.

Russell, E. W. (1995). The accuracy of automated and clinical detection of brain damage and lateralization in neuropsychology. *Neuropsychology Review, 5*(1), 1–68. doi:10.1007/BF02214929

Russell, E. W., Neuringer, C., & Goldstein, G. (1970). *Assessment of brain damage: A neuropsychological key approach.* New York, NY: Wiley-Interscience.

Russell, T. L., Ford, L., & Ramsberger, P. (2014). *Thoughts on the future of military enlisted selection and classification* (HumRRO Technical Report No. 053). Alexandria, VA: Human Resources Research Organization (HumRRO).

Russo, M., Fiedler, E., Thomas, M., & McGhee, J. (2005) Cognitive performance in operational environments. In *Strategies to maintain combat readiness during extended deployments—A human systems approach* (Report No. RTO-MP-HFM-124, paper 14, pp. 14-1–14-16). Neuilly-sur-Seine, France: North Atlantic Treaty Organization (NATO) Research and Technology Organization (RTO). doi:10.14339/RTO-MP-HFM-124

Salva, A. M., Alban, A. J., Wiederhold, M. D., Wiederhold, B. K., & Kong, L. (2009). Physiologically driven rehabilitation using virtual reality. In D. D. Schmorrow, I. V. Estabrooke, & M. Grootjen (Eds.), *Foundations of augmented cognition: Neuroergonomics and operational neuroscience* (Vol. 5638, pp. 836–845). doi:10.1007/978-3-642-02812-0_94

Samet, M., Geiselman, R. E., Zajaczkowski, F., & Marshall-Miles, J. (1986). *Complex Cognitive Assessment Battery (CCAB): Test descriptions.* Alexandria, VA: U.S. Army Research Institute.

Salisbury, D. B., Dahdah, M., Driver, S., Parsons, T. D., & Richter, K. M. (2016). Virtual reality and brain computer interface in neurorehabilitation. *Baylor University Medical Center Proceedings, 29*(2), 124–127.

Sands, W. A., Waters, B. K., & McBride, J. R. (Eds.). (1997). *Computerized adaptive testing: From inquiry to operation.* Washington, DC: American Psychological Association. doi:10.1037/10244-000

Sbordone, R. J. (1996). Ecological validity: Some critical issues for the neuropsychologist. In R. J. Sbordone & C. Long (Eds.), *Ecological validity of neuropsychological testing* (pp. 15–41). New York, NY: Charles Thomas.

Sbordone, R. J. (2008). Ecological validity of neuropsychological testing: Critical issues. In A. M. Horton Jr. & D. Wedding (Eds.), *The neuropsychology handbook* (3rd ed., pp. 367–394). New York, NY: Springer Publishing Company, LLC.

Schatz, P., & Browndyke, J. (2002). Applications of computer-based neuropsychological assessment. *The Journal of Head Trauma Rehabilitation, 17*(5), 395–410. doi:10.1097/00001199-2002100000003

Schaub, H. (2010). Assessment of military personnel for complex environment using human performance modeling. In *Human modelling for military application* (Report No. RTO-MP-HFM-202, paper 11, pp. 11-1–11-6). Neuilly-sur-Seine, France: North Atlantic Treaty Organization (NATO) Research and Technology Organization (RTO). doi:10.14339/RTO-MP-HFM-202-11-doc

Scherer, M. R., Weightman, M. M., Radomski, M. V, Davidson, L. F., & McCulloch, K. L. (2013). Returning service members to duty following mild traumatic brain injury: exploring the use of dual-task and multitask assessment methods. *Physical Therapy, 93*(9), 1254–1267. doi:10.2522/ptj.20120143

Schlegel, R. E., & Gilliland, K. (2007). Development and quality assurance of computer-based assessment batteries. *Archives of Clinical Neuropsychology, 22S*, S49–S61. doi:10.1016/j.acn.2006.10.005

Schultheis, M. T., & Chute, D. L. (1999). Development of a computerized, ecologically-valid driving assessment program: The Neurocognitive Driving Test (NDT). *Archives of Clinical Neuropsychology, 14*(8), 794–795. doi:10.1016/S0887-6177(99)80338-2

Schultheis, M. T., & Mourant, R. R. (2001). Virtual reality and driving: The road to better assessment for cognitively impaired populations. *Presence: Teleoperators and Virtual Environments, 10*(4), 431–439. doi:10.1162/1054746011470271

Scribner, D. R. (2016). Predictors of shoot–don't shoot decision-making performance: An examination of cognitive and emotional factors. *Journal of Cognitive Engineering and Decision Making, 10*(1), 3–13. doi:10.1177/1555343415608974

Segall, D. O, & Moreno, K. E. (1999). Development of the computerized adaptive testing version of the Armed Services Vocational Aptitude Battery. In F. Drasgow & J. B. Olson-Buchanan (Eds.), *Innovations in computerized assessment* (pp. 35–66). Mahwah, NJ: Lawrence Erlbaum Associates, Inc.

Seidel, R. J., & Chatelier, P. R. (Eds.) (1997). *Virtual reality, trainings future?: Perspectives on virtual reality and related emerging technologies.* New York, NY: Springer Science+Business Media. doi:10.1007/978-1-4899-0038-8

Semmes, J., Weinstein, S., Ghent, L., Meyer, J. S., & Teuber, H. L. (1963). Correlates of impaired orientation in personal and extrapersonal space. *Brain, 86*(4), 747–772. doi:10.1093/brain/86.4.747

Semmes, J., Weinstein, S., Ghent, L., &. Teuber, H. L. (1955). Spatial orientation in man after cerebral injury: 1. Analysis by locus of lesion. *Journal of Psychology, 39*, 227–243. doi:10.1080/00223980.1955.9916172

Serge, S. R., & Moss, J. D. (2015). Simulator sickness and the Oculus Rift: A first look. *Proceedings of the Human Factors and Ergonomics Society Annual Meeting, 59*(1), 761–765. doi:10.1177/1541931215591236

Sessoms, P. H. (2016, August). Enhancing warfighter readiness in a virtual environment. *Naval Medical Research and Development News, VIII*(8), 5-6. Retrieved from http://www.med.navy.mil/sites/nmrc/SiteCollectionDocuments/Aug%20%202016.pdf

Sessoms, P. H., Gottshall, K. R., Collins, J. D., Markham, A. E., Service, K. A., & Reini, S. A. (2015). Improvements in gait speed and weight shift of persons with traumatic brain injury and vestibular dysfunction using a virtual reality computer-assisted rehabilitation environment. *Military Medicine, 180*(Suppl. 3), 143–149. doi:10.7205/MILMED-D-14-00385

Sheehy, N., Chapman, A. J., & Conroy, W. A. (Eds.). (2002). Luria, Aleksandr Romanovich. In N. Sheehy, A. J. Chapman, & W. A. (Eds.), *Biographical dictionary of psychology* (pp. 365–366). New York, NY: Routledge.

Shin, H., & Kim, K. (2015). Virtual reality for cognitive rehabilitation after brain injury: A systematic review. *Journal of Physical Therapy Science, 27*(9), 2999–3002. doi:10.1589/ jpts.27.2999

Shingledecker, C. A. (1984). *A task battery for applied human performance assessment research* (Technical Report No. AFAMRL-TR-84-071). Wright-Patterson Air Force Base, OH: Air Force Aerospace Medical Research Laboratory.

Shively, S. B., & Perl, D. P. (2012). Traumatic brain injury, shell shock, and posttraumatic stress disorder in the military–Past, present, and future. *Journal of Head Trauma Rehabilitation, 27*(3), 234–239. doi:10.1097/HTR.0b013e318250e9dd

Sivan, A. D. (1992). *Benton Visual Retention Test* (5th ed.). New York, NY: The Psychological Corporation.

Slater, M. (2014). Grand challenges in virtual environments. *Frontiers in Robotics and AI, 1*(Article 3), 1–4. doi:10.3389/frobt.2014.00003

Smith, A. (1991). *Symbol Digit Modalities Test.* Los Angeles, CA: Western Psychological Services.

Staal, M. A., Bolton, A. E., Yaroush, R. A., & Bourne, L. E. (2008). Cognitive performance and resilience to stress. In B. J. Lukey & V. Tepe (Eds.), *Biobehavioral resilience to stress* (pp. 259–299). Boca Raton, FL: CRC Press, Taylor & Francis Group. doi:10.1201/97814 20071788.ch10

Stanney, K. M., & Cohn, J. V. (2012). Virtual environments. In J. A. Jacko (Ed.), *Human–computer interaction handbook: Fundamentals, evolving technologies, and emerging applications,* (3rd Edition; pp. 643–668). Boca Raton, FL: CRC Press, Taylor & Francis Group. doi:10.1201/b11963-32

Stanney, K. M., Hale, K. S., & Zyda, M. (2015). Virtual environments in the twenty-first century. In K. S. Hale & K. M. Stanney (Eds.), *Handbook of virtual environments: Design, implementation, and applications* (2nd Edition; pp. 3–22). Boca Raton, FL: CRC Press, Taylor & Francis Group. doi:10.1201/b17360-3

Steinmetz, J. P., Brunner, M., Loarer, E., & Houssemand, C. (2010). Incomplete psychometric equivalence of scores obtained on the manual and the computer version of the

Wisconsin Card Sorting Test? *Psychological Assessment, 22*(1), 199–202. doi:10.1037/a0017661

Strong, E. K., Jr., & Hankes, E. J. (1947). A note on the Hankes test scoring machine. *Journal of Applied Psychology, 31*(2), 212–214.

Stroop, J. R. (1935). Studies of interference in serial verbal reactions. *Journal of Experimental Psychology, 18*(6), 643–662. doi:10.1037/h0054651

Swiercinsky, D. P. (1978, September). *Computerized SAINT: System for analysis and interpretation of neuropsychological tests.* Paper presented at the meeting of the American Psychological Association, Toronto, Canada.

Szalma, J. L., Schmidt, T. N., Teo, G. W. L., & Hancock, P. A. (2014). Vigilance on the move: Video game-based measurement of sustained attention. *Ergonomics, 57*(9), 1315–1336. doi:10.1080/00140139.2014.921329

Taylor, J. L., O'Hara, R., Mumenthaler, M. S., & Yesavage, J. A. (2000). Relationship of CogScreen-AE to flight simulator performance and pilot age. *Aviation, Space, and Environmental Medicine, 71*(4), 373–380.

Teel, E., Gay, M., Johnson, B., & Slobounov, S. (2016). Determining sensitivity/specificity of virtual reality-based neuropsychological tool for detecting residual abnormalities following sport-related concussion. *Neuropsychology, 30*(4), 474–483. doi:10.1037/neu0000261

Terman, L. M. (1916). *The measurement of intelligence: An explanation of and a complete guide for the use of the Stanford revision and extension of the Binet-Simon intelligence scale.* Cambridge, MA: The Riverside Press.

Terman, L. M. (1918). The use of intelligence tests in the army. *Psychological Bulletin, 15*(6), 177–187. doi:10.1037/h0071532

Thomas, J. R., & Schrot, J. (1988). *Naval Medical Research Institute Performance Assessment Battery (NMRI-PAB) documentation* (Report No. NMRI 88-7). Bethesda, MD: Naval Medical Research Institute.

Thorne, D., Genser, S., Sing, H. C., & Hegge, F. W. (1985). The Walter Reed Performance Assessment Battery. *Neurobehavioral Toxicology and Teratology, 7*(4), 415–418.

Tucker, L. R. (1953, October). Use of electronic computing machines for testing problems. In W. N. Durost (Chair), *Proceedings of the invitational conference on testing problems* (pp. 151–153), New York, NY. Retrieved from http://files.eric.ed.gov/fulltext/ED173434.pdf

Tucker, L. R., & MacCallum, R. C. (1997). Factor fitting by statistical functions. In L. R. Tucker & R. C. MacCallum, *Exploratory factor analysis,* (pp. 256–315). Unpublished manuscript. Retrieved from https://www.unc.edu/~rcm/book/ch9.pdf

Uhlaner, J., & Bolanovich, D. (1952). *Development of the Armed Forces Qualification Test and predecessor Army screening tests, 1946–1950* (PRS Report 976). Retrieved from the Defense Technical Information Center (DTIC) website: http://www.dtic.mil/dtic/tr/fulltext/ u2/000191.pdf

U.S. Congress, Office of Technology Assessment (1994). *Virtual reality and technologies for combat simulation—Background paper* (OTA-BP-ISS-136). Washington, DC: U.S. Government Printing Office.

U.S. Congress, Office of Technology Assessment (1995). *Distributed interactive simulation of combat* (OTA-BP-ISS-151). Washington, DC: U.S. Government Printing Office.

U.S. Department of the Army (1962). Scoring Army tests. In *Army personnel tests and measurement* (pp. 84–90). Retrieved from http://www.ssi.army.mil/ncoa/AGS_SLC_ALC_ REGS/PAM%206112.pdf

van der Eerden, W. J., Otten, E., May, G., & Even-Zohar, O. (1999). CAREN—Computer Assisted Rehabilitation Environment. In J. D. Westwood, H. M. Hoffman, R. A. Robb, & D. Stredney (Eds.), *Studies in health technology and informatics: Vol. 62. Medicine meets virtual reality 7* (pp. 373–378). doi:10.3233/978-1-60750-906-6-373

van der Meer, R. (2014). Recent developments in computer assisted rehabilitation environments. *Military Medical Research, 1*(22), 1–7. doi:10.1186/2054-9369-1-22

Wald, J., & Liu, L. (2001). Psychometric properties of the driVR: A virtual reality driving assessment. In J. D. Westwood, H. M. Hoffman, G. T. Mogel, D. Stredney, & R. A. Robb (Eds.), *Studies in health technology and informatics: Vol. 81. Medicine meets virtual reality 2001* (pp. 564–566). doi:10.3233/978-1-60750-925-7-564

Wechsler, D. (2008). *Wechsler Adult Intelligence Scale—Fourth edition.* San Antonio, TX: Pearson.

Williams, J. E., & McCord, D. M. (2006). Equivalence of standard and computerized versions of the Raven Progressive Matrices Test. *Computers in Human Behavior, 22*(5), 791–800. doi:10.1016/j.chb.2004.03.005

Woo, E. (2008). Computerized neuropsychological assessments. *CNS Spectrums, 13,* 14–17. doi:10.1017/S1092852900026985

Wood, B. D. (1936, October). *Bulletin of information on the international test scoring machine.* New York, NY: The Cooperative Test Service of the American Council on Education.

Wright, W. G., McDevitt, J., Tierney, R., Dumont, M., Dumont, A., & Appiah-Kubi, K. (2014). *Virtual Environment TBI Screen* (VETS; Annual Report, Accession No. ADA613250). Retrieved from the Defense Technical Information Center (DTIC) website: http://oai.dtic. mil/oai/oai?verb=getRecord&metadataPrefix=html&identifier=ADA613250

Wrigley, C. (1957). Electronic computers and psychological research. *American Psychologist, 12*(8), 501–508. doi:10.1037/h0047607

Wu, D., Courtney, C. G., Lance, B. J., Narayanan, S. S., Dawson, M. E., Oie, K. S., & Parsons, T. D. (2010). Optimal arousal identification and classification for affective computing using physiological signals: Virtual Reality Stroop Task. *IEEE Transactions on Affective Computing, 1*(2), 109–118. doi:10.1109/T-AFFC.2010.12

Wu, D., Lance, B. J., & Parsons, T. D. (2013). Collaborative filtering for brain-computer interaction using transfer learning and active class selection. *PLoS ONE 8*(2), 1–18. doi:10.1371/journal.pone.0056624

Wu, D., & Parsons, T. D. (2011a). Active class selection for arousal classification. *Lecture Notes in Computer Science, 6975,* 132–141. doi:10.1007/978-3-642-24571-8_14

Wu, D., & Parsons, T. D. (2011b). Inductive transfer learning for handling individual differences in affective computing. *Lecture Notes in Computer Science, 6975,* 142–151. doi:10.1007/978-3-642-24571-8_15

Wu, D., & Parsons, T. D. (2012, August). Customized cognitive state recognition using minimal user-specific data. *Proceedings of the Military Health Systems Research Symposium,* Fort Lauderdale, FL.

Yerkes, R. M. (Ed.). (1921). *Psychological examining in the United States Army.* Washington, DC: Government Printing Office.

Yerkes, R. M., Bridges, J. W., & Hardwick, R. S. (1915). *A point scale for measuring mental ability.* Baltimore, MD: Warwick & York.

Yesavage, J. A., Jo, B., Adamson, M. M., Kennedy, Q., Noda, A., Hernandez, B., . . . Taylor, J. L. (2011). Initial cognitive performance predicts longitudinal aviator performance. *The Journals of Gerontology, Series B: Psychological Sciences and Social Sciences, 66*(4), 444–453. doi:10.1093/geronb/gbr031.

Yoakum, C. S., & Yerkes, R. M. (Eds.). (1920). *Army mental tests.* New York, NY: Henry Holt and Company.

Zangwill, O. L. (1945). A review of psychological work at the Brain Injuries Unit, Edinburgh, 1941–1945. *The British Medical Journal, 2*(4416), 248–251. doi:10.1136/bmj.2.4416.248

Zusman, M., & Golden, C. (2015). The relationship between the CPT-II and a driving simulator task. *Archives of Clinical Neuropsychology, 30*(6), 569. doi:10.1093/arclin/acv047.220

# 9

# Virtual Reality for Assessment of Episodic Memory in Normal and Pathological Aging

Gaën Plancher and Pascale Piolino

## Episodic Memory

Memory is one of the most important cognitive functions in a person's life. Memory is essential for recalling personal memories and for performing many everyday tasks, such as reading, playing music, returning home, and planning future actions, and, more generally, memory is crucial for interacting with the world. Determining how humans encode, store, and retrieve memories has a long scientific history, beginning with the classical research by Ebbinghaus in the late 20th century (Ebbinghaus, 1964). Since this seminal work, the large number of papers published in the domain of memory testifies that understanding memory is one of the most important challenges in cognitive neurosciences. With population growth and population aging, understanding memory failures both in the healthy elderly and in neurological and psychiatric conditions is a major societal issue.

A substantial body of evidence, mainly from double dissociations observed in neuropsychological patients, has led researchers to consider memory not as a unique entity but as comprising several forms with distinct neuroanatomical substrates (Squire, 2004). With reference to long-term memory, *episodic memory* may be described as the conscious recollection of personal events combined with their phenomenological and spatiotemporal encoding contexts, such as recollecting one's wedding day with all the contextual details (Tulving, 2002). Episodic memory is typically opposed to *semantic memory*, which is viewed as a system dedicated to the storage of facts and general decontextualized knowledge (e.g., Paris is the capital of France), including also the mental lexicon. Episodic memory was initially defined by Tulving as a memory system specialized in storing specific experiences in terms of what happened and where and when it happened (Tulving, 1972). Later, phenomenological processes were associated with the retrieval of memories (Tulving, 2002). Episodic memory is assumed to depend on the self, and involves mental time travel and a sense of reliving the original encoding context that includes autonoetic awareness (i.e., the awareness that this experience happened to oneself, is not happening now, and is part of one's personal history). More recently, the multiple components of memory (central and contextual information) that together form a complete episodic memory are thought to be linked through a process known as "binding" (Kessels, Hobbel, & Postma, 2007; Shimamura & Wickens, 2009). The neuronal substrates of episodic memory are widely distributed in the brain, from the medial temporal lobe, including the hippocampus (Davachi, 2006; Eichenbaum, Sauvage, Fortin, Komorowski, & Lipton, 2012), to the frontal lobe (Habib, Nyberg, & Tulving, 2003) and the parietal cortex (Cabeza, Ciaramelli, Olson, & Moscovitch, 2008).

Due to its large neuronal distribution, episodic memory is highly vulnerable. While episodic memory is considered to be the form of long-term memory that displays the greatest degree of age-related decline (Bäckman, Small, & Fratiglioni, 2001), its impairment is the most important deficit in Alzheimer's disease (AD) and constitutes a hallmark of early clinical manifestations (Hodges, 2006). Impairments in episodic memory function have also been described in individuals with mild cognitive impairment (MCI), Huntington's disease, Parkinson's disease, and psychiatric diseases, including schizophrenia, major depression, and dissociative disorders.

For decades, extensive research has been conducted on memory. While this research has led to a better understanding of memory, the majority of studies do not correspond to realistic situations close to daily life.

To further our understanding of memory, a sophisticated assessment is required, and hence the tools used to measure memory become crucial. The present chapter demonstrates how a new technology—virtual reality (VR)—can offer a relevant tool for the fundamental and clinical evaluation of memory. The discussion particularly focuses on episodic memory for two reasons: episodic memory is highly vulnerable to disease, and due to its complexity (what, where, when, and binding) it is the form of memory for which an ecological evaluation is of prime importance. The notion of *ecological validity* refers to the extent to which behavior indicative of cognitive functioning measured in one environment can be taken as characteristic of an individual's cognitive processes in a range of other environments (Barker, 1978; Bronfenbrenner, 1979). The discussion first addresses why VR provides features relevant for episodic memory assessment. Second, studies using VR for the fundamental comprehension of episodic memory are presented. Third, research on normal aging and on pathology is described. Finally, in conclusion some future perspectives are outlined.

## Contribution of Virtual Reality to Memory Assessment

To respect the need to work with well-controlled laboratory paradigms, the majority of studies have used verbal material. As pointed out by Tulving: "Words to the memory researcher are what fruit flies are to the geneticist: a convenient medium through which the phenomena and processes of interest can be explored and elucidated" (1983, p. 146). In verbal paradigms, participants typically study a list of words and are then tested on that list. Each word is assumed to constitute an event. In this traditional conception, the focus is placed on the number of items remaining in the store and accessible to memory. Neisser (1976) pointed out discontinuities between the spatial, temporal, and intermodal continuities of real objects and events characteristic of laboratory-based research, suggesting that: "It is almost as if ecological invalidity were a deliberate feature of the experimental design" (1976, p. 34).

A more naturalistic approach to memory has led to studies focusing on the quality of memory, giving rise to work on false memory and to studies assessing self-relevant and everyday life material. In particular, research on autobiographical memory tries to remain very close to everyday memory: a typical method is to provide participants with a verbal cue (e.g., *a journey*) and ask them to recall a personal memory from this cue (Piolino, Desgranges, & Eustache, 2009). These different approaches have advantages and disadvantages—while the former can be criticized for its weak ecological validity, the latter can be criticized for its weak experimental control (Koriat & Goldsmith, 1996).

We claim that different criteria have to be respected for episodic memory evaluation, in accordance with other views (McDermott, Szpunar, & Christ, 2009; Pause et al., 2013). To guarantee the best experimental control, episodic memories have to be induced in the laboratory; the encoding of memories must be incidental, in order to prevent semantic processes from taking place, and must remain totally episodic; the test should preferably involve a one-trial learning event, as is the case in real life; and, last, the episodic memory measure must include measures of what, where, and when (i.e., feature binding)

Tests based on VR represent an acceptable compromise between the experimental control required by all laboratory research and an everyday-memory-like assessment of episodic memory. Much of what people remember in everyday life refers to complex events, including visual information and actions that have been performed. Consequently, when we remember an event, typically we remember what happened, where and when it happened, and the multimodal details associated with it. Due to the infinite possibilities afforded by VR, one can investigate the memory of complex events, i.e., the memory for central and perceptual details, spatiotemporal contextual elements, and binding of the multidimensional information.

In a clinical neuropsychological approach, the assessment of cognition in an ecological fashion is crucial. During a rehabilitation program, if patients observe a difference between the forms of memory targeted by memory rehabilitation techniques and memory for general life experiences, the program won't offer patients meaningful forms of improvement, which might decrease their motivation. Because tests are sometimes far removed from patients' daily life experiences, it has also been observed that performance on standard neuropsychological tests does not predict patients' behavior in the real world (Bowman, 1996; Farias, Harrell, Neumann, & Houtz, 2003; Sbordone & Long, 1996; Schultheis, Himelstein, & Rizzo, 2002). In addition, a number of studies evaluating subjects' complaints of everyday memory problems have found weak associations with results on verbal memory tests (Jacoby, Jennings, & Hay, 1996; Pearman & Storandt, 2004; Plancher, Tirard, Gyselinck, Nicolas, & Piolino, 2012; Reid & Maclullich, 2006).

The ecological validity of studies conducted in neuropsychology has been criticized and the need for a neuropsychological assessment 3.0 has been formulated (Bohil, Alicea, & Biocca, 2011; Bowman, 1996; Farias et al., 2003; Parsons, 2015; Sbordone & Long, 1996; Schultheis et al., 2002). The lack of technological progress in the standardized testing industry has been pointed out by Sternberg (1997), and current standardized tests differ weakly from tests used throughout the last century. It is probably time to move from traditional paper-and-pencil batteries toward more ecologically valid tools, such as virtual environments (VEs; Parsons, 2015).

Classical neuropsychological tools used to assess episodic memory are far from encompassing its complexity (Table 9.1). In traditional neuropsychological assessment, the memory measure focuses most of the time on the core content (what) of episodic memory and uses verbal material, such as words or sentences (Grober & Buschke, 1987; Logical Memory Test, Wechsler, 1997). For visuospatial memory evaluation, the material used generally concerns abstract or concrete figures (e.g., Rey-Osterrieth Complex Figure, Meyers & Meyers, 1995; Family Pictures Test, Weschler, 1997), which bear little resemblance to everyday visuospatial memory.

TABLE 9.1  Comparison Between Standard Neuropsychological Tests and Virtual Reality Regarding Episodic Memory

| Criteria for episodic memory tests | Standard neuropsychological tests | Virtual reality tests |
| --- | --- | --- |
| Controlled laboratory studies | +++ | +++ |
| Recollection | + | +++ |
| Self-relevant events | − | ++ |
| Multimodality | + | +++ |
| Phenomenological context | + | ++ |
| Spatiotemporal context | + | +++ |
| Binding | − | +++ |
| Motivation | + | +++ |
| Transfer to reality | + | +++ |
| Predictive power in daily life | + | +++ |

+++: very high; ++: high; +: medium; −: low.

VR is gaining popularity as a tool in cognitive psychology and neuropsychology because it enables researchers and clinicians to create naturalistic and controlled situations with different levels of immersion (Bohil et al., 2011; Mueller et al., 2012; Zawadzki et al., 2013). According to Fuchs and colleagues (Fuchs, Moreau, Berthoz, & Vercher, 2006), the purpose of VR is to allow users to carry out cognitive and sensorimotor activities in an artificial world, i.e., a person immersed in the virtual world perceives and acts physically through the intermediary of sensory and motor interfaces. The virtual world is based on computer-generated three-dimensional (3D) images. It can be imaginary or symbolic, or it can simulate aspects of the real world.

When participants are immersed in the virtual world, they control their own displacements in the environment and they can have a real feeling of immersion (Mestre & Fuchs, 2006). A sensation of presence, or "being there," in the environment is important, as memory performance has been correlated with presence ratings for the experience in the VE (Schomaker, Roos, & Meeter, 2014). While the feeling of presence does not necessarily depend on the degree of realism or details of the VE, in order to achieve a VR experience, it is important to truly represent a real-world situation, instead of a simple video experience. Different levels of immersion can be achieved depending on the system (García-Betances, Arredondo Waldmeyer, Fico, & Cabrera-Umpiérrez, 2015). The non-immersive system involves a conventional computer, keyboard, and mouse; joysticks or gamepads may replace the mouse. Semi-immersive VR systems involve more sophisticated graphics, typically with a larger flat surface. A fully immersive VE consists of large surrounding projection surfaces, or 3D displays, such as head-mounted displays (HMDs), that place the patient inside the VE (e.g., a city, an apartment, a kitchen, a garden, etc.).

Neuropsychology as a discipline clearly stands to benefit from VR techniques. VR is flexible: an infinity of environments and experimental tasks can be created. Furthermore, VR offers the possibility of creating multimodal environments that stimulate all of the senses (vision, audition, olfaction, proprioception, tactile sensation, etc.). Lastly, it offers an alternative to rehabilitation in real-life situations that could be dangerous, costly, and hard to control. By creating rich multimodal environments and letting participants interact with them, memory assessment with VR can allow experiences closer to those of daily life than standard computer interfaces or paper-and-pencil tests.

## Virtual Reality Studies Assessing Memory in Young Adults

With an approach geared toward clinical neuropsychology, Parsons and Rizzo (2008) designed an experimental VR-based object memory and learning test (the Virtual Reality Cognitive Performance Assessment Test). Participants were asked to learn and recall objects across three free recall trials as a learning measure.

Subsequently, they navigated through five zones of a virtual city and for each zone, two items previously presented in the learning phase were presented again. Then the participants performed a delayed free recall task. The authors observed that performance on the VR test was consistent with that recorded by traditional paper-and-pencil measures involving learning and memory, thus validating the reliability of the virtual assessment of memory.

Because a main characteristic of VR is the possibility of creating a large-scale environment, many studies using VR have investigated spatial memory and navigation (Aguirre & D'Esposito, 1997; Brooks, Attree, Rose, Clifford, & Leadbetter, 1999; Gras, Gyselinck, Perrussel, & Orriols, 2013; Tlauka, Keage, & Clark, 2005; Wallet et al., 2011; Weniger, Ruhleder, Wolf, Lange, & Irle, 2009). These investigations show great rehabilitation promise, as it has been demonstrated for example that immersion in the virtual version of a city helped participants to transfer their spatial knowledge from the VE to the real world (Wallet et al., 2011). In addition, because it is convenient with this technology to directly compare active and passive exploration by keeping all other things equal, the question of how active learning enhances memory quickly arose. This kind of question fits with the framework of embodied cognition theories, for which "the mind must be understood in the context of its relationship to a physical body that interacts with the world" (Wilson, 2002). Memory should then be comprehended as a way to create meaning in the service of action (Glenberg, 1997).

Brooks and colleagues (1999) used a VE to compare the effects of active and passive conditions on recall of spatial layout, virtual objects, and their correct locations. Active participants used a joystick to navigate through a set of rooms. Passive participants watched the active participants' progress. At the same time, all participants had to look for an object. Active participants recalled the spatial layout better than passive participants. The authors attributed this benefit to an additional motor trace that increases the specificity of the memory. Different empirical findings suggest that active learning is important for memory (Nilsson, 2000; Carassa, Geminiani, Morganti, & Varotto, 2002; Nilsson, 2000; Zimmer et al., 2001). However, research using VR has yielded inconsistent results. Action is a complex cognitive construct; in a complex environment, action depends on the degree of interaction with the environment and freedom in the planning of an itinerary. Indeed, action has been defined as an intention to interact with the environment, rather than just a movement (Berthoz, 2003). The notion of planning thus appears as important as motion when investigating the effect of action on memory.

These hypotheses were tested by disentangling the interaction and planning components of action to examine whether each enhances factual and spatial memory (Plancher, Barra, Orriols, & Piolino, 2013). Participants explored a virtual town in one of three experimental conditions: a passive condition where participants were immersed as the passenger of the car (no interaction, no planning); a planning-only condition (the subject chose the itinerary but did not drive the car); and an interaction-only condition (the subject drove the car but the itinerary was fixed by the experimenter) (see Figure 9.1). The virtual

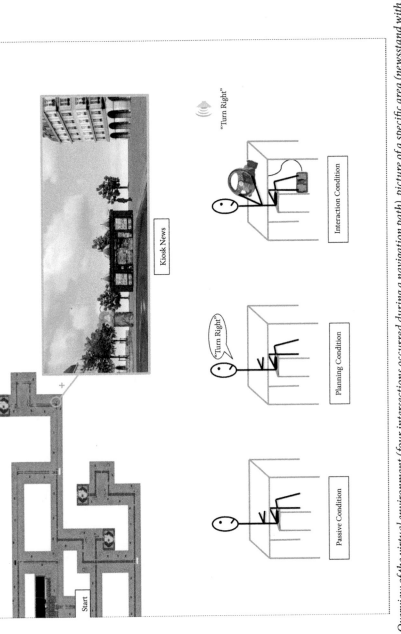

Start

Kiosk News

Passive Condition

Planning Condition

"Turn Right"

Interaction Condition

"Turn Right"

FIGURE 9.1 *Overview of the virtual environment (four intersections occurred during a navigation path), picture of a specific area (newsstand with a woman on the right and a statue on the left) and illustration of the three conditions. Passive condition: participants neither drove nor planned their itinerary. They watched the video of one participant who had driven the car in another condition. Planning condition: The experimenter drove the car; participants told the experimenter whether to turn left or right. Interaction condition: Participants drove the car, but the experimenter told them to turn left or right at each intersection. The experimenter's instructions to each subject in this third condition were based on the decisions of one subject in the planning condition. Since intersection, the participants saw the same elements regardless of what direction they turned in. From Plancher et al., 2013.*

equipment consisted of a computer-generated 3D model of an artificial environment built with novel in-house 3D software to create virtual urban environments and scenarios (Editomem & Simulamem, Memory and Cognition lab., Paris Descartes University; for an example, see https://www.youtube.com/watch?v=KfF7fv4L7pc). The program was run on a PC laptop computer and the VE was explored with a virtual car using a "real" steering wheel, gas pedal, and brake pedal. The VE was projected using a video projector onto a screen 85 cm high and 110 cm wide. Participants were seated in a comfortable chair and the VE was projected 150 cm in front of them. Free recall of the elements of the scenes (e.g., a girl, the train station, a no-entry sign) and a visuospatial memory test (drawing a map and locating elements on it; locating elements on a prepared map) were recorded. While itinerary choice and motor control both enhanced spatial memory, factual memory was impaired by online motor control. The benefit of action for spatial memory is here attributable to both interaction with the environment and route planning. The action enhancement previously observed in some VR studies could be due to the fact that the participants were able to navigate freely in the environment and to plan their itinerary. The negative impact of motion on factual memory can be explained by the costly attentional demands of motor control in VR environments.

Sauzéon and collaborators also investigated the differences between active and passive navigation on different measures of memory (Sauzéon et al., 2011). Using a 3D simulated apartment (HOMES test: Human Object Memory for Everyday Scenes), they aimed to investigate robust laboratory-based memory effects that provide clinically relevant information relative to learning, proactive interference, strategic processing, and false recognitions (as in a neuropsychological reference test, the California Verbal Learning Test (CVLT); Delis, Kramer, Kaplan, & Ober, 2000), and to study the possible influence of sensorimotor activity on these effects. They observed the expected effects of the four memory components classically obtained on standard paper-and-pencil memory tests (i.e., learning, proactive interference, memory strategies, and false memories). They also showed an active superiority effect on three measures (learning, retrieval strategy, and false memories) but not on active forgetting, encoding strategies, and gist-based false recognitions. According to the authors, their results demonstrate the important role of active navigation in strengthening distinctive memory traces and enriching source memory, but not in memory measures influenced by relational processing.

VR has also been used to determine the neural bases of episodic memory by discriminating factual and spatial components. Burgess and collaborators (Burgess, 2002; Burgess, Maguire, & O'Keefe, 2002; Burgess, Maguire, Spiers, & O'Keefe, 2001; King, Hartley, Spiers, Maguire, & Burgess, 2005) as well as Rauchs et al. (2008) used a VE to investigate the substrates of episodic memory with fMRI. In the study by Burgess et al. (2001), young participants followed a route with a joystick, in the course of which they encountered a number of people in different locations. Each person handed them an object. The memory of the objects, and of where and from whom they were received, was then assessed under functional neuroimaging. The authors observed that parahippocampal areas were specifically involved in the retrieval of spatial information, but not in the retrieval of object information, which involves more the parietal and prefrontal areas implicated by neuroimaging of retrieval of conventional laboratory stimuli. Recently, Park and collaborators (2014) directly measured neural oscillations involved in encoding novel environments in the human hippocampus during spatial navigation in a VE. Epileptic patients with implanted intracranial hippocampal depth electrodes performed a VE navigation and were instructed to remember the location of the objects during different blocks. The researchers observed that delta, theta, and low-gamma oscillations were associated with environmental novelty but that high-gamma oscillations were crucial for the successful encoding of the environmental novelty.

The above-mentioned studies have demonstrated that VR is relevant for the fundamental comprehension of memory in young adults. Because of the large-scale environment it offers, it enables an interesting investigation of the different components of episodic memory and the binding between the components; in addition, it makes it possible to examine the effect of action on episodic memory.

## Virtual Reality Studies Assessing Memory in Normal Aging

Due to its complexity, episodic memory is very sensitive to normal aging and neurodegenerative disorders (Aggleton & Pearce, 2001). In normal aging, the memory measures showing the highest effect are typically those involving strategic components requiring auto-initiated processes, such as free recall (Luo & Craik, 2008; Old & Naveh-Benjamin, 2008). When the core and contextual components of episodic memory are assessed, it is found that a decrease in memory performance affects mainly the spatiotemporal context and binding, indicating a source memory deficit (e.g., Chalfonte & Johnson, 1996; Kessels et al., 2007; Spencer & Raz, 1995). Episodic memory performance declines early in normal aging and this process is accentuated in AD. It is thus necessary to have sensitive tools for the cognitive stimulation of declining memory, to slow down the autonomy and cognition loss in elderly people and to improve well-being and quality of life during the aging process. The quality of the tools used to assess memory is also essential for diagnosis of a potential pathology. The prevention of cognitive and memory deficiencies could also be directed toward AD, particularly in older adults who have already begun to experience cognitive decline, namely, those with MCI, a category of persons who represent a preferential target of preventive interventions. We used VR to investigate episodic memory in normal aging (Plancher, Gyselinck, Nicolas, & Piolino, 2010; Plancher, Nicolas, & Piolino, 2008). We explored the effects of normal aging on the main aspects of episodic memory—what, where, and when—and on feature binding in an urban VE. Participants explored the virtual town via simulation of driving a car and saw several distinctive elements during their immersion (e.g., a fountain, the train station, a car accident). After a delay, participants were asked to freely recall and then recognize as much of the information encountered during the encoding phase as possible, specifying the perceptual details, the spatial and the temporal context of each factual element recalled. The main findings were that memory for spatiotemporal contexts decreases with aging, in accordance with previous studies (Chalfonte & Johnson, 1996; Kessels et al., 2007; Spencer & Raz, 1995), while memory for elements and perceptual details does not. In addition, we explored the influence of the mode of learning, intentional versus incidental. The majority of memory operations in daily life are incidental as opposed to intentional. However, neuropsychological tests seldom use incidental learning because it can be difficult to measure recall when encoding is not controlled. Previous experimental studies have demonstrated that participants perform better in memory tasks when they intentionally learn items, that is, when they make a conscious effort to memorize them, than when they learn the items incidentally and are not informed that their memory will be tested (Greene, 1986; Neill, Beck, Bottalico, & Molloy, 1990; Old & Naveh-Benjamin, 2008). We confirmed this finding with young adults, but found that older adults did not benefit as much as younger adults from effortful strategies. The fact that the deficit of memory with aging appeared mainly under intentional encoding is consistent with studies suggesting that deficits are observed in the context of tasks involving effortful processing, leaving more automatic processing unaffected (Hasher & Zacks, 1979; Old & Naveh-Benjamin, 2008).

We also tried to benchmark VE findings collected with older adults against data recorded in classical verbal memory tests, as well as clinical assessment of memory complaints. The subjective Cognitive Difficulties Scale (CDS; McNair & Kahn, 1983) was used to assess memory complaints in daily life. The CDS is a 39-item self-report measure of memory and general cognitive complaints using a Likert-type scale. For each item (e.g., Do you have difficulties in remembering the names of the people you know?), the participants have to choose among five responses, from "never" to "very often." We found that correlations existed between the score on the CDS and the following scores captured by our VR test: binding scores, detail recalls, and recognitions, whereas no correlation was observed between the CDS and the verbal memory test. This suggests that scores on our VR test are especially sensitive to everyday memory complaints in normal aging. The VR test reflects both objective and subjective cognitive deficits, in contrast to the classical verbal learning test. By testing rarely explored aspects of memory and by testing memories formed without deliberate memorization, VR-based assessment can contribute to the search for an ecological neuropsychology (Parsons, 2015; Schultheis et al., 2002).

One way to improve episodic memory in aging is to give older participants encoding instructions that favor the link between content and its context (Glisky & Kong, 2008; Naveh-Benjamin et al., 2004, 2005). It is also possible to add an environmental support at encoding that can serve as a compensatory strategy for deficient memory processing (for reviews, see Naveh-Benjamin et al., 2002, and Luo & Craik, 2008). As already demonstrated, an encoding strategy considered one of the most effective consists of enhancing memory by linking the information to be remembered with personal actions (Madan & Singhal, 2012; Zimmer et al. 2001). Using the enactment paradigm, comparison of active encoding (the encoding of action sentences by subject-performed tasks) with verbal encoding, showed a benefit of active encoding in both young and older adults (Feyereisen, 2009).

Using the virtual HOMES test, Arvind-Pala et al. (2014) investigated memory with several measures. They confirmed poor recall, but better recognition, and intact clustering and proactive interference effects for item memory in older adults. In a second study in young and older adults, they looked at the effect of active exploration on learning, proactive interference, semantic clustering, recognition hits, and false recognitions (Sauzéon, N'Kaoua, Arvind Pala, Taillade, & Guitton, 2015). Participants either actively navigated or passively followed the computer-guided tour of an apartment. The researchers observed in both groups that active exploration increased recognition hits, consistent with their previous result (Sauzéon et al., 2011), even if they did not replicate the effect on all scores. According to the authors, this indicates that active encoding strengthens distinctive memory traces and enriches source memory even in aging. However, a differential effect of active navigation was observed for young and older adults: while it reduced false recognitions in younger adults, it increased those made by older adults. Older adults are typically more prone to false memories (Plancher, Guyard, Nicolas, & Piolino, 2009; Rémy, Taconnat, & Isingrini, 2008), which is consistent with a source-monitoring deficit with aging.

The benefit of active navigation was assumed to result from the enrichment of item-specific processing (Plancher et al., 2013; Sauzéon et al., 2011), and the addition of perceptive-motor traces at encoding for a specific memory task (Brooks et al., 1999; Wallet et al., 2011), while the detrimental effect could depend on the level of complexity of the active navigation (Gaunet, Vidal, Kemeny, & Berthoz, 2001; Wilson & Peruch, 2002; Wolbers & Hegarty, 2010). Indeed, active navigation may sometimes require additional cognitive resources that are not fully available for the encoding process, leading to a detrimental effect on some aspects of memory (Plancher et al., 2013).

Jebara, Orriols, Zaoui, Berthoz, and Piolino (2014) tested in an urban VE how different components of action (active navigation and decision) may influence episodic memory performance (item plus context) and the effect of aging. They compared a passive condition (where the subject was just immersed as the passenger of a car, i.e., no active navigation, no decision); an itinerary condition (the subject was immersed as a passenger and chose the itinerary but did not drive the car); a low active navigation condition (the subject moved the car on rails, but the itinerary was fixed); and a high active navigation condition (the subject drove the car using a steering wheel and pedals, but the itinerary was fixed). The latter two navigation conditions differed in the degree of interactive sensorimotor engagement, but also in the degree of attentional load. Higher navigation control adds sensorimotor interaction, which could help memory, but it also makes driving more complex in the VE, requiring a higher level of attentiveness (Blankertz et al., 2010) and thus could be detrimental for memory, especially in older adults. It has been shown that age-related memory differences after active navigation are mediated by executive functions (Taillade et al., 2013). The findings showed that both the low active navigation condition and the choice of the itinerary enhanced the central component and the binding between the what–where–when components in young and older participants. These results can be explained by the fact that the conditions engage a lower amount of cognitive resources at encoding than the high active condition, but involve a higher environmental support than the passive condition. This study provides new evidence for the positive influence of decision making on feature binding (Bakdash et al., 2008; Plancher et al., 2013).

How can we explain this benefit? Integrating multimodal codes is important for binding, and applies not only to sensorimotor processing but also to action planning (Hommel, 2004). Voss, Gonsalves, Federmeier, Tranet, and Cohen (2011) also suggested that "volitional control" may improve the performance in memory thanks to the interplay between distinct neural systems related to planning, attention, and item processing. They argued that such control improves episodic memory performance because the hippocampus is not only concerned with relational feature binding (Eichenbaum, 2000; Ergorul & Eichenbaum, 2004), but also with planning (Bird & Burgess, 2008; Viard, Doeller, Hartley, Bird, & Burgess, 2011). The study by Jebara et al. (2014) suggests that navigational and decisional activity during real-life events should be useful in aging to boost memory. Encouraging older adults to use their own actions, both via active navigation and decisional control, could improve memory performance. A new challenge is to use VR to assess episodic memory to differentiate healthy older adults from pathological aging.

## Virtual Reality Studies Assessing Episodic Memory in Pathological Aging

Numerous studies have demonstrated that episodic memory impairment is one of the hallmarks of early clinical manifestations of AD (Hodges, 2006) and amnesic mild cognitive impairment (aMCI) (Petersen et al., 2001, 1999). This deficit has been explained by a reduced volume in the neural substrates of episodic memory, the hippocampus and in other brain regions, such as the parahippo-campal gyrus and cingulate cortex, in both AD and aMCI patients (Chételat et al., 2002; De Leon et al., 2006; Dickerson et al., 2001; Fox and Schott, 2004; Gerardin et al., 2009; Risacher et al., 2009). Notably, 50% of older adults with a focal mild episodic memory impairment compared to normal aging will develop AD in the following 4 years (Trojanowski et al., 2010). This subgroup of older adults has been shown to present intermediate brain characteristics between those of AD patients and healthy controls (Chételat et al., 2009; Evans et al., 2010; Gerardin et al., 2009). Reliable diagnosis of dementia as early as possible is thus crucial for treatment and rehabilitation of patients with suspected AD, such as the aMCI patients. Yet, the neurological tests used for early diagnosis are often time-consuming and expensive (e.g., amyloid plaques measured by PET scan, hippocampus volume measured by MRI, cephalorachidian fluid puncture) and the cognitive tests often present a weak sensitivity for early forms of the disease (Pike & Savage, 2008).

Various clinical memory tests used in dementia generally measure only one aspect of episodic memory in isolation, rather than offering a complete measure of its components, such as memory for what, where, and when, and binding between components. To improve the diagnosis and the rehabilitation of aMCI and AD patients, studies took advantage of VR to develop paradigms capable of early detection of functional changes in cognitive abilities and of presenting conditions that resemble daily life. Some studies with aMCI patients (Cushman, Stein, & Duffy, 2008) have found a close relationship between performance in virtual and real environments. Moreover, other studies with AD patients (Burgess, Trinkler, King, Kennedy, & Cipolotti, 2006; Drzezga et al., 2005; Zakzanis, Quintin, Graham, & Mraz, 2009) have specifically found allocentric spatial impairments. Widmann, Beinhoof, and Riepe (2010) immersed AD patients and healthy participants in a VE, a virtual version of Philadelphia, to assess the learning of verbal material in situations that imitate natural conditions. Participants sat passively and watched the film of the VE. The experimenter instructed participants that they were going on a shopping trip through the city. While jewelry shops were presented on the left and on the right sides of the street, participants were asked to read the shops' names out loud and to try to remember them. They were also told to remember the path they took. There were a total of 12 shop names to remember and the route consisted of seven virtual city blocks and three turns. AD patients were found to be impaired in free memory recall of shop names and in spatial memory compared to healthy participants, and the impairment was more marked than that observed with classical list learning. The authors concluded that classical list-learning paradigms wrongly estimate the memory capacities of patients in everyday situations.

We used a VE similar to that used in studying normal aging (Plancher et al., 2010) to characterize episodic memory profiles in an ecological fashion. The constructs researched included memory for central and perceptual details, spatiotemporal contextual elements, and binding (Plancher et al., 2012). Three different populations were contrasted: healthy older adults, patients with aMCI, and patients with early to moderate AD. The participants were successively immersed in two VEs: the first, as the driver of a virtual car (active exploration), and the second, as the passenger in that car (passive exploration). We sought to determine whether environmental factors that can affect encoding (active vs. passive exploration) influence memory performance also in pathological aging. Subjects were instructed to intentionally encode all the elements of the environment as well as the associated spatiotemporal contexts. Following each immersion (see Figure 9.2), we assessed the patient's recall and recognition of central information (i.e., the elements of the environment), contextual information (i.e., temporal, egocentric, and allocentric spatial information), and lastly, the quality of binding (number of types of contextual information associated to central elements, i.e., what-where-when). We found that the AD patients' performances were poorer than those of the aMCI group and even more so than those of the healthy aged group, in line with the progression of hippocampal atrophy reported in the literature.

Binding recall administered 20 minutes after the immersion and spatial allocentric memory assessments were found to be particularly useful for distinguishing aMCI patients from healthy older adults, a result that has been since confirmed (see Serino, Cipresso, Morganti, & Riva, 2014, for a review). In

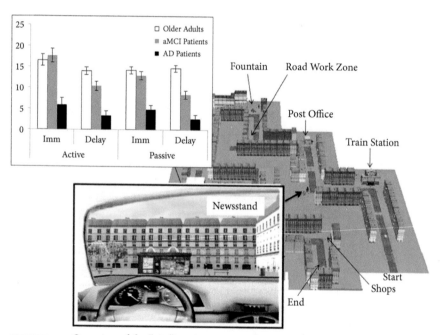

FIGURE 9.2 *Overview of the "city" environment and picture of a specific area (newsstand with a man and a bench on the right) and binding recall performance for normal healthy adults, aMCI and AD. From Plancher et al. (2012).*

particular, Morganti, Riva, and Stefanini (2013), using a VR-Maze and a VR-Road Map task, found a specific reduction in performing allo- to egocentric spatial tasks in AD, which is consistent with the early degeneration of the hippocampus and retrosplenial cortex underlying the ability to move between allocentric and egocentric reference frames. In addition, VR paradigms are able to discriminate pathological populations. Lee et al. (2014) observed that a significant spatial reference memory impairment was found in the aMCI group that converted to AD as compared to the nonconverter group, and Tu et al. (2015) found that spatial orientation performance assessed with a virtual supermarket task discriminated AD and frontotemporal dementia patient groups. We extended these results, revealing the relevance of the long-term feature binding assessment in ecological conditions for early detection of AD.

Confirming other VR studies in young and healthy older persons (Jebara et al., 2014; Plancher et al., 2013; Sauzéon et al. 2011, 2015), Plancher et al. (2012) observed that active exploration yielded enhanced recall of central and allocentric spatial information, as well as binding, in healthy aging but also in pathological populations (aMCI and AD). The beneficial effect of active encoding on populations showing a strong decline in episodic memory could be explained by relatively well-preserved frontal and motor brain functions implicated in procedural abilities or self-referential effects. Typically, AD patients exhibit a normal nondeclarative memory, at least when the disease is not too advanced (Lipinska & Bäckman, 1997; Van Halteren-van Tilborg, Scherder, & Hulstijn, 2007), as they can still play the piano or ride a bicycle and even can learn a new procedure. In addition, it has been demonstrated that AD patients can still experience some self-reference effects (Gutchess, Kensinger, & Schacter, 2010; Lalanne, Rozenberg, Grolleau, & Piolino, 2013). Interestingly, the patients' daily memory complaints were more highly correlated with their performance on the virtual test than with their performance on the classical memory test.

With a view to assessing multiple processes of episodic memory functioning embedded within contexts closely related to real life, Sauzéon and collaborators (2014) likewise investigated everyday memory from their VR apartment (HOMES test) in aging and in AD. As expected, they observed that AD patients exhibited poorer clustering, learning, and recognition performance than healthy older participants. They also observed that the HOMES indices were related to mnesic complaint, supporting the fact that the VR-based memory test is an appropriate device to capture the AD effect with respect to both in situ and laboratory settings. Taken together, these studies highlight specific cognitive differences found between AD and healthy populations that may provide additional insight into the early diagnosis and rehabilitation of pathological aging. In particular, neuropsychological studies would benefit from using virtual tests and a multicomponent approach to assess episodic memory, and to encourage the active encoding of information in patients suffering from mild or severe age-related memory impairment.

# Conclusion

In summary, in recent years, several criticisms have been leveled at the validity of neuropsychological tests for measuring episodic memory dysfunctions and predicting decline in daily life. With current developments and the decreasing cost of VR technology, an ecologically valid but nonetheless objective and well-controlled assessment of episodic memory has become possible. This noninvasive, nonpharmacological cognitive evaluation has gained increasing attention in recent years (Cotelli, Manenti, Zanetti, & Miniussi, 2012; García-Betances et al., 2015), addressing the challenge of MCI and AD diagnosis, as well as starting to assess pathology in pediatric patients (Abram, Cuny, Picard, & Piolino, 2014; Picard, Abram, Orriols, & Piolino, 2015), epileptic patients (Grewe et al., 2014; Rosas, Parrón, Serrano, & Cimadevilla, 2013), and schizophrenic patients (Spieker, Astur, West, Griego, & Rowland, 2011; Weniger & Irle, 2008).

VR provides an excellent opportunity for investigating memory in the context of embodied and situated cognition, especially the links between memory, perception, and action (Hommel, 2004). The domain needs to be developed in future research such as prospective memory (Canty et al., 2014; Debarnot et al., 2015; Kalpouzos et al., 2010; Sweeney, Kersel, Morris, Manly, & Evans, 2010) and interactions between working and long-term memory systems (Gras et al., 2013) and extended to other types of memory and associated functions (e.g., attention, executive functions, affective and social functions). The results indicating an improvement in episodic memory with active exploration of VE (at least when it is not too effortful) suggest that sensorimotor and decisional activity during real-life events should be useful to boost episodic memory. It could encourage older adults and patients with early dementia to use their own actions, both via active navigation and decisional control, to boost the encoding of complex events in their daily life or with VR training programs. Overall, this recent research opens up new avenues in the fundamental understanding of memory and clinical neuropsychology.

Even if VR offers a vast number of possibilities in clinical neuropsychology, improvements are still possible. Studies sometimes do not take full advantage of VEs with high levels of immersion and interaction. Increasing the immersion level induces a higher intensity of the subjective sense of presence experienced by patients and affects their behavioral responses (Slobounov, Ray, Johnson, Slobounov, & Newell, 2015). However, some devices, such as HMDs, can provoke cyber-sickness, a visually induced motion sickness, which should be avoided in clinical settings (Bohil et al., 2011). Finally, in clinical neuropsychology, it is important that VR applications be normed in large healthy populations as current standard tests. It is also crucial that this technic becomes easily and affordably transferable to clinical structures but also to home to transform the patient's environment in a place where cognitive training can be performed in an intensive and properly controlled way, and potentially open it to social networks.

# Acknowledgments

We thank Eric Orriols for the technical development of our virtual environments, and Maria Abram, Ursula Debanot, Doriane Gras, Valérie Gyselinck, Najate Jebara and Laurence Picard for their contribution to the conception and realization of the Memory and Cognition lab's studies using virtual reality. Finally, we thank all the participants in these studies for their time, and Elizabeth Rowley-Jolivet for the English corrections.

# References

Abram, M., Cuny, M. L., Picard, L., & Piolino, P. (2014). A double dissociation in virtual reality based episodic memory abilities: Case studies of two adolescents with medial temporal and frontal brain lesions. *European Journal of Neurology, 21*(SI), 561.

Aggleton, J. P., & Pearce, J. M. (2001). Neural systems underlying episodic memory: Insights from animal research. *Philosophical Transactions of the Royal Society of London. Series B, Biological Sciences, 356*, 1467–1482.

Aguirre, G. K., & D'Esposito, M. (1997). Environmental knowledge is subserved by separable dorsal/ventral neural area. *Journal of Neuroscience, 17*, 2512–2518.

Arvind-Pala, P., N'Kaoua, B., Mazaux, J. M., Simion, A., Lozes, S., Sorita, E., & Sauzéon, H. (2014). Everyday-like memory and its cognitive correlates in healthy older adults and in young patients with traumatic brain injury: A pilot study based on virtual reality. *Disability and Rehabilitation, Assistive Technology, 9*, 463–473. doi:10.3109/17483107.2014.941952

Bäckman, L., Small, B. J., & Fratiglioni, L. (2001). Stability of the preclinical episodic memory deficit in Alzheimer's disease. *Brain, 124*, 96–102.

Bakdash, J. Z., Linkenauger, S. A., & Proffitt, D. (2008). Comparing decision-making and control for learning a virtual environment: Backseat drivers learn where they are going. *Proceedings of the Human Factors and Ergonomics Society Annual Meeting, 52*, 2117–2121. doi:10.1177/154193120805202707

Barker, R. (1978). *Ecological psychology*. Stanford, CA: Stanford University Press.

Berthoz, A. (2003). *La décision*. Paris, France: Odile Jacob.

Bird, C. M., & Burgess, N. (2008). The hippocampus and memory: Insights from spatial processing. *Nature Review Neurosciences, 9*, 182–194. doi:10.1038/nrn2335

Blankertz, B., Tangermann, M., Vidaurre, C., Fazli, S., Sannelli, C., Haufe, S., et al. (2010). The Berlin brain–computer interface: Non-medical uses of BCI technology. *Frontiers Neurosciences, 4*, 198. doi:10.3389/fnins.2010.00198

Bohil, C. J., Alicea, B., & Biocca, F. A. (2011). Virtual reality in neuroscience research and therapy. *Nature Review Neurosciences, 12*, 752–762. doi:10.1038/nrn3122

Bowman, M. L. (1996). Ecological validity of neuropsychological and other predictors following head injury. *Clinical Neuropsychologist, 10*, 382–396.

Bronfenbrenner, U. (1979). *The ecology of human development*. Cambridge, MA: Harvard University Press.

Brooks, B. M., Attree, E. A., Rose, F. D., Clifford, B. R., & Leadbetter, A. G. (1999). The specificity of memory enhancement during interaction with a virtual environment. *Memory, 7*, 65–78. doi:10.1080/741943713

Burgess, N. (2002). The hippocampus, space, and viewpoints in episodic memory. *The Quarterly Journal of Experimental Psychology A, 55,* 1057–1080.

Burgess, N., Maguire, E. A., & O'Keefe, J. (2002). The human hippocampus and spatial and episodic memory. *Neuron, 35,* 625–641. doi:10.1016/S0896-6273(02)00830-9

Burgess, N., Maguire, E. A., Spiers, H. J., & O'Keefe J. (2001). A temporoparietal and prefrontal network for retrieving the spatial context of lifelike events. *Neuroimage, 14,* 439–453. doi:10.1006/nimg.2001.0806

Burgess, N., Trinkler, I., King, J., Kennedy, A., & Cipolotti, L. (2006). Impaired allocentric spatial memory underlying topographical disorientation. *Reviews in the Neurosciences, 17,* 239–251.

Cabeza, R., Ciaramelli, E., Olson, I. R., & Moscovitch, M. (2008). The parietal cortex and episodic memory: An attentional account. *Nature Review Neuroscience, 9,* 613–625.

Canty, A. L., Fleming, J., Patterson, F., Green, H. J., Man, D., & Shum, D. H. (2014). Evaluation of a virtual reality prospective memory task for use with individuals with severe traumatic brain injury. *Neuropsychological Rehabilitation, 24,* 238–265. doi:10.1080/09602011.2014.881746.

Carassa, A., Geminiani, G., Morganti, F., & Varotto, D. (2002). Active and passive spatial learning in a complex virtual environment: The effect of efficient exploration. *Cognitive Process, 3–4,* 65–81.

Chalfonte, B. L., & Johnson, M. K. (1996). Feature memory and binding in young and older adults. *Memory & Cognition, 24,* 403–416. doi:10.3758/BF03200930

Chételat, G., Desgranges, B., de la Sayette, V., Viader, F., Eustache, F., & Baron, J. C. (2002). Mapping gray matter loss with voxel-based morphometry in mild cognitive impairment. *Neuroreport, 13,* 1939–1943.

Chételat, G., Villain, N., Desgranges, B., Eustache, F., & Baron, J. C. (2009). Posterior cingulate hypometabolism in early Alzheimer's disease: What is the contribution of local atrophy versus disconnection? *Brain, 132,* e133.

Cotelli, M., Manenti, R., Zanetti, O., & Miniussi, C. (2012). Non-pharmacological intervention for memory decline. *Frontiers in Human Neuroscience, 6,* 1–17. doi:10.3389/fnhum.2012.00046

Cushman, L. A., Stein, K., & Duffy, C. J. (2008). Detecting navigational deficits in cognitive aging and Alzheimer disease using virtual reality. *Neurology, 71,* 888–95. doi:10.1212/01.wnl.0000326262.67613.fe

Davachi, L. (2006). Item, context and relational episodic encoding in humans. *Current Opinion in Neurobiology, 16,* 693–700.

Debarnot, U., Crépon, B., Orriols, E., Abram, M., Charron, S., Lion, S., ... Piolino, P. (2015). Intermittent theta burst stimulation over left BA10 enhances virtual reality-based prospective memory in healthy aged subjects. *Neurobiology of Aging, 36,* 2360–2369. doi:10.1016/j.neurobiolaging.2015.05.001

De Leon, M., DeSanti, S., Zinkowski, R., Mehta, P., Pratico, D., Segal, S., et al. (2006). Longitudinal CSF and MRI biomarkers improve the diagnosis of mild cognitive impairment. *Neurobiology of Aging, 27,* 394–401.

Delis, D. C., Kramer, J., Kaplan, E., & Ober, B. A. (2000). *California Verbal Learning Test—Second Edition.* San Antonio, TX: Psychological Corporation.

Dickerson, B. C., Goncharova, I., Sullivan, M. P., Forchetti, C., Wilson, R. S., Bennett, D. A., et al. (2001). MRI derived entorhinal and hippocampal atrophy in incipient and very mild Alzheimer's disease. *Neurobiology of Aging, 22*, 747–754.

Drzezga, A., Grimmer, T., Peller, M., Wermke, M., Siebner, H., Rauschecker, J. P., et al. (2005). Impaired cross-modal inhibition in Alzheimer disease. *PLoS Medicine, 2*, e288.

Ebbinghaus H. (1964). *Memory: A contribution to experimental psychology.* New York, NY: Dover Publications.

Eichenbaum, H. (2000). A cortical-hippocampal system for declarative memory. *Nature Review Neuroscience, 1*, 41–50. doi:10.1038/35036213

Eichenbaum, H., Sauvage, M., Fortin, N., Komorowski, R., & Lipton, P. (2012). Towards a functional organization of episodic memory in the medial temporal lobe. *Neuroscience and Biobehavioral Reviews, 36*, 1597–1608. doi:10.1016/j.neubiorev.2011.07.006

Ergorul, C., & Eichenbaum, H. (2004). The hippocampus and memory for "what," "where," and "when." *Learning and Memory, 11*, 397–405. doi:10.1101/lm.73304

Evans, M. C., Barnes, J., Nielsen, C., Kim, L. G., Clegg, S. L., Blair, M., et al. (2010). Volume changes in Alzheimer's disease and mild cognitive impairment: Cognitive associations. *European Radiology, 20*, 674–682.

Farias, S. T., Harrell, E., Neumann, C., & Houtz, A. (2003). The relationship between neuropsychological performance and daily functioning in individuals with Alzheimer's disease: Ecological validity of neuropsychological tests. *Archives of Clinical Neuropsychology, 18*, 655–672.

Feyereisen, P. (2009). Enactment effects and integration processes in younger and older adults' memory for actions. *Memory 17*, 374–385.

Fox, N., & Schott, J. (2004). Imaging cerebral atrophy: Normal ageing to Alzheimer's disease. *Lancet, 363*, 392–394.

Fuchs, P., Moreau, G., Berthoz, A., & Vercher, J. L. (2006). Le traité de la réalité virtuelle— Vol. 1. L'homme et l'environnement virtuel. [Treaty of virtual reality—Vol. 1. Man and the virtual environment]. Paris, France: Presses de l'Ecole des Mines de Paris.

García-Betances, R. I., Arredondo Waldmeyer, M. T., Fico, G., & Cabrera-Umpiérrez, M. F. (2015). A succinct overview of virtual reality technology use in Alzheimer's disease. *Frontiers in Aging Neuroscience, 7*, 80. doi:10.3389/fnagi.2015.00080

Gaunet, F., Vidal, V., Kemeny, A., & Berthoz, A. (2001). Active, passive and snapshot exploration in a virtual environment: Influence on scene memory, reorientation and path memory. *Cognitive Brain Research, 11*, 409–420.

Gerardin, E., Chételat, G., Chupin, M., Cuingnet, R., Desgranges, B., Kim, H. S., et al. (2009). Multidimensional classification of hippocampal shape features discriminates Alzheimer's disease and mild cognitive impairment from normal aging. *NeuroImage, 47*, 1476–1486.

Glenberg, A.M. (1997). What memory is for. *Behavioral and Brain Sciences, 20*, 1–55. http://dx.doi.org/10.1017/S0140525X97000010.

Glisky, E. L., & Kong, L. L. (2008). Do young and older adults rely on different processes in source memory tasks? A neuropsychological study. *Journal of Experimental Psychology: Learning, Memory and Cognition, 34*, 809–822. doi:10.1037/0278-7393.34.4.809

Gras, D., Gyselinck, V., Perrussel, M., & Orriols, E. (2013). The role of working memory components and visuospatial abilities in route learning within a virtual environment. *Journal of Cognitive Psychology, 25*, 38–50.

Greene, R. L. (1986). Word stems as cues in recall and completion tasks. *The Quarterly Journal of Experimental Psychology, 38A*, 663–673.

Grewe, P., Lahr, D., Kohsik, A., Dyck, E., Markowitsch, H. J., Bien, C., Botsch, M., & Piefke, M. (2014). Real-life memory and spatial navigation in patients with focal epilepsy: Ecological validity of a virtual reality supermarket task. *Epilepsy and Behavior, 31*, 57–66. doi:10.1016/j.yebeh.2013.11.014

Grober, E., & Buschke, H. (1987). Genuine memory deficits in dementia. *Developmental Neuropsychology, 3*, 13–36.

Gutchess, A. H., Kensinger, E. A., & Schacter, D. L. (2010). Functional neuroimaging of self-referential encoding with age. *Neuropsychologia, 48*, 211–219.

Habib, R., Nyberg, L., & Tulving, E. (2003). Hemispheric asymmetries of memory: The HERA model revisited. *Trends in Cognitive Sciences, 7*(6), 241–245. doi:10.1016/S1364-6613(03)00110-4

Hasher, L., & Zacks, R. T. (1979). Automatic and effortful processes in human memory. *Journal of Experimental Psychology: General, 108*, 356–388.

Hodges, J. R. (2006). Alzheimer's centennial legacy: Origins, landmarks and the current status of knowledge concerning cognitive aspects. *Brain, 129*, 2811–2822.

Hommel, B. (2004). Event files: Feature binding in and across perception and action. *Trends in Cognitive Sciences, 8*, 494–500. doi:10.1016/j.tics.2004.08.007

Jacoby, L. L., Jennings, J. M., & Hay, J. F. (1996). Dissociating automatic and consciously controlled processes: Implications for diagnosis and rehabilitation of memory deficits. In D. J. Herrmann, C. L. McEvoy, C. Hertzog, P. Hertel, & M. K. Johnson (Eds.), *Basic and applied memory research: Theory in context* (Vol. 1, pp. 161–193). Mahwah, NJ: Erlbaum.

Jebara, N., Orriols, E., Zaoui, M., Berthoz, A., & Piolino, P. (2014). Effects of enactment in episodic memory: A pilot virtual reality study with young and elderly adults. *Frontiers in Aging Neuroscience, 6*, 338. doi:10.3389/fnagi.2014.00338

Kalpouzos, G., Eriksson, J., Sjolie, D., Molin, J., & Nyberg, L. (2010). Neurocognitive systems related to real-world prospective memory. *PLoS One, 5*, e13304.

Kessels, R. P., Hobbel, D., & Postma, A. (2007). Aging, context memory and binding: A comparison of "what, where and when" in young and older adults. *International Journal of Neurosciences, 117*, 795–810.

King, J. A., Hartley, T., Spiers, H. J., Maguire, E. A., & Burgess, N. (2005). Anterior prefrontal involvement in episodic retrieval reflects contextual interference. *NeuroImage, 15*, 256–267.

Koriat, A., & Goldsmith, M. (1996). Memory metaphors and the real-life/laboratory controversy: Correspondence versus storehouse conceptions of memory. *The Behavioral and Brain Sciences, 19*, 167–228.

Lalanne, J., Rozenberg, J.,Grolleau, P., & Piolino, P. (2013). The self-reference effect on episodic memory recollection in young and older adults and Alzheimer's disease. *Current Alzheimer Research, 10*, 1107–1117. doi:10.2174/1567205011310660175

Lee, J. Y., Kho, S., Yoo, H. B., Park, S., Choi, J. S., Kwon, J. S., Cha, K. R., & Jung, H. Y. (2014). Spatial memory impairments in amnestic mild cognitive impairment in a virtual radial arm maze. *Neuropsychiatric Disease and Treatment, 10,* 653–660. doi:10.2147/NDT.S58185

Lipinska, B., & Backman, L. (1997). Encoding–retrieval interactions in mild Alzheimer's disease: The role of access to categorical information. *Brain and Cognition, 34,* 274–286.

Luo, L., & Craik, F. I. M. (2008). Aging and memory: A cognitive approach. *La Revue Canadienne de Psychiatrie, 53,* 346–353.

Madan, C. R., & Singhal, A. (2012). Motor imagery and higher-level cognition: Four hurdles before research can sprint forward. *Cognitive Process, 13,* 211–229. doi:10.1007/s10339-012-0438-z

McDermott, K. B., Szpunar, K. K., & Christ, S. E. (2009). Laboratory-based and autobiographical retrieval tasks differ substantially in their neural substrates. *Neuropsychologia, 47*(11), 2290–2298. doi:10.1016/j.neuropsychologia.2008.12.025

McNair, D., & Kahn, R. (1983). Self-assessment of cognitive deficits. In T. Crook, S. Ferris, & R. Bartus (Eds.), *Assessment in geriatric psychopharmacology* (pp. 137–143). New Canaan, CT: Powley.

Mestre, D. R., & Fuchs, P. (2006). Immersion et présence. In P. Fuchs, G. Moreau, A. Berthoz, & J. L. Vercher (Eds.), *Le traité de la réalité virtuelle* (pp. 309–338). Paris: Ecole des Mines de Paris.

Meyers, J. E., & Meyers, K. R. (1995). *Rey Complex Figure Test and Recognition Trial.* Lutz, FL: Psychological Assessment Resources.

Morganti, F., Stefanini, S., & Riva, G. (2013). From allo- to egocentric spatial ability in early Alzheimer's disease: A study with virtual reality spatial tasks. *Cognitive Neuroscience, 4,* 171–180. doi:10.1080/17588928.2013.854762

Mueller, C., Luehrs, M., Baecke, S., Adolf, D., Luetzkendorf, R., Luchtmann, M., et al. (2012). Building virtual reality fMRI paradigms: A framework for presenting immersive virtual environments. *Journal of Neuroscience Methods 209,* 290–298. doi:10.1016/j.jneumeth.2012.06.025

Naveh-Benjamin, M., Craik, F. I. M., & Lilach Ben-Shaul, L. (2002). Age-related differences in cued recall: Effects of support at encoding and retrieval. *Aging, Neuropsychology, and Cognition, 9,* 276–287.

Naveh-Benjamin, M., Guez, J., & Shulman, S. (2004). Older adults' associative deficit in episodic memory: Assessing the role of decline in attentional resources. *Psychonomic Bulletin and Review, 11,* 1067–1073. doi:10.3758/BF03196738

Naveh-Benjamin, M., Craik, F. I., Guez, J., & Kreuger, S. (2005). Divided attention in younger and older adults: Effects of strategy and relatedness on memory performance and secondary task costs. *Journal of Experimental Psychology: Learning Memory and Cognition, 31,* 520–537.

Neill, W. T., Beck, J. L., Bottalico, K. S., & Molloy, R. D. (1990). Effects of intentional versus incidental learning on explicit and implicit tests of memory. *Journal of Experimental Psychology: Learning, Memory, and Cognition, 16,* 457–463.

Neisser, U. (1976). *Cognition and reality.* San Francisco, CA: Freeman.

Nilsson, L.-G. (2000). Remembering actions and words. In F. I. M. Craik & E. Tulving (Eds.), *Oxford handbook of memory* (pp. 137–148). Oxford: Oxford University Press.

Old, S. R., & Naveh-Benjamin, M. (2008). Differential effects of age on item and associative measures of memory: A meta-analysis. *Psychology and Aging, 23,* 104–118.

Park, J., Lee, H., Kim, T., Park, G. Y., Lee, E. M., Baek, S., ... & Kang, J. K. (2014). Role of low- and high-frequency oscillations in the human hippocampus for encoding environmental novelty during a spatial navigation task. *Hippocampus, 24,* 1341–1352.

Parsons, T. D. (2015). Ecological validity in virtual reality-based neuropsychological assessment. In Mehdi Khosrow-Pour (Ed.), *Encyclopedia of information science and technology* (3rd ed., pp. 214–223). Hershey: IGI Global.

Parsons, T. D., & Rizzo, A. A. (2008). Initial validation of a virtual environment for assessment of memory functioning: Virtual reality cognitive performance assessment test. *Cyberpsychology and Behavior, 11,* 17–25. doi:10.1089/cpb.2007.9934

Pause, B. M., Zlomuzica, A., Kinugawa, K., Mariani, J., Pietrowsky, R., & Dere, E. (2013). Perspectives on episodic-like and episodic memory. *Frontiers in Behavioral Neuroscience, 7,* 33. doi:10.3389/fnbeh.2013.00033

Pearman, A., & Storandt, M. (2004). Predictors of subjective memory in older adults. *Journal of Gerontology, Series B: Psychological Sciences and Social Sciences, 59,* 4–6.

Petersen, R. C., Doody, R., Kurz, A., Mohs, R. C., Morris, J. C., Rabins, P. V., et al. (2001). Current concepts in mild cognitive impairment. *Archives of Neurology, 58,* 1985–1992.

Petersen, R. C., Smith, G. E., Waring, S. C., Ivnik, R. J., Tangalos, E. G., & Kokmen, E. (1999). Mild cognitive impairment: Clinical characterization and outcome. *Archives of Neurology, 56,* 303–308.

Picard, L., Abram, M., Orriols, E., & Piolino, P. (2016). Virtual reality as an ecologically valid tool for assessing multifaceted episodic memory in children and adolescents. *International Journal of Behavioral Development.* doi:10.1177/0165025415616198

Pike, K. E., & Savage, G. (2008). Memory profiling in mild cognitive impairment: Can we determine risk for Alzheimer's disease? *Journal of Neuropsychology, 2,* 361–372.

Piolino, P., Desgranges, B., & Eustache, F. (2009). Episodic autobiographical memories over the course of time: Cognitive, neuropsychological and neuroimaging findings. Special issue on episodic memory in honour of Endel Tulving. *Neuropsychologia, 47,* 2314–2329

Plancher, G., Barra, J., Orriols, E., & Piolino, P. (2013). The influence of action on episodic memory: A virtual reality study. *Quarterly Journal of Experimental Psychology, 66,* 895–909. doi:10.1080/17470218.2012.722657

Plancher, G., Guyard, A., Nicolas, S., & Piolino, P. (2009). Mechanisms underlying the production of false memories for famous people's names in aging and Alzheimer's disease. *Neuropsychologia, 47,* 2527–2536. doi:10.1016/j.neuropsychologia.2009.04.026

Plancher, G., Gyselinck, V., Nicolas, S., & Piolino, P. (2010). Age effect on components of episodic memory and feature binding: A virtual reality study. *Neuropsychology, 24,* 379–390. doi:10.1037/a0018680

Plancher, G., Tirard, A., Gyselinck, V., Nicolas, S., & Piolino, P. (2012). Using virtual reality to characterize episodic memory profiles in amnestic mild cognitive impairment and Alzheimer's disease: Influence of active and passive encoding. *Neuropsychologia, 50,* 592–602. doi:10.1016/j.neuropsychologia.2011.12.013

Plancher, G., Nicolas, S., & Piolino, P. (2008). Apport de la réalité virtuelle en neuropsychologie de la mémoire: Étude dans le vieillissement. *Psychologie et Neuropsychiatrie Du Vieillissement, 6,* 7–22.

Rauchs, G., Orban, P., Balteau, E., Schimdt, C., Degueldre, C., Luxen, A., . . . Peigneux, P. (2008). Partially segregated neural networks for spatial and contextual memory in virtual navigation. *Hippocampus, 18,* 503–518.

Reid, L. M., & Maclullich, A. M. (2006). Subjective memory complaints and cognitive impairment in older people. *Dementia and Geriatric Cognitive Disorders, 22,* 471–485.

Rémy, P., Taconnat, L., & Isingrini, M. (2008). Effects of aging and attention-demanding tasks on false recognition induced by photographs: Differences between conceptually and perceptually modified lures. *Experimental Aging Research, 34,* 220–231. doi:10.1080/03610730802070118

Risacher, S. L., Saykin, A. J., West, J. D., Shen, L., Firpi, H. A., & McDonald, B. C. (2009). Baseline MRI predictors of conversion from MCI to probable AD in the ADNI cohort. *Current Alzheimer Research, 6,* 347–361.

Rosas, K., Parrón, I., Serrano, P., & Cimadevilla, J. M. (2013). Spatial recognition memory in a virtual reality task is altered in refractory temporal lobe epilepsy. *Epilepsy & Behavior, 28,* 227–231.

Sauzéon, H., Arvind Pala, P., Larrue, F., Wallet, G., Déjos, M., Zheng, X., Guitton, P., & N'Kaoua, B. (2011). The use of virtual reality for episodic memory assessment: Effects of active navigation. *Experimental Psychology, 59,* 99–108. doi:10.1027/1618-3169/a000131

Sauzéon, H., N'Kaoua, B., Arvind-Pala, P., Taillade, M., Auriacombe, S., & Guitton, P. (2016). Everyday-like memory for objects in ageing and Alzheimer's disease assessed in a visually complex environment: The role of executive functioning and episodic memory. *Journal of Neuropsychology, 10,* 33–58. doi:10.1111/jnp.12055.

Sauzéon, H., N'Kaoua, B., Arvind Pala, P., Taillade, M., & Guitton, P. (2016). Age and active navigation effects on episodic memory: A virtual reality study. *British Journal of Psychology, 107,* 72–94.

Sbordone, R. J., & Long, C. J. (1996). *Ecological validity of neuropsychological testing.* Delray Beach, FL: St. Lucie Press.

Schomaker, J., Roos, R., & Meeter, M. (2014). Expecting the unexpected: The effects of deviance on novelty processing. *Behavioral Neuroscience, 128,* 146.

Schultheis, M. T., Himelstein, J., & Rizzo, A. R. (2002). Virtual reality and neuropsychology: Upgrading the current tools. *Journal of Head Trauma and Rehabilitation, 17,* 379–394. doi:10.1097/00001199-200210000-00002

Serino, S., Cipresso, P., Morganti, F., & Riva, G. (2014). The role of egocentric and allocentric abilities in Alzheimer's disease: A systematic review. *Ageing Research Reviews, 16,* 32–44.

Shimamura, A. P., & Wickens, T. D. (2009). Superadditive memory strength for item and source recognition: The role of hierarchical relational binding in the medial temporal lobe. *Psychological Review, 116,* 1–19. doi:10.1037/a0014500

Slobounov, S. M., Ray, W., Johnson, B., Slobounov, E., & Newell, K. M. (2015). Modulation of cortical activity in 2D versus 3D virtual reality environments: An EEG study. *International Journal of Psychophysiology, 95,* 254–260. doi:10.1016/j.ijpsycho.2014.11.003

Spencer, W. D., & Raz, N. (1995). Differential effects of aging on memory for content and context: A meta-analysis. *Psychology and Aging, 10,* 527–539.

Spieker, E.A., Astur, R.S., West, J.T., Griego, J.A., & Rowland, L. M. (2012). Spatial memory deficits in a virtual reality eight-arm radial maze in schizophrenia. *Schizophrenia Research, 135,* 84–89. doi: 10.1016/j.schres.2011.11.014.

Squire, L. R. (2004). Memory systems of the brain: A brief history and current perspective. *Neurobiology of Learning and Memory, 82,* 171–177.

Sternberg, R. J. (1997). Intelligence and lifelong learning: What's new and how can we use it? *The American Psychologist, 52,* 1134–1139. doi:10.1037/0003-066X.52.10.1134 PMID:9329294

Sweeney, S., Kersel, D., Morris, R. G., Manly, T., & Evans, J. J. (2010). The sensitivity of a virtual reality task to planning and prospective memory impairments: Group differences and the efficacy of periodic alerts on performance. *Neuropsychological Rehabilitation, 20,* 239–263.

Taillade, M., Sauzéon, H., Arvind-Pala, P., Déjos, M., Larrue, F., Gross, C., et al. (2013). Age-related wayfinding differences in real large-scale environments: Detrimental motor control effects during spatial learning are mediated by executive decline? *PLoS ONE, 8,* e67193. doi:10.1371/journal.pone.0067193

Tlauka, M., Keage, H., & Clark, C. R. (2005). Viewing a map versus reading a description of a map: Modality-specific encoding of spatial information. *Cognitive Science, 29,* 807–818.

Trojanowski, J. Q., Vandeerstichele, H., Korecka, M., Clark, C. M., Aisen, P. S., Petersen, R. C., et al. (2010). Update on the biomarker core of the Alzheimer's disease neuroimaging initiative subjects. *Alzheimers Dementia, 6,* 230–238.

Tu, S., Wong, S., Hodges, J. R., Irish, M., Piguet, O., & Hornberger, M. (2015). Lost in spatial translation—A novel tool to objectively assess spatial disorientation in Alzheimer's disease and frontotemporal dementia. *Cortex, 67,* 83–94.

Tulving, E. (1983). *Elements of episodic memory.* New York, NY: Oxford University Press.

Tulving, E. (1972). Episodic and semantic memory. In E. Tulving & W. Donaldson (Eds.), *Organisation and memory.* New York, NY: Academic Press.

Tulving, E. (2002). Episodic memory: From mind to brain. *Annual Review of Psychology, 53,* 1–25

Van Halteren-van Tilborg, I. A., Scherder, E. J., & Hulstijn, W. (2007). Motor-skill learning in Alzheimer's disease: A review with an eye to the clinical practice. *Neuropsychology Review, 3,* 203–212.

Viard, A., Doeller, C. F., Hartley, T., Bird, C. M., & Burgess, N. (2011). Anterior hippocampus and goal-directed spatial decision making. *Journal of Neurosciences, 31,* 4613–4621. doi:10.1523/JNEUROSCI.4640-10.2011

Voss, J. L., Gonsalves, B. D., Federmeier, K. D., Tranel, D., & Cohen, N. J. (2011). Hippocampal brain-network coordination during volitional exploratory behaviour enhances learning. *Nature Neuroscience, 14,* 115–122. doi:10.1038/nn.2693

Wallet, G., Sauzéon, H., Arvind Pala, P., Larrue, F., Zheng, X., & N'Kaoua, B. (2011). Virtual/real transfer of spatial knowledge: Benefit from visual fidelity provided in a virtual environment and impact of active navigation. *Cyberpsychology, Behavior, and Social Networking, 14,* 417–423.

Weschler, D. (1997). *Weschler Adult Intelligence Scale,* 3rd ed. San Antonio, TX: The Psychological Corporation.

Weniger, G., & Irle, E. (2008). Allocentric memory impaired and egocentric memory intact as assessed by virtual reality in recent-onset schizophrenia. *Schizophrenia Research, 101,* 201–209. doi: 10.1016/j.schres.2008.01.011.

Weniger, G., Ruhleder, M., Wolf, S., Lange, C., & Irle, E. (2009). Egocentric memory impaired and allocentric memory intact as assessed by virtual reality in subjects with unilateral parietal cortex lesions. *Neuropsychologia, 47,* 59–69.

Widmann, C. N., Beinhoff, U., & Riepe, M. W. (2010). Everyday memory deficits in very mild Alzheimer's disease. *Neurobiology of Aging, 33,* 297–303.

Wilson, P. N., & Péruch, P. (2002). The influence of interactivity and attention on spatial learning in a desktop virtual environment. *Cahiers de Psychologie Cognitive, 21,* 601–633.

Wilson, M. (2002). Six views of embodied cognition. *Psychonomic Bulletin & Review, 9,* 625–636.

Wolbers, T., & Hegarty, M. (2010). What determines our navigational abilities? *Trends in Cognitive Sciences, 14,* 138–146. doi:10.1016/j.tics.2010.01.001

Zakzanis, K. K., Quintin, G., Graham, S. J., & Mraz, R. (2009). Age and dementia related differences in spatial navigation within an immersive virtual environment. Medical Science Monitor. *International Medical Journal of Experimental and Clinical Research, 15,* 140–150.

Zawadzki, J. A., Girard, T. A., Foussias, G., Rodrigues, A., Siddiqui, I., Lerch, J. P., et al. (2013). Simulating real world functioning in schizophrenia using a naturalistic city environment and single-trial, goal-directed navigation. *Frontiers in Behavioral Neurosciences, 7,* 180. doi:10.3389/fnbeh.2013.00180

Zimmer, H. D., Cohen, R. L., Guynn, M., Engelkamp, J., Kormi-Nouri, R. & Foley, M. N. (2001). *Memory for action.* New York, NY: Oxford University Press.

# 10

# Factors Affecting Aging Services Technology Use in the Aging Population

Joyce W. Tam and Maureen Schmitter-Edgecombe

Age-related changes in physical health and cognitive functions can negatively affect quality of life as well as increase caregiver burden and societal healthcare costs. While aging services technologies (ASTs) have the potential to facilitate functional independence, they have been underutilized in the aging population due to various factors, including awareness and access. ASTs were defined in the 2009 American Recovery and Reinvestment Act as "health technology that meets the health-care needs of seniors, individuals with disabilities, and the caregivers of such seniors and individuals" (Public Law 111-5). For the purpose of this chapter, tools or devices not discussed in the context of older adult use are referred to as assistive technologies (ATs). Both ATs and ASTs span a spectrum from low-tech to high-tech devices. Low-tech devices are often simple, easy to operate, and economical. Magnifying glasses, pill boxes, daily planners, and canes are all considered low-tech devices. In contrast, high-tech devices are computerized, often require additional training to learn and to operate, and are more costly. Computers, tablets, smartphone software or assistive apps, wearable sensors, and smart homes are some examples of high-tech tools.

An assortment of ASTs are available to address both physical changes (e.g., changes in vision or mobility) and cognitive limitations (e.g., memory decline). The devices can be used to address issues that arise from normal aging as well as symptoms associated with neurological disorders, including memory, motor, and autoimmune disorders (Cattaneo, de Nuzzo, Fascia, Macalli, Pisoni, Cardini, 2002; Constantinescu, Leonard, Deeley, & Kurlan, 2007; Padilla, 2011). In a randomized controlled study, Mann and colleagues (1999) recruited older adults who were in need of ASTs (e.g., receiving in-home services, participating in a hospital rehabilitation program) and assigned them to usual standard of care or treatment. Participants in the treatment group received an 18-month intervention that included ongoing functional assessment as well as recommendations for ASTs and home modifications. The treatment group participants also received AST training. In comparison to standard care, the results showed that the intervention was efficacious in increasing the number of AST devices acquired and in slowing functional decline.

A body of literature documenting the benefits of AST use is beginning to accumulate. More specifically, a recent review of ASTs for low vision concluded that low-vision ASTs improve users' ability to perform everyday activities, especially when combined with training that was geared toward personalized goals (Liu, Brost, Horton, Kenyon, & Mears, 2013). Similarly, support was established for the use of ATs to facilitate cognitive functions (e.g., attention, organization, and planning) based on a systematic review of ATs for cognition (Gillespie, Best, & O'Neill, 2012). Physical and psychological benefits of using other assistive devices, including mobility, fall prevention, and transferring tools, have also been documented (Bateni & Maki, 2005; Chase, Mann, Wasek, & Arbesman, 2012; Zhuang, Stobbe, Hsiao, Collins, & Hobbs, 1999). Despite the fact that AST use has been found to be associated with a reduction in informal care and healthcare costs (Agree, Freedman, Cornman, Wolf, & Marcotte, 2005; Mann et al., 1999), ASTs remain significantly underutilized among older adults (U.S. Department of Health and Human Services, 2012).

The underutilization of ASTs may be due to a number of factors, both individual (e.g., individual expectation and belief) and systemic (e.g., product design, insurance coverage). Knowledge and understanding of the factors would allow healthcare providers, including neuropsychologists, to address the issues and to reduce barriers to AST adoption. As advocated by Scherer (2012), neuropsychologists are in a unique position to increase and to promote AST awareness and use. Neuropsychologists can provide holistic recommendations appropriate for a given individual to prevent, compensate for, and/or slow physical and cognitive changes (Atkinson et al., 2007; Auyeung et al., 2008; Rosano et al., 2005; Wang, Larson, Bowen, & van Belle, 2006) based on a comprehensive evaluation.

The primary goal of this chapter is to raise awareness regarding issues related to AST acceptance and adoption in the field of neuropsychology. Several reviews have been written concerning factors related to specific AST devices, AST domains, AST use within specific clinical groups, or AST nonuse (e.g., Baxter, Enderby, Evans, & Judge, 2012; Demiris & Hensel, 2008; Kraskowsky & Finlayson, 2000; Topo, 2008; Wessels, Dijcks, Soede, Gelderblom, & De Witte, 2003). The chapter focuses on specific factors that contribute to the underutilization and to the adoption of ASTs, as well as future research directions and clinical applications to increase AST acceptance and use. The following questions are addressed:

1. What approaches have been taken to evaluate technology acceptance and adoption?
2. What demographic factors contribute to AST use?
3. What individual variables (e.g., user characteristics, user's perception) contribute to AST acceptance and adoption?

4. What are some of the social factors and systemic issues that affect AST acceptance and use?
5. How can an understanding of technology acceptance research inform clinical practice and future AT research with the aging and clinical populations?

## Approaches Taken to Evaluate Technology Acceptance

Assistive technology (AT) research can be conceptualized as an extension of a larger body of research on technology acceptance. Studies on technology acceptance and use have evaluated everyday technologies, from ATMs, computers, and Internet use (e.g., Jamieson & Rogers, 2000; Slegers, van Boxtel, & Jolles, 2007, & Xie, 2003) to medical devices and technologically more advanced systems, including augmentative and alternative communication tools, sensors, and residential technologies (Ahn, Beamish, & Goss, 2008; Blaschke, Freddolino, & Mullen, 2009; Demiris et al., 2004; Demiris, Oliver, Dickey, Skubic, & Rantz, 2008; Hickman, Rogers, & Fisk, 2007). Within the context of AT, studies have evaluated individuals across the lifespan as well as medical populations with and without cognitive or intellectual disabilities (Agree & Freedman, 2003; Palmer, Wehmeyer, Davies, & Stock, 2012; Parsons, Daniels, Porter, & Robertson, 2008; Pressler & Ferraro, 2010). Various research designs, participant samples, and survey instruments have been used to further expand understanding of the diverse and complex issues related to AST acceptance and adoption. A broad overview of the methodologies used in the AT literature is included here to provide a context for the findings related to AST acceptance and use summarized in the chapter.

### RESEARCH DESIGN

Technology adoption and utilization have been operationalized differently across studies. Some have evaluated perspectives pertaining to specific AT devices (Baxter, Enderby, Evans, & Judge, 2012; Landau, Werner, Auslander, Shoval, & Heinik, 2010; Shone Stickel, Ryan, Rigby, & Jutai, 2002), while others have approached the topic more generally, to include everyday technologies without specifying a particular device (Mitzner et al., 2010). Researchers have also taken a variety of approaches to data collection. The methodologies have included qualitative data-gathering processes (e.g., individual and group interviews, focus groups), quantitative approaches to statistical analyses (Horowitz, Brennan, Reinhardt, & Macmillan, 2006), quasi-experimental designs (Czaja et al., 2006; Vishwanath, Brodsky, Shaha, Leonard, & Cimino, 2009), and randomized controlled clinical trials (Mann et al., 1999). Although less commonly, longitudinal designs have also been adopted (Boise et al., 2013).

## PARTICIPANT SAMPLES/STUDY SETTINGS

The characteristics of study participants in the articles reviewed also varied widely across studies and settings. Study samples included individuals with specific acute or chronic physical or cognitive difficulties as well as cognitively intact individuals across the lifespan and various cultures. For example, studies have focused on individuals participating in cognitive rehabilitation after acquired brain injuries (de Joode, van Boxtel, Verhey, & van Heugten, 2012), adults with intellectual disabilities (Parsons, Daniels, Porter, & Robertson, 2008), patients with chronic medical conditions (Horowitz et al., 2006; Pressler & Ferraro, 2010), as well as current and potential users of more narrowly defined technologies (tele-health, health monitoring, fall detection, or smart home technologies; Coughlin, D'Ambrosio, Reimer, & Pratt, 2007; Courtney, Demiris, & Hensel, 2007). Other studies considered the experience of current older adult users of AST regardless of functional change, specific types of AST used, or settings of AST use (e.g., work, home, health, and adult day services; Mitzner et al., 2010; Parsons et al., 2008). Furthermore, other populations of interest were nonusers (Landau et al., 2010), caregivers or family members (Palmer et al., 2012; Rosenberg, Kottorp, & Nygard, 2011), and healthcare professionals or treatment providers (de Joode et al., 2012; Vishwanath, Brodsky, Shaha, Leonard, & Cimino, 2009; Yarbrough & Smith, 2007).

## EVALUATION INSTRUMENTS

The length and purpose of surveys used varied by instruments. In a comprehensive approach to data collection, information regarding participant demographics, disability status, depressive symptoms, and hours of assistance received (e.g., rehabilitation), in addition to AST perception and use were frequently gathered (Gitlin et al., 1996; Horowitz et al., 2006). A number of studies utilized The National Health Survey to understand AST needs and utilization (Agree & Freedman, 2003; Cornman, Freedman, & Agree, 2005; Hartke, Prohaska, & Furner, 1998). The Functional Independence Measure (Granger & Hamilton, 1992) and the International Classification of Function (World Health Organization, 2001) were among other measures commonly used to assess functional and/or disability status. Several questionnaires were developed and validated to gather relevant information associated with general and specific AST use (e.g., quality of life, Agree & Freedman, 2011; user satisfaction, Demers, Weiss-lambrou, & Ska, 2002; psychosocial impact, Jutai & Day, 2002; also see Lenker, Scherer, Fuhrer, Jutai, & DeRuyter, 2005 for a review), while nonstandardized instruments were also used to elicit study-specific information (e.g., prepurchase decision making, intention to use; Martin, Martin, Stumbo, & Morril, 2011; Roelands, Van Oost, Depoorter, & Buysse, 2002). Questionnaires were completed in some cases by study participants (Hartke, Prohaska, & Furner, 1998) and in other cases by informants (Gitlin et al., 1996), which included caregivers and professionals.

## SUMMARY

Various AST research approaches have been used to broaden our understanding of factors affecting AST acceptance. While experimental designs allow for the manipulation of independent variables (e.g., intervention vs. standard care assignment; Mann et al., 1999), qualitative data gathered through focus groups may enable the identification of critical variables in a relatively efficient and cost-effective manner (Kitzinger, 1994; Powell & Single, 1996). The latter approach may also enable deeper understanding of factors affecting AST acceptance in a timely manner when relatively little information is available on a complex research topic. Investigating AST acceptance with different sample groups can also serve a similar purpose. The potential influence of sampling bias is important to consider, given that the goal of this line of research is to understand factors contributing to AST nonuse in a population that may be uninterested in, or resistant to, participating in studies regarding ASTs. For example, in a study that used a web-based questionnaire, older age and lower socioeconomic status (SES) were found to be associated with poorer participation in research (Ahn et al., 2008). In fact, when response rates in Ahn and colleagues' study are compared, there were far fewer individuals in age groups of 75 to 84 (< 10%) and 85 and older (< 1%) than in the group age 55 to 64 (about 60%). Furthermore, their data also suggested that the study participants had a high SES (e.g., higher household income and number of home owners). Although sample bias can never be completely eliminated, it is important to continue to reach out to populations that may be less interested in, or have more restricted access to, technology.

In addition to sampling issues, the selection of questionnaires and surveys also requires thoughtful consideration. Selection of study instruments will likely depend on the nature of use and the questions to be answered (e.g., clinical assessment and epidemiological studies, specific AT use vs. general AST use, etc), psychometric properties of measures, and instruments available (Agree & Freedman, 2011). Although similar questionnaires will likely provide a comparable pattern of information, it should be noted that questionnaire selection can significantly affect results depending on the topic of interest (Cornman et al., 2005). It is also important to note that the number of validated questionnaires that evaluate factors associated with AST acceptance and use is limited. Further development and use of standardized measures will allow for comparisons across studies and a better understanding of AST constructs within this area of research.

## Factors Affecting Technology Acceptance and Use

Various models and theories have postulated factors that predict human behavior; these factors have informed our understanding of general technology and AST acceptance and utilization. For example, social cognitive theory (SCT;

Bandura, 1986) is a well-established theory that considers the bidirectional effects of social/environmental and cognitive factors on behavior. Some of the core constructs of SCT, including self-efficacy, expectations, and social factors, have been evaluated in AST studies (e.g., Roelands, Van Oost, Depoorter et al., 2002). Other models were initially developed specifically for technology use. The technology acceptance model (TAM; David, 1989), for instance, conceptualized that perceived usefulness and perceived ease of use predict intention to use technology, which in turn affect actual technology use. More recently, the model has been revised (i.e., TAM2; Venkatesh & Davis, 2000) to include additional factors that modulate perceived usefulness and intention to use (e.g., experience, subjective norm, etc.). The Matching Person and Technology model (MPT; Scherer, 1998), commonly seen in the rehabilitation literature, takes a comprehensive approach to determine assistive device use. As its name suggests, the model proposes that successful technology adoption is dependent upon an appropriate fit among the user, the device, and the user's environment. In the following sections, proposed factors and research findings related to the influence of demographic variables, individual factors, and social and systemic factors are presented.

## DEMOGRAPHIC VARIABLES

Demographic variables have been given additional consideration in more recent models of technology acceptance (for a review, see Chen & Chan, 2011). Demographic factors (e.g., age and gender) are often broadly incorporated into models (e.g., TAM). Research has found that demographic variables, including age, education, marital status, gender, race, and income, are associated with technology acceptance and use as well as with attitudes regarding a broad spectrum of technology and computer-related technology (Ahn et al., 2008; Czaja et al., 2006; Hartke, Prohaska, & Furner, 1998). In general, youth, higher educational level, higher SES, single status, male gender, and Caucasian race are individual characteristics that have typically been found to be associated with increased general technology use. However, results regarding the relationship between age and AST use are not always consistent. While some studies found that AST users tended to be older than nonusers (Hartke et al., 1998; Horowitz et al., 2006), others found that the oldest-old age group (80+ years old) had a slower AST adoption rate (Pressler & Ferraro, 2010). Yet, others found that the relationship between age and AST adoption may be moderated by technology type (i.e., low-tech vs. high-tech devices; Kaye, Yeager, & Reed, 2008). More specifically, older individuals were found to be more inclined to use low-tech, but not high-tech, devices. In addition, it was reported that the influence of age was limited after accounting for the number and the type of disability (Kaye et al., 2008).

The relationship between AST use and level of education is equivocal. While some studies reported that AT use was associated with higher level of education irrespective of age, especially for devices that are in the medium- to high-tech ranges (Kaye et al., 2008), others found that lower education was associated with more AST use in an older adult sample (Hartke et al., 1998). Some of the observed differences may be modulated by health status or race (Hartke et al., 1998; Loggins, Alston, & Lewis, 2013). Several studies suggested that women were more likely than men to adopt assistive devices (Hartke et al., 1998; Kaye et al., 2008; Loggins et al., 2013). In addition, single women with poorer health status were found to be the most likely to use more than one AST device (Hartke et al., 1998). Minority status has been shown to be associated with less AST use, which was thought to be due to various factors, including cultural factors, limited access, and lower healthcare utilization (Kaye et al., 2008; Loggins et al., 2013). While individuals from minority groups or lower SES/education level were found to use AST less, they often have higher health needs than Caucasians or individiauls with higher SES or educational attainment (Hartke et al., 1998; LaPlante, Hendershot, & Moss, 1992). In contrast, the reverse was observed in a more recent study that included individuals who resided in Guam, Puerto Rico, and the U.S. Virgin Islands in addition to U.S. residents (Loggins et al., 2013). More specifically, it was reported that African Americans reported higher rates of AT use than their white counterparts. Furthermore, most of the African American AT users were from lower SES, less educated, reported less healthcare coverage, and expressed more concerns with medical cost.

## Summary

Demographic variables have been found to affect AST acceptance and use in different ways. Specifically, the relationships between AST use and age as well as education seem to be dynamic and nonlinear. While women and individuals with higher SES are more likely to adopt ASTs, minorities are generally less likely to adopt ASTs, which may be related to both SES and cultural factors. Findings regarding the impact of demographic variables on AST acceptance across studies may be difficult to compare because of the different ASTs evaluated. Although demographic factors are important to consider in AST acceptance, the impact of these factors may not always be the most pertinent determinants of AST use. For example, expectation to use, but not demographic variables (age, race, gender, and living situation), accounted for significant variance of device use at one month postdischarge and was a unique predictor of use among patients with diagnoses of cerebrovascular accident, orthopedic deficit, or lower limb amputation (Gitlin, Schemm, Landsberg, & Burgh, 1996). Regardless, AST use likely increases with age, as developmental physical and cognitive changes are inevitable. It is important to recognize that older individuals may be more comfortable using low-tech ASTs and that age may significantly affect findings of studies that evaluate use of low-tech versus high-tech devices. The relationship between demographic variables and AST use will likely continue to change with future cohorts of older adults who are much more confident and comfortable with technology. In addition, some of the observed trends will probably shift with changes in societal and cultural norms. Furthermore, given that technological level of ASTs modulated the relationship between AST use and several demographic variables, it would be beneficial to further investigate these factors with a more systematic approach. More specifically, it would be helpful to compare rates of AST acceptance across the technology spectrum of a specific AST domain using a within-subject design with a diverse group of participants.

### INDIVIDUAL VARIABLES

Individual variables that may impact AST acceptance and use include a heterogeneous number of factors such as beliefs about ASTs and self as well as situational factors (e.g., health condition). In the next section, individual variables related to AST specific beliefs and attitudes, personal beliefs and expectations about self and ASTs, and health and functional status will be discussed.

## AST-Specific Beliefs/Attitudes/Perception

Individual beliefs, attitudes, and/or perceptions have been implicated in several behavioral as well as technology acceptance models and theories (e.g., TAM, Theory of Planned Behavior; Ajzen, 1991). Included in this section is a review of studies evaluating older adults' general attitudes toward ASTs, perception regarding the usability and use of ASTs, and perceived advantages of using ASTs. It is critical to understand an individual's belief and perception about AST in order to increase individual AST use, develop effective intervention, and improve AST development.

Despite the common general perception that older adults are less open to new experience and more resistant to the use of technology, research findings seem to indicate the contrary. When asked to problem-solve hypothetical scenarios involving home-management needs, older adults more readily proposed the use of tools and techniques for assistance compared to other possible solutions (Kelly, Fausset, Rogers, & Fisk, 2012). Furthermore, several focus group studies suggested that older adults generally held a positive attitude toward a wide spectrum of ASTs (Demiris et al., 2004; McCreadie & Tinker, 2005; Mitzner et al., 2010). While older adults often expressed that ASTs could promote functional independence, some acknowledged that ASTs were not without limitations, because personal assistance or additional training/practice may be required. (Blaschke et al., 2009; Kelly et al., 2012; Roelands, Van Oost, Buysse, & Depoorter, 2002). Although older adults generally welcomed the use of ASTs, they also reported issues that can hinder AST use (e.g., usability, costs).

The perception of the usefulness of AST (i.e., perceived usefulness) to promote and maintain functional independence as well as the perceived degree of effort required to use an AST (i.e., perceived ease of use) have been found to be important factors in AST acceptance (e.g., Ahn et al., 2008; de Joode et al.,

2012; de Joode, van Heugten, Verhey, & van Boxtel, 2010; Mitzner et al., 2010; Roelands, Van Oost, Buysse, et al., 2002). Across studies, older adults identified that they generally valued AST products that promote safety and autonomy as well as product designs that were efficient, durable, and reliable (Courtney et al., 2007; Landau et al., 2010; Roelands, Van Oost, Buysse, et al., 2002). Others indicated that portability, functionality, and relative advantage over aids that serve a similar purpose were important when evaluating ASTs for cognitive rehabilitation (e.g., PDAs vs. low-tech compensatory aids; de Joode et al., 2012). While perception of usefulness may vary based on individual needs and prior experiences (Courtney et al., 2007), findings generally indicate that older adults are more accepting of ASTs when they regard ASTs as usable based on the products' reliability, effectiveness, and ability to promote and maintain safety (McCreadie & Tinker, 2005). In contrast, inconveniences and unhelpful features, as well as security and reliability concerns, have been associated with negative attitudes regarding ASTs (Mitzner et al., 2010).

The degree of effort required to use an AST (i.e., ease of use) has been suggested as one of the most critical factors in purchasing decisions across age groups; however, ease of use and postpurchase customer service support have also been found to be particularly important to older adults (Ahn et al., 2008; Mitzner et al., 2010). A lack of user friendliness of an AST lowers perceived ease of use, which negatively affects AST acceptance and utilization (Demiris et al., 2004). This generalization may be less relevant for individuals with a higher level of technology acceptance (Ahn et al., 2008). Although derived from a review of barriers to communication tool utilization among older adults, older adults' skeptical beliefs about general communicative technology (e.g., emails, computer, video chat, etc.; Blaschke et al., 2009), including issues related to safety, reliability, complexity, and self-confidence, are likely generalizable to other high-tech AT devices.

## Personal Beliefs and Expectations About Self and ASTs

One's beliefs and expectations about ability to use ASTs may contribute to perception and attitude toward ASTs, which in turn affects AST use and acceptance. Expectation plays a role in technology adoption. Krantz (2012) defined AST expectation as an individual's thoughts and attitudes prior to use of an AST about the appropriateness of the match between the needs of the individual and the functionality of the AST to enable participation in previously restricted activities. A hierarchical regression analysis from a longitudinal study of recently discharged patients age 55 and older showed that individuals' expectation regarding the need for ASTs while hospitalized was the strongest predictor of AST use one month postdischarge (Gitlin et al., 1996).

Personal value and perceived meaning of AST may tie closely with expectations, and they also affect AST adoption. Thoughts and attitudes regarding ASTs may be shaped by prior experiences as well as social and environmental factors. Individuals who value social acceptance may be more reluctant to use ASTs that are not accepted by his or her social group (Louise-Bender, Kim, & Weiner, 2002). In addition, a qualitative evaluation of comments by individuals with cerebrovascular accident suggested that use of ASTs can elicit feelings of ambivalence (i.e., feelings of loss vs. independence and well-being) that affect AST acceptance and adoption (Gitlin et al., 1996). Therefore, interventions that could adjust potential users' expectations or resolve any ambivalence or cognitive dissonance regarding AST use would likely lead to higher AST acceptance.

Historically, self-efficacy has been a well-established factor that contributes to behavioral change (Bandura, 1986). In the context of AST use, self-efficacy can be evaluated in a more general sense (e.g., general AST use) or can be assessed within a more specific domain (e.g., computerized devices). According to the self-efficacy theory, it is reasonable to expect that self-efficacy would be associated with AST acceptance and use. Consistently, older adults were found to be more resistant to adopting AST when they did not believe that they had adequate knowledge or experience with an AST (de Joode et al., 2012). Similarly, Roelands and colleagues (2002) found that self-efficacy was a unique predictor of intention to use. Apart from exposure and prior experience with ASTs, AST self-efficacy may also be specific to the type of device being evaluated (i.e., low-tech vs. high-tech; de Joode et al., 2012; Roelands, Van Oost, Buysse, et al., 2002).

The variability of self-efficacy across the AST technology spectrum may be associated with computer-related self-efficacy. Czaja et al. (2006) found that computer self-efficacy, mediated by computer anxiety, was associated with computer experience and exposure, which affected one's confidence and perceived ability in using computers and related tools (e.g., emailing and web browsing). Computer self-efficacy has also been found to be moderated by demographic factors, namely old age, minority status, and lower level of education (Czaja et al., 2006). In addition, computer self-efficacy can contribute to rates of AST acceptance and use. For example, "innovators" were found to be earlier adopters of technology than their peers (Saladin & Hansmann, 2008; Yi, Jackson, Park, & Probst, 2006). While various factors may contribute to the worsening of computer anxiety, computer self-efficacy may be enhanced through appropriate training and instruction. In a study of adults with cognitive complaints ($M = 53.5$; $SD = 12$), participants indicated on a questionnaire that instruction could enhance their ability to use ASTs like PDAs (de Joode et al., 2012).

## Health and Functional Status

Perceptions and beliefs about AST may be informed or altered by physical changes. With regard to health status and AST use, in a large sample of community-dwelling older adults, users of ASTs were found to be more likely to self-report poorer health, more restricted activity level, more days in bed, and higher frequency of medication utilization than participants who were nonusers (Hartke et al., 1998). Consistent with this finding, Ahn and colleagues (2008) found that individuals on both ends of the health-status spectrum (i.e., individuals who reported either poor or excellent health) were more accepting of household technologies, including health monitoring, than those who were in the middle of the continuum. This may suggest that individuals who are healthier may be more health-conscious and may be more interested in, or willing to consider, strategies that could promote health and well-being, while individuals who have more health issues have a higher need. In addition, the middle group may feel that monitoring could reduce their perception of independence and indicate difficulties that they do not want to acknowledge, or they could view monitoring as having little relevance to their needs.

Changes in health status often affect functional status, although they do not necessarily share a causal relationship. A decline in functional status has been shown to be associated with increased intensity of AST use, a higher number of AST devices used, and more reliance on personal care among community-dwelling older adults (Agree & Freedman, 2011; Hartke et al., 1998). Furthermore, individuals who experienced a higher level of disability were more likely to require personal assistance when using ASTs (Agree & Freedman, 2003). Thus, the relationship between functional status and AST use is likely nonlinear. Although there may be a negative correlation initially between functional status and AST use, over time, as functional status decreases, AST use may also decline due to increased reliance on personal assistance, difficulty with AST use, or the AST device failure to meet the user's changed needs.

Apart from health and functional status, research also suggests that medical diagnosis and the onset and duration of disability may play a role in AST adoption. More specifically, lower-body deficits and obesity were both independently associated with consistent AST use (Gitlin et al., 1996; Pressler & Ferraro, 2010). In contrast, a higher number of individuals with cerebrovascular accident than those with orthopedic deficits and lower-limb amputation did not use ASTs after discharge, despite being provided with at least one AST (Gitlin et al., 1996). However, the explanations of the differences in AST use across medical diagnoses are likely multifactorial. For example, when an illness or disability was diagnosed at birth or at a younger age, individuals were more inclined to adopt ATs and to consider more technologically advanced equipment than when assistive needs emerged in old age (Kaye et al., 2008). Furthermore, research suggests that individuals in some medical groups may be more willing to accept and use ASTs temporarily during a recovery period (e.g., individuals with orthopedic deficits; Haworth, 1983; Haworth & Hopkins, 1980).

Other medical diagnoses, including psychiatric disorders, may also affect AST use. Despite limited studies evaluating the effect of mental health factors on AST use, there is some evidence to suggest that a higher level of depression is associated with AST use, especially for individuals less than 75 years old (Okoro, Strine, Balluz, Crews, & Mokdad, 2010). In addition, in a study that evaluated vision impairment in a group of older adults, the use of ASTs that enhance vision (e.g., magnifiers), but not devices that compensate for vision loss (e.g., talking books, large-print material), was found to be correlated with a reduction of depressive symptoms and disability over time (Horowitz et al., 2006). Findings from these studies suggest that the higher levels of depression associated with AST use may be an indicator of impairment severity. In fact, data showed that greater disability at baseline was found to be a predictor of increased depression over time (Horowitz et al., 2006). Unlike the AT use trends observed in individuals with depression, individuals who were anxious were found to be much less likely to use ATs after discharge, as their ability to learn to use ATs may be affected by their anxiety (Wielandt, Mckenna, Tooth, & Strong, 2006). Further understanding of the impact of psychological factors on AST use outcome is needed.

## Summary

Several individual variables contribute to AST adoption and use. While some of these factors may be more difficult to control (e.g., health or functional status), others are likely modifiable (e.g., AST expectations, beliefs, self-efficacy). For example, one way to increase AST acceptance and use may be through providing AST information to help adjust expectations and shape personal views of ASTs. On an Internet survey, current AST users indicated that knowing about different options, soliciting other users' perspectives, and discussion with healthcare professionals were factors that contributed to feeling informed about ASTs (Martin et al., 2011). In contrast, not knowing available options or where to seek additional information, as well as feeling that a decision was dictated by funding sources, contributed to feeling uninformed. More importantly, results from the same study demonstrated that feeling informed, but not length of AST use, was associated with AST satisfaction. In addition, continued education and training with ASTs may be one way to increase older adults' AST self-efficacy, as technology is constantly changing and advancing. In addition to providing education and training, it is equally critical to establish and to evaluate different approaches that may be effective in increasing motivation and/or adherence to AST use as well as adjusting perceptions of self and ASTs.

### SOCIAL FACTORS AND OTHER SYSTEMIC ISSUES

Individual users of ASTs operate within a macrosystem. Therefore, social factors and systemic issues related to AST use likely affect a person's perception of, and experience with, ASTs. Some of the social and systemic factors highlighted in the literature that can significantly affect AST use and adoption are stigma, cost, and design issues.

## Social Factors

Social influence can significantly affect behavior and behavioral change, including older adults' decisions about AST use. While some older adults may be interested in current users' opinions when making decisions about AST use (Martin

et al., 2011), others may place more emphasis on their primary care providers' recommendations over nurses' or peers' opinions (Roelands, Van Oost, Depoorter,
et al., 2002). Family members' input (i.e., children and spouses) have also been
found to be important to older adults' consideration of AST adoption across studies (Chen & Chan, 2011; Roelands, Van Oost, Depoorter, et al., 2002). In a recent
study, while current AST users reported testing out devices prior to purchasing,
they also indicated that they considered input from durable medical equipment
(DME) supply staff, healthcare providers, family members, and peers in making
decisions about AST purchases (Martin et al., 2011). In contrast, customers' and
professionals' reviews were not commonly used during the information gathering process. It is also important to note that the utilization of consultation or the
type of consultation solicited may vary depending on the AST of interest. For
example, with regard to hearing devices, consultations with healthcare professionals were found to be more common than consultations with DME supply
staff (Martin et al., 2011), and individuals who used scooters were much less likely
than electric wheelchair users to consult with a healthcare professional prior to
making a purchase (Edwards & McCluskey, 2010).

Intertwined with social influence, stigma or image is another component
that contributes to AST acceptance (Coughlin et al., 2007; Krantz, 2012). There
is often a negative connotation to AST use, although the level of stigma may vary
depending on the device, and research has shown that negative social image due
to AST use is associated with a higher level of resistance to AST acceptance and
adoption (Coughlin et al., 2007; Courtney et al., 2007). A social image inconsistent with an individual's perception of his or her self-image or health status
may also result in greater resistance to AST use. For example, an individual who
does not self-identify as an older adult may be more resistant to ASTs that are
perceived to be made for the frail oldest-old (Courtney et al., 2007). Similarly,
the level of stigma associated with a medical diagnosis may also affect an individual's willingness to adopt an AST (Gitlin et al., 1996). Negative perceptions
could reduce technology acceptance and compliance, making ASTs less effective
and beneficial (Demiris et al., 2004). Although not often explicitly distinguished,
stigma can include social stigma (e.g., society's view regarding individuals who
use ASTs) and/or self-stigma (e.g., a user's perspective about the use of ASTs),
which can interact and reinforce one another (see Wallhagen, 2010). In a supportive social environment, individuals were more likely to use ASTs (Wessels
et al., 2003). Interventions and public policies that target reduction of the stigma
related to AST use would likely increase the population's rate of AST acceptance
and use.

## Systemic Issues

In addition to social perceptions of ASTs, other systemic issues can hinder AST
adoption. Cost is often a factor affecting AST acceptance, although its influence

can vary greatly across individuals and needs. While some participants indicated cost as a prohibitive factor (Steele, Lo, Secombe, & Wong, 2009), others placed less emphasis on financial burden in their decision making (Ahn et al., 2008; Roeland, Van Oost, Buysse, et al., 2002). The differences may be attributable to beliefs held by the older adult. More specifically, monetary cost had less salience when participants believed that there was a need for the AST device (Roelands, Van Oost, Depoorter, et al., 2002) or if they held a more accepting attitude about general household technology (Ahn et al., 2008). Concerns regarding cost are likely magnified when considering a higher-tech system like a smart home (Courtney et al., 2007) or smart wearable systems (Chan, Estève, Fourniols, Escriba, & Campo, 2012). In general, users of ASTs indicated that benefits outweigh costs (e.g., Mitzner et al., 2010). Regarding responsibility for payment, a web-based study showed that it is common for older adults to cover the expenses of ASTs, although some devices were more likely to be covered by insurance (e.g., mobility or respiratory devices; Martin et al., 2011).

Aside from monetary cost, loss of privacy has also been indicated as a potential cost of AST use, especially with high-tech devices that collect health information. Privacy concerns include personal information, obtrusiveness of a device (e.g., invasion of personal space), and perception of how the device may affect one's life (e.g., change of daily routine, confinement to a specific way of doing things, etc.; Courtney et al., 2008). While privacy and confidentiality concerns have been identified by staff and policy advocates as reasons for resistance to smart home technology (Coughlin et al., 2007), most older adults in a residential care facility who required some assistance with daily activities indicated in a focus group that the amount of privacy they expected would depend on their need for the technology (Courtney, 2008).

In addition to various factors that have been discussed in AST models, other systemic issues are barriers to AST acceptance and use and hinder AST adoption: lack of insurance coverage; product design issues; the lack of support and training for healthcare professionals, users, and caregivers; and the lack of research and development. When finances are a limiting factor in adopting ASTs, delayed or refused insurance claims make ASTs even more difficult to obtain (de Joode et al., 2012). Facilitating access to ASTs is essential to increasing AST acceptance and use (Xie, 2003). In addition, physical environments, including public areas, that are not conducive to AST use hinder AST acceptance and utilization (Seplaki et al., 2014; Wessels et al., 2003). In addition to access and environmental factors, design issues can contribute to nonuse of technology by older adults (e.g., small print). It is important for manufacturers to tailor AST devices to meet the needs of the aging population based on physical, sensory, and cognitive changes. For example, AST devices should have user-friendly language/instructions in age-appropriate fonts, simple, large button controls, and simple designs with centralized information (for a review, see Blaschke et al., 2009).

As mentioned, the lack of training available for healthcare professionals is also a barrier to AST acceptance and utilization in the older adult population. While the legislation continues to promote AST awareness and access through organizations like the Rehabilitation Engineering and Assistive Technology Society of North America (RESNA), training related to AST devices for healthcare providers, including neuropsychologists, remains limited. Although neuropsychologists often work with individuals who can benefit from ASTs, AST use by patients (e.g., smart pen for note-taking and audio recording) and by caregivers (e.g., sensor alerts for wandering) has not been widely considered in neuropsychological evaluation or treatment recommendations. Traditionally in neuropsychology, treatment and training in rehabilitation have largely focused on cognitive rehabilitation. Providers' perception and level of familiarity with ASTs can affect the potential users' adoption of AST. Staff who were less exposed to technology or held a less favorable view of it were less likely to recommend or encourage clients to consider ASTs (Baxter et al., 2012; de Joode et al., 2012). Similarly, older adult users also indicated the need for training and support, especially for more complex or technologically advanced devices (de Joode et al., 2012; Wessels et al., 2003). Providers with limited training and access to AST-related resources may find it difficult to make appropriate referrals or to provide suitable recommendations. Appropriate training and support for healthcare providers, users, and caregivers can in turn promote AST awareness and facilitate acceptance and utilization, thereby helping older individuals compensate for physical and cognitive changes.

Inadequate AST training may be partially related to a general lack of empirical support for AST efficacy, despite it being a burgeoning field of research (Blaschke et al., 2009; Demiris & Hensel, 2008), which could also inhibit AST awareness and acceptance. Furthermore, Rodgers and colleagues (2012) provided a summary from a workshop on technologies that called for increased interdisciplinary collaboration, active involvement of users in research and development, and further understanding of underlying mechanisms behind some of the age-related issues (e.g., falls) to refine the development of ASTs. Education of healthcare professional, patients, and caregivers will expand knowledge of AST needs and development and the efficacy of AST devices, as well as increase awareness of the clinical utility of ASTs.

## Summary

Based on several models, such as ICF, MPT, Value and Meaning in Human Occupations (for review, see Krantz, 2012), successful AST implementation is conceptualized as an appropriate match and/or efficient interaction between ASTs and the individual's needs or goals and/or environment. Research findings have provided support for this notion. For example, responses from a semistructured interview of a group of older adults age 70 and over suggested that the perceived need for ASTs may be dependent upon the individual's characteristics and his or her environment (McCreadie & Tinker, 2005). Similarly, some of the older adult participants from a study evaluating rehabilitation utilization, AST use, and social engagement who chose not to participate in the rehabilitation study indicated that they did not wish to modify their home environment (Lilja, Bergh, Johansson, & Nygård, 2003). However, the amount of home modification may also depend on the clinical issue at hand. For example, there is some evidence to suggest that minor adjustments (e.g., increased lighting, concealed door knobs, modification of home décor in a hallway) can be made to facilitate behavioral management of individuals with Alzheimer's disease (for a review, see Letts et al., 2011). To enhance the match between users and ASTs, social factors, cost, privacy, design issues, and appropriate training for users should be considered. Support and training for healthcare professionals and caregivers, collaboration with manufacturers, modification of the environment, and empirical support for AST outcome will also likely increase AST usability. In addition, further research is needed to illuminate the social and systemic factors that enhance AST outcomes. Validated interventions that would reduce social or self-perceived stigma would also be beneficial. While focus groups have identified general AST needs and perceptions from users and caregivers, it would also be beneficial to identify specific needs and recommendations regarding product designs. In addition, professional input into ways to improve product design or functionality to facilitate treatment and to better match clients' needs is important.

## Conclusion

A review of the AST literature showed a complex area of research that involves a number of different tools and devices spanning a wide spectrum of technology levels across diverse participant samples. Therefore, it is challenging to compare studies, given that ASTs were operationalized differently, participant characteristics were diverse, and cohort effects were likely present across study samples, as were cultural differences. It is also difficult to determine the relative importance of the varying factors reviewed to AST acceptance and use, since different factors were evaluated across models. However, it is also likely that the significance of the different factors varies across individuals and circumstances. Clearly, many individual, social, and systemic factors, as well as the interactions among the factors, can contribute to AST acceptance and use. Some of the factors included user's functional status, perceptions, and beliefs (including perceived ease of use and perceived usefulness); users' expectations and self-efficacy; stigma; cost; and privacy issues associated with AST use. While theoretical models continue to serve as a useful foundation for empirical research, the AST literature may benefit from a unified model drawing from the similarities and relevant unique factors among models. This would also allow for a more systematic approach to evaluating AST acceptance and use in future work.

## IMPLICATION OF CURRENT FINDINGS

Both personal and environmental factors are important to consider when developing new technologies and interventions for older adults and patients with neurological challenges. Increased research and clinical collaboration, effective education and training, and advocacy to increase AST acceptance and utilization are all essential to facilitating AST acceptance and use.

### New Technologies Development

Development of ASTs using a holistic approach to facilitate aging in place could benefit older adults (Levy & Waksvik, 1979). Until recently, most ASTs have largely been developed in isolation for specific needs. Given that most older adults desire to age in place and to utilize more than one AST (Bayer & Harper, 2000), it is important to continue to further develop both stand-alone devices and more comprehensive smart home technologies and/or smart wearable systems that meet the aging population's needs while promoting functional independence and overall well-being. Research findings demonstrated that, in addition to taking a comprehensive approach to AST development, a holistic perspective may maximize the benefit of AST use: for example, an approach incorporating health education, exercise, medication, and home modification can reduce fall risk (see Chase et al., 2012). Further research is needed to establish effective protocols for prevention and for management of age-related cognitive and physical changes, protocols that could also have clinical implications for the management of symptoms resulting from neurological disorders.

Currently, ASTs are available for individuals with cognitive difficulties as well as their caregivers. Recent studies have demonstrated that ATs, including smart technologies, are effective in monitoring household appliances to enhance safety (Mrazovac, Bjelica, Teslic, & Papp, 2011). In addition, there are a number of promising smart technology prototypes available for dementia care, although additional effort is needed to establish efficacy in this clinical population (Bharucha et al., 2009; Demiris & Hensel, 2008). Table 10.1 provides examples of devices commonly used by individuals with cognitive impairment and their caregivers (see also Daniel, Cason, & Ferrell, 2009; LoPresti, Mihailidis, & Kirsch, 2004). When used appropriately, ASTs (e.g., GPS tracking devices, lockable gas shut-off) can provide a sense of safety and reduce caregiver burden, especially when caregivers are away from their care-receivers (Landau et al., 2010; Wherton & Monk, 2008). While ATs and smart technologies have the potential to promote safety and functional independence, they are not without limitations. Neuropsychologists

TABLE 10.1  Examples of ASTs for Individuals with Cognitive Impairment and Their Caregivers

| | Individual with Cognitive Problems | Caregivers |
|---|---|---|
| Promote safety | • Night lights<br>• Timers<br>• Detectors (flood, carbon monoxide)<br>• Alarms (e.g., fire, burglar)<br>• Outlet switch-off devices | • Alerts<br>• Motion senors<br>• Pressure monitors<br>• Remote monitoring<br>• Wandering technology<br>• Tracking technologies (GPS) |
| Memory enhancer | • Planners/calendars/notes/to-do lists<br>• Reminder watch/alarms<br>• Electronic calendars<br>• Memory notebook<br>• Object finders<br>• Pill box reminders<br>• Recording devices<br>• Camera (e.g., Autographers, sensecam)<br>• Smartphones; Personal digital assistants (PDAs) | • Message board/to-do list<br>• Verbal reminders/reminder devices/cues<br>• Medication management devices |
| Support daily activities | • Motion-sensor faucets<br>• Bidets<br>• Intelligent prompting/cueing technologies (e.g., smart grab bars, planning & executing) | • Step-by-step instruction guide<br>• Intelligent prompting |
| Provide emotional support and information | • Picture button phones<br>• Support groups<br>• Tele-support<br>• Biofeedback devices | • Support groups<br>• Chat rooms<br>• Internet & telephone-based support groups<br>• Videoconferencing |

providing AST recommendations will have to consider individual strengths and weaknesses, as ASTs can present difficulties, depending on the level and area of cognitive deficits (Malinowsky, Almkvist, Kottorp, & Nygård, 2010). In addition, the cognitive effort required to effectively operate assistive devices may vary across individuals, which may hinder the successful utilization of ASTs (Bateni & Maki, 2005). Therefore, prescribing providers should work closely with the patient and family members/caregivers to determine the optimal use of ASTs and the amount of assistance or monitoring that individuals with cognitive impairment may require. Additional research is needed to further evaluate the effectiveness and limitations of ASTs across individuals with varying cognitive deficits and among various clinical populations.

Several authors have advocated that developers solicit and consider users' input, both during and beyond the production process, to ensure and increase AST usability and acceptance by developing a deeper understanding of users' needs and goals (de Joode et al., 2010; Demiris et al., 2004; Mitzner et al., 2010; Mynatt & Rogers, 2001; Rogers & Fisk, 2010). Doing so could reduce user frustration related to mismatch between user characteristics (e.g., physical and cognitive limitations) and features of AST devices. In addition, design issues (e.g., safety, durability, fonts, ease of use, etc.) must also be addressed to further reduce barriers to technology adoption. In a review of user experience of smart home technologies, it was recommended that interface designs should be intuitive and easy to learn (Kim, Oh, Cho, Lee, & Kim, 2012). Such a recommendation is applicable to other ASTs, especially medium- and high-tech devices. To design products that are developmentally appropriate, developers should consider the sensory, motor, and cognitive changes commonly experienced by older adults or the clinical populations that the devices are intended for (Mynatt & Rogers, 2001). Additionally, multimodal interfaces should be considered when applicable to meet different user needs and to facilitate encoding (Kim et al., 2012). Neuropsychologists can also serve as informed advocates to provide feedback to developers, because they are knowledgeable about physical and cognitive changes commonly involved in aging and in neurological pathology.

## Assistive Technology Awareness and Recommendation

To promote AST awareness, it is important to consider the medium favorable for introducing AST information to older adults (e.g., online information vs. printed materials), which may differ across cohorts of older adults. It is also important to continue to explore innovative ways to access populations who are less likely to respond and to take part in research, which limits our understanding of their needs and widens the gap between user needs and product functionality. In addition, it will be particularly beneficial to highlight factors that were found to be important in older adults' decision making. For example, it would be effective to underscore the safety benefits of, and increased efficiency with, AST use (Roelands, Van Oost, Buysse, et al., 2002).

Interdisciplinary collaboration is also essential to promote AST awareness and adoption. Collaboration among various healthcare providers, including medical doctors, nursing staff, neuropsychologists, physical therapists, occupational therapists, and speech therapists, should be encouraged. Neuropsychologists may find collaboration with physical, occupational, and/or speech therapists to be particularly fruitful in helping patients incorporate ASTs into their daily routine. While recommendations from healthcare providers are not always well understood or appreciated by patients (Scherer, 1996), neuropsychologists may be able to address or reinforce some of the issues through a biopsychosocial perspective. Similarly, it is important to consider patient and family members' opinions and to actively involve them in the process of AST decisions and implementation in order to increase user satisfaction and compliance (Baxter et al., 2012). When considering these factors, it is also important to reconcile differences that may occur between the client's/patient's perspectives and the caregivers' opinions (e.g., contradicting views regarding financial burden and the suitability of ASTs; de Joode et al., 2012). Addressing these issues openly can help the users and their caregivers to form realistic expectations about ASTs, which in turn facilitate AST acceptance and adoption (Gitlin et al., 1996).

To provide appropriate referrals/recommendations, clinicians must have a working understanding of the ASTs available and how they meet the needs of the client/patient. When prescribing ASTs, it is important to recommend devices that meet patients' physical and cognitive needs. In addition, it is equally critical to consider personal and familial factors, cultural heritage, and the social impact of AST use (Louise-Bender et al., 2002). Given the multilevel factors contributing to AST acceptance, neuropsychologists hold a unique position in facilitating the match between client needs and ASTs available, based on knowledge of a client's cognitive and psychosocial functions (Gillespie, Best, & O'Neill, 2012; Scherer, 2012).

## Education, Training, and Public Policy

Education is an effective method for increasing awareness and knowledge in the general public. Information regarding different types of ASTs and their associated benefits will increase knowledge as well as promote self-efficacy by increasing a perceived feeling of being informed (Martin et al., 2011; Mitzner et al., 2010). Education about AST use can encourage the perception that ASTs may not necessarily be needed as part of a treatment protocol, but may be helpful as preventive measures (a good example is grab bars in the bathroom to prevent falls). In addition, proper use of ASTs is required to maximize the effectiveness and efficiency of AST features. Krantz (2012) conjectured that the negative impact of improper AST use is worse than not using one at all. In fact, data suggest that inappropriate use of mobility devices may increase fall risk (Bateni & Maki, 2005). Therefore, training for users, caregivers, and healthcare providers is important to facilitate proper use (de Joode et al., 2012; Scherer, 1996). In addition, to maximize its benefits, training needs to be conducted in a manner that is appropriate to the target audience (Demiris et al., 2004). Training approaches that enhance the learner's ability to retain information are optimal. One study found that individuals who received and were able to recall AT training while hospitalized were more likely to use ATs postdischarge (Wielandt et al., 2006). Therefore, recommendations from neuropsychologists regarding the best training approach based on an individual's cognitive profile can be particularly beneficial.

Efforts should also be directed toward implementing environmental adjustments to enable the successful use of ASTs at home and in public (Layton, 2012). The Australian study by Layton (2012) found the perception that government funding and healthcare policies are often inadequate to support needs in this area. Furthermore, as participants expressed in the same study, a lack of efficient public transportation is also limiting for individuals who may have mobility, vision, and cognitive difficulties.

## Future Directions

Despite an accumulating body of literature supporting AST devices, there is still limited research evaluating the efficacy of AST use in the aging population (Horowitz et al., 2006). Several authors have advocated for more outcome research, especially randomized controlled studies with large samples that evaluate the efficacy of AST functions (de Joode, van Heugten, Verhey, & van Boxtel, 2010b; Gillespie et al., 2012; Lenker et al., 2010). Researchers conducting outcome studies should consider the guidelines put forth by Lenker and colleagues (2010) that highlight the importance of clear identification of the independent and dependent variables as well as the predicted relationships and the underlying mechanisms of AT outcomes (also see Lenker & Paquet, 2003, for a review of conceptual models for AST outcome research and practice). Interventions targeted at factors discussed in this chapter (e.g., adjusting one's expectations, reducing perceived stigma, etc.) would increase AST acceptance and use. In addition, attention should also focus on increasing AST awareness, given the lack of awareness of available assistive devices among older adults, caregivers, and healthcare professionals (Roelands, Van Oost, Buysse, et al., 2002). More specifically, additional work is needed to identify the optimal approach and methodology to increase awareness (e.g., written materials vs. demonstrative videos) and the format in which the information is delivered (e.g., individual vs. group, in-person vs. online). The effectiveness of approaches and methodologies across various clinical settings (e.g., inpatient vs. outpatient) and target populations (e.g., users vs. caregivers) should also be evaluated.

Recently, efforts have been made to develop effective approaches to increase AST awareness. For example, Sellers and Markham (2012) showed that an educational program that included brainstorming current assistive device use, demonstrating different ATs, and providing additional information related to ATs (e.g., cost, funding source) was effective in increasing AT knowledge in a sample from the general public ($N = 872$, age range = 21 to 96, $SD = 14.88$). The authors reported that about half (i.e., 40%) of a subset of the participants who completed a six-month follow-up ($N = 52$) purchased an AT or made home modifications. Similarly, Hill and colleagues (2009) demonstrated that older adults who watched a video on fall prevention reported a higher level of knowledge of fall risk, formulated more prevention strategies, and indicated a higher level of motivation to avoid falls than inpatients who read a workbook with identical information.

Extending the above work, to increase awareness and use of ASTs by older adults, caregivers, and healthcare professionals, including neuropsychologists, our laboratory, together with collaborators, recently developed an eight-video series on ASTs. Each video is 8- to 12-min long, and the topics covered are memory, daily living, medication management, mobility, fall prevention, hearing, vision, and communication. The videos can be accessed through our project's website, www.tech4aging.wsu.edu. Additional information about ASTs, including keywords, pricing information, national AT support information through RESNA, and other AST websites, is also available on the website. Our goal is to increase awareness and use of ASTs through the video program, as well as to further understand individual factors that may contribute to AST use/intention to use from a social cognition perspective (i.e., awareness, attitude, self-efficacy, subjective norm, and functional status; Roelands, Van Oost, Depoorter, et al., 2002). Consistent with this goal, our recent work showed that the program, which consisted of three selected videos, was effective in increasing AST knowledge, promoting more positive AST attitude, and reducing AST stigma in a sample of older adults (N = 231; Tam, Van Son, Dyck, & Schmitter-Edgecombe, under review). Not only were the reported effects sustained over a four-week follow-up, our data also showed that reducing AST stigma was a significant predictor of increased intention to engage in AST use. Therefore, we believe the materials developed through our research program are a valuable resource for neuropsychologists and their patients.

To further facilitate AST adoption, interventions to increase motivation, minimize barriers to adoption, and to facilitate an individual's progression from intention to use to AST adoption and use are needed. Increasingly, efforts have been made to further elucidate factors that may be important in enhancing learning in older adults (Callahan, Kiker, & Cross, 2003; Hickman et al., 2007). However, continued investigation to identify effective training approaches for older adults with and without cognitive impairment for different devices along the technology spectrum is also critical to successful AST implementation. Outcome research should also provide empirical support for intervention strategies and training paradigms for professionals, including neuropsychologists, and caregivers to increase AST utilization. Evaluation of interventions and training approaches that target different devices on the technology spectrum (e.g., low-tech vs. high-tech), clinical populations (e.g., individuals with mild cognitive impairment and/or psychiatric disorders), and context of use (e.g., essential use vs. voluntary use; see Brown, Massey, Montoya-weiss, & Burkman, 2002) will also likely be beneficial. Interdisciplinary collaboration, including input from users, is highly encouraged in this line of research.

# References

Agree, E. M., & Freedman, V. A. (2003). A comparison of assistive technology and personal care in alleviating disability and unmet need. *The Gerontologist, 43*(3), 335–344. Retrieved from http://www.ncbi.nlm.nih.gov/pubmed/12810897

Agree, E. M., & Freedman, V. A. (2011). A quality-of-life scale for assistive technology: Results of a pilot study of aging and technology. *Physical Therapy, 91*(12), 1780–1788. doi:10.2522/ptj.20100375

Agree, E. M., Freedman, V. A., Cornman, J. C., Wolf, D. A., & Marcotte, J. E. (2005). Reconsidering substitution in long-term care: When does assistive technology take the place of personal care? *Journal of Gerontology: Social Sciences, 60B*(5), 272–280.

Ahn, M., Beamish, J. O., & Goss, R. C. (2008). Understanding older adults' attitudes and adoption of residential technologies. *Family and Consumer Sciences Research Journal, 36*(3), 243–260. doi:10.1177/1077727X07311504

Ajzen, I. (1991). The theory of planned behavior. *Organizational Behavior and Human Decision Processes, 50*, 179–211.

Atkinson, H. H., Rosano, C., Simonsick, E. M., Williamson, J. D., Davis, C., Ambrosius, W. T., . . . Kritchevsky, S. B. (2007). Cognitive function, gait speed decline, and comorbidities: The Health, Aging and Body Composition study. *The Journal of Gerontology. Series A, Biological Sciences and Medical Sciences, 62*(8), 844–850. Retrieved from http://www.ncbi.nlm.nih.gov/pubmed/17702875

Auyeung, T. W., Kwok, T., Lee, J., Leung, P. C., Leung, J., & Woo, J. (2008). Functional decline in cognitive impairment—The relationship between physical and cognitive function. *Neuroepidemiology, 31*(3), 167–173. doi:10.1159/000154929

Bandura, A. (1986). The explanatory and predictive scope of self-efficacy theory. *Journal of Social and Clinical Psychology, 4*(3), 359–373. doi:10.1521/jscp.1986.4.3.359

Bateni, H., & Maki, B. E. (2005). Assistive devices for balance and mobility: Benefits, demands, and adverse consequences. *Archives of Physical Medicine and Rehabilitation, 86*(1), 134–145. doi:10.1016/j.apmr.2004.04.023

Bayer, A. H., & Harper, L. (2000). *Fixing to stay: A national survey of housing and home modification issues.* Washington, DC: AARP.

Baxter, S., Enderby, P., Evans, P., & Judge, S. (2012). Barriers and facilitators to the use of high-technology augmentative and alternative communication devices: A systematic review and qualitative synthesis. *International Journal of Language & Communication Disorders/Royal College of Speech & Language Therapists, 47*(2), 115–129. doi:10.1111/j.1460-6984.2011.00090.x

Bharucha, A. J., Anand, V., Forlizzi, J., Dew, M. A., Reynolds, C. F., Stevens, S., & Wactlar, H. (2009). Intelligent assistive technology applications to dementia care: current capabilities, limitations, and future challenges. *The American Journal of Geriatric Psychiatry: Official Journal of the American Association for Geriatric Psychiatry, 17*(2), 88–104. doi:10.1097/JGP.0b013e318187dde5

Blaschke, C. M., Freddolino, P. P., & Mullen, E. E. (2009). Ageing and technology: A review of the research literature. *British Journal of Social Work, 39*(4), 641–656. doi:10.1093/bjsw/bcp025

Boise, L., Wild, K., Mattek, N., Ruhl, M., Dodge, H. H., & Kaye, J. (2013). Willingness of older adults to share data and privacy concerns after exposure to unobtrusive home monitoring. *Gerontechnology, 11*(3), 428–435.

Brown, S. A., Massey, A. P., Montoya-weiss, M. M., & Burkman, J. R. (2002). Do I really have to? User acceptance of mandated technology. *European Journal of Information Systems, 11*(4), 283–295. doi:10.1057/palgrave.ejis.3000438

Callahan, J. S., Kiker, D. S., & Cross, T. (2003). Does method matter? A meta-analysis of the effects of training method on older learner training performance. *Journal of Management, 29*(5), 663–680. doi:10.1016/S0149-2063

Cattaneo, D., de Nuzzo, C., Fascia, T., Macalli, M., Pisoni, I., & Cardini, R. (2002). Risks of falls in subjects with multiple sclerosis. *Archives of Physical Medicine and Rehabilitation, 83* (6), 864–867. doi:10.1053/apmr.2002.32825

Chan, M., Estève, D., Fourniols, J.-Y., Escriba, C., & Campo, E. (2012). Smart wearable systems: Current status and future challenges. *Artificial Intelligence in Medicine, 56*(3), 137–156. doi:10.1016/j.artmed.2012.09.003

Chase, C. A., Mann, K., Wasek, S., & Arbesman, M. (2012). Systematic review of the effect of home modification and fall prevention programs on falls and the performance of community-dwelling older adults. *The Journal of Occupational Therapy, 66,* 284–291. Doi:10.5014/ajot.2012.005017

Chen, K., & Chan, A. H. S. (2011). A review of technology acceptance by older adults. *Gerontechnology, 10*(1). doi:10.4017/gt.2011.10.01.006.00

Constantinescu, R., Leonard, C., Deeley, C., & Kurlan, R. (2007). Assistive devices for gait in Parkinson's disease. *Parkinsonism & Related Disorders, 13* (3), 133–138. doi:10.1016/j.parkreldis.2006.05.034

Cornman, J. C., Freedman, V. A., & Agree, E. M. (2005). Measurement of assistive device use: Implications for estimates of device use and disability in late life. *The Gerontologist, 45*(3), 347–58. Retrieved from http://www.ncbi.nlm.nih.gov/pubmed/15933275

Coughlin, J. F., D'Ambrosio, L. A., Reimer, B., & Pratt, M. R. (2007). Older adult perceptions of smart home technologies: Implications for research, policy & market innovations in healthcare. *Proceedings of the 29th Annual International Confeence of the IEEE EMBS, France, 1810-1815.*

Courtney, K. L. (2008). Privacy and senior willingness to adopt smart home information technology in residential care facilities. *Methods of Information in Medicine, 47*(1), 76–81.

Courtney, K. L., Demiris, G., & Hensel, B. K. (2007). Obtrusiveness of information-based assistive technologies as perceived by older adults in residential care facilities: A secondary analysis. *Medical Informatics and the Internet in Medicine, 32*(3), 241–249. doi:10.1080/14639230701447735

Czaja, S. J., Charness, N., Fisk, A. D., Hertzog, C., Nair, S. N., Rogers, W. A., & Sharit, J. (2006). Factors predicting the use of technology: Findings from the Center for Research and Education on Aging and Technology Enhancement (CREATE). *Psychology and Aging, 21*(2), 333–352. doi:10.1037/0882-7974.21.2.333

Daniel, K., Cason, C., & Ferrell, S. (2009). Assistive technologies for use in the home to prolong independence. In *Proceedings of the 2nd International Conference on Pervasive Technologies Related to Assistive Environments.* ACM, Greece. doi:10.1145/1579114.1579140

David, F. D., Bagozzi, R. P., & Warshaw, P. R. (1989). User acceptance of computer technology: A comparison of two theoretical models. *Management Science, 35*(8): 982–1003. doi:10.1287/mnsc.35.8.982

de Joode, E. A., van Boxtel, M. P. J., Verhey, F. R., & van Heugten, C. M. (2012). Use of assistive technology in cognitive rehabilitation: Exploratory studies of the opinions and expectations of healthcare professionals and potential users. *Brain Injury, 26*(10), 1257–1266. doi:10.3109/02699052.2012.667590

de Joode, E., van Heugten, C., Verhey, F., & van Boxtel, M. (2010). Efficacy and usability of assistive technology for patients with cognitive deficits: A systematic review. *Clinical Rehabilitation, 24*(8), 701–714. doi:10.1177/0269215510367551

Demers, L., Weiss-lambrou, R., & Ska, B. (2002). The Quebec User Evaluation of Satisfaction with Assistive Technology (QUEST 2. 0): An overview and recent progress. *Technology and Disability, 14,* 101–105.

Demiris, G., & Hensel, B. K. (2008). Technologies for an aging society: A systematic review of "smart home" applications. *Yearbook of Medical Informatics,* 33–40. Retrieved from http://www.ncbi.nlm.nih.gov/pubmed/18660873

Demiris, G., Oliver, D. P., Dickey, G., Skubic, M., & Rantz, M. (2008). Findings from a participatory evaluation of a smart home application for older adults. *Technology and Health Care: Official Journal of the European Society for Engineering and Medicine, 16*(2), 111–8. Retrieved from http://www.ncbi.nlm.nih.gov/pubmed/18487857

Demiris, G., Rantz, M., Aud, M., Marek, K., Tyrer, H., Skubic, M., & Hussam, A. (2004). Older adults' attitudes towards and perceptions of "smart home" technologies: A pilot study. *Medical Informatics and the Internet in Medicine, 29*(2), 87–94. doi:10.1080/14639230410001684387

Edwards, K., & McCluskey, A. (2010). A survey of adult power wheelchair and scooter users. *Disability and Rehabilitation. Assistive Technology, 5*(6), 411–419. doi:10.3109/17483101003793412

Gillespie, A., Best, C., & O'Neill, B. (2012). Cognitive function and assistive technology for cognition: A systematic review. *Journal of the International Neuropsychological Society: JINS, 18*(1), 1–19. doi:10.1017/S1355617711001548

Gitlin, L. N., Schemm, R. L., Landsberg, L., & Burgh, D. (1996). Factors predicting assistive device use in the home by older people following rehabilitation. *Journal of Aging and Health, 8*(4), 554–575. doi:10.1177/089826439600800405

Granger, C. V., & Hamilton, B. B. (1992). The uniform data system for medical rehabilitation report of first admissions for 1990. *American Journal of Physical Medicine and Rehabilitation, 71*,108–113.

Hartke, R. J., Prohaska, T. R., & Furner, S. E. (1998). Older adults and assistive devices: Use, multiple-device use, and need. *Journal of Aging and Health, 10*(1), 99–116.

Haworth, R. J. (1983). Use of aids during the first three months after total hip replacement. *British Journal of Rheumatology, 22*,29–35.

Haworth, R. J., & Hopkins, J. (1980). Use of aids following total hip replacement. *British Journal of Occupational Therapy, 43*, 398–400.

Hickman, J. M., Rogers, W. A., & Fisk, A. D. (2007). Training older adults to use new technology. *The Journals of Gerontology. Series B, Psychological Sciences and Social Sciences, 62*(Spec. I), 77–84. Retrieved from http://www.ncbi.nlm.nih.gov/pubmed/17565168

Hill, A.-M., McPhail, S., Hoffmann, T., Hill, K., Oliver, D., Beer, C., . . . Haines, T. P. (2009). A randomized trial comparing digital video disc with written delivery of falls prevention education for older patients in hospital. *Journal of the American Geriatrics Society, 57*(8), 1458–1463. doi:10.1111/j.1532-5415.2009.02346.x

Horowitz, A., Brennan, M., Reinhardt, J. P., & Macmillan, T. (2006). The impact of assistive device use on disability and depression among older adults with age-related vision impairments. *The Journals of Gerontology. Series B, Psychological Sciences and Social Sciences, 61*(5), S274–280. Retrieved from http://www.ncbi.nlm.nih.gov/pubmed/16960241

Jamieson, B. A., & Rogers, W. A. (2000). Age-related effects of blocked and random practice schedules on learning a new technology. *The Journals of Gerontology. Series B, Psychological Sciences and Social Sciences, 55*(6), P343–353. Retrieved from http://www.ncbi.nlm.nih.gov/pubmed/11078104

Jutai, J., & Day, H. (2002). Psychosocial Impact of Assistive Devices Scale (PIADS). *Technology and Disability, 14*, 107–111.

Kaye, H. S., Yeager, P., & Reed, M. (2008). Disparities in usage of assistive technology among people with disabilities. *Assistive Technology: The Official Journal of RESNA, 20*(4), 194–203. doi:10.1080/10400435.2008.10131946

Kelly, A. J., Fausset, C. B., Rogers, W., & Fisk, A. D. (2014). Responding to home maintenance challenge scenarios: The role of selection, optimization, and compensation in aging-in-place. *Journal of Applied Gerontology, 33*(8), 1018–1042. doi:10.1177/0733464812456631

Kim, M. J., Oh, M. W., Cho, M. E., Lee, H., & Kim, J. T. (2012). A critical review of user studies on healthy smart homes. *Indoor and Built Environment, 22*(1), 260–270. doi:10.1177/1420326X12469733

Kitzinger, J. (1994). The methodology of focus groups: The importance of interaction between research participants. *Sociology of Health and Illness, 16*(1), 103–121. doi:10.1111/1467-9566.ep11347023

Krantz, O. (2012). Assistive devices utilisation in activities of everyday life—A proposed framework of understanding a user perspective. *Disability and Rehabilitation. Assistive Technology, 7*(3), 189–198.

Kraskowsky, L. H., & Finlayson, M. (2000). Factors affecting older adults' use of adaptive equipment: Review of the literature. *The American Journal of Occupational Therapy, 55*(3), 303–310.

Landau, R., Werner, S., Auslander, G. K., Shoval, N., & Heinik, J. (2010). What do cognitively intact older people think about the use of electronic tracking devices for people with dementia? A preliminary analysis. *International Psychogeriatrics/IPA, 22*(8), 1301–1309. doi:10.1017/S1041610210001316

LaPlante, M. P., Hendershot, G. E., & Moss, A. J. (1992). *Assistive technology devices and home accessibility features: Prevalence, payment, need, and trends* (pp. 1–12). Advance data from vital and health statistics, No. 217.

Layton, N. (2012). Barriers and facilitators to community mobility for assistive technology users. *Rehabilitation Research and Practice, 2012,* 1–9. doi:10.1155/2012/454195

Lenker, J. A., Fuhrer, M. J., Jutai, J. W., Demers, L., Scherer, M. J., & DeRuyter, F. (2010). Treatment theory, intervention specification, and treatment fidelity in assistive technology outcomes research. *Assistive Technology: The Official Journal of RESNA, 22*(3), 129–138; quiz 139–140. doi:10.1080/10400430903519910

Lenker, J. A., & Paquet, V. L. (2003). A review of conceptual models for assistive technology outcomes research and practice. *Assistive Technology: The Official Journal of RESNA, 15*(1), 1–15.

Lenker, J. A., Scherer, M. J., Fuhrer, M. J., Jutai, J. W., & DeRuyter, F. (2005). Psychometric and administrative properties of measures used in assistive technology device outcomes research. *Assistive Technology: The Official Journal of RESNA, 17*(1), 7–22. doi:10.1080/10400435.2005.10132092

Letts, L., Minezes, J., Edwards, M., Berenyi, J., Moros, K., O'Neill, C., & O'Toole, C. (2011). Effectiveness of interventions designed to modify and maintain perceptual abilities in people with Alzheimer's disease and related dementias. *American Journal of Occupational Therapy, 65*(5), 505–513. doi:10.5014/ajot.2011.002592

Levy, R., & Waksvik, K. (1979). Reflections on designing special devices for the disabled: Towards a holistic approach. *Physiotherapy Canada, 31*(6), 313–317.

Lilja, M., Bergh, A., Johansson, L., & Nygård, L. (2003). Attitudes towards rehabilitation needs and support from assistive technology and the social environment among elderly people with disability. *Occupational Therapy International*, 10(1), 75–93. Retrieved from http://www.ncbi.nlm.nih.gov/pubmed/12830320

Liu, C-J., Brost, M. A., Horton, V. E., Kenyon, S. B., & Mears, K. E. (2013). Occupational therapy interventions to improve performance of daily activities at home for older adults with low vision: A systematic review. *The American Journal of Occupational Therapy*, 67, 279–287. doi:10.5014/ajot.2013.005512

Loggins, S., Alston, R., & Lewis, A. (2014). Utilization of assistive technology by persons with physical disabilities: An examination of predictive factors by race. *Disability and Rehabilitation. Assistive Technology*, 9(2014), 1–6. doi:10.3109/17483107.2013.836683

LoPresti, E. F., Mihailidis, A., & Kirsch, N. (2004). Assistive technology for cognitive rehabilitation: State of the art. *Neuropsychological Rehabilitation*, 14(1–2), 5–39. doi:10.1080/09602010343000101

Louise-Bender, P. T., Kim, J., & Weiner, B. (2002). The shaping of individual meanings assigned to assistive technology: A review of personal factors. *Disability and Rehabilitation*, 24(1–3), 5–20. Retrieved from http://www.ncbi.nlm.nih.gov/pubmed/11827155

Malinowsky, C., Almkvist, O., Kottorp, A., & Nygård, L. (2010). Ability to manage everyday technology: A comparison of persons with dementia or mild cognitive impairment and older adults without cognitive impairment. *Disability and Rehabilitation. Assistive Technology*, 5(6), 462–469. doi:10.3109/17483107.2010.496098

Mann, W. C., Ottenbacher, K. J., Fraas, L., Tomita, M., & Granger, C. V. (1999). Effectiveness of assistive technology and environmental interventions in maintaining independence and reducing home care costs for the frail elderly. A randomized controlled trial. *Archives of Family Medicine*, 8(3), 210–217. Retrieved from http://www.ncbi.nlm.nih.gov/pubmed/10333815

Martin, J. K., Martin, L. G., Stumbo, N. J., & Morrill, J. H. (2011). The impact of consumer involvement on satisfaction with and use of assistive technology. *Disability and Rehabilitation. Assistive Technology*, 6(3), 225–242. doi:10.3109/17483107.2010.522685

McCreadie, C., & Tinker, A. (2005). The acceptability of assistive technology to older people. *Ageing and Society*, 25(1), 91–110. doi:10.1017/S0144686X0400248X

Mitzner, T. L., Boron, J. B., Fausset, C. B., Adams, A. E., Charness, N., Czaja, S. J., . . . Sharit, J. (2010). Older adults talk technology: Technology usage and attitudes. *Computers in Human Behavior*, 26(6), 1710–1721. doi:10.1016/j.chb.2010.06.020

Mrazovac, B., Bjelica, M. Z., Teslic, N., & Papp, I. (2011). Towards ubiquitous smart outlets for safety and energetic efficiency of home electric appliances. *IEEE International Conference on Consumer Electronics—Berlin (ICCE-Berlin)*, 322–326.

Mynatt, E. D., & Rogers, W. A. (2001). Developing technology to support the functional independence of older adults. *Ageing International*, 27(1), 24–41. doi:10.1007/s12126-001-1014-5

Okoro, C. A., Strine, T. W., Balluz, L. S., Crews, J. E., & Mokdad, A. H. (2010). Prevalence and correlates of depressive symptoms among United States adults with disabilities using assistive technology. *Preventive Medicine*, 50(4), 204–209. doi:10.1016/j.ypmed.2010.01.008

Palmer, S. B., Wehmeyer, M. L., Davies, D. K., & Stock, S. E. (2012). Family members' reports of the technology use of family members with intellectual and developmental disabilities. *Journal of Intellectual Disability Research: JIDR, 56*(4), 402–414. doi:10.1111/j.1365-2788.2011.01489.x

Padilla, R. (2011). Effectiveness of environment-based interventions for people with Alzheimer's disease and related dementias. *American Journal of Occupational Therapy, 65*(5), 514–522. doi:10.5014/ajot.2011.002600

Parsons, S., Daniels, H., Porter, J., & Robertson, C. (2008). Resources, staff beliefs and organizational culture: Factors in the use of information and communication technology for adults with intellectual disabilities. *Journal of Applied Research in Intellectual Disabilities, 21,* 19–33.

Powell, R. A., & Single, H. M. (1996). Focus groups. *International Journal for Quality in Health Care, 8*(5), 499–504.

Pressler, K. A., & Ferraro, K. F. (2010). Assistive device use as a dynamic acquisition process in later life. *The Gerontologist, 50*(3), 371–381. doi:10.1093/geront/gnp170

The American Recovery and Reinvestment Act of 2009, 42 U.S.C. §17903. Public Law 111-5. Roelands, M., Van Oost, P., Buysse, A., & Depoorter, A. (2002). Awareness among community-dwelling elderly of assistive devices for mobility and self-care and attitudes towards their use. *Social Science & Medicine (1982), 54*(9), 1441–1451. Retrieved from http://www.ncbi.nlm.nih.gov/pubmed/12058859

Roelands, M., Van Oost, P., Depoorter, A., & Buysse, A. (2002). A social-cognitive model to predict the use of assistive devices for mobility and self-care in elderly people. *The Gerontologist, 42*(1), 39–50. Retrieved from http://www.ncbi.nlm.nih.gov/pubmed/11815698

Rodgers, M. M., Cohen, Z. A., Joseph, L., & Rossi, W. (2012). Workshop on personal motion technologies for healthy independent living: Executive summary. *Archives of Physical Medicine and Rehabilitation, 93*(6), 935–939. doi:10.1016/j.apmr.2011.12.026

Rogers, W. A., & Fisk, A. D. (2010). Toward a psychological science of advanced technology design for older adults. *Journal of Gerontology: Psychological Sciences, 65B*(6), 645–653. doi:10.1093/geronb/gbq065.

Rosano, C., Simonsick, E. M., Harris, T. B., Kritchevsky, S. B., Brach, J., Visser, M., . . . Newman, A. B. (2005). Association between physical and cognitive function in healthy elderly: The Health, Aging, and Body Composition Study. *Neuroepidemiology, 24,* 8–14.

Rosenberg, L., Kottorp, A., & Nygard, L. (2011). Readiness for technology use with people with dementia: The perspectives of significant others. *Journal of Applied Gerontology, 31*(4), 510–530. doi:10.1177/0733464810396873

Saladin, S. P., & Hansmann, S. E. (2008). Psychosocial variables related to the adoption of video relay services among deaf or hard-of-hearing employees at the Texas School for the Deaf. *Assistive Technology: The Official Journal of RESNA, 20*(1), 36–47. doi:10.1080/10400435.2008.10131930

Seplak, C. L., Agree, E. M., Weiss, C. O., Szanton, S. L., Bandeen-Roche, K., Fried, L. P. (2014). Assistive devices in context: Cross-sectional association between challenges in the home environment and use of assistive devices for mobility. *The Gerontologist, 54* (4), 651–660. doi: 10.1093/geront/gnt030

Scherer, M. J. (1998). *Matching person and technology*. Webster, NY: Institute for Matching Person & Technology.

Scherer, M. J. (1996). Outcomes of assistive technology use on quality of life. *Disability and Rehabilitation, 18*(9), 439–448.

Scherer, M. J. (2012). *Assistive technologies and other supports for people with brain impairment*. New York, NY: Springer Publishing Company.

Sellers, D. M., & Markham, M. S. (2012). Raising awareness of assistive technology in older adults through a community-based, cooperative extension program. *Gerontology & Geriatrics Education, 33*(3), 287–313. doi:10.1080/02701960.2012.664589

Shone Stickel, M., Ryan, S., Rigby, P. J., & Jutai, J. W. (2002). Toward a comprehensive evaluation of the impact of electronic aids to daily living: Evaluation of consumer satisfaction. *Disability and Rehabilitation, 24*(1–3), 115–125. Retrieved from http://www.ncbi.nlm.nih.gov/pubmed/11827145

Slegers, K., van Boxtel, M. P. J., & Jolles, J. (2007). The effects of computer training and Internet usage on the use of everyday technology by older adults: A randomized controlled study. *Educational Gerontology, 33*(2), 91–110. doi:10.1080/03601270600846733

Steele, R., Lo, A., Secombe, C., & Wong, Y. K. (2009). Elderly persons' perception and acceptance of using wireless sensor networks to assist healthcare. *International Journal of Medical Informatics, 78*(12), 788–801. doi:10.1016/j.ijmedinf.2009.08.001

Tam, J., Van Son, C., Dyck, D., & Schmitter-Edgecombe, M. (under review). An educational video program to increase aging services technology awareness among older adults.

Topo, P. (2008). Technology studies to meet the needs of people with dementia and their caregivers: A literature review. *Journal of Applied Gerontology, 28*(1), 5–37. doi:10.1177/0733464808324019

U.S. Department of Health and Human Services, Assistant Secretary for Planning and Education, Office of Disability, Aging and Long-Term Care Policy. (2012). *Report to Congress: Aging Services Technology Study*. Retrieved from http://aspe.hhs.gov/daltcp/reports/2012/astsrptcong.shtml

Venkatesh, V., & Davis, F. D. (2000). A theoretical extension of the technology acceptance model: Four longitudinal field studies. *Management Science, 46*(2), 186–204. doi:10.1287/mnsc.46.2.186.11926

Vishwanath, A., Brodsky, L., Shaha, S., Leonard, M., & Cimino, M. (2009). Patterns and changes in prescriber attitudes toward PDA prescription-assistive technology. *International Journal of Medical Informatics, 78*(5), 330–9. doi:10.1016/j.ijmedinf.2008.10.004

Wallhagen, M. I. (2010). The stigma of hearing loss. *The Gerontologist, 50*(1), 66–75. doi:10.1093/geront/gnp107

Wang, L., Larson, E. B., Bowen, J. D., & van Belle, G. (2006). Performance-based physical function and future dementia in older people. *Archives of Internal Medicine, 166*(10), 1115–1120. doi:10.1001/archinte.166.10.1115

Wessels, R., Dijcks, B., Soede, M., Gelderblom, G. J., & De Witte, L. (2003). Non-use of provided assistive technology devices, a literature overview. *Technology and Disability, 15*, 231–238.

Wherton, J. P., & Monk, A. F. (2008). Technological opportunities for supporting people with dementia who are living at home. *International Journal of Human-Computer Studies, 66*(8), 571–586. doi:10.1016/j.ijhcs.2008.03.001

Wielandt, T., Mckenna, K., Tooth, L., & Strong, J. (2006). Factors that predict the post-discharge use of recommended assistive technology (AT). *Disability & Rehabilitation. Assistive Technology, 1*(1–2), 29–40. doi:10.1080/09638280500167159

World Health Organization. (2001). *International classification of functioning, disability and health: ICF.* Geneva, Switzerland: World Health Organization.

Xie, B. (2003). Older adults, computers, and the Internet: Future directions. *Gerontechnology, 2*(4), 289–305. doi:10.4017/gt.2003.02.04.002.00

Yarbrough, A. K., & Smith, T. B. (2007). Technology acceptance among physicians: A new take on TAM. *Medical Care Research and Review: MCRR, 64*(6), 650–672. doi:10.1177/1077558707305942

Yi, M. Y., Jackson, J. D., Park, J. S., & Probst, J. C. (2006). Understanding information technology acceptance by individual professionals: Toward an integrative view. *Information & Management, 43*(3), 350–363. doi:10.1016/j.im.2005.08.006

Zhuang, Z., Stobbe, T. J., Hsiao, J., Collins, J. W., & Hobbs, G. R. (1999). Biomechanical evaluation of assistive devices for transferring residents. *Applied Ergonomics, 30*(4), 285–294. doi:10. 1016/S0003-6870(98)000.5-0

# 11

# Using Smart Environment Technologies to Monitor and Assess Everyday Functioning and Deliver Real-Time Intervention

Maureen Schmitter-Edgecombe, Diane J. Cook, Alyssa Weakley, and Prafulla Dawadi

Technology is changing healthcare and our understanding of human behavior. To date, most of our theories about behavior, everyday activities, and cognitive health have been formed based on questionnaire data, laboratory tests and experiments, and placing observers within the environment to record human behavioral habits. Smart technologies offer an opportunity to passively collect data about human behavior within the everyday environment. The possibilities for using smart technologies that can adapt, sense, infer, learn, anticipate, and intervene for health monitoring and intervention are considered "extraordinary" (Department of Health, 2007). Our Smart Home group affiliated with the Center for Advanced Studies in Adaptive Systems (CASAS) and others have been studying the role of smart environments as a type of "cognitive prosthesis" in which the smart environment operates alongside humans in order to monitor, maintain, and enhance their health and functional capabilities and overcome their limitations.

For the clinical neuropsychologist, smart environment technologies offer opportunities for new methods of data collection, for both clinical and research purposes. Over the past decade, sensor technologies have become more mature. For example, sensor power and capacity have increased while sensor size and cost have decreased. Similarly, there has been significant progress in the areas of wireless networks, data processing, and machine learning. Data can now be automatically collected from sensor-filled smart homes (environmental or fixed devices), activity trackers (wearable devices), and smartphones (portable devices) in an unobtrusive manner while people perform their normal activities of daily living. The data can then be used to support everyday activities and to assist in rehabilitation and proactive interventions through real-time assistance and monitoring of real-world responses to intervention. The data can also be used to improve our understanding of the effects of cognitive impairment on everyday functioning as well as theories about behavior. The chapter begins with a discussion of research in the area of activity recognition, followed by application of this work to functional and health assessment and to activity-aware intervention.

## Activity Monitoring

Understanding everyday functioning and responses to intervention is important to the field of neuropsychology. Clinical neuropsychologists are often tasked with predicting everyday functioning from interview and cognitive testing data and with providing recommendations for intervention. Technologies that allow for automated modeling and monitoring of activities within the home and community environment have the potential to provide more continuous, detailed, and ecologically valid information about everyday functioning and response to interventions. However, in order to monitor activities from sensor data, methods for recognizing predefined activities (e.g., eating) and discovering activities (e.g., toy-making hobby) from unlabeled sensor data are needed. In addition, activity-learning methods must generalize beyond labeled training data to monitor activities for new individuals, in new settings, and with diverse sensor platforms. Work in the areas of activity recognition, activity discovery, and activity generalization serves as the basis for using smart environment technologies for functional assessment and intervention.

### ACTIVITY RECOGNITION

In a smart home environment, a variety of sensor types can be used to provide insight about everyday activities. The sensors may include passive infrared sensors, or motion sensors, that detect heat-based movement in their field of view. Such sensors provide insight about the location of individuals within a smart home. Other useful sensors include magnetic door sensors that indicate when a particular door or cabinet is open or shut, light sensors that report ambient light levels, temperature sensors, humidity sensors, and whole-home electricity consumption sensors. Sensors like vibration sensors and pressure sensors can also be attached to particular items within the home (e.g., a chair, a bed, a medicine dispenser) to indicate when the item is in use. One advantage of employing such ambient sensors is that they are passive. That is, the residents do not need to wear anything or perform activities in any particular manner for the smart home to gather information.

Sensors record event states that can be used in activity recognition. For example, motion sensors turn to an ON state when movement is detected and turn OFF when movement stops. Each ON/OFF state is recorded as a sensor event. The combination of sensor events can be learned by an activity-recognition algorithm and can be linked to predefined output activity labels (e.g., cooking, grooming, left house). The challenge of activity recognition is to map a sequence of sensor events, $x = <e_1 e_2 \ldots e_n>$, onto a value from a set of predefined activity labels. Activity recognition can be viewed as a type of supervised machine-learning problem.

Figure 11.1 shows the steps involved in activity recognition. First, raw sensor data are collected and preprocessed, then the data are divided into sensor subsequences of manageable size. Next, sensor-event features are extracted from the sub-sequences and are correctly labeled by an expert who can identify what was occurring when the sensor pattern emerged (e.g., cooking). This provides ground truth for the particular sensor event. The algorithm can than examine the particular ON/OFF sensor-event sequence and map it onto the expert-derived activity label for future recognition. Once the relationship is learned, the algorithm can automatically detect and label future occurrences of the activity without any expert intervention.

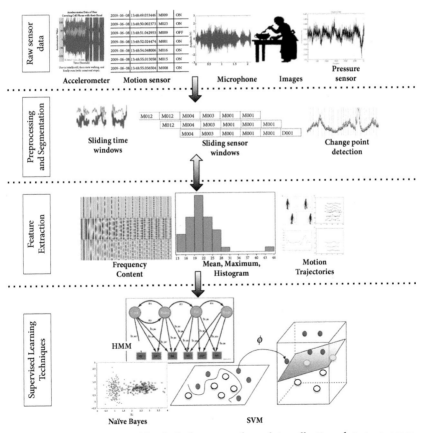

FIGURE 11.1 *Activity recognition includes stages of raw data collection, data preprocessing and segmentation, feature extraction, and supervised machine learning.*

A number of approaches have been explored for supervised activity recognition (Bulling, Blanke, & Schiele, 2014; Chen, Hoey, Nugent, Cook, & Yu, 2012; Lara & Labrador, 2013; Reiss, Stricker, & Hendeby, 2013; Vishwakarma & Agrawal, 2013). The machine-learning methods include probabilistic approaches, such as naïve Bayes classifiers, Markov models, conditional random fields, and dynamic Bayes networks, which perform well when a large amount of labeled training data is available (Cook, 2012; Singla, Cook, & Schmitter-Edgecombe, 2010; Zhang & Sawchuck, 2012). Alternatively, template-matching techniques, such as k-nearest neighbor classifiers, do not require a lot of training data and are very fast, but their performance depends heavily on the choice of features that are used. Finally, discriminative approaches that explicitly model the boundary between activity classes offer an effective alternative. These techniques include decision trees, meta classifiers based on boosting and bagging, support vector machines, and ensemble methods (Bulling, Ward, & Gellersen, 2012; Cook, 2012; Van Kasteren, Noulas, Englebienne, & Krose, 2008). While most of these recognize activities offline after the data are extensively analyzed, recent approaches offer the possibility of recognizing activities in real time as they occur by considering a fixed amount of the most recent sensor events when generating an activity label (Krishnan & Cook, 2014). The types of activities that are modeled, recognized, and monitored vary somewhat depending on the types of sensors and machine-learning algorithms that are utilized. Table 11.1 summarizes some of the activities that have been recognized in the literature using the techniques described above.

TABLE 11.1 Categories of Recognizable Activities

| ACTIONS | |
| --- | --- |
| Walk, run, cycle, jump, sit down, stand up | Lie down, fall down, ascend/descend stairs |
| Pick up/put down item, open/close door | Point, talk, gesture, chew, speak, swallow |

| ACTIVITIES | |
| --- | --- |
| **Clean House** | **Social** |
| Dust, vacuum, sweep, mop | Make phone call, talk on phone |
| Clear table, wash dishes, dry dishes | Entertain guests, leave/enter home |
| **Meals** | **Leisure** |
| Prepare/eat breakfast, lunch, dinner, snack | Play/listen to music, read |
| Set table | Watch television, play game |
| **Personal Hygiene/Health Maintenance** | **Exercise** |
| Bathe, shower, toilet | Lift weights, calisthenics |
| Brush teeth, floss, comb hair | Use treadmill, elliptical, cycle, rower |
| Take medicine, fill medicine dispenser | Dive, golf, swim, skate |
| **Sleep** | **Work** |
| Nightime sleep, naps, sleep out of beds | Work at computer, desk, table |

ACTIVITY DISCOVERY

When reasoning about human activities from sensor data, one approach is to identify activities that are important to track for clinical reasons, then model and recognize occurrences of those activities. However, modeling all of human behavior in a recognition-based approach faces a number of challenges and limitations. First, to model and recognize activities, a large amount of sensor data must be available that has already been prelabeled by an expert with the actual activities they represent (the "ground truth" labels). In most real-world everyday settings, such prelabeled data are not readily available.

Second, time spent engaging in commonly tracked activities, such as those from the Lawton Instrumental Activities of Daily Living Scale (e.g., preparing meals, doing housework, telephone use; Lawton, Moss, Fulcomer, & Kleban, 1982), is only a fraction of an individual's total everyday routine; thus, the largest category of tracked behavior would fall under the "other" category. The U.S. Bureau of Labor Statistics reports 462 activities that people perform in their daily lives. This number is likely much larger worldwide when we consider unique individual interests and the diversity of activities in different cultures. Even if all of the activities listed in common compendiums are tracked, they will still not account for time spent transitioning between activities and performing unique other activities. Therefore, modeling and tracking only preselected activities ignores the important insights that other activities can provide on behavior. This is particularly significant when we want to understand routine behaviors for individuals with cognitive impairment, the impact the behaviors have on their cognitive health and functional performance, and interventions that can be developed to assist them with functional independence.

Third, if the classes of activities shown in Table 11.1 are modeled by an activity recognition algorithm, the algorithm will be affected by the large other-activity class, resulting in a skewed class distribution. The problem of modeling activity classes with a skewed class distribution has vexed researchers for over a decade. As Aristotle said, "We are what we repeatedly do" (Durant, 1926). Our group has built on this idea to design unsupervised-activity discovery algorithms that automatically detect activities based on the frequency and complexity of recurring sensor event sequences. One activity- discovery challenge is yielding the desired level of complexity in the discovered-activity descriptions. Depending on the purpose of activity learning, the desired activities may be simple movements with short length/duration or complex activities that can themselves be described in terms of the shorter components. Ideally, then, a hierarchy of activities would be discovered that decompose into other activity patterns and collectively represent a majority of the original data.

Unlike other activity-discovery approaches (Coates, Karpathy, & Ng, 2012; Gu, Chen, Tao, & Lu, 2010; Wyatt, Philipose, & Choudhury, 2005), our activity-discovery method searches the space of sensor event sequences to find patterns that maximally compress the dataset, and therefore exhibit sufficient frequency and complexity to constitute a significant activity. We apply the compression-based activity discovery in an iterative manner, allowing for a hierarchy of activities to be discovered. First, the discovery algorithm searches the feature space for sensor event sequences to find significant activity patterns. The best sensor event patterns discovered are reported and then compressed. The compression procedure replaces all instances of the sensor event pattern by a single activity descriptor (e.g., yoga), which represents the pattern definition. We repeat the discovery process on the compressed data until all possible patterns are considered. We employ an edit distance measure (Levenshtein, 1996; Yang & Want, 2003; Zhou & Shan, 2013) to allow some minor variations in how the activity is performed.

We have found that activity-recognition accuracy can be improved by more than 10% when combined with activity discovery. Furthermore, when the discovery algorithm is applied to actual smart home data collected from individuals living in smart homes, the discovered activities highlight important patterns, such as the ones shown in Figure 11.2 (Cook, Crandall, Thomas, & Krishnan, 2012). In the figure, one of the discovered activities (on the left) highlights nightly transitions that take place between the living room and the bedroom as the resident prepares to go to sleep. The second discovered pattern (on the right) highlights a scrap-booking hobby that takes place in the guest bedroom. While neither of the patterns falls into a predefined activity category, they both represent important aspects of the resident's routine behavior that would need to be monitored for a holistic view of the individual and to provide a basis for detecting changes in the resident's routine.

ACTIVITY GENERALIZATION

In addition to developing learning algorithms that can discover new activity patterns in resident routines, our group has also been investigating methods for activity generalization. Most current technologies require that separate training data be provided for each person, home setting, and sensor platform. To make this technology practical and widely usable, however, it needs to generalize to new settings without requiring training data for each new application.

Part of this goal can be achieved by extracting sensor features that are not dependent on a particular home layout or sensor configuration. For example, extracted features could consist of generic information, such as the date and time of the sensor reading, the ambient light, temperature, and humidity levels, and recent prior activities performed by the smart home resident. Sensors whose location is important for activity monitoring can be indicated by their position in the house (e.g., "Kitchen: Sink", "Kitchen: Refrigerator"), and further linked to common everyday activities (e.g., cooking). In this way, activity models can be learned from a sample of testbeds and used to provide labels in new settings. Previous work using our CASAS in-home testbeds indicates that activity recognition can be applied in new settings without any new learning with greater

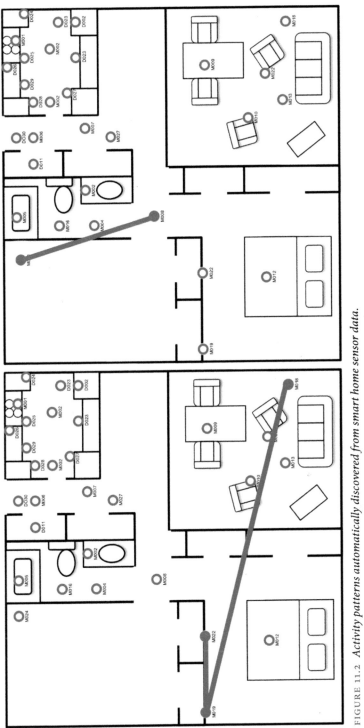

FIGURE 11.2 *Activity patterns automatically discovered from smart home sensor data.*

than 85% accuracy, depending on the type of activity and uniqueness of the new setting (Cook, 2012).

An alternative approach is to explicitly learn mapping from previous sites to a new site, using the mapping to transform activity models to the new setting. In the machine-learning literature, this is referred to as *transfer learning* (Cook, Feuz, & Krishana, 2013; Pan & Yang, 2010; Xu, Tao, & Xu, 2013). Up to this point, we have focused on monitoring activities from sensors found in a home environment. However, not only can transfer learning be used to reuse activity models for new homes, new residents, and new activities, but also it can be used to transfer activity information between a smart home and a smartphone or other sensor platform. Researchers have designed activity-learning methods that work on smartphones, wearable sensors, and video data. However, each of the platforms has a limited scope of use, which therefore limits the effectiveness of the monitoring and intervention technologies. While a person's home may be equipped with sensors, the home's ability to monitor and aid with activities stops when the individual leaves the house. Similarly, a clinician's office or lab may be equipped with depth cameras to assess motor function and activity performance, but the information cannot be used in a person's everyday setting unless the camera's models can be used by other sensor platforms in other settings. Because the number and diversity of devices with sensing and computing capabilities are increasing, technologies should ideally offer a personalized activity ecosystem. In this ecosystem, an individual's smart home, smartphone, smart vehicle, and smart lab all work together to monitor and enhance an individual's well-being.

One challenge we face in meeting this goal is that activity learning is typically limited to a single class of sensor devices. However, new research focuses on the design of transfer-learning techniques to handle collegial learning between different types of sensor devices. Transfer-learning algorithms apply knowledge learned from a previous task to a new, related task (Cook, Feuz, & Krishnan, 2013). As an example, consider the problem of activity recognition in a smart home. We can train a model to recognize an activity that occurs in a particular home based on data collected from motion sensors that were integrated into the environment. If the user also wants to start using a phone-based recognizer, the labeling-and-training process must be repeated. To overcome this problem, the CASAS Smart Home group developed omnidirectional interdevice multiview learning techniques, or collegial learning, to allow the existing smart home to act as a teacher for the new smartphone and for the phone to, in turn, boost the performance of the smart home model (Fuez & Cook, 2015). The implication for clinical research and practice is that technologies for activity monitoring and intervention can extend beyond an individual's home to offer a personalized assistive ecosystem.

## SUMMARY

Over the past decade, the maturing of sensor technologies and advances in wireless networks, data processing, and machine learning have shifted researchers' focus from low-level data collection and transmission to high-level information collection, inference, and recognition. The work described above indicates that it is possible to use sensor-derived data to gather information about everyday human behaviors and routines. The data can then be used to assist with an individual's healthcare, such as by monitoring for significant changes in everyday activities or routines. Smart environment data can also be used to increase understanding of human behavior and to develop better interventions. For example, transitions that occur in everyday functional abilities from normal aging through MCI and dementia could be mapped and methods for extending everyday functional independence could be developed.

Currently, clinical translation of the work requires that developed activity-recognition algorithms be validated in the real-world setting. As a step toward this goal, we are in the process of validating our activity-recognition and activity-discovery algorithms with residents living in CASAS smart homes. We have designed an automated phone system connected to the CASAS software that will determine the three activities most likely to be occurring at the time the call is placed. The phone system queries participants about which activity they are currently performing. If none of the labels fits the activity, then the participant can select "other activity" and provide a name for the current activity. By providing labels for activities that are not currently in the activity- recognition dictionary, the participant is allowing us to crowdsource data that dynamically expands our activity dictionary. The provided labels will then be automatically added to our database along with the training data in order to recognize an increased set of activities in new settings.

Privacy, confidentiality, and security of personal information collected from smart environments are also concerns that must be addressed as the work moves forward (Beringer et al.,2011; Courtney, Demiris, & Hensel, 2007). Researchers are investigating approaches to privacy that give individuals more control over when and where information is gathered and that can flexibly modify who has access to the data (Babbitt, 2006; Moncrieff, Venkatesh, & West, 2008). Research generally indicates that the population is open and accepting of smart home technologies and embraces further development (Coughlin, D'Ambrosio, Reimer, & Pratt, 2007; Davis, Freeman, Kaye, Vuckovic, & Buckley, 2014; Demiris et al., 2004; Wilson, Hargreaves, & Hauxwell-Baldwin, 2014).

## Assessment

Current assessment methods used by neuropsychologists to evaluate the cognitive, functional, and health status of patients are typically limited to measuring a small number of variables at a few discrete times in the clinician's office. Factors like a patient's mood, pain, sleep, medications, other health conditions, or negative life events can significantly influence data collected at discrete time points. In addition, the methods do not capture variability in daily functioning over time, which could better control for the effects of extraneous variables and be more representative of a patient's everyday functioning compared to absolute performance (Kaye, 2008). To understand the everyday effects of patient symptoms, neuropsychologists often rely on a patient's or care partner's report of symptom onset, duration, and course, which may be biased, insensitive to subtle changes, or inaccurate (Kaye, 2008). Smart technologies that make available continuous assessment data could assist neuropsychologists in interpreting test data and making diagnostic decisions by providing the neuropsychologist with more impartial, ecologically valid, and frequent measures of change in a patient's functioning.

## FUNCTIONAL ASSESSMENT

It has been argued that assessing individuals in their everyday environment will provide the most valid information about everyday functional status, especially when observing subtle changes in behaviors across extended periods of time (Marcotte, Scott, Kamat, & Heaton, 2010). This opens up important possibilities for developing smart technologies that can provide continuous data for understanding and assessing the quality of everyday activity performance. Currently, in the field of neuropsychology, informant-report and performance-based measures are most commonly used as proxies for real-world functioning because they typically show stronger relationships with objective cognitive decline than self-report measures (Miller, Brown, Mitchell, & Williamson, 2013; Mitchell et al., 2010; Tsang, Diamond, Mowszowski, Lewis, & Naismith, 2012). Both methods, however, have advantages and disadvantages. For example, although informant-report measures are subject to reporter biases, they can capture information about performances and activities across multiple unstructured environments and over an extended period of time (Dassel & Schmitt, 2008; for a review, see Sikkes, de Lange-de Klerk, Pijnenburg, Scheltens, & Uitdehaag, 2009). Concomitantly, although performance-based measures represent a single evaluation point and typically require completion of one task at a time in a controlled artificial laboratory, they provide a more objective measure of functional capacity (Marson & Herbert, 2006; for a review, see Moore, Palmer, Patterson, & Jeste, 2007). A body of data also suggests that informant-report and performance-based methods do not always correlate highly with each other (Burton, Strauss, Bunce, Hunter, & Hultsch, 2009; Finlayson, Havens, Holm, & Van Denend, 2003; Loewenstein et al., 2001; Schmitter-Edgecombe, Parsey & Cook, 2011; Tabert et al., 2002), and they may be capturing different aspects of everyday functioning (Schmitter-Edgecombe et al., 2011).

As evident from the information presented above, our current clinical approaches for assessing functional status are limited by restricted behavior sampling, data collection in a laboratory or physician office, and lack of a "gold standard" for measuring everyday functional abilities. In contrast to the body of work exploring activity recognition, less attention has been directed toward using smart home technologies to examine the quality of tasks being performed within a smart environment. As a first step, we had a large sample ($N = 349$) of younger adults, healthy older adults, individuals with mild cognitive impairment (MCI), and individuals with dementia complete single scripted activities and complex, multitasking activities in our controlled campus smart apartment testbed while under direct observation. In the smart home testbed, we have motion sensors that record an individual's location by indicating ON or OFF sensor events, door/cabinet sensors that index when a door or cabinet is open or closed, and item sensors that register whether an item placed on the sensor, such as medication, is present or absent. There are also sensors that measure water temperature, ambient temperature, and whether the stove burner is on or off. The layout of our smart apartment campus testbed and some sensor examples are shown in Figure 11.3. Each sensor entry is tagged with the date and time of the event, the ID of the sensor that generated the event, the activity associated with the sensor event, and the sensor reading.

For the single scripted activities, participants completed eight common IADLs, one at a time (e.g., sweep and dust, fill medication dispenser, water houseplants, cook). Prior to each activity, the experimenter provided the participant with a brief verbal instruction for the task and then the participant used the materials in the campus apartment to carry out the activity. For the complex, multitasking activity, participants completed the Day Out Task (Schmitter-Edgecombe, Schmitter-Edgecombe, McAlister, & Weakley, 2012; McAlister & Schmitter-Edgecombe, 2013). This task required participants to efficiently prepare for a day out by multitasking and interweaving eight subtasks that needed to be completed prior to leaving the house (e.g., gather correct change for bus ride, take motion sickness medication just prior to leaving, microwave a heating pad for 3 min to take on bus). A comprehensive direct observation coding system that recorded error types (e.g., omissions, inefficient actions), subtask accuracy, and sequencing scores was developed (see Schmitter-Edgecombe et al., 2011; Schmitter-Edgecombe et al., 2012). Participants also completed a medical interview, including the Clinical Dementia Rating Scale (Hughes, Berg, Danzinger, Coben, & Martin, 1982; Morris, 1993), and a 3-hour battery of standardized neuropsychological tasks that was used in diagnostic classification and to evaluate cognitive correlates of functional performance. Knowledgeable informants (e.g., spouse, adult child) were also interviewed and completed the Clinical Dementia Rating Scale.

Across both the single scripted and the more complex Day Out Task, we found poorer performances were a function of age and cognitive impairment. In addition, a behavioral pattern emerged in the data. More specifically, compared to younger adults, the performances of older adults were characterized by significantly greater task inefficiencies (e.g., multiple trips, searching behaviors), which were related to poorer executive abilities (Schmitter-Edgecombe et al., 2011;

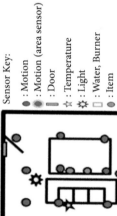

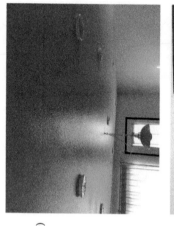

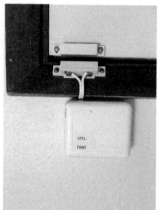

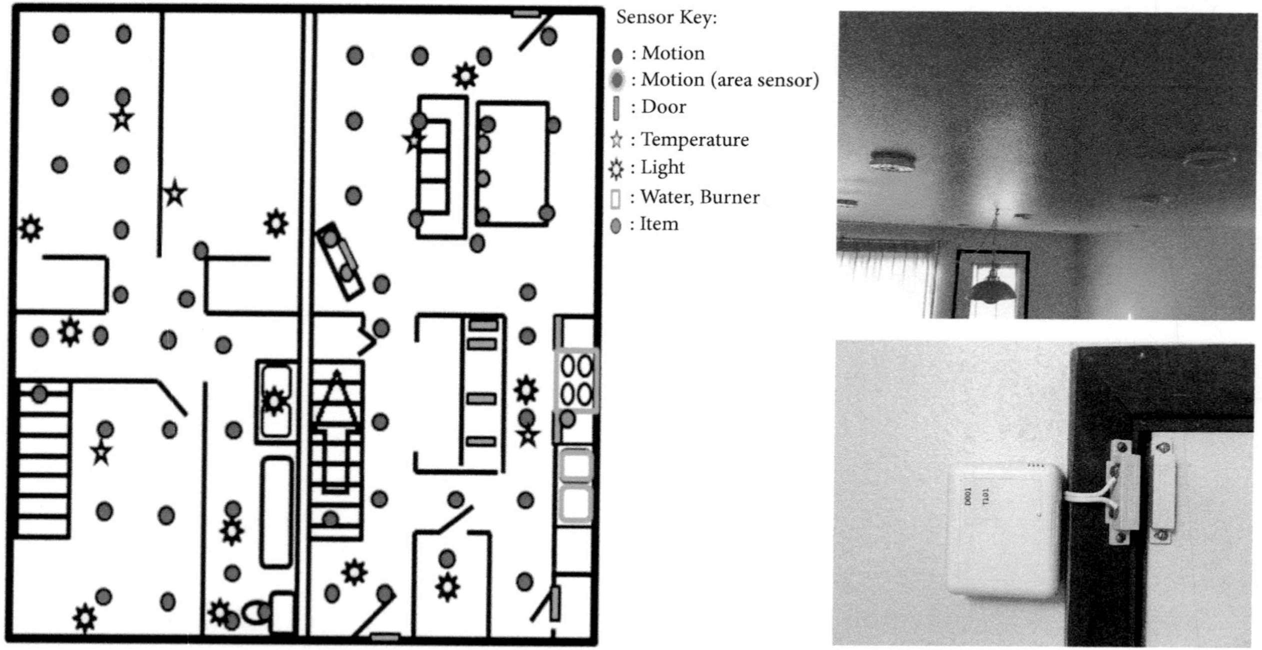

Sensor Key:

● ● ━━ : Motion
●          : Motion (area sensor)
      : Door
☆ : Temperature
�֍ : Light
▢ : Water, Burner
● : Item

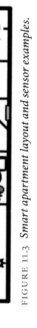

FIGURE 11.3 *Smart apartment layout and sensor examples.*

Schmitter-Edgecombe & Parsey, 2014, McAlister & Schmitter-Edgecombe, 2013). Relative to older adults, the performances of individuals with primarily amnestic MCI (single and multidomain) were characterized by significantly greater omission errors (e.g., not initiating a task step) and incomplete and/or inaccurate task completion, which reflected compromised memory (Schmitter-Edgecombe & Parsey, 2014; Schmitter-Edgecombe et al., 2012). Participants with dementia had significantly more errors across all coded categories, including substitutions (e.g., using a wrong item), when compared to older adults and individuals with MCI, with level of impairment correlating highly with general cognitive status (Schmitter-Edgecombe & Parsey, 2014). The findings revealed a differential pattern of clinically observable functional difficulties across the groups completing experiments in our campus testbed. The next question was whether the simultaneously collected smart environment sensor data would also be able to capture the differences.

To automate functional assessment (see Figure 11.4), we designed machine-learning algorithms that generated task scores from sensor-derived features (e.g., time spent on the entire activity, time spent on each step of the activity, triggered sensor events, unusual sensor events triggered). The scores were fed to an additional machine-learning algorithm and logistic regression to generate classification labels based on diagnosis (i.e., cognitively healthy, MCI, or dementia). Geometric mean (G-mean) and area under the receiver operating characteristic (ROC) curve (AUC) were used to evaluate classification accuracy. G-mean balances classification performance of imbalanced diagnostic groups and is defined as the product of the square root of sensitivity and specificity (Kubat & Matwin, 1997). AUC is the probability that a learning algorithm will rank a positive example higher than a negative one and is comparable to the Mann-Whitney *U* (Fawcet, 2006). Our results yielded an AUC (0.87) and G-mean (0.75) within an acceptable range for single scripted activities (Dawadi, Cook, Schmitter-Edgecombe, & Parsey, 2013).

We also used the information learned from the models to create functional-status scores for a new sample of 28 participants (14 healthy older adult controls, 14 individuals with MCI) matched in age and education. We compared the functional-status measures derived from the sensor data with activity accuracy scores derived from our direct observation coding system and obtained a significant moderate to high correlation ($r = .61$; Parsey, Dawadi, Schmitter-Edgecombe, & Cook, 2011). In addition, using data from the more complex Day Out Task that allowed multitasking of the activity steps yielded an automated diagnosis AUC of 0.94 and a G-mean of 0.99 (Dawadi, Cook, & Schmitter-Edgecombe, 2013). The data indicate that sensor-based data mining is capable of capturing information about how well activities are being performed. Furthermore, such models appeared more robust when the activities being performed had a higher degree of complexity.

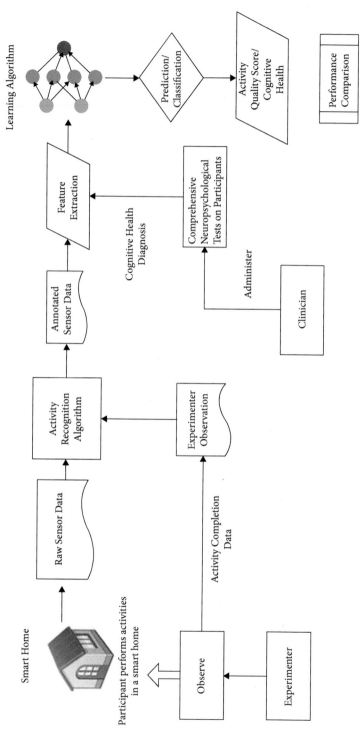

FIGURE 11.4 *Steps involved in performing sensor-assisted cognitive health assessment.*

## HEALTH ASSESSMENT

Although the on-campus apartment presents a unique opportunity to collect direct behavioral observation data within a naturalistic environment and to provide ground truth for sensor labeling, participants are not being tested in their own homes nor are repeated measurements of the same everyday activities being collected. By tracking trends in everyday activity performance in a person's home environment on a daily basis and comparing the findings with clinical data, smart environment technologies could be used to identify new markers that signal acute health-status changes. Furthermore, such information could contribute a missing, fundamental element to our knowledge of the natural history of functional change between healthy aging and dementia, as well as lead to innovative, proactive (as opposed to reactive) healthcare interventions.

As researchers have argued, merely checking laboratory values can ignore important trends where the indicator is markedly decreasing, increasing, or periodically fluctuating (Haimowitz & Kohane, 1993). Through unobtrusive monitoring we can design ways to visualize daily activity patterns for assessment of meaningful deviations. For example, Galambos, Skubic, Wang, and Rantz (2013) developed methods to visualize overall activity level in the home and time spent away from home. Gait, pillbox use, and computer use (Kaye, 2008) have also been successfully monitored over time, in addition to sleep and sleep quality (Paavilainen et al., 2005). While the previous methods provide a tool for understanding sensor data and variation in data, they rely on manual inspection of the data in order to make higher-level conclusions regarding daily routines.

Developing methods for detecting behavior change over time from continuously collected sensor-derived data is important, because it can lead to proactive interventions and the discovery of unique and distinguishable patterns. For example, in comparison to controls, variation on measures of walking speed and day-to-day activity were associated with a diagnosis of MCI (Hayes et al., 2008). Researchers have also correlated sensor measurements of sleep patterns, gait, activity rhythms, and indoor activities with everyday functioning and cognitive status. For example, Paavilainen and colleagues (2005) found a significant relationship between sensor-observed time spent in bed and self-reported functional ability as well as objective measures of cognitive status for older adults living in nursing homes. In other work, Robben and Krose (2013) found the location and transition patterns of an individuals' indoor mobility behavior strongly correlated with the Assessment of Motor and Process Skills scores (AMPS; Fisher, Merritt, Fisher, & Jones, 2012).

As described above, while other researchers have considered the relationship between activity level, transition patterns, sleep quality, computer use, and cognitive and functional health, research to date has not considered automatically quantified parameters reflecting performance of activities of daily living. In our initial in-home assessment study, we extracted features for automatically detected activities from sensor data collected in 18 smart homes over 24 months (Dawadi, Cook, & Schmitter-Edgecombe, 2014, 2016). Twice a year, we performed clinical assessments of the participants (5 females, 13 males; 73 years old or older, mean education level of 17.52). The sample consisted of healthy adults, individuals at risk for experiencing cognitive difficulties, and individuals with MCI and early-stage dementia. Statistical features that describe characteristics of a resident's daily activity performance were extracted from the sensor data. Sensor-derived measures of mobility included total distance traveled in the home and number of sensors triggered, while sleep was based on sleep duration and bed–toilet transition, as well as the number of sensor events in sleep and bed–toilet transition. Everyday activity was represented by the time involved in cooking, eating, relaxing, and personal hygiene. We then computed the correlation between in-home activity performance features (i.e., sensor-derived measures of mobility, sleep, and everyday activities) and clinical scores using a support vector machine with a linear kernel. We found a statistically significant correlation between our clinical measure of global cognitive health (i.e., Repeatable Battery for the Assessment of Neuropsychological Status; Randolph, Mohr, & Chase, 1998) and our sensor-derived measures of sleep and activities of daily living, but not mobility. In a finding suggesting some specificity in the sensor-derived data, we also found a relationship between sensor-derived mobility and leave-home measures and the clinical measure of mobility (i.e., Timed Up and Go; Podsiadlo & Richardson, 1991). The results are promising, as they indicate that smart home technologies have the potential to predict/assess the cognitive and physical health of patients. However, much more research is currently needed employing larger sample sizes (which is a challenge) and examining alternate modeling techniques, such as those that use the individuals as their own baselines, for analyzing the data.

## SUMMARY

With much continued research, smart environment technologies have the potential to enrich a client's clinical picture, augmenting the patient's and care partner's report data and clinical assessment data collected in the laboratory or office. At the same time, information learned from deploying the technologies in residents' homes can be used to inform the development of better clinical tests and interventions. The continuous data collection afforded by smart environments also provides an opportunity to see variability and trends or trajectories, rather than absolute values, and to identify how daily activities affect traditional measures. For example, smart home technologies could capture acute healthcare changes that require immediate intervention, syndromes that evolve slowly over time, and even changes that may be difficult for patients and/or knowledgeable informants to report.

To make such possibilities a reality, numerous challenges need to be overcome. One such challenge is to derive methodologies that will automatically identify anomalous or rare events that may indicate a cause for concern. Anomaly detection is less thoroughly understood in machine learning than recognizing instances of well-defined concepts. In addition, research is needed to better understand what health information clinicians would find useful. Healthcare providers have raised concerns about information overload, and the potential that irrelevant information and technology could detract from interpersonal care (Kang et al., 2010). A related issue is how to visualize collected data and health events in a way that can be easily digested by those who need to use the data. If information is to be of clinical use, it must be presented in an intuitive format for users (e.g., individual, caregiver, healthcare professional) and be valuable in clinical decision making. Thus, it will be important to involve all stakeholders in technology development and in assessment of the efficacy of the technology (Hwang, Troung, & Mihailidis, 2012; Kraskowsky & Finlayson, 2001). Furthermore, if smart environment data are to be used to make informed medical decisions, then it is important to demonstrate that the collected health data are both reliable and valid.

In ongoing work, we are evaluating the test–retest reliability and construct validity of sensor-derived algorithms for assessment of sleep parameters, activity level, socialization, and mood. We are pairing in-home environment sensor data collection with actigraphy and ecological momentary assessment (EMA) to obtain ground truth data. Actigraphy has been found to provide reliable and valid information about sleep parameters, physical activity, and sedentary behavior (Blackwell et al., 2008; Evans & Rogers, 1994; Hart, Swartz & Strath, 2011; Copeland & Eslinger, 2009). EMA is also considered a reliable measurement technique for recording events, subjective symptoms, and physiological and behavioral data multiple times per day in a natural setting (Smyth, 2003; Jones & Johnston, 2011; Kim, Kikuchi, & Yamamoto, 2013).

## Intervention

The work of clinicians could also be augmented by smart home technologies that deliver interventions in the real world at the time they are needed. For example, a resident with memory impairment could be reminded to record information in a memory notebook after a visitor has left, or a resident recovering from knee surgery could be monitored and reminded to engage in exercises for at least 10 min three times per day. By building on activity-recognition and activity-discovery algorithms, activity-aware smart home technology could be used to support initiation and completion of IADLs, promote healthy lifestyle behaviors, and provide real-time intervention to support faster recovery from surgery or trauma. It is becoming increasingly more pressing to develop innovative technologies that can support healthcare needs. For example, functional impairment has been associated with increased healthcare utilization, poorer quality of life, and conversion to dementia in the elderly (Fauth et al., 2013: Luck et al., 2011; Teng, Tassniyom, & Lu, 2012). Studies also indicate that physical activity, cognitive stimulation, social engagement, and good nutrition all have positive effects on well-being (Giles, Glonek, Luszcz, & Andrews, 2005; Purath, Buchholz, & Kark, 2009; Spector, Orrell, & Woods, 2010) and are associated with a reduction of risk of dementia. Similarly, routinely engaging in rehabilitation exercises has been found to support better functional outcomes (Lenze et al., 2004), enhanced cerebral plasticity (Fisher & Sullivan, 2001), and improved self-efficacy (Berkhuysen, Nieuwland, Buunk, Sanderman, & Rispens, 1999)

## PROMPTING TECHNOLOGIES

Prompting technologies, defined as any form of verbal or nonverbal intervention delivered to the user (Das, Chen, Seelye, & Cook, 2011), have been shown to increase adherence to instructions, decrease errors in completing everyday activities, and increase independence and activity engagement for individuals with cognitive impairment (Bewernitz, Mann, Dasler, & Belchior, 2009; Boger & Mihailidis, 2011; Boll, Heuten, Meyer, & Meis, 2010). In our intervention work, we have been experimenting with activity-aware prompting technologies, which are designed to learn the resident's routine and deliver prompts based on context (e.g., reminder to take medication with breakfast) as opposed to time (e.g., 7:00 AM alarm to take medication when resident is sleeping in). Furthermore, such activity-aware prompts only need to be provided if the resident forgets to take the daily medication with breakfast. In addition, once a prompt is delivered, the smart home can monitor whether the individual has followed through with the prompted activity and can repeat the prompt if necessary.

Simple prompting technologies include reminders, notifications, and alerts, which are typically time-based (reminder set for 2:00 PM) or location-based (alarm rings when close to a grocery store). While some limited context-based prompting methods have been explored for medication adherence and activity initiation (Hayes et al., 2009; Hoey, Von Bertoldi, Craig, Poupart, & Mihailidis, 2010; Kaushik, Intille, & Larson, 2008; Sohlberg, Ehlhardt, & Kennedy, 2005), these approaches do not employ knowledge of current and upcoming activities or detection of activity transitions when delivering prompts. In addition, while time-based or location-based prompting may help individuals use the aid more often, they typically require the user to do extra work to learn how to use the system and set the prompts (Epstein, Willis, Conners, & Johnson, 2001; Pollack et al., 2003; Wilson, Evans, Emslie, & Malinek, 1997), which may reduce use overall (Ferguson, Myles, & Hagiwara, 2005). Furthermore, a prompt that is unaware of current activities may be delivered when the person is taking a nap or actively engaged in another activity and will likely be ineffective (Hayes et al., 2009; Lundell, 2005). Similarly, a prompt delivered after the individual has already completed the task will result in annoyance.

## ACTIVITY PREDICTION

To provide interventions that are effective, we not only need to recognize activities as they are performed but also need to anticipate when they should, or do typically, occur. If we can accurately predict when an activity should occur, then we can use automated prompting as an effective real-time intervention. For example, if our algorithm learns that an individual takes medication every morning at 9:00 AM with breakfast, it may also be able to detect deviations from this pattern. Deviation in the pattern can signal that a prompt to take medication should be delivered in a context-appropriate manner. We have designed two activity-prediction algorithms. The purpose of the algorithms is to generate an estimate of when a particular activity will occur based on sensor data that was collected at a time that the desired activities did occur (the resident was performing activities either in an independent manner or with caregiver assistance).

Our algorithms are designed to forecast the time at which an activity will occur (e.g., breakfast) as well as which activity will occur next in the sequence (e.g., take medication; Gopalratnam & Cook, 2007; Krumm & Horvitz, 2006). This way, activity timings can be learned both for activities that occur at regular times and activities that occur in relation to another activity. This information can be combined with a prompting algorithm to deliver cues when an activity has not been initiated. Our first version of an activity-prompting algorithm (CASAS-AP) learned rules for each prompted activity (e.g., medication) as a function of another reference activity (e.g., breakfast), with which it is highly time correlated. Based on 8 months of historic data, CASAS-AP was observed to have an 85% predictive accuracy for 12 activities (Cook & Holder, 2013).

Our second version, CASAS-AP-forecasted, frames the prompt-timing problem as an activity-forecasting problem. Some approaches have been tested to predict upcoming activities based on sequential prediction (Alam, Reaz, & Ali, 2012; Das et al., 2011; Gopalratnam & Cook, 2003). However, the approaches all make assumptions that the current activities are labeled by an expert. Our approach makes no such assumptions, but instead partners the forecasting algorithm with our automated activity-recognition algorithm so that predictions can be made directly from the observed sensor data. Figure 11.5 shows actual values juxtaposed with CASAS-AP-forecasted values for the number of seconds until a bed–toilet transfer will occur again after being trained on 1 week of data. The *x*-axis shows the time of day over a 3-day span and the *y*-axis shows the number of time units until the next occurrence of the activity. The near-overlap of the red and blue lines indicates that CASAS-AP-forecasted is learning the timing of this activity with high accuracy.

## PROMPT CONTENT AND DELIVERY

Although activity-prompting technologies are being rapidly developed by researchers (e.g., Boger et al., 2006; Mihaildis, Fernie, & Barbenel, 2001), there

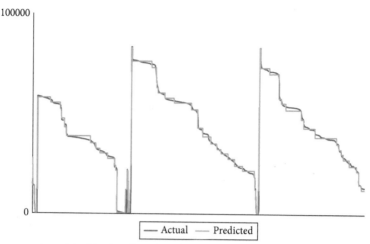

FIGURE 11.5 *Actual (red line) and predicted (blue line) number of seconds until the next occurrence of a bed–toilet transition activity, over 3 days in a CASAS smart home. Predictions are generated using a regression tree trained on 1 week of data.*

is currently no clear consensus regarding the most optimal prompt content, method of prompt delivery, or interface. We recently utilized cognitive rehabilitation principles to develop a graded hierarchy of technology-based prompts to assist with complex IADL initiation and completion. In studies completed in our campus smart apartment, cognitively healthy adults and individuals with MCI and dementia completed eight IADL, such as cooking oatmeal and changing a light bulb. When the experimenter detected an activity-completion error, a preprogrammed prompt was delivered (Seelye, Schmitter-Edgecombe, Cook, & Crandall, 2013). There were three levels of prompt. The first level, or indirect verbal prompt, was designed to orient the individual back to the task (e.g., the oatmeal will burn if the stove is left on). The second level, a direct verbal prompt, told the participants exactly what to do (e.g., turn the stove off now), while the third level was a multimodal prompt (i.e., visual with direct verbal prompt).

Activity-performance data as well as participant feedback revealed that individuals with MCI, like healthy adults, benefit from verbal indirect prompting technology to assist with IADL completion. In contrast, the more cognitively impaired participants require greater directive and multimodal prompting (Seelye, Schmitter-Edgecombe, & Cook, 2013). The data are consistent with research in other populations (Greber, Ziviani, & Rodger, 2007; Hume & Odom, 2007) and suggest that less-directive verbal cues may be effective when cognitive difficulties are mild, while more-directive and supportive cues will be needed as cognitive impairment progresses. The data further suggest that older adults and individuals with MCI can benefit from smart environment prompting technology, and this type of technology might keep these individuals functioning independently in their homes for longer periods of time.

## PROMPT TIMING

Detecting activity transitions and prompting during transition periods are integral to our prompt-timing approach. Research suggests that prompting when a user is not engaged in an activity may increase compliance to the first prompt and reduce errors that result from information overload (Ho & Intille, 2005; Iqbal & Baile, 2006; Modayll et al., 2008). Instances of information overload can occur when prompts are delivered during an activity (Ho & Intille, 2005). Furthermore, individuals (especially those with cognitive impairment) typically perform better if they perform one activity at a time (Byrne & Anderson, 2001; Strayer, Drews, & Johnston, 2003). Therefore, if prompting a user to initiate a new activity occurs while the user is engaged in another activity, time to complete and task accuracy of each activity may be affected. In a recent experiment in our smart home testbed with 42 undergraduate students, we showed that manually prompting participants during activity transitions significantly improved response time to prompts, produced higher adherence to the first prompt and more positive perceptions of the prompting system when compared to time-based prompts (Robertson, Rosasco, Feuz, Schmitter-Edgecombe, & Cook, 2015). In this study, prompts to write in a notebook were delivered manually by experimenters either during activity transition (transition-based condition) or every 5 min (time-based condition). Participants had the option to respond to each prompt either immediately, after a second prompt (given 1 min later), or not at all if the prompt felt unnatural and inconvenient.

To detect activity transitions, we have designed an unsupervised approach to finding activity transitions. The algorithm detects a "break in the action," or a change in the nature of the sensor-detected activity. This unsupervised activity-transition technique uses Relative Unconstrained Least Squares Importance Fitting (RuLSIF; Liu, Yamada, Collier, & Sugiyama, 2013). RuLSIF estimates the probability density distribution ratio between two sets of samples and, therefore, does not require ground truth training data containing examples of all possible activity transitions. The RuLSIF approach can identify activity transitions by detecting changes in the underlying probability distributions sampled before and after a transition point, using the assumption that the distribution changes as the activities change.

## ADAPTIVE REWARDS

Even if the timing and the content of the prompt work well, individuals may lose motivation to comply with repeated prompts. The relationship between participant adherence and intervention success is very clear (Lee et al., 2013). Insights from social cognitive theory and from persuasion theory (Bandura, 1997, 2000) highlight the fact that motivation via persuasion and reward can profoundly affect the use of a new technology and adoption of a new behavior. Intelligent-tutoring researchers have also found that the form of feedback highly influences user success (Aleven, Mclaren, Roll, & Koedinger, 2004; Jackson, 2011). Our own preliminary work highlights the observation that reward type can affect compliance (Simon et al., 2014). Despite the fact that increasing numbers of people are using apps to tap into mobile healthcare resources, the effectiveness of the apps is short-lived, often less than 30 days (Jackson, 2011). Our group has been motivated by the hypothesis that adapting rewards to each user will improve compliance. Incorporating static rewards is not ideal, because people may not know in advance the reward type that will motivate them (Chajewska, Koller, & Parr, 2000; Pu & Chen, 2009) and optimal rewards change over time (Allcott & Rogers, 2012). Therefore, we have been working toward developing adaptive rewards that will help motivate individuals to change behavior and increase intervention adherence.

## SUMMARY

Activity-aware prompting technologies that could be deployed in the home environment and delivered at the time cues are needed have the potential to reduce or delay functional disability, promote healthy lifestyle behaviors, augment recovery from trauma or surgery, decrease caregiver burden, and lessen health care costs associated with treatment. Our approach to activity-aware prompting builds on our activity recognition and activity discovery work by developing algorithms that can anticipate when activities should occur and provide automated prompting. Such technologies will likely prove especially efficacious for individuals with cognitive impairment and their caregivers, as the user would not be responsible for learning to use the prompting system and for setting the prompts.

As the above information highlights, in addition to developing suitable algorithms that can deliver activity-aware prompts in the real-world environment, many additional questions remain to be explored. They include questions related to the timing, content, and delivery of prompts. Regarding the type of prompt, adaptive methodologies will likely need to be developed that can provide prompts with the correct level of support needed for specific individuals and situations. For example, with the downward trajectory of cognitive abilities in persons developing dementia, more directive and supportive prompts will likely be required over time. In contrast, for a person recovering from a severe brain injury, less directive support may be required with time. In addition, prompting technologies will only be effective if individuals do not habituate to the prompts and there is good prompt adherence. Techniques to assist individuals in remaining motivated to comply with prompts, such as adaptive rewards or building on gaming techniques, remain to be explored.

In addition, the current version of our prompting technology is suited to prompt activity initiation. Developing prompting technologies that can detect errors in activities at the moment they occur and deliver an appropriate and accurate prompt presents numerous additional challenges. While we have experimented with detection of errors as they occur during the completion of everyday activities in our smart home testbed (Das et al., 2011; Cook & Schmitter-Edgecombe, 2009), there are definite challenges to detecting this level of specificity in activity errors. For example, we found that the algorithms were unable to identify the errors when specialized sensors were not available to detect the items involved in the steps of the task. Research is needed to determine the types of undetected errors that pose risks for functional independence and are important to monitor. Alternate approaches to activity-error detection may also be required and other methods have been experimented with, though these have generally been limited to specific tasks. For example, Boger and colleagues (2006) developed a prompting system called COACH that uses a video camera to monitor hand-washing activity progress and to provide audiovisual prompts when there is user departure from the appropriate sequence of steps.

Concerns have been raised that technology could be used to replace the caregiver–patient interaction, leading to decreased social contact for patients. Rather than replacing human care, the goal of technologies is to help individuals maintain their quality of life, highest level of independence, and physical and mental autonomy (Ching-Show, 2008). Designed with these concerns in mind, prompting technologies could be developed in ways that actually enhance social contact. For example, individuals with memory impairment could be prompted to use a picture-based phone as a way to enhance social interaction beyond what is being received from a primary caregiver. Technology may also have the psychological benefits of increasing independence and self-respect (Cohen-Mansfield & Biddison, 2007). For example, data suggest that people associate the use of technology with a lower level of dependence than with using other people for help in care (Penhale & Manthorpe, 2001).

## Conclusion

Technology is changing healthcare and is providing new tools for understanding human behavior. Smart technologies have the potential to offer health innovations for home-based prevention, early detection, functional assessment, independent living, safety, behavioral intervention, and caregiving. The technologies also offer neuropsychologists opportunities to unobtrusively study human behavior and everyday functioning within the everyday environment. Given that clinical neuropsychologists are experts in working with cognitively impaired patients in the areas of assessment, intervention, and cognitive rehabilitation, they are in a unique position to aid in the development, evaluation, use, and dissemination of these technologies in the health arena. For example, empirically supported cognitive rehabilitation techniques, such as memory notebook training, could be built into, or synergistically combined with, smart environment technologies to support the everyday functioning of individuals with memory impairment.

One exciting advantage of smart environment technologies is their ability to capture more ecologically valid, impartial, and frequent measures of change when evaluating patient everyday functioning. For example, such technologies could provide information about variability and trends or trajectories, rather than absolute values captured at discrete time points. Subtle changes in participants' everyday functioning (e.g., change in walking pattern through the house, slowing in activity completion) might also be captured even before residents or family members are aware of such changes, thereby leading to earlier and more proactive interventions. To improve test interpretation and diagnostic decision making, sensor data could also be combined with clinical assessments conducted in the office and with symptoms reported by patients. Furthermore, sensors could provide an unobtrusive method for individuals and clinicians to examine an individual's health and everyday habits and even provide individuals with an unbiased means for examining the health effects of their decisions (Stanley & Osgood, 2011).

Another exciting opportunity afforded by smart environment technologies is the ability to unobtrusively monitor compliance with pharmaceutical regimens and rehabilitation programs, resulting in better patient outcomes. For example, if a patient misses taking a dose of medication or experiences difficulty putting into place a treatment intervention, such as daily walking or using a computerized cognitive training program, the clinician could be alerted immediately rather than at the next scheduled appointment. This in turn could reduce lost time in a patient's treatment, leading to accelerated recovery or preventing health conditions from deteriorating to the point of requiring hospital admittance. Evaluation of a patient's everyday functioning before, during, and after receiving an intervention could also be used in treatment planning to better monitor progress and to tailor interventions to individual needs and preferences.

Smart environment technologies also have the potential to support real-time interventions. For example, the development of activity-aware prompting technologies that learn a resident's routine and deliver prompts based on context have the potential to augment recovery, reduce or delay functional disability, and lessen healthcare costs. Because such approaches can provide prompt-based interventions with minimal effort on the part of the user, the technologies offer a solution that can easily be adapted to most homes and used by individuals experiencing cognitive difficulties. Technologies that allow for optimal timing of prompts in the everyday environment with suitable rewards could lead to enhanced compliance with interventions and improved quality of life for patients. Neuropsychologists have an important role to play in the development and evaluation of such interventions.

In addition, smart environment technologies have the potential to keep individuals functioning independently in their homes while also supporting caregivers. For example, prompting technologies can be used to help individuals engage in preventive healthcare measures (e.g., regular exercise, good sleep habits). In addition, sensor technologies that can track everyday functional activity accomplishments and prompt memory-impaired residents to initiate everyday activities, such as bathing, could benefit caregivers. This is underscored by the finding that tracking and assisting with everyday activities are frequently overwhelming duties that negatively affect the caregiver's own health (Vitaliano, Echeverria, Phillips, Young, & Siegler, 2005).

Data from numerous studies suggest that both older and younger adult populations are accepting of smart environment technologies and support continued development (Coughlin et al., 2007; Davis et al., 2014). Despite the potential value that smart environment technologies hold for clinical use, many challenges remain in bringing smart technologies into the healthcare arena (Kang et al., 2010). For example, many sensors that could be used to monitor behavioral and physiological health have a short battery life (i.e., only weeks or days) and standards are needed to facilitate interdevice communication and control. In addition, the reliability, validity, and efficacy of algorithms designed to monitor health behaviors will need to be demonstrated. While the challenges are vast, ranging from technical issues to privacy issues, to concerns about replacing caregiver–human contact, they are not insurmountable. The. challenges will, however, require computer scientists, engineers, healthcare professionals, and other disciplines to work synergistically. In addition, users must continuously be involved in the development and evaluation of the smart health technologies (Kraskowsky & Finlayson, 2001). Furthermore, it will be important that healthcare professionals remain aware of new technologies and their potential benefits so that they can assist patients and families in identifying technologies that will best meet their needs.

# Acknowledgments

This work was partially supported by grants from the National Institutes of Biomedical Imaging and Bioengineering (Grants #R01 EB009675; #R01 EB015853), the National Science Foundation (Grant DGE-0900781), and the National Institute of Aging (Grant #R25 AG046114). No conflicts of interest exist.

Correspondence concerning the publication should be addressed to Maureen Schmitter-Edgecombe, Department of Psychology, Washington State University, Pullman, Washington 99164-4820. Electronic mail may be sent to schmitter-e@ wsu.edu.

# References

Alam, M. R., Reaz, M. B. I., & Ali M. A. M. (2012). A review of smart homes—Past, present, and future. *IEEE Transactions on Systems, Man,and Cybernetics Part C, 42,* 1190–1203.

Allcott, H., & Rogers, T. (2014). The short-run and long-run effects of behavioral interventions: Experimental evidence from energy conservation. *The American Economic Review, 104*(10), 3003–3037.

Aleven, V., McLaren, B., Roll, I., & Koedinger, K. (2004, August). Toward tutoring help seeking. In *Proceedings of the International Conference on Intelligent Tutoring Systems* (pp. 227–239). Springer: Berlin Heidelberg.

Babbitt, R. (2006, September). Information privacy management in smart home environments: Modeling, verification, and implementation. In *Proceedings of the 30th Annual International Computer Software and Applications Conference (COMPSAC'06).*

Bandura, A. (1997). *Self-efficacy: The exercise of control.* Gordonsville, VA: WH Freeman & Co.

Bandura, A. (2000). Exercise of human agency through collective efficacy. *Current Directions in Psychological Science, 9,* 75–78.

Beringer, R., Sixsmith, A., Campo, M., Brown, J., & McCloskey, R. (2011, June). The "acceptance" of ambient assisted living: Developing an alternate methodology to this limited research lens. In *International Conference on Smart Homes and Health Telematics* (pp. 161–167). Springer: Berlin Heidelberg.

Berkhuysen, M. A., Nieuwland, W., Buunk, B. P., Sanderman, R., & Rispens, P. (1999). Change in self-efficacy during cardiac rehabilitation and the role of perceived overprotectiveness. *Patient Education and Counseling, 38,* 21–32.

Bewernitz, M. W., Mann, W. C., Dasler, P., & Belchior, P. (2009). Feasibility of machine-based prompting to assist persons with dementia. *Assistive Technology, 21,* 196–207.

Blackwell, T., Redline, S., Ancoli-Israel, S., Schneider, J. L., Surovec, S., Johnson, N. L., . . . & Study of Osteoporotic Fractures Research Group. (2008). Comparison of sleep parameters from actigraphy and polysomnography in older women: The SOF study. *Sleep, 31,* 283–291.

Boger, J., & Mihailidis, A. (2011). The future of intelligent assistive technologies for cognition: Devices under development to support independent living and aging-with-choice. *Neurorehabilitation, 28,* 271–280.

Boger, J., Hoey, J., Poupart, P., Boutilier, C., Fernie, G., & Mihailidis, A. (2006). A planning system based on Markov decision processes to guide people with dementia through activities of daily living. *IEEE Transactions on Information Technology in Biomedicine, 10,* 323–333.

Boll, S., Heuten, W., Meyer, H. M., & Meis, M. (2010). Development of a multimodal reminder system for older persons in their residential homes. *Informatics for Health and Social Care, 35,* 104–124.

Bulling, A., Blanke, U., & Schiele, B. (2014). A tutorial on human activity recognition using body-worn inertial sensors. *ACM Computing Surveys, 46,* 107–140.

Bulling, A., Ward, J. A., & Gellersen, H. (2012). Multimodal recognition of reading activity in transit using body-worn sensors. *ACM Transactions on Applied Perception, 9,* 2:1–2:21.

Burton, C. A., Strauss, E., Bunce, D., Hunter, M. A., & Hultsch. D. F. (2009). Functional abilities in older adults with mild cognitive impairment. *Gerontology, 55,* 570–581.

Byrne, M. D., & Anderson, J. R. (2001). Serial modules in parallel: The psychological refractory period and perfect time-sharing. *Psycholoigcal Review, 108,* 847–869.

Chajewska, U., Koller, D., & Parr, R. (2000). Making rational decisions using adaptive utility elicitation. In *Proceedings of the National Conference on Artificial Intelligence* (pp. 363–369). Austin, Texas.

Chen, L., Hoey, J., Nugent, C. D., Cook, D. J., & Yu, Z. (2012). Sensor-based activity recognition. *IEEE Transactions on Systems, Man, and Cybernetics Part C, 42,* 790–808.

Ching-Show, L. (2008). Technology for care. *Gerontechnology, 7,* 349–350.

Coates, A., Karpathy, A., & Ng, A. Y.(2012). Emergence of object-selective features in unsupervised feature learning. In *Proceedings of the Inernational Conference on Neural Information Processing Systems* (pp. 1–9).

Cohen-Mansfield, J., & Biddison, J. (2007). The scope and future trends of gerontechnology: Consumers' opinions and literature survey. *Journal of Technology in Human Services, 25,* 1–19.

Cook, D. (2012). Learning setting-generalized activity models for smart spaces. *IEEE Intelligent Systems, 27,* 32–38.

Cook, D. J., Crandall, A., Thomas, B., & Krishnan, N. (2012). CASAS: A smart home in a box. *IEEE Computer, 46,* 1–15.

Cook, D. J., Feuz, K., & Krishnan, N. (2013). Transfer learning for activity recognition: A survey. *Knowledge Information Systems, 36,* 537–556.

Cook, D. J., & Holder, L. (2013). Automated activity-aware prompting for activity initiation. *Gerontechnology, 11,* 534–544.

Cook, D. J., & Schmitter-Edgecombe, M. (2009). Assessing the quality of activities in a smart environment. *Methods of Information in Medicine, 48,* 480–485.

Copeland, J. L., & Esliger, D. W. (2009) Accelerometer assessment of physical activity in active, healthy older adults. *Journal of Aging Physical Activity, 17,* 17–30.

Coughlin, J. F., D'Ambrosio, L. A., Reimer, B., & Pratt, M. R. (2007, August). Older adult perceptions of smart home technologies: Implications for research, policy & market innovations in healthcare. In *Proceedings of the 29th Annual International Conference of the IEEE Engineering in Medicine and Biology Society* (pp. 1810–1815).

Courtney, K. L., Demiris, G., & Hensel, B. K. (2007). Obtrusiveness of information-based assistive technologies as perceived by older adults in residential care facilities: A secondary analysis. *Informatics for Health and Social Care, 32,* 241–249.

Das, B., Chen, C., Seelye, A. M., & Cook, D. J. (2011, June). An automated prompting system for smart environments. In *International Conference on Smart Homes and Health Telematics* (pp. 9–16). Springer: Berlin Heidelberg.

Davis, M. M., Freeman, M., Kaye, J., Vuckovic, N., & Buckley, D. I. (2014). A systematic review of clinician and staff views on the acceptability of incorporating remote monitoring technology into primary care. *Telemedicine and e-Health, 20,* 428–438.

Dassel, K. B., & Schmitt, F. A. (2008). The impact of caregiver executive skills on reports of patient functioning. *The Gerontological Society of America, 48,* 781–792.

Dawadi, P., Cook, D., Schmitter-Edgecombe, M., & Parsey, C. (2013). Automated assessment of cognitive health using smart home technologies. *Technology and Health Care, 21,* 323–343.

Dawadi, P., Cook, D., & Schmitter-Edgecombe, M. (2013). Automated cognitive health assessment using smart home monitoring of complex tasks. *IEEE Transactions on Systems, Man, and Cybernetics: Systems, 43,* 1302–1313.

Dawadi, P., Cook, D. J., & Schmitter-Edgecombe, M. (2014, September). Smart home-based longitudinal functional assessment. In *Proceedings of the 2014 ACM International Joint Conference on Pervasive and Ubiquitous Computing: Adjunct Publication* (pp. 1217–1224).

Dawadi, P. N., Cook, D. J., & Schmitter-Edgecombe, M. (2016). Automated cognitive assessment from smart-home based behavior data. *IEEE Journal of Biomedical and Health Informatics, 20*(4), 1188–1194.

Demiris, G., Rantz, M. J., Aud, M. A., Marek, K. D., Tyrer, H. W., Skubic, M., & Hussam, A. A. (2004). Older adults' attitudes towards and perceptions of "smart home" technologies: A pilot study. *Informatics for Health and Social Care, 29*, 87–94.

Department of Health. (2007). Speech by the Rt Hon Patricia Hewitt MP, Secretary of State for Health. In *Proceedings of the Long-term Conditions Alliance Annual Conference, 2007.*

Durant, W. (1926). *The story of philosophy: The lives and opinions of the world's greatest philosophers.* New York, NY: Washington Square Press.

Epstein, N., Willis, M. G., Conners, C. K., & Johnson, D. E. (2001). Use of technological prompting device to aid a student with attention deficit hyperactivity disorder to initiate and complete daily tasks: An exploratory study. *Journal of Special Education Technology, 16*, 19–28.

Evans, B. D., & Rogers, A. E. (1994). 24-hour sleep/wake patterns in healthy elderly persons. *Applied Nursing Research, 7*, 75–83.

Fauth, E. B., Schwartz, S., Tschanz, J. T., Østbye, T., Corcoran, C., & Norton, M. C. (2013). Baseline disability in activities of daily living predicts dementia risk even after controlling for baseline global cognitive ability and depressive symptoms. *International Journal of Geriatric Psychiatry, 28*, 597–606.

Fawcett, T. (2006). An introduction to ROC analysis. *Pattern Recognition Letters, 27*, 861–874.

Feuz, K., & Cook, D. J. (2014). Transfer learning across feature-rich heterogeneous feature spaces via feature-space remapping. *ACM Transactions on Intelligent Systems and Technology, 6*(1), 3.

Ferguson, H., Myles, B. S., & Hagiwara, T. (2005). Using a personal digital assistant to enhance the independence of an adolescent with Asperger syndrome. *Education and Training in Mental Retardation and Developmental Disabilities, 40*, 60–67.

Finlayson, M., Havens, B., Holm, M. B., & Van Denend, T. (2003). Integrating a performance-based observation measure of functional status into a population-based longitudinal study of aging. *Canadian Journal on Aging, 22*, 185–195.

Fisher, A. G., Merritt, B. K., Fisher, A. G., & Jones, K. B. (2012). Current standardization sample, item and task calibration values, and validity and reliability of the AMPS. *Assessment of Motor and Process Skills, 1*, 15–11.

Fisher, B. E., & Sullivan, K. J. (2001). Activity-dependent factors affecting poststroke functional outcomes. *Topics in Stroke Rehabilitation, 8*, 31–44.

Galambos, C., Skubic, M., Wang, S., & Rantz, M. (2013). Management of dementia and depression utilizing in-home passive sensor data. *Gerontechnology, 11*, 457–468.

Giles, L. C., Glonek, G. F., Luszcz, M. A., & Andrews, G. R. (2005). Effect of social networks on 10-year survival in very old Australians: The Australian Longitudinal Study of Aging. *Journal of Epidemiology and Community Health, 59*, 574–579.

Gopalratnam, K., & Cook, D. J. (2004). Active LeZi: An incremental parsing algorithm for sequential prediction. *International Journal on Artificial Intelligence Tools, 13*(04), 917–929.

Gopalratnam, K., & Cook, D. J. (2007). Online sequential prediction via incremental parsing: The Active LeZi algorithm. *IEEE Intelligent Systems, 22*, 52–58.

Greber, C., Ziviani, J., & Rodger, S. (2007). The four quadrant model of facilitated learning: A clinically based action research project. *Australian Occupational Therapy Journal, 54*, 149–152.

Gu, T., Chen, S., Tao, X., & Lu, J. (2010). An unsupervised approach to activity recognition and segmentation based on object-use fingerprints. *Data Knowledge in Engineering, 69*, 533–544.

Haimowitz, I. J., & Kohane, I. S. (1993). An epistemology for clinically significant trends. In *Proceedings of the 10th National Conference on Artificial Intelligence* (pp. 176–181). AAAI Press, Menlo Park.

Hart, T. L., Swartz, A. M., & Strath, S. J. (2011). How many days of monitoring are needed to accurately estimate physical activity in older adults? *International Journal of Behavioral Nutrition and Physical Activity, 8*, 62–69.

Hayes, T. L., Abendtroth, F., Adami, A., Pavel, M., Zitzelberger, T. A., & Kaye, J. A. (2008). Unobtrusive assessment of activity patterns associated with mild cognitive impairment. *Alzheimer's & Dementia, 4*, 395–405.

Hayes, T. L., Cobbinah, K., Dishongh, T., Kaye, J. A., Kimel, J., Labhard, M., . . . & Vurgun, S. (2009). A study of medication-taking and unobtrusive, intelligent reminding. *Telemedicine and e-Health, 15*, 770–776.

Ho, J., & Intille, S. S. (2005, April). Using context-aware computing to reduce the perceived burden of interruptions from mobile devices. In *Proceedings of the SIGCHI Conference on Human Factors in Computing Systems* (pp. 909–918).

Hoey, J., Von Bertoldi, A., Craig, T., Poupart, P., & Mihailidis, A. (2010). Automated handwashing assistance for persons with dementia using video and a partially observable Markov decision process. *Computer Vision and Image Understanding, 114*, 503–519.

Hughes, C. P., Berg, L., Danzinger, W. L., Coben, L. A., & Martin, R. L. (1982). A new clinical scale for the staging of dementia. *The British Journal of Psychiatry, 140*, 566–572.

Hume, K., & Odom, S. (2007). Effects of an individual work system on the independent functioning of students with autism. *Journal of Autism and Developmental Disorders, 37*, 1166–1180.

Hwang, A. S., Truong, K. N., & Mihailidis, A. (2012, May). Using participatory design to determine the needs of informal caregivers for smart home user interfaces. In *Proceedings of the 6th International Conference on Pervasive Computing Technologies for Healthcare (PervasiveHealth) and Workshops* (pp. 41–48).

Iqbal, T., & Baile, T. P. (2006). Leveraging characteristics of task structure to predict costs of interruption. In *Proceedings of the SIGCHI Conference on Human Factors in Computing Systems* (pp. 741–750).

Jackson, S. (2011). Online rewards key to effectiveness of apps for your hospital's patients. Retrieved from www.fiercemobilehealthcare.com/story/online-rewards-key-effectiveness-apps-your-hospitals-patients/2011-06-27

Jones, M., & Johnston, D. (2011). Understanding phenomena in the real world: The case for real time data collection in health services research. *Journal of Health Services Research & Policy, 16*, 172–176.

Kaushik, P., Intille, S., & Larson, K. (2008). User-adaptive reminders for home-based medical tasks: A case study. *Methods of Information in Medicine, 47*, 203–207.

Kaye, J. (2008). Home-based technologies: A new paradigm for conducting dementia prevention trials. *Alzheimer's & Dementia, 4*, S60–S66.

Kim, J., Kikuchi, H., & Yamamoto, Y. (2013). Systematic comparison between ecological momentary assessment and day reconstruction method for fatigue and mood states in healthy adults. *British Journal of Health Psychology, 18*, 155–167.

Kang, H. G., Mahoney, D. F., Hoenig, H., Hirth, V. A., Bonato, P., Hajjar, I., & Lipsitz, L. A. (2010). In situ monitoring of health in older adults: Technologies and issues. *Journal of the American Geriatrics Society, 58*, 1579–1586.

Kraskowsky, L. H., & Finlayson, M. (2001). Factors affecting older adults' use of adaptive equipment: Review of the literature. *American Journal of Occupational Therapy, 55*, 303–310.

Krishnan, N., & Cook, D. J. (2014). Activity recognition on streaming sensor data. *Pervasive and Mobile Computing, 10*, 138–154.

Krumm, J., & Horvitz, E. (2006, September). Predestination: Inferring destinations from partial trajectories. In *International Conference on Ubiquitous Computing* (pp. 243–260). Springer Berlin Heidelberg.

Kubat, M., & Matwin, S. (1997). Addressing the curse of imbalanced training set: One-sides selection. In *Proceedings of the Fourteenth International Conference on Machine Learning* (pp. 179–186).

Lara, O. D., & Labrador, M. A. (2013). A survey on human activity recognition using wearable sensors. *Communications Surveys & Tutorials, IEEE, 15*, 1192–1209.

Lawton, M., Moss, M., Fulcomer, M., & Kleban, M. (1982). A research and service oriented multilevel assessment instrument. *Journal of Gerontology, 37*(1), 91–99.

Lee, S. I., Ghasemzadeh, H., Mortazavi, B., Lan, M., Alshurafa, N., Ong, M., & Sarrafzadeh, M. (2013, November). Remote patient monitoring: What impact can data analytics have on cost? In *Proceedings of the 4th Conference on Wireless Health* (p. 4).

Lenze, E. J., Munin, M. C., Quear, T., Dew, M. A., Rogers, J. C., Begley, A. E., & Reynolds, C. F. III. (2004). Significance of poor patient participation in physical and occupational therapy for functional outcome and length of stay. *Archives of Physical Medicine and Rehabilitation, 85*, 1599–1601.

Levenshtein, V. I. (1966). Binary codes capable of correcting deletions, insertions, and reversals. *Soviet Physics Doklady, 10*, 707–710.

Liu, S., Yamada, M., Collier, N., & Sugiyama, M. (2013). Change-point detection in time-series data by relative density-ratio estimation. *Neural Networks, 43*, 72–83.

Loewenstein, D. A., Argüelles, S., Bravo, M., Freeman, R. Q., Argüelles, T., Acevedo, A., & Eisdorfer, C. (2001). Caregivers' judgments of the functional abilities of the Alzheimer's disease patient: A comparison of proxy reports and objective measures. *The Journals of Gerontology Series B: Psychological Sciences and Social Sciences, 56*, P78–P84.

Luck, T., Luppa, M., Angermeyer, M. C., Villringer, A., König, H.-H., & Riedel-Heller, S. G. (2011). Impact of impairment in instrumental activities of daily living and mild cognitive impairment on time to incident dementia: Results of the Leipzig Longitudinal Study of the Aged. *Psychological Medicine, 41*, 1087–1097.

Lundell, J. (2005). Ubiquitous computing to support older adults and informal caregivers. *From Smart Homes to Smart Care, 15*, 11–22.

Marcotte, T. D., Scott, J. C., Kamat, R., & Heaton, R. K. (2010). Neuropsychology and the prediction of everyday functioning. In T. D. Marcotte & I. Grant (Eds.), *Neuropsychology of Everyday Functioning* (pp. 5–38). New York: The Guilford Press.

Marson, D., & Hebert, K. (2006). Functional assessment. In D. Attix. & K. Welsh-Bohmer (Eds.), *Geriatric neuropsychology assessment and intervention* (pp. 158–189). New York, NY: Guilford Press.

McAlister, C., & Schmitter-Edgecombe, M. (2013). Naturalistic assessment of executive function and everyday multitasking in healthy older adults. *Aging, Neuropsychology and Cognition, 20*, 735–756.

Mihaildis, A., Fernie, G. R., & Barbenel, J. C. (2001). The use of artificial intelligence in the design of an intelligent cognitive orthosis for people with dementia. *Assistive Technology, 13*, 23–39.

Miller, L. S., Brown, C. L., Mitchell, M. B., & Williamson, G. M. (2013). Activities of daily living are associated with older adult cognitive status: Caregiver versus self-reports. *Journal of Applied Gerontology, 32*, 3–30.

Mitchell, M., Miller, L. S., Woodard, J. L., Davey, A., Martin, P., Burgess, M., & Poon, L. W. (2010). Regression-based estimates of observed functional status in centenarians. *The Gerontologist, 51*, 179–189.

Modayil, J., Levinson, R., Harman, C., Halper, D., & Kautz, H. A. (2008, November). Integrating Sensing and Cueing for More Effective Activity Reminders. In *AAAI Fall Symposium: AI in Eldercare: New Solutions to Old Problems* (Vol. 216).

Moncrieff, S., Venkatesh, S., & West, G. (2008). Dynamic privacy assessment in a smart house environment using multimodal sensing. *ACM Transactions on Multimedia Computing, Communications, and Applications, 5*, 10.

Moore, D. J., Palmer, B. W., Patterson, T. L., & Jeste, D. V. (2007). A review of performance-based measures of functional living skills. *Journal of Psychiatric Research, 41*, 97–118.

Morris, J. C. (1993). The Clinical Dementia Rating (CDR): Current version and scoring rules. *Neurology, 43*, 2412–2414.

Paavilainen, P., Korhonen, I., Lötjönen, J., Cluitmans, L., Jylhä, M., Särelä, A., & Partinen, M. (2005). Circadian activity rhythm in demented and non-demented nursing-home residents measured by telemetric actigraphy. *Journal of Sleep Research, 14*, 61–68.

Parsey, C., Sawadi, P., Schmitter-Edgecombe, M., & Cook, D. (2011). Measures of Everyday Functioning in a Smart Environment. Presented at the *Festival of International Conferences on Caregiving, Disability, Aging and Technology, Toronto, Canada*.

Pan, S. J., & Yang, Q. (2010). A survey on transfer learning. *IEEE Transactions on Knowledge and Data Engineering, 22*, 1345–1359.

Penhale, B., & Manthorpe, J. (2001). Using electronic aids to assist people with dementia. *Nursing and Resident Care, 3*, 586–589.

Podsiadlo, D., & Richardson, S. (1991). The timed "Up & Go": A test of basic functional mobility for frail elderly persons. *Journal of the American Geriatrics Society, 39*, 142–148.

Pollack, M. E., Brown, L., Colbry, D., McCarthy, C. E., Orosz, C., Peintner, B., . . . & Tsamardinos, I. (2003). Autominder: An intelligent cognitive orthotic system for people with memory impairment. *Robotics and Autonomous Systems, 44*, 273–282.

Pu, P., & Chen, L. (2009). User-involved preference elicitation for product search and recommender systems. *AI Magazine, 29*, 93.

Purath, J., Buchholz, S., & Kark, D. (2009). Physical fitness assessment of community-dwelling older adults. *Journal of the American Academy Nurse Practitioners, 21*, 101–107.

Randolph, C., Tierney, M. C., Mohr, E., & Chase, T. N. (1998). The Repeatable Battery for the Assessment of Neuropsychological Status (RBANS): Preliminary clinical validity. *Journal of Clinical and Experimental Neuropsychology, 20,* 310–319.

Reiss, A., Stricker, D., & Hendeby, G. (2013, May). Towards robust activity recognition for everyday life: methods and evaluation. In *Proceedings of the 7th International Conference on Pervasive Computing Technologies for Healthcare and Workshops* (pp. 25–32).

Robben, S., & Kröse, B. (2013, May). Longitudinal residential ambient monitoring: correlating sensor data to functional health status. In *Proceedings of the 7th International Conference on Pervasive Computing Technologies for Healthcare* (pp. 244–247).

Robertson, K., Rosasco, C., Feuz, K., Schmitter-Edgecombe, M., & Cook, D. (2015). Prompting technologies: A comparison of time-based and context-aware transition-based promoting. *Technology and Health Care, 23,* 745–756.

Singla, G., Cook, D. J., & Schmitter-Edgecombe, M. (2010). Recognizing independent and joint activities among multiple residents in smart environments. *Ambient Intelligence and Humanized Computing Journal, 1,* 57–63.

Schmitter-Edgecombe, M., McAlister, C., & Weakley, A. (2012). Naturalistic assessment of everyday functioning in individuals with mild cognitive impairment: The Day Out Task. *Neuropsychology, 26,* 631–641.

Schmitter-Edgecombe, M., & Parsey, C. (2014). Assessment of functional change and cognitive correlates in the progression from normal aging to dementia. *Neuropsychology, 28,* 881–893.

Schmitter-Edgecombe, M., & Parsey, C. (2014). Cognitive correlates of functional abilities in individuals with mild cognitive impairment: Comparison of questionnaire, direct observation and performance-based measures. *The Clinical Neuropsychologist, 28,* 726–746.

Schmitter-Edgecombe, M., Parsey, C., & Cook, D. J. (2011). Cognitive correlates of functional performance in older adults: Comparison of self-report, direct observation, and performance-based measures. *Journal of the International Neuropsychological Society, 17,* 853–864.

Seelye, A. M., Schmitter-Edgecombe, M., Cook, D. J., & Crandall, A. (2013). Naturalistic assessment of everyday activities and prompting technologies in mild cognitive impairment. *Journal of the International Neuropsychological Society, 19,* 442–452.

Seelye, A., Schmitter-Edgecombe, M., & Cook, D. J. (2013). Technology based prompting for instrumental activities of daily living in healthy aging, mild cognitive impairment and dementia. Presentation at the International Neuropsychological Society.

Sikkes, S. A. M., de Lange-de Klerk, E. S. M., Pijnenburg, Y. A. L., Scheltens, P., & Uitdehaag, B. M. J. (2009). A systematic review of instrumental activities of daily living scales in dementia: Room for improvement. *Journal of Neurology, Neurosurgery & Psychiatry, 80,* 7–12.

Simon, C., Cain, C., Hajiammini, S., Saeedi, R., Schmitter-Edgecombe, M., & Cook, D. (2014, September). Digital memory notebook: Experimental evaluation of motivational reward strategies. In *Proceedings of the 2014 ACM International Joint Conference on Pervasive and Ubiquitous Computing: Adjunct Publication* (pp. 1201–1208).

Smyth, J. M. (2003). Ecological momentary assessment research in behavioral medicine. *Journal of Happiness Studies, 4,* 35–52.

Sohlberg, M., Ehlhardt, L., & Kennedy, M. (2005). Instructional techniques in cognitive rehabilitation: A preliminary report. *Seminars in Speech and Language, 26*, 268–279.

Spector, A., Orrell, M., & Woods, B. (2010). Cognitive stimulation therapy (CST): Effects on different areas of cognitive function for people with dementia. *International Journal of Geriatric Psychiatry, 25*, 1253–1258.

Stanley, K. G., & Osgood, N. D. (2011). The potential of sensor-based monitoring as a tool for health care, health promotion, a research. *Annals of Family Medicine, 9*, 296–298.

Strayer, D. L., Drews, F. A., & Johnston, W. A. (2003). Cell phone induced attention in simulated driving. *Journal of Experimental Psychology, 9*, 23–32.

Tabert, M. H., Albert, S. M., Borukhova-Milov, L., Camacho, Y., Pelton, G., Liu, X., . . . Devanand, D. P. (2002). Functional deficits in patients with mild cognitive impairment: Prediction of AD. *Neurology, 58*, 758–764.

Teng, E., Tassniyom, K., & Lu, P. H. (2012). Reduced quality-of-life ratings in mild cognitive impairment: Analyses of subject and informant responses. *American Journal of Geriatric Psychiatry, 20*, 1016–1025.

Tsang, R. S. M., Diamond, K., Mowszowski, L., Lewis, S. J. G., & Naismith, S. L. (2012). Using informant reports to detect cognitive decline in mild cognitive impairment. *International Psychogeriatrics, 24*, 967–973.

Van Kasteren, T., Noulas, A., Englebienne, G., & Kröse, B. (2008, September). Accurate activity recognition in a home setting. In *Proceedings of the 10th International Conference on Ubiquitous Computing* (pp. 1–9).

Vishwakarma, S., & Agrawal, A. (2013). A survey on activity recognition and behavior understanding in video surveillance. *The Visual Computer, 29*, 983–1009.

Vitaliano, P., Echeverria, D., Yi, J., Phillips, P., Young, H., & Siegler, I. (2005). Psychophysiological mediators of caregiver stress and differential cognitive decline. *Psychology and Aging, 20*, 402–411.

Wilson, B. A., Evans, J. J., Emslie, H., & Malinek, V. (1997). Evaluation of NeuroPage: A new memory aid. *Journal of Neurology, Neurosurgery, & Psychiatry, 63*, 113–115.

Wilson, C., Hargreaves, T., & Hauxwell-Baldwin, R. (2014). Smart homes and their users: A systematic analysis and key challenges. *Personal and Ubiquitous Computing, 19*, 1–14.

Wyatt, D., Philipose, M., & Choudhury, T. (2005). Unsupervised activity recognition using automatically mined common sense. In *Proceedings of the National Conference in Artificial Intelligence* (Vol. 5, pp. 21–27).

Xu, C., Tao, D., & Xu, C. (2013). A survey on multi-view learning. *arXiv preprint*.

Yang, J., & Wang, W. (2003, March). CLUSEQ: Efficient and effective sequence clustering. In *Proceedings of the 19th International Conference in Data Engineering* (pp. 101–112).

Zhang, M., & Sawchuk, A. A. (2012, January). Motion primitive-based human activity recognition using a bag-of-features approach. In *Proceedings of the 2nd ACM SIGHIT International Health Informatics Symposium* (pp. 631–640).

Zhou, H. Y., & Shan, J. S. (2013). Time sequence clustering based on edit distance. *Applied Mechanics and Materials, 401*, 1428–1431.

# PART IV

# Integrating Cognitive Assessment with Biological Metrics

# 12

# Technological Innovations to Enhance Neurocognitive Rehabilitation

Anthony J.-W. Chen, Fred Loya, and Deborah Binder

## Introduction

In an instant, a brain injury can cause changes that affect a person for a lifetime. Although traumatic brain injury (TBI) can result in almost any neurological deficit, the most common and persistent deficits tend to affect neurocognitive functioning. Functional issues may produce a tremendous chronic burden on individuals, families, and healthcare systems (Thurman, Alverson, Dunn, Guerrero, & Sniezek, 1999; Yu et al., 2003). The far-reaching impact of these seemingly "invisible" deficits is often not recognized. Individuals who have suffered a TBI may also be at increased risk for developing cognitive changes later in life (Mauri et al., 2006; Schwartz, 2009; Van Den Heuvel, Thornton, & Vink, 2007). Military veterans report even higher rates of persistent issues, especially in the context of posttraumatic stress (PTS) (Polusny et al., 2011). Despite their importance, chronic neurocognitive dysfunctions are often poorly addressed. A long-term view on care-oriented research and development is needed (Chen & D'Esposito, 2010).

Even as we get deeper into the 21st century, there continue to be many gaps in the rehabilitation of neurocognitive functioning after brain injury. There is a need for increased effort to advance rehabilitation care and delivery. There are two major gaps in care that could benefit from neuroscience research and technology-assisted intervention development. First, there remains a major need for theory-driven approaches to cognitive training, accompanied by the development of innovative tools to support learning of useful skills and their generalization to help achieve real-life goals. Second, major gaps in the delivery and coordination of rehabilitation must be addressed in order to provide care to the many people with brain injury who lack access to services due to barriers imposed by distance, financial constraints, and disability.

This chapter introduces and illustrates some technology-assisted innovations that may help to advance neurocognitive rehabilitation care. Examples of using technology to reach into the community via tele-rehabilitation, as well as examples of reaching students in a manner aligned with their scholastic goals, are discussed.

Much of the research described in this chapter is based on a rehabilitation neuroscience approach to intervention development. A neurocognitive framework helps to elucidate intervention targets and measurements to guide intervention development and testing. Rehabilitation interventions may provide powerful tools to probe neural-behavioral mechanisms of plasticity. It is hoped that defining mechanisms of neural plasticity will lead to new potential targets for treatment. The chapter discusses an evolving series of intervention development work, with the unifying target being a person's ability to *regulate their brain states to achieve goals*.

Some of the most common and long-lasting consequences of brain injury affect the highest levels of cognition, disrupting functions vital for goal achievement. Brain injury can lead to persistent difficulty with selectively processing important information and taking necessary actions for achieving goals, with particular vulnerability to cognitive-emotional dysregulation. An individual's ability to regulate attention (to be able attend to, hold in mind, and process information, especially in the setting of distractions) provides a vital 'gateway' to the most efficient and effective pathways of goal-directed functioning. These functions are important for learning and adaptation in personal life, and unaddressed deficits can therefore have far-reaching effects (Chen & D'Esposito, 2010; Chen & Novakovic-Agopian, 2012). Training that improves core functioning could be quite valuable in helping individuals with brain injury.

### GOAL-DIRECTED FUNCTIONING WITH TBI-PTS—THE IMPORTANCE OF COGNITIVE-EMOTIONAL FUNCTIONING

In considering intervention research and development, it is worthwhile to explicitly address the combination of TBI and PTS, given its importance to military veterans, the special challenges in treating the combined conditions (Chen & Novakovic-Agopian, 2012), and the paucity of research directly addressing the topic (Cooper et al., 2015). It is currently estimated that as many as one in five service members of the recent conflicts in the Middle East sustained a TBI during their deployment, of which as many as 40% also experience clinically significant symptoms of PTS (Carlson et al., 2011; Hoge et al., 2008). One of the most common and debilitating consequences of TBI, with or without co-occurring symptoms of PTS, is difficulty with goal-directed functioning. This stems from problems with regulating cognitive-emotional states, characterized by difficulty with managing distractions (from internal and external sources), with holding important information in mind, and, ultimately, with following through to accomplish multistep goals (Dean & Sterr, 2013; Vanderploeg, Curtiss, & Belanger, 2005; Vasterling, Bryant, & Keane,

2012). These impairments are associated with poor community outcomes, such as unemployment (Ponsford et al., 2014; van Velzen, van Bennekom, Edelaar, Sluiter, & Frings-Dresen, 2009) and problems in school (Church, 2009; Kennedy, Krause, & Turkstra, 2008). Dysfunctions associated with TBI and PTS tend to interact, exacerbating difficulties (Vasterling et al., 2012) and resulting in presentations that require special consideration for treatment. Strengthening regulation of cognitive-emotional states may help improve goal-directed functioning for those experiencing combined TBI and PTS. Interactions between TBI and PTS, including implications for treatment, have been previously addressed elsewhere (Chen & Novakovic-Agopian, 2012). Here, considerations regarding the formulation and design of interventions, and how technology can contribute to addressing the challenges in this area, are discussed in more depth.

## TARGETING CORE SELF-REGULATORY CONTROL FUNCTIONS INVOLVED IN TBI-PTS

Interactions in cognitive-emotional functioning are particularly relevant to intervention development. Both TBI and PTS tend to affect the regulation of cognitive-emotional functions.

Dorsolateral prefrontal cortex and ventromedial prefrontal cortex interact in the regulation of emotions, with modulation by the amygdala (Phelps, Delgado, Nearing, & LeDoux, 2004). The interactions of cognition and emotion are complex, but certain aspects of functional interactions become especially clear in a goal framework, and considering cognition-emotion in this framework leads to particular treatment considerations. The pathway to any goal involves continuous and dynamic regulation of internal (brain) states, from initiation of goal pursuit through all of the potential challenges to goal achievement. Without the necessary goal-directed regulation of brain/cognitive-emotional states, goal pursuit may be derailed.

Emotional and cognitive control are directly tied together, in that the underlying neural systems interact significantly in achieving the self-regulatory control necessary for goal-directed behavior. For example, individuals experiencing overly severe anxiety and/or distress will be less able to effectively complete tasks that require overcoming challenges and solving problems. Similarly, it is likely that reduced cognitive control contributes to difficulties with emotional control. For example, an inability to filter out information and demands that are not directly related to a current goal may lead to increased feelings of being overwhelmed. Given the limitations of neural processing resources, it is expected that an increase in load, whether from cognitive or emotional sources, would lead to less efficient overall functioning.

In sum, the combined syndrome of TBI-PTS is common, complex, debilitating, and requires special consideration. The issues from TBI-PTS include disruption of core cognitive-emotional self-regulation mechanisms that are essential for goal-directed functioning in daily life. Interventions that target cognitive-emotional self-regulatory functions in a goal framework may be particularly valuable in treating combined TBI-PTS (Chen & Novakovic-Agopian, 2012). Such interventions may provide a gateway to enhance success in achieving goals in multiple settings. For example, this may open the way to success with other aspects of therapy, school, and other settings in which learning goals are to be achieved (Chen & Novakovic-Agopian, 2012).

### INCREASING ACCESS TO CARE THROUGH INNOVATIONS IN SERVICE DELIVERY

In addition to delineating appropriate therapeutic targets to address as part of intervention development, there is a great need to establish effective ways to provide services to veterans and other individuals who lack access to rehabilitation. One major impediment to service access is the barrier imposed by distance. Many rural veterans, who comprise over a third of all enrollees in the Veterans Affairs (VA) system and 30% of servicemen in the recent wars in Iraq and Afghanistan (Veterans Affairs Office of Rural Health, 2014), live a significant distance from hospitals or treatment centers (Weeks, Wallace, West, Heady, & Hawthorne, 2008). However, even for those with more ready access to care, an additional barrier is a general lack of TBI rehabilitation specialists, a situation worsened by a further lack of clinicians with expertise in managing combined TBI-PTS (Alfers & Heady, 2014). The need for expanded care is especially urgent given that more than one million Americans are expected to transition to veteran status in the next 5 years, many of whom will be returning to their rural communities (Veterans Affairs Office of Rural Health, 2015). This pattern of limited access to services characterizes the civilian healthcare sector as well.

Success in education is a major goal for many veterans and other individuals with TBI. In 2013, the GI Bill supported 1,091,044 student veterans (Department of Veterans Affairs, 2014). However, the effects of TBI and PTS can create major challenges for students. Thus, helping students is another important goal of neurocognitive rehabilitation. Treatment approaches that are integrated into scholastic settings might better reach and help students.

As addressed below, there are challenges in maximizing the benefits of neurocognitive rehabilitation through training of neurocognitive skills, including increasing access to this care. Thus, the line of work aimed at enhancing rehabilitation with the assistance of technology, bringing together best clinical practices, neuroscience, and learning theory, is important. Patient-oriented design, development, and testing of training systems is also critical to improving goal-directed functioning. Technology can be designed and utilized to provide opportunities for guided experiential learning of key neurocognitive skills, and this approach can assist with the learning and transfer of skills to everyday goal pursuit. The approach may also help address gaps in the continuum of brain injury care, through its ability to reach those in need more directly in their home communities.

## Brain State Regulation—A Fundamental Target for Improving Goal-Directed Functioning

### TARGETING GATEWAY FUNCTIONS THAT UNDERLIE SUCCESSFUL GOAL-DIRECTED FUNCTIONING

What are the most fundamental and generalizable skills for improving goal-directed cognitive functioning? One key to improving goal-directed cognitive functioning is to improve the ability to regulate one's brain state so that it is optimal for guiding attention, processing information, learning, adapting, and taking action in the context of one's current goal and situation.

At any given moment, the brain is characterized by a functional state of networks of neurons. Cognitive actions always occur in the context of a pre-existing brain state. Some brain network states are associated with enhanced learning, memory, motivation, and self-control (Filevich, Kuhn, & Haggard, 2012; Seager, Johnson, Chabot, Asaka, & Berry, 2002; Stellar, 1980). The ability to regulate one's baseline state likely influences performance during goal-directed cognitive tasks (Fox, Snyder, Zacks, & Raichle, 2006; Kitzbichler, Henson, Smith, Nathan, & Bullmore, 2011; Papo, 2013). One way to characterize brain state is by parameters of functional brain networks. For example, the functional organization of brain networks into modules has been theorized to support learning and plasticity by enhancing the adaptivity, robustness, and evolvablity of network function (Bassett & Bullmore, 2006; Meunier, Achard, Morcom, & Bullmore, 2009; Meunier, Lambiotte, & Bullmore, 2010). Parameters of brain state like modularity may 'tune' how the brain handles tasks, influencing the responsiveness, efficiency, and, potentially, the plasticity of brain networks in response to experiences.

People vary in their ability to regulate brain states. When brain states are not regulated as needed for a current task or goal, individuals are more prone to being distracted, having difficulties processing or remembering goal-relevant information, being taken off track, or getting overwhelmed. Ultimately, the end result of this suboptimal state is a lower likelihood of accomplishing a goal. Dysregulated states are more common in individuals with TBI-PTS, and, consequently, training to enhance state regulation skills may be particularly beneficial for persons with these conditions.

The regulation of information processing is integrally related to aspects of brain state and deserves special emphasis. Selective processing of goal-relevant information, a central component of executive control, is a crucial gateway that filters what information gains access to more in-depth processing (Awh & Vogel,

2008; Baddeley, 2001; Cowan & Morey, 2006; Repovs & Baddeley, 2006; Vogel, McCollough, & Machizawa, 2005). The integrity of information processing, from perception through other steps to action, requires mechanisms of selection, maintenance, and protection from disruption during working memory, learning, decision making, and/or problem solving. The protection of information processing from distractions anywhere along this pathway is crucial to efficient and effective goal attainment, especially when extended time or multiple steps are required.

As one test of the potential importance of brain network state in moderating learning with cognitive training, we examined the extent to which network modularity might explain variability in response to cognitive training for patients with acquired brain injury (Arnemann et al., 2015). We acquired functional MRI (fMRI) data from brief (5 min) pretraining assays of brain state regulation. We examined the predictive value of baseline modularity for pre- to posttraining changes in measures of attention and executive control. Pretraining brain modularity predicted the degree of improvement in attention and executive functioning following training, such that those individuals with higher baseline modularity exhibited greater treatment response. The results provided preliminary support for the hypothesis that the regulation of functional brain network organization may influence learning.

## What Skills Need to be Trained to Improve Goal-Directed Functioning?

Some approaches to training state regulation were discovered millennia ago, and are being rediscovered now. Approaches like mindfulness and meditation training can be very valuable in achieving improved state regulation. However, these approaches are typically learned in optimal situations (quiet, calm environments), whereas the skills are actually most needed (and least likely to be activated) in the moment during challenges in personal life. Furthermore, some approaches have traditionally been limited by the need for a high level of pre-existing self-regulation, motivation, and perseverance, a particular problem when individuals suffer from brain injury (and would thus traditionally be considered poor candidates for training). Even for healthy individuals, it can take years of training with these approaches to accomplish mastery—in particular, the far-end goal of successful transfer of skill application to improve functioning during actual real-life challenges.

For brain injury rehabilitation, successful skill use in challenge situations (when a person is distracted, overwhelmed, or distressed) is an explicit proximal rather than distal goal of training. We argue that concrete, clearly delineated learning activities, with effective guidance to learn self-regulation skills during these activities, are vital for effective learning for these individuals.

## How Might We Train the Ability to Regulate
## Brain State to Best Achieve Goals?

There can be major gaps between the explanations and guidance provided by trainers in traditional therapy sessions and successful application of useful skills and strategies in an individual's personal life. It is clear that advice or didactics alone, without useful learning experiences, is often not sufficient. For example, simply advising someone to make a change that would be "good for you" (e.g., lose weight, quit smoking) famously leads to limited progress (Baranowski, Cullen, Nicklas, Thompson, & Baranowski, 2003). Even if behavior can be improved in training contexts, cognitive skills may not be utilized and applied to greatest benefit in various situations by individuals with brain injury. For example, an individual may successfully regulate attention to accomplish a clear, simple task with unambiguous instructions in a quiet setting, but then fail to successfully regulate attention in the context of a complex, multistep task in a setting with multiple distractions (i.e., personal life). In the latter situation, performance of the main tasks may be disrupted by any of a range of distractions, from background noise or conversations up to cell phone rings or even direct disruption by other individuals who may have questions or other demands. The individual may not anticipate or notice in-the-moment attentional dysregulation in the first place, and so will miss opportunities to apply skills to improve functioning.

This chapter describes how state regulation can be approached as a learnable step-wise process that involves stopping current activity, followed by regulation of the current state, and then redirecting attention to the task at hand. More generally, the last step is that of goal-directed cognition that is facilitated by effective state regulation. Goal-directed cognitive actions can include refocusing, redirecting attention, retrieving information, or re-activating goal-relevant action plans.

There are certain essential "stepping stones" important for bridging the initial learning of skills to the successful application of skills outside the training setting, in support of goals and in the context of being challenged.

State-regulation skills need to be extensively practiced to achieve a degree of automaticity in their application. In order to increase the likelihood of initiating state regulation, it is valuable to use a motif that is easy to learn and remember. We have emphasized Stop-Regulate motifs, such as Stop-Relax-Refocus (SRR). This can be practiced in different contexts to increase the automaticity of a regulation response.

It may also be necessary for an individual to understand the rationale underlying skill use, to recognize opportunities for skill application (e.g., avoiding distraction while listening to a lecture), and actually to be prepared to make use of skills when certain challenges arise. Having a clear goal framework supports a degree of self-knowledge and self-awareness that facilitates the recognition or even anticipation of challenges to goal direction. Goals frame and guide the initiation, monitoring, evaluating, and adjusting of self-regulation (Locke & Latham, 2002). The successful application of regulation skills requires identifying situations for strategic skill application, and this is supported by clear and accessible goals, self-knowledge, and self-awareness. We cannot know if we are going off track unless we have a sense of where the track is and where it is going. We also need to be able to identify when our internal state or features of our environment threaten goal direction. An "if/then" plan can then maximize the effective initiation of state regulation in these situations. Thus, increasing the clarity and accessibility of goals and intentions is an essential part of state-regulation training, especially as highlighted by the issue of goal neglect (Duncan, Emslie, Williams, Johnson, & Freer, 1996).

Without these stepping stones, skills might be learned at a basic level, but there will be limited application to benefit the individual outside the training context. Indeed, issues of learning and transfer are especially important for individuals with cognitive impairments due to brain injury. Even when these individuals seem to do well during training, they may miss opportunities to apply skills in personal life. Given the special challenges our patients face, it is paramount to fully address the potential gaps in learning and skill application.

## What Would the Ideal Training Approach Look Like? Building Generalizable Neurocognitive Skills in a Nonideal World

One training approach might be training directly in challenging contexts in personal life, with 'coaching' in the moment and in situ to provide guidance on useful skills and strategies, with real-time monitoring and feedback. This is achievable in cases where therapists can work directly with individuals in their homes, at school, or in work environments. However, there are practical as well as theoretical limitations to this approach. Some limitations are obvious—for example, time and effort limit the availability of such training. More often, therapists can provide some instruction in a clinical setting, but it is less clear to what extent patients actually follow through when in the community.

Other limitations may affect the value of learning opportunities in these settings. For example, life challenges may be unpredictable in frequency and difficulty, as well as in the severity of consequences. A typical encounter with a boss who is requesting multiple assignments with high-pressure deadlines isn't necessarily the most ideal environment for initial learning of cognitive skills. In addition, learning may be more effective with a graded approach to challenges. For example, patients may benefit from practicing to handle work assignments that require holding in mind smaller amounts of information before working up to high information loads. Similarly, patients may develop skills more effectively if they have the opportunity to work on goal-based tasks without distractions before learning to handle disruptions that take them away from the main task.

Once distractions are introduced, patients may benefit from learning to handle a range of different distractions and disruptions, from background conversation to the boss's disrupting the performance of a task. All of these features of training are difficult to consistently achieve with traditional modalities of rehabilitation for individuals in the community.

On different a front, some might think a drill-and-practice approach is the key to learning. Indeed, there has been much emphasis on training using simple but challenging cognitive tasks. We argue that practice on simple tasks alone is not sufficient for improving goal-directed functioning, however. Training in repetitive simple tasks often leads to major gains—in those simple tasks and contexts, but little beyond. By analogy, having someone drill and practice hamstring curls may result in strong hamstrings, but by itself won't make that person better at scoring goals against an aggressive defense during a soccer game. Why would it be any simpler to train and improve higher-order neurobehavioral functions important for achieving complex goals in challenging situations? The training experiences need to be more sophisticated to provide the best possible learning experiences. For training experiences to be useful for skill acquisition and transfer of skill use to complex challenges in personal life, they need to be challenging, complex, and varied across a range of contexts.

We therefore argue that active, guided experiential learning is the best way to help someone learn transferable skills to improve goal-directed cognitive functioning. An ideal system would involve experiential learning through the intensive practice of core skills, with personalized, progressive increases in challenges across a wide range of simple to complex contexts. The training system would provide active guidance for the learner through the steps of learning and transfer. Thus, the interventions described in this chapter have been designed to provide active experiential learning of skills while guiding learners to deepen learning and achieve successful transfer of skills to the situations when and where the skills are needed most.

## Potential Contributions of Technology to Enhancing Skill Training and Addressing Service Delivery: How Might Games be Useful in Augmenting Cognitive Training?

### TECHNOLOGY TO AID IN APPLICATION AND TRANSFER OF SKILL USE

In particular, gaming technology can provide interactive experiences that augment the potential of coaching. Overall, learning opportunities can be designed into interactive digital games to assist with the objectives of cultivating experiential understanding of cognitive processes, such as attention regulation, working memory, and goal maintenance (especially weaknesses or failures in these areas), and promoting application of skills and strategies to improve functioning in appropriate situations. Patients can make use of game experiences to learn skills as well as the strategic application of skills that are broadly applicable in different cognitive contexts and generalizable across contexts into personal life. Extensive practice with broadly applicable skills across a variety of contexts may help individuals with brain injury apply skills more effectively in personal contexts.

## TECHNOLOGY CAN SUPPORT TRAINING ACROSS A RANGE OF COGNITIVE CONTEXTS

It may be beneficial for an individual to train in a range of scenarios (across contexts), with calibrated challenges and intense practice while guided by coaching. Opportunities for supporting learning are feasible in the design of digital games, because interactive gaming scenarios provide a range of contexts in which particular cognitive processes can be engaged and challenged. Games can challenge the integrated functions of attention, working memory, and other processes in diverse contexts that engage these functions in different ways. Furthermore, the occurrence and progression of challenges can be controlled and adjusted, and supportive feedback can be provided during challenging experiences.

## EXPERIENCE DELIVERED THROUGH DIGITAL TECHNOLOGY CAN SUPPORT INTENSITY AND CALIBRATION OF TRAINING

It is advantageous to increase the intensity of training. As mentioned, real-world situations are not always optimal learning opportunities, but game scenarios can be designed to create a bridge of opportunities with specific learning goals. The ability to calibrate the experiences to be more optimal for learning is possible in digital games, with the potential for personalizing difficulty in chosen domains of functioning (e.g., working memory load, goal complexity, and/or experiences with distractions).

## TECHNOLOGY ASSISTANCE CAN SUPPORT SCENARIO-BASED EXPERIENTIAL LEARNING

Technology supported scenario-based training can add value to therapist guidance or coaching by providing concrete experiences that 'illustrate' particular processes or challenges for coaching. In other words, trainees can learn through experiences while experiences also provide specific opportunities for coaching and guidance.

## DIGITAL SCENARIO-BASED GAME EXPERIENCES CAN AUGMENT THE POWER OF COACHING

As tools to maximize the benefits of coaching, games could expand opportunities for trainers to observe patients, query and reinforce conceptual understanding, monitor actual application of skills and strategies, and provide valuable coaching that extends from game to real-life experiences. Furthermore, having a range of scenarios readily available can provide useful opportunities for a therapist to observe, model, and provide feedback, more effectively guiding and shaping skill learning and application.

## TECHNOLOGY CAN EXTEND THERAPIST REACH
## AND PATIENT ACCESS

Technology could be used to extend the reach of the therapist beyond traditional settings and improve access to training for patients, helping to deal with barriers like distance, impediments to travel, and lack of specialists, as well as associated costs. All of the features above also help to address important needs for remote service delivery through tele-rehabilitation.

This chapter discusses training interventions that utilize digital game scenarios to allow intensive practice of skills, with the key target being a person's ability to regulate the state of his/her brain to be as optimal as possible for the current situation and accomplishing a goal. That is, the training works to strengthen the individual's ability to adjust attention, emotion, and energy to make the best of the task at hand, and to regulate that state as required through all the steps to achieving a complex goal. This is neither as simple as asking an individual to 'go home and try it' nor as simple as sending someone off to practice game tasks.

## BRAIN-TRAINING GAMES AS A STAND-ALONE APPROACH
## TO COGNITIVE TRAINING

It may be informative to contrast our approach with that of using brain-training games alone as training. This contrast helps to highlight some considerations important for developing patient-oriented training systems.

Although the potential application of stand-alone computer games in brain injury rehabilitation was first noted several decades ago following the advent of home computers and gaming consoles (Lynch, 2002), it has gained increased attention in recent years. The ascendancy of this approach to cognitive training has been inspired largely by theories of neuroplasticity and the premise that intensive, repetitive practice on progressively challenging cognitive tasks may strengthen the associated neural circuitry on which task performance is based (Berlucchi, 2011; Kolb & Muhammad, 2014). This training approach has been heralded by studies showing cognitive improvements following computerized brain training among older adults (Anguera et al., 2013; Ballesteros et al., 2014; Mayas, Parmentier, Andrés, & Ballesteros, 2014), children (Klingberg et al., 2005; van der Oord, Ponsioen, Geurts, Ten Brink, & Prins, 2014), and, in some instances, clinical populations with associated cognitive problems (Lebowitz, Dams-O'Connor, & Cantor, 2012).

There are several reasons to question whether stand-alone brain games are sufficient to achieve rehabilitative goals for those with brain injury. Many game-based approaches to brain training provide isolated task-based practice activities (using 'gamified' versions of cognitive tasks originally designed to isolate particular cognitive processes). By design, game situations differ considerably from the complex real-life settings that often cause persons with brain injury difficulty. However, consistent evidence from studies of skill learning spanning multiple modalities have shown that repetition alone often leads to learning that is highly task specific and rarely transferable to other domains (see Green & Bavelier, 2008). Moreover, many patients find it difficult to make the connections from game to life. This may explain why many available brain games involving repetitive play have produced short-term, specific effects that do not appear to generalize (Melby-Lervag & Hulme, 2013; Owen et al., 2010; Shipstead, Hicks, & Engle, 2012; Shipstead, Redick, & Engle, 2012). Thus, it is critical that the conceptualization of games for neurorehabilitation move beyond practice on simple tasks alone.

There are also considerations specific to rehabilitation of persons with brain injury that must be addressed. For instance, current treatment guidelines for executive dysfunction, which includes impaired attentional processes and goal-directed functioning, emphasize raising metacognitive awareness and training goal-based strategies as valuable therapeutic elements. Individualized feedback, coaching, and collaborative problem solving are critical to training these abilities to be of practical benefit in the lives of individuals with brain injury. Indeed, in clinical contexts, the relevance of stand-alone games in the absence of explicit skills training may not be clear to persons with brain injury. Direct coaching is likely required in order to connect training experiences to personal goals and general life lessons, particularly in patients prone to concrete thinking.

Game-based approaches rarely provide any guidance in the goal-directed self-regulatory skills that we argue are of great generalizable value for improving a person's functioning. Some individuals may be able to learn by chance that self-regulation of brain state helps them improve and persist in practicing these activities (especially when the tasks get difficult or tedious), but many individuals, especially those who have deficits in self-regulation, problem solving, and adaptation, will not learn this lesson.

## Technology-Assisted Training Systems for Guided Experiential Learning of Goal-Directed Brain State Regulation

The following sections introduce the rationale, design, development, and testing process for training systems that integrate scenario-based experiential learning via games into the guided experiential learning of attention regulation, bridging skill use to personal life. Game scenarios based on patient experiences were built to train skill application across contexts with progressive challenges to goal direction. The discussion highlights key design elements important for skill acquisition and transfer, honed through patient-oriented, collaborative design, testing, and feedback.

Technology can be designed and incorporated into training to support at least two elements essential for skill learning and real-life skill application (Burke & Hutchins, 2007; Gollwitzer & Sheeran, 2006; Toglia, Johnston, Goverover, & Dain, 2010). First, technology-assisted training can provide varied opportunities for experiential skill learning, allowing for trained skills to be practiced and developed in the face of myriad types of well-calibrated cognitive challenges and contexts. Second, technology-assisted training experiences can help facilitate individualized coaching efforts by providing concrete means to illustrate and foster conceptual understanding of the rationale and opportunities for strategic skill application. Technology-assisted training allows for the modeling of skills and provision of corrective and timely feedback on skill application, as well as aids in the identification of individual vulnerabilities and key situational challenges (e.g., managing distractions) where skill use might be beneficial.

Beyond the initial acquisition of trained skills (including understanding the underlying rationale for skill use), one critical obstacle rehabilitation specialists face is helping persons with brain injury transfer skills to real-life situations where and when they are most needed. To be maximally effective, training must address common disruptions to frontal cognitive functioning, such as concrete thinking, reduced self-awareness, and goal neglect (Duncan et al., 1996; Robertson & Schmitter-Edgecombe, 2015; Ropacki, Rickards, Barrera, & Yutsis, 2014)—factors that undermine and impede training efforts. For instance, concrete thinking may prevent individuals with brain injury from seeing the parallels between training contexts, such as between game-based skills training and real life, resulting in missed opportunities for skill application. An individual with reduced self-awareness may also not notice or anticipate situations likely to result in dysregulated internal states in the moment, and consequently may not initiate strategic use of trained skills to appropriately resolve the situation. Further, a person who suffers from goal neglect may have limited recognition of going off-task and so not see the need for applying trained skills at these moments.

Well-designed game-based scenarios that align with learning goals may help bridge skill building to benefit patients outside the training context. Gaming scenarios can be designed to reflect common difficulties experienced by individuals with brain injury and to be clearly relevant to real-life concerns. They can be further utilized to practice and refine strategic application of trained skills with the direct assistance of trainer coaching, readying a person to take on real-life challenges. Practice in game-based scenarios may also increase the automaticity of skill use, so that skills will be applied with greater consistency and ease outside the training environment. Personal guidance can help with skill development, as well as directly address barriers to transfer through fostering goal orientation and helping trainees appreciate the broad range of life contexts where trained skills may be useful and relevant.

We have developed a series of interventions to promote improvements in goal-directed functioning (Chen et al., 2011; Loya et al., 2014; Novakovic-Agopian et al., 2011; Rodriguez et al., 2014). The training emphasizes learning state-regulation skills and the goal-directed application of the skills across multiple challenge contexts. To promote the strategic application of state-regulation skills, participants are trained in applying the SRR strategy to stop activity when distracted or overwhelmed, relax, and redeploy attentional resources for the task at hand. To facilitate the transfer of these skills to daily life, we developed scenarios that allow for greater intensity of skill practice across a wide range of challenging contexts. In designing the training experiences, we drew from real-life situations where the target brain functions are often challenged and developed underlying software architecture to allow adjustments of cognitive challenges to optimize learning. The scenarios were implemented in digital game format to increase access to well-designed and calibrated learning opportunities, while trainers provide intensive, individualized coaching that maximizes each patient's conceptual understanding of trained skills, strengthens skill use, and develops the ability to strategically apply the skills in situations outside the training environment. In sum, challenging experiences are integrated with coaching to provide intensive guided experiential learning.

## Summary of Training Approach

The general approach involves coaching integrated with extensive practice in strategic application of skills in digital game and real-life experiences (see Figure 12.1). Through game scenarios, trainees experience a range of contexts requiring attention regulation, working memory, and higher-order goal direction (e.g., coordinating multiple tasks), and this provides an important bridge to the effective application of skills in personal life. We use game technologies to present learners with a variety of specially designed challenges in a storyline arc, using a training protocol that bridges skill learning to application in personal life, especially for challenges in school or work. Without intensive bridging experiences, new skills may not be learned very well, and even if they are learned to a first level, they may not be used to effectively help in the moments when an individual needs the most help.

Digital games provide opportunities for experiential learning, with coaching reinforcing learning through observation and feedback in the moment, as well as through "after action review." Coaching also fosters generalization of trained skills by helping the trainee understand the why, when, where, and how of skill use, from the game world into personal life. Experiences in game environments help raise self-awareness for areas of cognitive strength and weakness by

**Guided Experiential Learning of Brain State Regulation to Improve Goal-directed Functioning**

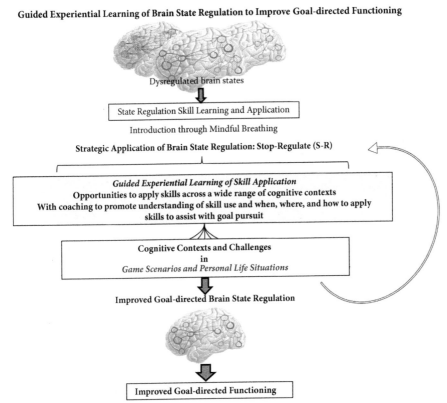

FIGURE 12.1 *Overview of training schema.*

providing direct experience of challenges to these abilities, with opportunities to assess and learn from missed opportunities and failures. Skill building with these tools helps to increase self-efficacy in applying skills across a range of situations.

The major part of training highlights opportunities to strategically apply regulation skills in both game and real-life contexts. In order to help the trainee strategically apply regulation skills in situations in which they are most needed (e.g., to achieve an optimal state for attending to important information and handling distractions, or when otherwise challenged and overwhelmed), the trainee is instructed in applying simple-to-remember metacognitive Stop-Regulate (SR) strategies to stop activity at key junctures (e.g., prior to starting a task, when distracted, when switching to a side task, or when overwhelmed) and to regulate state as appropriate for the current situation. We have previously found that SR strategies help patients regulate attentional state, particularly when distracted and/or overwhelmed (Chen et al., 2011; Novakovic-Agopian et al., 2011). A variety of extensions of the basic SR technique are taught and are applied to various game and real-life contexts where an individual needs the frontal lobe functions of goal direction.

In sum, in order for trainees to most effectively learn, apply, and transfer the new, adaptive target skill of goal-directed brain-state regulation, it is best to link together self-regulation skills (which requires learning through repeated practice, enriched or informed by a range of experiences and deepening understand through guidance) with a simple strategic self-regulatory action sequence (e.g., SRR, executable in the moment and in situations when most needed), training in self-cuing (with associations with markers that counteract goal-pursuit failures and otherwise support goal attainment) and implementation intentions (if/then plans that directly support self-cuing, triggering the strategic, executable self-regulatory behavior via SRR), and a framework of clear, accessible goals.

## Principles of the Design of Technology-Assisted Neurocognitive Skill Training

Our technology-assisted cognitive training systems support guided experiential learning of goal-directed self-regulatory skills via the integration of skill instruction, intensive skill practice across contexts ranging from game scenarios to real life, and direct coaching on skill implementation. Throughout training, a consistent emphasis is placed on promoting transfer of skills to the trainee's individual goals and everyday pursuits. To help achieve this objective, the trainer actively guides the trainee through a progression of steps important for skill learning and transfer (Burke & Hutchins, 2007; Gollwitzer & Sheeran, 2006; Toglia et al., 2010) to help promote an understanding of the rationale for utilizing skills to improve goal-directed functioning, to assist with the development and refinement of skill usage via active coaching and feedback on skill application, to identify and raise awareness of life situations where skills might be helpful, and to support the trainee's intentions to implement skills in daily life.

Our main approach to training strategic skill application is based upon our prior work on improving goal-directed functioning for persons with brain injury (Chen et al., 2011; Novakovic-Agopian et al., 2011). Pursuing and achieving goals is a complex process, dependent upon the regulation and coordination of a range of component cognitive processes. Relevant information must first be selectively attended to for more in-depth processing within working memory and then organized and maintained over time in order to guide behaviors to accomplish goals (Awh & Vogel, 2008; Baddeley, Chincotta, & Adlam, 2001; Chen et al., 2011). Protecting goal-relevant information along this pathway is of paramount importance, since goal attainment can be undermined by distractions and/or disruptions anywhere along the continuum of processes. Strengthening goal-directed self-regulatory skills is hypothesized to help the trainees direct and sustain attention toward goal-relevant information, selectively maintain this information over time, suppress irrelevant distractions, and redirect attention back toward goals if distracted. We designed game and training activities (see below) to provide the trainee with multiple and varied opportunities to practice the strategic application of self-regulatory skills.

At another level, training involves cultivating "goal-mindedness" to help address problems of goal neglect (Duncan et al., 1996; Manly & Murphy, 2012), which are common among persons with TBI. Goal-mindedness involves developing a "habit of mind" in which goals and goal-related representations (e.g., values, priorities, plans) directly influence behavior and provide cognitive and motivational ballast against distractions (Aarts, Custers, & Holland, 2007). Establishing and maintaining clear goals provides an organizing framework for regulating attention, enabling the trainee to compare and evaluate information and behaviors against a concrete standard. The process of regularly reviewing and updating goals is also intended to help strengthen mental representations of goals, making this information more accessible to working memory and less susceptible to attention capture by distractions (Mecklinger, von Cramon, Springer, & Matthes-von Cramon, 1999). Strengthening goals in working memory may increase the likelihood the trainee will be alert to goal-related opportunities, monitor the environment for goal relevance, and check for markers of goal progress during goal pursuit.

Two related approaches to training strategic application of goal-directed self-regulatory skills are highlighted throughout training. The greatest emphasis is on the strategic use of SR strategies during active goal pursuit and/ or when having difficulty focusing or feeling overwhelmed. The SR technique involves stopping activity, relaxing, and then refocusing on the present goal. Strategic application of the technique is practiced across varied contexts and is linked to the multiple levels of goal-directed functioning discussed above in order to effectively guide self-regulation when needed most. Use of SR strategies has been shown to help regulate attentional state and manage distractions (Chen et al., 2011; Novakovic-Agopian et al., 2011). As an initial pathway to strategic application of SR strategies, a more general self-regulation technique is also taught. The trainee is instructed in mindful breathing, which involves maintaining a relaxed focus on the act of breathing, noticing instances of mind wandering, and redirecting attention back to the breath when distracted. Regular practice in brief mindful breathing is associated with reduced autonomic arousal (Larson, Steffen, & Primosch, 2013) and greater efficiency in allocating cognitive resources involved in regulating attention (Moore, Gruber, Derose, & Malinowski, 2012; Tang et al., 2007). This basic practice is extended to more targeted and goal-directed SR use.

To help guide the strategic application of these skills and to increase the likelihood of their use during goal pursuit, training includes instruction in setting and clarifying goals, partitioning goals into subgoals, plans, and tasks, monitoring goal progress, and updating goals and plans as needed (Levine et al., 2000; Novakovic-Agopian et al., 2011). The trainer assists the trainee with identifying and anticipating key junctures along the pathway to achieving goals that are vulnerable to disruption, such as when switching between subgoals, and forming implementation intentions (Burke & Hutchins, 2007) to apply trained skills at these moments. Trainees are taught the if/then formulation: if [a difficulty at a key juncture arises], then apply SR strategies. Overall, training cultivates goal-mindedness, in which the trainee's internal state, behavior, and environment are considered in terms of important goals.

## Theory-Driven, Patient-Centered Intervention Development

Using the above background to inform intervention development, we have developed a series of interventions designed to train the goal-directed regulation of brain state.

First, we designed a protocol for training goal-oriented attentional self-regulation (GOALS) in a group-based intervention that takes into account the links connecting brain state and goal-based direction of behavior required for complex, real-life goals (Duncan, Burgess, & Emslie, 1995; Duncan et al., 1996; Novakovic-Agopian et al., 2011; Novakovic-Agopian et al., 2010). The experimental training protocol was based on interventions applied to patients with brain injury as well as other populations (D'Zurilla & Goldfried, 1971; Levine et al., 2000, 2007; Nezu, Nezu, & D'Zurilla, 2007; Rath, Simon, Langenbahn, Sherr, & Diller, 2003; Mai, 1991), with a special emphasis on the strategic application of attention-regulation skills to everyday situations and complex, project-based functional tasks. At a broad level, GOALS training emphasizes two key components: applied mindfulness-based state-regulation training, and goal-management strategies applied to participant-defined goals. In order to trigger state regulation, participants are trained in applying the SRR strategy to stop activity when distracted or overwhelmed, to relax, and to redeploy attentional resources for the task at hand. Trainees practice skills in daily life and in application to self-generated complex goals. In an initial study, sixteen individuals with acquired brain injury and chronic executive dysfunction (primarily non-veterans) completed training or a brief education intervention (Novakovic-Agopian et al., 2011). Goals participants showed improvements on neuropsychological measures of complex attention and executive functions, as well as on a functional measure approximating real-life goal pursuit. We have been applying this intervention in a study of veterans with TBI, and preliminary data thus far show effects consistent with the previous study. The main ingredients in this intervention have formed the basis for further intervention development to increase the intensity and range of application of goal-directed state-regulation skills.

## AUGMENTING TRAINING WITH TECHNOLOGY-ASSISTED LEARNING EXPERIENCES (THE NEURAL PATHFINDER SERIES)

In order to augment core aspects of training in goal-directed state regulation, we developed a series of digital game training scenarios to increase the intensity and range of skill application experience. The project nickname "Pathfinder" refers to the importance of the targeted brain functions in helping an individual find (and stay on) the best path to goal achievement. In one storyline in our Neural Pathfinder Project, "Apprentice," trainees work their way up as an employee in a company. In a follow-up training system, "Startup-to-CEO," the game-world storyline revolves around the trainee's establishing an exciting new food truck business—a step toward independence that challenges frontal brain functions. With the digital games, trainees use a first-person perspective and interact with scenarios via touch screen or PC interface to accomplish varying goal-based activities in a range of different cognitive contexts. Training is designed to help patients stengthen goal-directed state-regulation skills to become adept at applying the skills across multiple contexts, from the game world to personal life. Game-world and real-world experiences provide learning opportunities, supported by intensive coaching to maximize conceptual understanding, acquisition of skills, strengthening of skill application, and transfer of skill use to settings outside of training. The game experiences were thus integrated with a full training protocol to provide intensive guided experiential learning.

## Working Your Way Up as an Apprentice in Cognitive Rehabilitation

In the design and development process for a training system that integrates game scenarios into guided experiential learning of goal-directed state regulation, it was important to incorporate principles important for skill learning, transfer, application of skills, and generalization of benefits.

We designed learning opportunities in the form of scenarios. We set out to design game experiences drawn from real-life situations, with explicit features to support training goals while addressing the needs of individuals with brain injury and cognitive deficits. We designed an underlying architecture to the game experiences that engages cognitive processes important for goal-directed task completion—focusing on the ability to attend to, hold in mind, and process information, particularly in the presence of distractions. We specifically sought to strengthen state-regulation skills and to promote broad application of these skills across multiple contexts, taking advantage of game scenarios for providing extensive exposure to tasks that require selective attention and working memory.

In designing the game experiences, we incorporated the following principles in order to connect game-design features with training goals (Chen & Novakovic-Agopian, 2012; D'Esposito & Chen, 2006): experiences in multiple contexts for training, in the form of a range of scenarios as well as a range of cognitive demands within each scenario, where the cognitive experiences included (a) experiences working on naturalistic tasks with a range of working memory demands, requiring efforts to attend to, hold in mind, and process information and then translate this information into action plans and actual task execution, and (b) experiences with naturalistic distractor challenges, pulling attention away from the central task, with a range of different distractors; progression of experiences with the above tasks and distractors within simpler to more complex contexts, carried along a storyline; recognizable phases of goal-directed cognition embedded within naturalistic sequences, including encoding, planning, execution, and switching, to support teachable moments for coaching; and game experiences that are analogous to real-world situations, to facilitate coaching the relevance of trained skills to real-life contexts. Ideas for the scenarios, tasks, and distractors were translated from common experiences of patients with brain injury, with game design allowing for parameterization, calibration, and control of the training experiences. In addition, a first-person perspective was chosen in order to enhance likelihood of transfer. Overall, the game scenarios were designed to be integrated into the training system as opportunities for guided experiential learning.

The patient-centered approach continued from design into the iterative development process. The primary target audience for patient-centered development was individuals with a history of brain injury, with an emphasis on veterans of military service. Extensive patient-oriented feedback was obtained throughout the development process (with over 90 user/testers, primarily veterans and other individuals with brain injury.)

In brief, the development process included the following steps: games were designed based on common difficulties in personal life reported by patients; prototypes were developed and user tested by patients; the user interface, mechanics, and central task activities and instructions were user tested by patients; information-processing loads were parameterized for each game scenario and user tested; the distractor elements were categorized into distractions (sensory events not relevant to, but potentially distracting from, main task goals) and disruptions (events requiring the player to redirect attention, make decisions, and fulfill tasks separate from the main task goals), and player experience of distractors was tested by patients; and training protocol elements to guide coaching were reviewed by clinicians and tried by patients to collect feedback, then revised for clarity and optimal integration of game experiences into the protocol. In later stages of the design and development process, we tested components of the training experience, including querying users' understanding of attention-regulation skills and how these skills could usefully be applied to game tasks and in their personal lives.

The end result of this patient-oriented development process was a training system that integrates game experiences with trainer-guided coaching to improve goal-directed cognitive functioning. There were four game-world scenarios that allow for over 30 different cognitive contexts with different cognitive demands, all with parameterized challenges for attention regulation and information processing. Game scenarios were designed for deployment via PC and touch screen devices.

## GAME SCENARIOS

Each scenario includes a main task that requires some form of working memory, from simple (requiring just maintenance) to complex or executive (requiring manipulation of information, such re-ordering, sequencing, switching, and/or prioritizing; see Figure 12.2). Each task requires information to be held or processed via working memory in order to guide an action or series of actions. Task-relevant information may be presented in auditory or visual modalities. In sum, a range of cognitive contexts for the practice of attention-regulation skills is provided by a range of game scenarios and differing levels of working memory load. Engagement of working memory forms a base during which play may require management of distractions or disruptions to the goal-directed main task.

In the game-world storyline, the trainee/player is offered a job and progresses through increasingly demanding job assignments (in different environments or scenarios), to work up a corporate ladder at "Pathfinder, Inc." Each scenario provides cognitive contexts in which tasks central to the main job engage goal-directed control processes. Each scenario is designed to engage slightly different cognitive processes in the central tasks. Manipulations of particular task parameters alter the engagement and challenge of working memory processes within simpler to more complex task contexts. Working memory load is adjusted upward based on task performance. The game contexts provide a varied and progressive range of situations where skills and strategies for goal-directed attention regulation may be applied and practiced when distractors occur.

## DISTRACTIONS AND DISRUPTIONS

An important aspect of all the scenarios is the inclusion of distractors designed to challenge trainees' abilities to regulate attention and maintain goal-centered activity. Distractors were designed and implemented for each game scenario, as discrete game elements superimposed on the central tasks (see Figure 12.2, right). Distractions were categorized based on qualitatively different characteristics as types D1 to D3, and disruptions were categorized into types D4 to D6. Disruptions were designed to challenge attention regulation to varying degrees, because the player needs to direct attention to the disruptive task and redirect attention back to accomplish the main task. The highest level of disruption requires the player

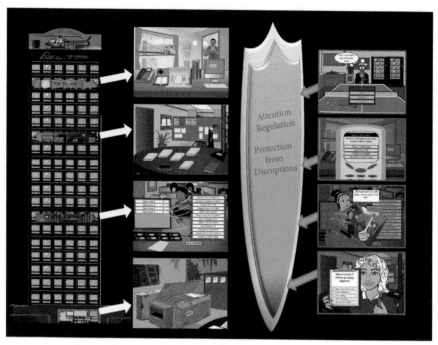

FIGURE 12.2 *Apprentice game scenarios. In the storyline arc, the player is hired at the bottom rung of a large corporation and works his/her way up through four scenarios to a high-level position (from bottom to top alongside the office building: "Copy Technician," "Binder Design Specialist," "Call Center Specialist," and "Top Floor Executive Assistant.") Each game scenario provides opportunities to practice attention regulation as different distractions and disruptions occur in the various job contexts (examples from bottom to top on the right: directing a delivery to the correct location in the company while in the middle of designing binders, helping to find something from a bin for an employee while routing calls, responding to a cell phone call while performing executive tasks in the top floor office, and being challenged to a game of table tennis during the work day).*

to leave the main game action and spend a period of time engaged in a side task on another screen before returning to the primary task.

### TRAINING PROTOCOL

The games were integrated into a training protocol composed of six supervised training sessions spanning 5 to 6 weeks, with home practice between sessions. Training sessions lasted between 1 and 2 hours, and included structured questioning during and after sessions, as well as trainer observation of game play. During game play, trainees were presented with many opportunities to apply strategies taught in the training session. The opportunities allowed trainers to observe trainees play the game, conduct behavioral analysis of play, and provide modeling of how to apply strategies within the game.

The main themes, introduced in the early sessions and extended across training sessions, include increasing awareness and understanding of key cognitive processes and states that affect goal attainment, an explicit goal-based approach to ground use of skills and strategies within the wider context of achieving goals, the importance of cultivating a state of "relaxed readiness" for optimal goal-directed attention regulation, and consideration of a range of contexts in which skills can be applied.

Specific skills taught in the supervised sessions included mindful breathing as a way to enter a relaxed and ready state, with exercises prior to each game round and in personal life. Trainees are then taught to use the SRR technique to help trigger this state of relaxed readiness in the moment in a range of challenging situations in game play and in real life. SRR was taught as a generalizable prompt to engage state regulation, especially in situations where information needs to be learned, attention needs to be shifted, and distractions and disruptions challenge goal-directed activity. Variations on SR are practiced for a range of contexts.

The combinations of different scenarios, central tasks, working memory loads and distractor events provide a varied and progressive range of cognitive contexts in which skills of goal-directed self-regulation may be applied and practiced. Game activities are designed to be naturalistic but include identifiable task junctions that are good potential opportunities for practicing strategies and engaging target state-regulation skills.

The junctions occur at key points in tasks where the individual is especially vulnerable to insufficiencies in cognitive processes that can undermine goal achievement, such as insufficient encoding of task information, forgetting what needs to be done, becoming distracted, or feeling overwhelmed. When applied at these key junctures, the skills and strategies serve to reinstate a regulated state that strengthens the ability to stay on track to goal completion. Such junctures include right before starting a new task, when important task-related information is being presented, switching back and forth among tasks, and when task progression is disrupted.

Trainees are taught specific strategies, the principles underlying strategy use, and the contexts in which the strategies may be especially useful. For example, in the Top Floor game scenario (see Figure 12.3), trainees are taught to use SRR before the boss appears to give instructions, the principle being to optimize one's attentional state—to be relaxed and ready—for an upcoming task. Then, as the boss is making task requests, trainees are taught to maintain a relaxed focus to encode and then lock-in task information, increasing the likelihood the information will be accessible during task execution. The boss's requests often involve performance of multiple tasks, and trainees are taught to use SR prior to switching to the next task, thus regulating their attentional state and refreshing working memory for goal-relevant information. At unpredictable intervals the trainee may have to address a disruptive side task before returning to the main action. Trainees are taught to briefly use SR and to lock-in the main task

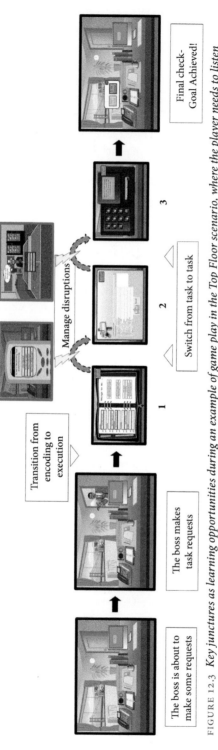

FIGURE 12.3 *Key junctures as learning opportunities during an example of game play in the Top Floor scenario, where the player needs to listen to requests from the boss, encode this information, plan an action sequence, and execute the actual tasks, while subject to possible distractions or disruptions.*

The boss is about to make some requests

The boss makes task requests

Transition from encoding to execution

Manage disruptions

1

Switch from task to task

2

3

Final check-Goal Achieved!

before redirecting attention to the disruption. The underlying principle here is to regulate attentional state (SR) and to reinforce representations of the main task (lock-in) before redirecting attention to a disruptive event, the better to re-access goal-related information when returning to the main task. Following the disruption, trainees then have an opportunity to practice redirecting attention and retrieving information needed to complete the main tasks.

The learning opportunity junctions may not be easily or immediately identified by game players in the naturalistic experience of play. The nature and importance of the junctions is highlighted in after-play coaching, and opportunities for strategy application at the junctions are a major emphasis of coaching. Actual strategy application is observed and queried, as well as modeled during coaching. We train individuals to form situation/response associations that trigger regulatory processes, with an emphasis on learning common situations associated with executive dysfunction: (a) internal states (such as feeling distracted or overwhelmed) and (b) recurrent external challenges (key everyday situations that tend to challenge cognitive processes, such as when one is given important task-related information, starting a new task, disruption, and/or task switching). The coaching then turns to helping trainees understand and delineate analogous situations in personal life—junctions at which use of the trained skills and strategies could be useful.

In the final stage of testing, participants included eight individuals with history of brain injury (> 6 months postinjury) and chronic cognitive deficits. All had symptoms related to difficulties with attention, memory, multitasking, and/or organization, but with differing levels of functioning, from mild dysfunction (e.g., able to work or attend school but at a lower level than baseline) to more severe (e.g., disorganized, distractible, unemployable, with poor engagement in rehabilitation therapies). We addressed a series of questions pertinent to the objectives of training—that is, to what extent did the training system support progress toward transfer and generalization of trained skills to personal life?

## TO WHAT EXTENT WERE INDIVIDUALS WITH BRAIN INJURY ABLE TO LEARN BASIC GAME PLAY?

Participants were able to learn basic game play (mechanics and rules) for each of the games with no significant difficulties despite the relative complexity of the game scenarios, personal cognitive deficits, and varying levels of familiarity with computer use and digital games. With effective learning of basic game play, additional training could proceed.

## TO WHAT EXTENT DID PARTICIPANTS DEMONSTRATE UNDERSTANDING OF TARGET COGNITIVE PROCESSES?

During supervised sessions, trainers asked participants to explain concepts and skills taught during the supervised sessions. All eight participants were able to correctly answer direct questions relating to the concepts of attention, working memory, and goal maintenance by the end of the second training session. Game play helped to illustrate the concepts and contributed to the experiential understanding of the importance of these functions during performance of tasks, as well as an understanding of factors that challenge these functions. Participants were also able to verbally explain the basics of skills and strategies taught (e.g., mindful breathing, SRR) by the end of the second training session. Participants were not necessarily able to fully explain how and when the skills would best be applied.

### TO WHAT EXTENT DID PARTICIPANTS DEMONSTRATE USE OF THE TRAINED SKILLS DURING GAME PLAY?

Trainers directly observed and queried to what extent participants were able to recognize in-game opportunities for application of the skills. Ability to recognize situations where skill application could be useful did not occur immediately, and benefited from after-play queries and reviews. Overall, recognition solidified by the time of the third training session as participants learned through the combination of experience and coaching the nature of the cognitive challenges and opportunities. There was another gap between this level of understanding and the accomplishment of actual self-initiated strategy application during the opportunities. Initially, significant cuing was required. There was particular variability across individuals, with individuals with more severe dysfunction requiring more cuing. Overall, self-initiated strategy application tended to increase from the third session onward. In particular, participants began to utilize the SRR strategy when switching between tasks and when managing the disruptive effects of the distractors. Overall, participants were able to verbalize when and where to appropriately apply training strategies, without trainer prompting, by the fourth week of training.

### TO WHAT EXTENT DID PARTICIPANTS FIND THE DISTRACTORS DISRUPTIVE?

Although some participants found the distractions (distractor types D1 to D3) to be disruptive, many participants found that sensory distractions were easy to ignore (i.e., did not significantly detract from attention to the main tasks) after relatively little practice experience. All participants found the disruptions (distractor types D4 to D6) to be disruptive of the main task, and, with assistance from coaching, participants were able to recognize that these were opportunities for application of attention-regulation skills. Participants reported that application of the SRR strategy was helpful in managing the disruptions (i.e., being able to switch to addressing the disruption and redirect back to the main task).

## WERE TRAINEES ABLE TO PROSPECTIVELY GENERATE REAL-LIFE SITUATIONS WHERE SKILLS AND STRATEGIES COULD BE APPLIED?

It was observed that participants required significant coaching to generate ideas regarding specific situations in their personal lives that might benefit from improved attention regulation. By the final session, participants were able to identify situations in their own lives where application of skills taught in-game could be beneficial. For example, one patient stated that applying SRR while shopping at the grocery store (with tasks that used to overwhelm him) would help him remain calm and focused. Another participant identified other potentially stressful situations where training strategies could be applied, including when driving, when meeting new people, and when coming up with a plan and prioritizing. Still another patient expressed motivation to use mindful breathing, SRR, and goal setting/planning skills in his daily bicycle rides, including preparing for and planning the ride as well as monitoring his surroundings and using SRR to remain attentive while on his bicycle. General ideas benefited from coaching to identify more specific junctions clear enough for cuing strategy application.

## DID TRAINEES REPORT APPLYING SKILLS AND STRATEGIES TO REAL-LIFE SITUATIONS?

Participants reported applying training strategies during real-life situations by the final session to varying degrees. For example, participant 3 reported using SRR in daily life, such as when developing marketing ideas, communicating with someone, switching from one task to another, and when transitioning from home to work. Participant 4 reported that he used SRR when he needed to transition from a project he was working on to address something for his child, and then return to his project. Participant 5 stated that he was surprised to find that he was multitasking successfully again, managing multiple contractor appointments in the same day even when they overlapped. Participant 6 described using SRR to help switch between working on a project and helping customers as they called for his attention. He also reported that by applying the trained skills, he managed to be efficient and productive on a day when his workplace was understaffed, when he would typically feel overwhelmed.

In addition, some participants described use of the trained skills in emotionally overwhelming situations in personal life. For example, Participant 2 reported applying a version of SRR when talking to an upset friend. Participant 6 reported using SRR during a heated confrontation with his manager, so that he was able re-approach the situation, consider his goal, and think about how best it could be accomplished.

## TO WHAT EXTENT DID EACH PARTICIPANT PERCEIVE
## CHANGES IN PERSONAL GOAL-RELATED FUNCTIONING?

Participants rated self-perceived change in various areas related to aspects of goal processing. Four questions related to areas directly addressed in training—aspects of attention, working memory, and task execution. Although the responses need to be interpreted at the individual level for each case, the following summary was observed. Seven respondents reported perception of positive change in response to two items: "Your ability to stop and relax during stressful times" and "Your ability to get back on track if you are distracted from a task." In response to the other two items, six participants reported positive change and one participant reported no change for each area of functioning. These items were: "Your ability to hold important information in mind in a distracting environment (e.g., a noisy place)" and "Your ability to ignore sounds, noise, or other things going on around you, while working on a task."

### THE APPRENTICE PROJECT

The pilot experiences support the feasibility of game integration into training and provide preliminary qualitative and anecdotal data that suggest that elements of such training may promote transfer and generalization. Over the course of training experiences, patients demonstrated increased understanding of the target cognitive skills, as well as why/how/when/where to strategically apply these skills. They also demonstrated appropriately applying strategies during game challenges, were able to identify analogous real-life situations, and reported utilizing attention-regulation skills in real-life situations.

It was only with further experiences in combination with coaching that individuals reported significant and helpful application in personal life. Overall, the pilot experiences support the contention that integrating games with rehabilitation may help patients to develop a conceptual understanding of different strategies and their rationale, as well as promote self-knowledge and self-awareness, to facilitate application of skills across contexts, including in personal life. The trainers' experiences from this project highlighted that game scenarios may be especially useful in allowing trainers to observe how individuals handle particular situations.

The qualitative data suggest that game scenarios may be useful as a form of experiential learning in the training of applied self-regulation skills. One of the major limitations in the learning of self-regulation skills for patients with brain injury is the limited application of these skills across contexts, such as in the midst of a stressful circumstance. The pilot project suggests that increased learning experiences made possible by game play may help establish the use of these skills, providing a stepping stone to support transfer of use into other life contexts.

Some observations were pertinent to the design of game elements for training the management of disruptions of attention. Distractions of the more typical form (sensory distractions, such as sounds or voices) could be disruptive (i.e., redirect attention) for some individuals, but were generally relatively easy to ignore after a small amount of training. The disruptions we developed, which required explicit redirection of attention in order to accomplish a secondary task, were clearly more disruptive and were reported to be more useful motivators for the use of trained skills and strategies. This feedback may help inform efforts at designing game elements to enhance training. In any case, different individuals experienced different levels of disruption from the various distractor elements, and parameterization of distractor elements in game design may be a useful approach for tailoring training to different individuals.

In sum, this project highlights potential contributions of a game-assisted approach for guided experiential learning of state regulation, with potential benefits for enhancing transfer and generalization to personal life. This illustrates how the careful design of games as an integrated part of a training system can address factors important for learning, behavioral change, transfer, and generalization. The training system illustrated was developed as a potential segment in a longitudinal training program, so that the initial apprenticeship could be followed by additional training in more complex game-world contexts as well as with real-world projects. Although the effects of training using this focused package would be expected to be limited relative to a more extensive or multifaceted training intervention, we argue that it is worthwhile to determine the potential contribution of each component alone before determining the optimal combination of components into a longer or more complex training system.

## Moving from Start-up to CEO

We developed an additional training system, the Start-up-to-CEO game (CEO for short), with a new set of scenarios to expand the range of experiences. The same fundamental themes in training introduced above were extended into CEO, with additional opportunities for intensive skill practice. The primary objective of training was to maximize the effective use of self-regulation skills when and where they are needed most—especially in the context of challenges.

### GAME DESIGN TO FACILITATE STRATEGIC SKILL APPLICATION

CEO was designed to provide the trainee with a range of calibrated cognitive tasks that engage and challenge goal-directed functioning. The scenarios require the integration of higher-order cognitive abilities commonly affected by TBI, including working memory, prospective memory, planning, and organization. The scenarios provide contexts for opportunities to practice strategic skill application. Game scenarios provide concrete examples to anchor teaching of abstract training concepts as well as opportunities for modeling, practicing, and refining their application. They were also designed to help facilitate discussions on how skills might be applied in analogous situations or junctures in the trainee's personal life.

At the level of story narrative, the central premise of CEO is the establishment of a food truck business, with the core game task involving fulfilling multiple customers' orders following a brief on-screen presentation. Order complexity and information load are continually adjusted based upon performance to promote engagement and to ensure play occurs at the upper bounds of the trainee's working memory capacity. The menu also expands as play progresses to include items requiring multistep assembly and cooking time, providing opportunities for planning (sequencing orders within and across customers) and optimizing efficiency. Over the course of training, CEO gameplay increases in complexity to include the simultaneous management of multiple scenarios requiring increased planning and monitoring efforts. Specifically, the trainee's responsibilities expand to include managing an urban farm, where select menu items are grown and harvested, and assembling and baking pies to be sold in the food truck. The additional sequences require trainees to continuously monitor their food supply, plan accordingly, and coordinate tasks across multiple contexts in order to meet customers' changing demands. (Figure 12.4 illustrates these contexts and their interrelationships.)

One facet of gameplay involves the trainee's establishing a superordinate goal, providing the trainee opportunities to practice prioritizing and making goal-based decisions. Certain customers are eligible for item upgrades via special ingredients concealed from view. In order to run the business in the most goal-oriented manner, the trainee needs to proactively alter previous, basic default actions to take advantage of the goal-congruent opportunities. Since default behaviors might be utilized more frequently when the trainee is anxious, flustered, or stressed, training involves coaching on establishing a goal-minded approach through the application of SR strategies. This game feature also allows for tracking of goal-congruent behaviors during training, providing data that can be utilized to help guide learning.

## COACHING OPPORTUNITIES IN CEO

CEO provides numerous opportunities for coaching the application of self-regulation skills to improve functioning (see Figure 12.5). On one level, game scenarios are utilized to highlight contexts where goal-directed functioning is susceptible to disruption and where skill use might be helpful. At another level, game-based experiences are used to facilitate discussions about skill application

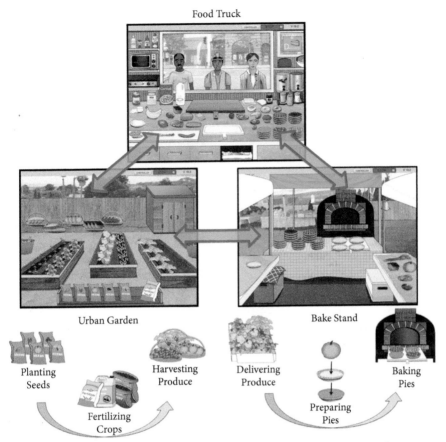

FIGURE 12.4 *Game world scenarios. The top panel shows the initial scenario of managing a food truck, with the primary goal of accurately fulfilling customers' orders. The bottom right panel depicts the second scenario, in which the trainee prepares pies at a bake stand to supply the food truck. The bottom left panel illustrates the third scenario, requiring the trainee to tend an urban garden and grow a supply of produce to be used later in preparing pies. Action sequences involved with the bake stand and urban garden contexts are displayed underneath each of their respective panels. The coordinated management of the contexts requires the trainee to organize and execute multiple steps across varied scenarios.*

in trainees' personal lives. Throughout this process, trainees are coached on considering their current state or situation in the context of their goals to guide strategic skill application, a practice which is reflected in CEO's increasingly complex goal hierarchy.

To encourage SRR application during game challenges, use of a "Stop" button is cued during initial phases of training. The trainee is instructed to utilize this Stop whenever applying self-regulation skills during gameplay, which provides a source of feedback to guide learning. Gameplay data are reviewed during sessions

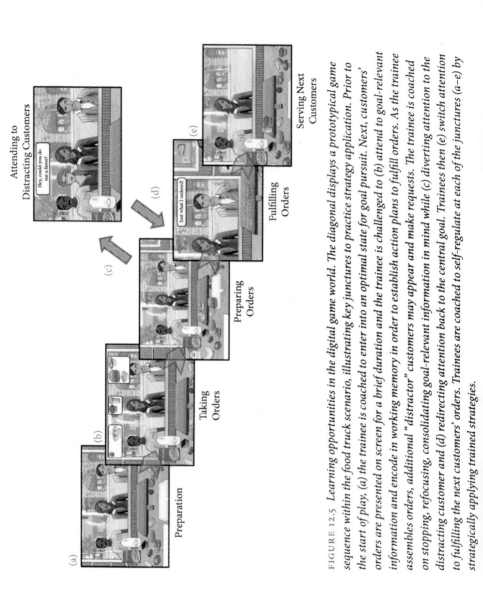

FIGURE 12.5 Learning opportunities in the digital game world. The diagonal displays a prototypical game sequence within the food truck scenario, illustrating key junctures to practice strategy application. Prior to the start of play, (a) the trainee is coached to enter into an optimal state for goal pursuit. Next, customers' orders are presented on screen for a brief duration and the trainee is challenged to (b) attend to goal-relevant information and encode in working memory in order to establish action plans to fulfill orders. As the trainee assembles orders, additional "distractor" customers may appear and make requests. The trainee is coached on stopping, refocusing, consolidating goal-relevant information in mind while (c) diverting attention to the distracting customer and (d) redirecting attention back to the central goal. Trainees then (e) switch attention to fulfilling the next customers' orders. Trainees are coached to self-regulate at each of the junctures (a–e) by strategically applying trained strategies.

to increase the trainee's awareness of vulnerabilities and to reinforce skill application. Overall, this allows the trainee to experiment with skill use to better learn where and why self-regulation skills can be applied to improve functioning.

## ONGOING STUDIES OF GUIDED EXPERIENTIAL LEARNING WITH CEO

We have been performing studies to evaluate the potential effects of training using the CEO technology-assisted training protocol. Training has been administered in one-to-one in-person sessions and via televideo, as well as in a for-credit course offered to students (at the University of California, Berkeley) with and without history of brain injury (Only data from participants with history of TBI is included in the discussion that follows). In all studies, training followed a fully manualized protocol spanning seven training sessions and approximately 30 minutes of daily game practice as well as application to personally defined goals in daily life. Participants in both in-person and televideo training also received twice weekly semistructured phone check-ins to review and clarify training materials, discuss skill application within the context of at-home gameplay and in personal life, provide motivational support, and resolve any technical issues that occurred. Student participants received analogous check-ins via email reminders and in-person consultation in the form of office hours.

All participants had a history of chronic TBI (> 6 months), confirmed via review of medical records as well as clinical interview. Participants also self-reported cognitive complaints that interfered with daily functioning. Below we highlight a range of quantitative and qualitative data with respect to the impact of training for multiple metrics, including changes to objective indices of cognitive performance and self-perceived functioning as well as experiences with the training system. The data represent a synthesis of multiple projects, with both common and unique measurements. Additional data are mentioned separately as pertinent to tele-rehabilitation and college-integrated training.

## TRAINING EXPERIENCE

Across studies, participants endorsed the value of practicing the strategic application of trained self-regulatory skills during game-based scenarios and in the context of personally defined goals. Regular feedback within the game as well in coaching sessions appeared helpful for highlighting the relevance of skills and reinforcing their use during gameplay and in daily life. Direct in-game feedback as well as weekly review of at-home game practice enabled the participants to see the direct benefits of skill application on a range of game metrics, including increased accuracy with fulfilling customers' orders, increased working memory capacity (as reflected in increased order complexity and items served), an improved ability to manage distractions, and taking greater advantage of goal-congruent opportunities.

Feedback further provided opportunities for participants to experiment with skill application at various task junctures, which occurred through comparing performance during instances in which skills were and were not applied. As one illustrative example, several participants were initially skeptical of applying self-regulatory strategies early during gameplay because it slowed down the rate of their play. Rather, they insisted that fulfilling orders as quickly as possible would result in a superior performance. Comparing improved performance on trials in which trained vs. trained strategies were utilized helped reinforce the relevance and potential benefit of skill use.

In addition, review of weekly questionnaires completed by participants enrolled in both individualized forms of training (in-person and televideo) indicated that participants' comprehension of key training concepts and the rationale for skill use, as well as their ability to identify and anticipate situations in which skill use was potentially beneficial, improved over the course of training. Further, participants reported increased application of trained strategies during gameplay and in personal life over the course of training. Success with applying strategies appeared to contribute to skill mastery and improve participants' sense of self-efficacy regarding cognitive challenges.

## CHANGES TO COGNITIVE PERFORMANCE

Participants in all pilot studies underwent pre–post neuropsychological testing to assess the impact of training on nontrained cognitive tasks. We selected a test battery consisting of well-validated neuropsychological tests routinely administered in clinical settings. Selection of tests included domains hypothesized to be directly affected by training (working memory/executive functions) as well as others commonly affected by brain injury but not the specific focus of training (processing speed/learning and memory).

Preliminary analyses have documented pre–post intervention improvements for 21 participants on composite scores of complex attention and working memory (standardized effect size $d = +0.67$), verbal learning and memory ($d = +0.84$), and processing speed ($d = +0.39$). In addition, participants undergoing classroom-based training were assessed with computerized psychometric tasks and showed improvements on computerized neuroscience-based measures of sustained attention ($d = +1.64$) and working memory span (i.e., holding information in mind in the context of distractions; $d = +1.62$).

## SELF-REPORTED BENEFITS OF TRAINING

Overall, participants reported to have benefited from training and to have experienced improvements in a range of cognitive abilities. Participants provided Likert-scale ratings (0 = much worse function, 5 = no change, 10 = much better) with respect to self-perceived changes to their cognitive functioning following training across nine distinct cognitive domains. Participants reported improvements in their abilities to plan (*Mdn* [median] rating = 7.1), initiate tasks (*Mdn* = 6.5), attend to and manipulate information in working memory (*Mdn* = 7.2), problem solve (*Mdn* = 6.9), self-monitor behaviors (*Mdn* = 6.6), learn from past experiences (*Mdn* = 6.8), sequence task (*Mdn* = 6.5), execute tasks (*Mdn* = 6.8), and accurately estimate how well they will perform on a task prior to starting it (*Mdn* = 7.0).

The self-perceived changes are consistent with participants' reports of how training positively affected their daily lives. All participants enrolled in individualized forms of training (i.e., in-person and via televideo) reported they used and benefited from applying self-regulatory strategies in their personal life by the end of training. Instances in which strategy use was noted to be helpful included starting a new activity (*n* = 3), switching between tasks or subcomponents within tasks (*n* = 3), when feeling stressed and/or overwhelmed (*n* = 8), and when distracted (*n* = 6).

Examples of strategy use in personal life included helping to manage symptoms of posttraumatic stress (such as feeling overwhelmed in public places), to concentrate at work in the context of multiple distractions, to remain calm in order to formulate plans for dealing with a car accident, to stay focused when navigating a spousal separation, and to manage teaching responsibilities. For students who participated in classroom-based training, 34 of 39 reported using strategies to redirect attention when distracted from their coursework.

Taken together, the preliminary data suggest that participants responded favorably to participation in technology-assisted guided experiential training, preliminarily showing improvements on nontrained tasks, and applied skills in daily life, resulting in enhanced functioning. Overall, the training system shows promise for brain injury rehabilitation by providing an important bridge between skills training and strategic application during everyday goal pursuit.

## Implications of Guided Experiential Learning

As games are increasingly applied to rehabilitation settings, it is particularly important in the research and development process to consider factors that support transfer of learning. Significant barriers to transfer are especially prominent with cognitive deficits associated with brain injury (D'Esposito & Gazzaley, 2006; D'Esposito & Chen, 2006; Landa-Gonzalez, 2001; Park & Ingles, 2001; Toglia, 1991; Ylvisaker, Turkstra, & Coelho, 2005). The project described here provides an initial illustration of how game elements may be integrated into training design to support the connections between skill learning and transfer of trained skills to personal life for individuals with brain injury. Games may be utilized not only for practice of tasks, but also for supporting a patient in achieving certain stepping stones likely to be important for transfer of trained skills to personally relevant goals. We argue for a particular use of digital game scenarios in rehabilitation, where the games are developed to provide opportunities for guided experiential learning, with experiences aligned to directly support the learning goals of coaching.

An integrated training system—composed of game scenarios and personal guidance—can provide intense practice to strengthen strategic use of state-regulation skills, as well as provide an experiential basis for enhancing conceptual understanding and self-awareness via coaching to promote broad applicability of skills and strategies to personally relevant contexts. The trainee can learn to apply these skills across multiple contexts both in the game and in personal life. This contributes to the generalizability of skill use, so that individuals with brain injury are better equipped to effectively regulate their internal state in almost any situation.

And then, very importantly, we wanted the trainees to have experience applying their skills across different working memory loads. Different memory loads result in different task conditions, which we designed to be adjustable to individual capacity and performance. As working memory load increased, to include high working memory loads where trainees might be overwhelmed, they then could apply state-regulation skills to learn to better manage task demands in the presence of high or even overwhelming working memory load.

The use of working memory goes beyond simple information maintenance, and involves the manipulation and sequencing of information to form action plans, and then to maintain and update that information across tasks. A unique feature of our design was the addition of distractions and disruptions to the context of working memory demands, to help trainees develop the ability to manage disruptive challenges to working memory while engaged in goal-directed tasks.

Games integrated into training may enhance understanding and awareness of a range of contexts where cognitive abilities are challenged and where trained skills could be helpful. Game scenarios can provide experiential illustrations of otherwise difficult to understand concepts (e.g., state regulation, working memory, and other aspects of goal-directed cognitive functioning), and provide contexts to support the application and practice of useful skills for improving functioning. It may be especially valuable to emphasize repeated application of useful skills across situations, with training cues that are common across multiple contexts and how to explicitly draw connections to real-life contexts. In the setting of these rehabilitation goals, it is valuable for patient-oriented game design to take into consideration the types of real-life situations that are particularly challenging for patients, extract the core challenges of these situations, and design these challenges into the game world as learning opportunities. This approach stands in contrast to the design of training games based on simplified cognitive tasks isolated from important life contexts.

# Reaching Farther: Technology in Support of Service Delivery in Neurocognitive Rehabilitation

## A TECHNOLOGY-BASED COGNITIVE TRAINING SYSTEM TO MEET INDIVIDUAL NEEDS

An additional advantage of the technology-based cognitive training systems discussed here is the versatility in application, both to address the needs of different clinical populations as well as to address different service delivery needs in different training settings. Training has been successfully implemented for veterans with TBI-PTS and other comorbidities, for veterans and non-veterans with other forms of brain injury, as well as for college students. In addition, versions of training have been offered as individual face-to-face training sessions, via televideo, and in small groups as part of a for-credit college course. The integration of technology into training helps extend the trainer's interactive reach and provides valuable opportunities for individualized guidance and feedback on skill application.

### TELE-REHABILITATION

Many individuals with brain injury lack access to intensive cognitive training. For them, cognitive rehabilitation services are simply nonexistent in the areas where they live, or issues such as significant travel time, cost, or limited mobility make accessing rehabilitation impractical. In addition to logistical considerations, remote rehabilitation is limited by a lack of effective approaches and tools to train cognitive skills (as opposed to providing assistance with compensatory methods, such as external aids). While tele-rehabilitation has the potential to address many of these obstacles and provide intensive cognitive training, remote interactions are limited without the development of training tools and approaches that support skill learning and transfer.

Unfortunately, much of the research on the use of televideo technologies to address cognitive difficulties for individuals with brain injury has focused on diagnosis and assessment rather than on the provision of tele-rehabilitation (Girard, 2007; Hailey, Roine, Ohinmaa, & Dennett, 2013). In one recent review of tele-rehabilitation for neurological conditions, Hailey and colleagues (Hailey et al., 2013) cited just three controlled studies, of which only one study (Fish et al., 2007) actually featured training to develop cognitive skills. Thus, little clinical guidance is available to inform remote cognitive training efforts. In particular, little work has been done to address limitations of tele-rehab for skill learning and transfer. For instance, remote interactions typically limit a trainer's ability to provide instruction on tasks (e.g., following through on multistep tasks in the presence of distractions) or in environments that many report as challenging (e.g., office setting). It is thus important to consider what innovations are needed in brain injury tele-rehabilitation to support intensive skill training and promote skill transfer to daily life.

The technology-assisted training described above can be delivered by televideo to enable remote training (see Figure 12.6). The technical set-up required for remote deployment consists of separate computer terminals at each site equipped with a web-camera and microphone, an additional auxiliary document camera,

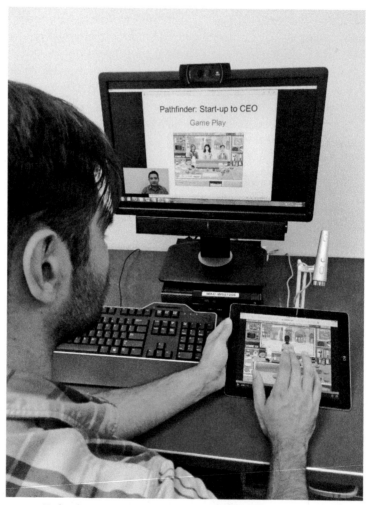

FIGURE 12.6  *Technology set-up for remote cognitive training. Hardware consists of a computer equipped with web camera, a secondary USB camera, and a touchscreen tablet loaded with CEO game at both the trainer's and trainee's sites. Training materials reflecting key training concepts are presented on the trainee's computer screen alongside live video of the trainer. The secondary desk camera is positioned to capture live gameplay, enabling the trainer to both model and observe gameplay and strategy application. Real-time observations allow for detailed and individualized coaching and feedback.*

speakers, video-teleconferencing software that allows for screen sharing (many freely available televideo tools can support this interaction, but clinicians should consider software that provides secure and encrypted connections to ensure patient confidentiality), and game software running on a tablet or computer. The document camera serves to relay trainer and participant gameplay, allowing for real-time modeling, observations, and individualized feedback on skill application. Gameplay observations, training materials, and detailed feedback on weekly game performance are shared via online presentation tools.

An example of a tested technical set-up is illustrated in Figure 12.6. Skill learning is guided through at least three different levels of interactions operating synergistically. Verbal instruction and guidance on skill application both within game contexts and real-life settings occur over televideo. The interactions are further supported by visual displays of summaries of key training points, which are also provided to the trainee as handouts. Trainees are encouraged to take notes during training sessions to reinforce conceptual understanding and learning as well as for a reference to use out of session. Finally, transmitting real-time gameplay allows for the trainer both to model skill application during different game challenges and to observe trainees' use of skills in order to provide timely and corrective feedback. The exchanges provide a rich and multilayered foundation for coaching use of skills in trainees' daily lives.

## FEASIBILITY OF IMPLEMENTATION AND PLAUSIBILITY OF BENEFITS

In a preliminary sample testing the feasibility of remote deployment of this training system, 18 individuals with history of brain injury and chronic cognitive complaints were assigned to training via televideo ($n = 8$) or to treatment as usual ($n = 10$). No participant had any major psychiatric, substance use, or other neurological condition that limited participation, although most participants experienced clinically meaningful symptoms of depression and PTS. All participants also reported that current cognitive difficulties interfered with their responsibilities at work or school or with caregiving. The sample was well matched across demographic and injury variables, with the exception that treatment-as-usual participants were older.

Training was administered utilizing two Dell laptop computers and a tablet (iPad running iOS) with game software. Remote sessions were conducted over a secure network, and each terminal was equipped with Cisco Jabber Video for Telepresence software, a Logitech B910 web-camera, and an iPevo point-2-view USB document camera. Training was conducted either between separate VA locations, or between VA and University of California. The trainer had no in-person contact with the trainee.

All portions of the training protocol were successfully implemented (i.e., manualized instruction and guidance, interpersonal interactions over televideo, remote visualization of game activities, data viewing and feedback, semistruc-tured phone check-ins). Overall, trainers and participants responded favorably to the visualization and discussion of gameplay in real time, including modeling, observing, and provision of feedback on skill application. All participants were highly engaged during tele-video sessions. The most frequent technical issue encountered related to inconsistent Internet connectivity, which resulted in some temporary delays, but participants tolerated the disruptions and the delays inter-fered only minimally with training. While the disruptions were not intentionally built into training, trainers utilized the experiences as additional opportunities to practice state-regulation skills for tolerating frustrations.

Training participants demonstrated greater pre–post intervention changes than treatment as usual on our primary outcome composite measure of complex attention and executive functions ($d$ = 1.38), as well as a trend toward greater improvements on measures of verbal learning and memory ($d$ = 0.91). While other differences in pre–post change score did not reach the threshold for statis-tical significance, many of the effect sizes of the. differences were in the medium range. This included greater training-associated improvements on an ecologi-cally valid functional measure ($d$ = 0.42) as well as self-reported functioning on tasks requiring working memory ($d$ = 0.71) and organization/planning ($d$ = 0.67). Persons in the training intervention also reported greater metacognitive aware-ness ($d$ = 0.41) and less fatigue ($d$ = 0.38).

Training participants were largely compliant with at-home game practice and accumulated substantial experiential practice with SR use during gameplay (num-ber of Stop button presses: $Mdn$ = 722, IQR (interquartile range) = 1772; proportion of total gameplay spent in Stop mode: $Mdn$ = 33.1%, IQR = 35.4%). In line with our intention of designing game-based scenarios to augment training, all participants reported that gameplay provided multiple and varied opportunities to practice stra-tegic skill application. Further, most participants reported understanding the ratio-nale for practicing strategy application within the context of gameplay as a means to facilitate their use of state-regulation skills in pursuit of their individual goals. Review of gameplay data, particularly the impact of Stop button use on multiple game metrics, appeared helpful with training use of state-regulation skills on an individual basis. Finally, all participants indicated they would recommend training to others with brain injury who experience difficulties with state regulation.

Regular feedback within the game as well in coaching sessions was helpful for highlighting the relevance of skills and reinforcing their use during gameplay and in daily life. For instance, at the start of training, all participants expressed skepticism about the potential utility of applying SR strategies during gameplay. They felt that because strategy use slowed down their rate of play, it would inter-fere with their overall performance. The availability of game data allowed for this assumption to be tested through direct experimentation: participants were able to compare their performance during rounds where they did and did not employ SR strategies to learn how to optimally use utilize skills to their own benefit.

Participants were encouraged to assume an active role in their learning process and to experiment with strategies to verify for themselves the potential benefit of strategy use. This approach helped raise participants' awareness of situations in which strategies could be profitably applied, such as game junctures where they were particularly susceptible to disruption. For instance, one participant observed the accuracy of his performance improve when he utilized mindful breathing prior to starting tasks as well as SR strategies while encoding customers' orders and managing distractions. He also identified a tendency to get overwhelmed when customers' faces changed to express their dissatisfaction with his service. Based upon these observations, he was able to construct if/then plans for applying SR strategies to manage this aspect of the game. These experiences were then utilized to facilitate discussions of potentially similar situations in his personal life where SR strategies might be helpful. For example, he established a practice of applying mindful breathing for at least 5 min in his car before entering work, as well as at points during the day when he noticed himself becoming frustrated by his co-workers. By the end of training, he reported utilizing mindful breathing and SR strategies routinely, and he felt they had contributed to his being more productive and engaged at work. Specifically, he reported feeling less overwhelmed and better able to manage his work responsibilities.

Experimenting with strategy use and experiencing positive outcomes may have contributed to the transfer of skills to personal life. For example, several participants observed, and confirmed via objective feedback on their performance, that use of SR strategies improved their ability to manage game distractions and to multitask. During gameplay, they consistently practiced applying SR strategies to refresh goal-relevant information in working memory (i.e., remaining customers' orders) and update their plans before diverting attention to distracting customers. With the help of these training experiences, participants reported developing confidence in their ability to apply these strategies in pursuit of other goals. For instance, one participant reported establishing plans for applying SR strategies at moments he found himself distracted, frustrated, or losing focus while preparing for a conference presentation. He further expressed anxiety about networking at the event, due to his difficulty remembering people's names. He was coached on applying SR in these instances and rehearsing names in working memory before diverting attention to another person or topic (as he had done during gameplay). He reported that he successfully utilized these experiences at the conference, which he felt contributed to a better overall experience. Overall, the experience of successful skill application with a positive outcome strengthened a sense of self-efficacy.

## IMPLICATIONS FOR TELE-REHABILITATION

Using technology in the form of digital game experiences to guide skill learning is a practical and feasible way to provide experiential learning opportunities via televideo. The combination of game experiences, timely feedback, and guidance can help trainees' achieve a conceptual understanding of the rationale for strategies, increase awareness of personal vulnerabilities to distraction and dysregulation, identify situations where strategy use might be beneficial, and develop a sense of self-efficacy with skill use. Therefore, the training system can help trainees generalize and transfer their learning experiences to a range of contexts within their personal lives.

Remote deployment of this self-regulation training system would extend its potential benefits to individuals with limited access to care. The development of tools to aid with remote training represents an important step in enhancing care for individuals with brain injury, PTS, and other neurobehavioral health conditions. Providing guided experiential learning opportunities that are challenging, calibrated, individually tailored, and varied may help tele-rehabilitation realize its full potential.

### REACHING VETERANS IN SCHOOL

Many in the current generation of veterans are interested in continuing to serve in their own ways, on the home front. Many have shared that their goals include returning to school—of course, with the intent of succeeding. The GI Bill has supported over 1 million beneficiaries with over $12 billion in payments in 2013 alone (Department of Veterans Affairs, 2014). Higher education is recognized as an important bridge to a successful career. Symptoms related to TBI and PTS, common among veterans of recent conflicts, can have a significant negative impact on the neurobehavioral functions that form an essential foundation for scholastic success. There remains a paucity of rehabilitation intervention work that addresses the neurocognitive issues that most commonly affect the current generation of veterans (Cooper et al., 2015), with combined TBI-PTS being a hallmark problem for this generation (Carlson et al., 2011; Chen & Novakovic-Agopian, 2012). Of note, the extant literature does not address veterans who are students, and consequently, there remains a significant need for the development of interventions specifically designed to improve functioning to enhance success in school and beyond.

A system for the guided experiential learning of self-regulation skills can be adapted for the classroom setting, in a small group, seminar-type format. The major adaptation is integrating goals from student lives into the training. An initial implementation at the college level in the University of California has received much positive feedback. A study involving students in the University of California system is ongoing. The application of tele-rehabilitation approaches also raises the potential for reaching students via online learning, while addressing some of the limitations of online learning in terms of guidance, engagement, interaction, and practice experiences.

# Conclusion

The use of technology-assisted training, with guided skill learning augmented by game-assisted experiential learning, has great potential to increase access to cognitive rehabilitation in both VA and civilian settings. Technology assistance can potentially add not only to the effectiveness of learning but also to versatility of service delivery. Training could potentially be administered by a wide range of clinicians (e.g., neuropsychologists, speech and language therapists, recreation therapists), while providing key features to support remote training and classroom settings as well, allowing access to specialized training for more patients.

# References

Aarts, H., Custers, R., & Holland, R. W. (2007). The nonconscious cessation of goal pursuit: When goals and negative affect are coactivated. *Journal of Personality and Social Psychology, 92*(2), 165–178.

Alfers, J. A., & Heady, H. R. (2014). Rural veterans: A special concern for rural health advocates. Retrieved from http://www.ruralhealthweb.org/index.cfm?objectid= 70A65A88-3048-651A-FEC6F164AD6ADE87

Anguera, J. A., Boccanfuso, J., Rintoul, J. L., Al-Hashimi, O., Faraji, F., Janowich, J., . . . Gazzaley, A. (2013). Video game training enhances cognitive control in older adults. *Nature, 501*(7465), 97–101.

Arnemann, K. L., Chen, A. J., Novakovic-Agopian, T., Gratton, C., Nomura, E. M., & D'Esposito, M. (2015). Functional brain network modularity predicts response to cognitive training after brain injury. *Neurology, 84*(15), 1568–1574.

Awh, E., & Vogel, E. K. (2008). The bouncer in the brain. *Nature Neuroscience, 11*(1), 5–6.

Baddeley, A., Chincotta, D., & Adlam, A. (2001). Working memory and the control of action: Evidence from task switching. *Journal of Experimental Psychology: General, 130*(4), 641–657.

Baddeley, A. D. (2001). Is working memory still working? *American Psychologist, 56*(11), 851–864.

Ballesteros, S., Prieto, A., Mayas, J., Toril, P., Pita, C., Ponce de León, L., . . . Waterworth, J. (2014). Brain training with non-action video games enhances aspects of cognition in older adults: A randomized controlled trial. *Frontiers in Aging Neuroscience, 6*, 277.

Baranowski, T., Cullen, K. W., Nicklas, T., Thompson, D., & Baranowski, J. (2003). Are current health behavioral change models helpful in guiding prevention of weight gain efforts? *Obesity Research, 11*(Suppl.), 23S–43S.

Bassett, D. S., & Bullmore, E. (2006). Small-world brain networks. *Neuroscientist, 12*(6), 512–523.

Berlucchi, G. (2011). Brain plasticity and cognitive neurorehabilitation. *Neuropsychological Rehabilitation, 21*(5), 560–578.

Burke, L. A., & Hutchins, H. M. (2007). Training transfer: An integrative literature review. *Human Resource Development Review, 6*(3), 263–296.

Carlson, K. F., Kehle, S. M., Meis, L. A., Greer, N., MacDonald, R., Rutks, I., . . . Wilt, T. J. (2011). Prevalence, assessment, and treatment of mild traumatic brain injury and posttraumatic stress disorder: A systematic review of the evidence. *The Journal of Head Trauma Rehabilitation, 26*(2), 103–115.

Chen, A., & Novakovic-Agopian, T. (2012). Intervening to improve cognitive functioning after neurotrauma. In J. Tsao (Ed.), *Traumatic brain injury: A neurologic approach to diagnosis, management and rehabilitation*: New York: Springer.

Chen, A. J.-W., & D'Esposito, M. (2010). Traumatic brain injury: From bench to bedside to society. *Neuron, 66*(1), 11–14.

Chen, A. J.-W., Novakovic-Agopian, T., Nycum, T. J., Song, S., Turner, G. R., Hills, N. K., . . . D'Esposito, M. (2011). Training of goal-directed attention regulation enhances control over neural processing for individuals with brain injury. *Brain, 134*(Pt. 5), 1541–1554.

Church, T. E. (2009). Returning veterans on campus with war related injuries and the long road back home. *Journal of Postsecondary Education and Disability, 22*(1), 43–52.

Cooper, D., Bunner, A., Kennedy, J., Balldin, V., Tate, D., Eapen, B., & Jaramillo, C. (2015). Treatment of persistent post-concussive symptoms after mild traumatic brain injury: A systematic review of cognitive rehabilitation and behavioral health interventions in military service members and veterans. *Brain Imaging & Behavior, 9*(3), 403–420.

Cowan, N., & Morey, C. C. (2006). Visual working memory depends on attentional filtering. *Trends in Cognitive Sciences, 10*(4), 139–141.

D'Esposito, M., & Chen, A. J.-W. (2006). Neural mechanisms of prefrontal cortical function: Implications for cognitive rehabilitation. *Progess in Brain Research, 157*, 123–139.

D'Esposito, M., & Gazzaley, A. (2006). Neurorehabilitation and executive function. In M. Selzer, L. Cohen, F. Gage, S. Clarke, & P. Duncan (Eds.), *Neural Rehabilitation and Repair* (pp. 475–487). Cambridge, U.K: Cambridge University Press.

D'Zurilla, T. J., & Goldfried, M. (1971). Problem solving and behavior modification. *Journal of Abnormal Psychology, 78*, 107–126.

Dean, P. J., & Sterr, A. (2013). Long-term effects of mild traumatic brain injury on cognitive performance. *Frontiers in Human Neuroscience, 7*, 30. doi:10.3389/fnhum.2013.00030

Departments of Veterans Affairs. (2014). *Veterans Benefit Administration Annual Benefits Report Fiscal Year 2014*. Washington, D.C.: Author. 2014. Retrieved from http://benefits.va.gov/REPORTS/abr/ABR-Combined-FY14-11052015.pdf.

Duncan, J., Burgess, P., & Emslie, H. (1995). Fluid intelligence after frontal lobe lesions. *Neuropsychologia, 33*(3), 261–268.

Duncan, J., Emslie, H., Williams, P., Johnson, R., & Freer, C. (1996). Intelligence and the frontal lobe: The organization of goal-directed behavior. *Cognitive Psychology, 30*(3), 257–303.

Filevich, E., Kuhn, S., & Haggard, P. (2012). Intentional inhibition in human action: The power of 'no'. *Neuroscience & Biobehavioral Reviews, 36*(4), 1107–1118.

Fish, J., Evans, J. J., Nimmo, M., Martin, E., Kersel, D., Bateman, A., . . . Manly, T. (2007). Rehabilitation of executive dysfunction following brain injury: "Content-free" cueing improves everyday prospective memory performance. *Neuropsychologia, 45*(6), 1318–1330.

Fox, M. D., Snyder, A. Z., Zacks, J. M., & Raichle, M. E. (2006). Coherent spontaneous activity accounts for trial-to-trial variability in human evoked brain responses. *Nature Neuroscience, 9*(1), 23–25.

Girard, P. (2007). Military and VA telemedicine systems for patients with traumatic brain injury. *Journal of Rehabilitation Research and Development, 44*(7), 1017–1026.

Gollwitzer, P. M., & Sheeran, P. (2006). Implementation intentions and goal achievement: A meta-analysis of effects and processes. *Advances in Experimental Social Psychology, 38*, 69–119.

Green, C. S., & Bavelier, D. (2008). Exercising your brain: A review of human brain plasticity and training-induced learning. *Psychology and Aging, 23*(4), 692–701.

Hailey, D., Roine, R., Ohinmaa, A., & Dennett, L. (2013). The status of telerehabilitation in neurological applications. *Journal of Telemedicine and Telecare, 19*(6), 307–310.

Veterans Affairs Office of Rural Health. (2014). Fact Sheet: Information about the Office of Rural Health and Rural Veterans. Washington, DC: Author. Retrieved from http://www.ruralhealth.va.gov/docs/factsheets/ORH_General_FactSheet_2014.pdf.

Veterans Affairs Office of Rural Health. (2015). The rural connection. Washington, D.C: Author. Retrieved from http://www.ruralhealth.va.gov/docs/news/ORH_The_Rural_Connection_Newsletter_winter2015.pdf

Hoge, C. W., McGurk, D., Thomas, J. L., Cox, A. L., Engel, C. C., & Castro, C. A. (2008). Mild traumatic brain injury in U.S. soldiers returning from Iraq. *New England Journal of Medicine, 358*(5), 453–463.

Kennedy, M. R., Krause, M. O., & Turkstra, L. S. (2008). An electronic survey about college experiences after traumatic brain injury. *NeuroRehabilitation, 23*(6), 511–520.

Kitzbichler, M. G., Henson, R. N., Smith, M. L., Nathan, P. J., & Bullmore, E. T. (2011). Cognitive effort drives workspace configuration of human brain functional networks. *Journal of Neuroscience, 31*(22), 8259–8270.

Klingberg, T., Fernell, E., Olesen, P. J., Johnson, M., Gustafsson, P., Dahlström, K., . . . Westerberg, H. (2005). Computerized training of working memory in children with ADHD—A randomized, controlled trial. *Journal of the American Academy of Child and Adolescent Psychiatry, 44*(2), 177–186.

Kolb, B., & Muhammad, A. (2014). Harnessing the power of neuroplasticity for intervention. *Frontiers in Human Neuroscience, 8*, 377. doi:10.3389/fnhum.2014.00377

Landa-Gonzalez, B. (2001). Multicontextual occupational therapy intervention: A case study of traumatic brain injury. *Occupational Therapy International, 8*(1), 49–62.

Larson, M. J., Steffen, P. R., & Primosch, M. (2013). The impact of a brief mindfulness meditation intervention on cognitive control and error-related performance monitoring. *Frontiers in Human Neuroscience, 7*, 308.

Lebowitz, M. S., Dams-O'Connor, K., & Cantor, J. B. (2012). Feasibility of computerized brain plasticity-based cognitive training after traumatic brain injury. *Journal of Rehabilitation Research and Development, 49*(10), 1547–1556.

Levine, B., Robertson, I. H., Clare, L., Carter, G., Hong, J., Wilson, B. A., . . . Stuss, D. T. (2000). Rehabilitation of executive functioning: An experimental-clinical validation of goal management training. *Journal of the International Neuropsychological Society, 6*(3), 299–312.

Levine, B., Stuss, D. T., Winocur, G., Binns, M. A., Fahy, L., Mandic, M., . . . Robertson, I. H. (2007). Cognitive rehabilitation in the elderly: Effects on strategic behavior in relation to goal management. *Journal of the International Neuropsychological Society,* *13*(1), 143–152.

Locke, E. A., & Latham, G. P. (2002). Building a practically useful theory of goal setting and task motivation. A 35-year odyssey. *American Psychologist, 57*(9), 705–717.

Loya, F., Rodriguez, N., Binder, D., Buchanan, B., Novakovic-Agopian, T., & Chen, A. J. W. (2014, March). *'From start-up to CEO': Development of game-assisted training for persons with brain injury to improve higher order functional cognition.* Poster presented at the Tenth World Congress on Brain Injury, San Francisco, CA.

Lynch, B. (2002). Historical review of computer-assisted cognitive retraining. *Journal of Head Trauma Rehabilitation, 17*(5), 446–457.

Manly, T., & Murphy, F. C. (2012). Rehabilitation of executive function and social cognition impairments after brain injury. *Current Opinion in Neurology, 25*(6), 656–661

Mauri, M., Sinforiani, E., Bono, G., Cittadella, R., Quattrone, A., Boller, F., & Nappi, G. (2006). Interaction between apolipoprotein epsilon 4 and traumatic brain injury in patients with Alzheimer's disease and mild cognitive impairment. *Functional Neurology, 21*(4), 223–228.

Mayas, J., Parmentier, F. B. R., Andrés, P., & Ballesteros, S. (2014). Plasticity of attentional functions in older adults after non-action video game training: A randomized controlled trial. *PloS One, 9*(3), e92269.

Mecklinger, A. D., von Cramon, D. Y., Springer, A., & Matthes-von Cramon, G. (1999). Executive control functions in task switching: Evidence from brain injured patients. *Journal of Clinical and Experimental Neuropsychology, 21*(5), 606–619. doi:10.1076/jcen.21.5.606.873

Melby-Lervag, M., & Hulme, C. (2013). Is working memory training effective? A meta-analytic review. *Developmental Psychology, 49*(2), 270–291.

Meunier, D., Achard, S., Morcom, A., & Bullmore, E. (2009). Age-related changes in modular organization of human brain functional networks. *Neuroimage, 44*(3), 715–723.

Meunier, D., Lambiotte, R., & Bullmore, E. T. (2010). Modular and hierarchically modular organization of brain networks. *Frontiers in Neuroscience, 4,* 200.

Moore, A., Gruber, T., Derose, J., & Malinowski, P. (2012). Regular, brief mindfulness meditation practice improves electrophysiological markers of attentional control. *Frontiers in Human Neuroscience, 6,* 18.

Nezu, A. M., Nezu, C. M., & D'Zurilla, T. J. (2007). *Solving life's problems.* New York: Springer Publishing Company.

Novakovic-Agopian, T., Chen, A. J., Rome, S., Abrams, G., Castelli, H., Rossi, A., . . . D'Esposito, M. (2011). Rehabilitation of executive functioning with training in attention regulation applied to individually defined goals: A pilot study bridging theory, assessment, and treatment. *Journal of Head Trauma Rehabilitation, 26*(5), 325–338.

Owen, A. M., Hampshire, A., Grahn, J. A., Stenton, R., Dajani, S., Burns, A. S., . . . Ballard, C. G. (2010). Putting brain training to the test. *Nature, 465*(7299), 775–778.

Papo, D. (2013). Why should cognitive neuroscientists study the brain's resting state? *Frontiers in Human Neuroscience, 7,* 45.

Park, N. W., & Ingles, J. L. (2001). Effectiveness of attention rehabilitation after acquired brain injury: A meta-analysis. *Neuropsychology, 15,* 199–210.

Phelps, E. A., Delgado, M. R., Nearing, K. I., & LeDoux, J. E. (2004). Extinction learning in humans: Role of the amygdala and vmPFC. *Neuron, 43*(6), 897–905.

Polusny, M., Kehle, S., Nelson, N., Erbes, C., Arbisi, P., & Thuras, P. (2011). Longitudinal effects of mild traumatic brain injury and posttraumatic stress disorder comorbidity on postdeployment outcomes in National Guard soldiers deployed to Iraq. *Archives of General Psychiatry, 68*(1), 79–89.

Ponsford, J. L., Downing, M. G., Olver, J., Ponsford, M., Acher, R., Carty, M., & Spitz, G. (2014). Longitudinal follow-up of patients with traumatic brain injury: Outcome at two, five, and ten years post-injury. *Journal of Neurotrauma, 31*(1), 64–77.

Rath, J., Simon, D., Langenbahn, D. M., Sherr, R., & Diller, L. (2003). Group treatment of problem-solving deficits in outpatients with traumatic brain injury: A randomised outcome study. *Neuropsychological Rehabilitation, 13*(4), 461–488.

Repovs, G., & Baddeley, A. (2006). The multi-component model of working memory: Explorations in experimental cognitive psychology. *Neuroscience, 139*(1), 5–21.

Robertson, K., & Schmitter-Edgecombe, M. (2015). Self-awareness and traumatic brain injury outcome. *Brain Injury,* (29)7–8, 848–858.

Rodriguez, N., Loya, F., Binder, D., Buchanan, B., Novakovic-Agopian, T., Murphy, M., . . . Chen, A. (2014, March). *'Working your way up' from simple to complex situations in game-assisted training of attention regulation for individuals with brain injury.* Poster presented at the Tenth World Congress on Brain Injury, San Francisco, CA.

Ropacki, S., Rickards, T., Barrera, K., & Yutsis, M. (2014). The relationship between self-awareness and functional outcomes in brain injury rehabilitation. *Archives of Clinical Neuropsychology, 29*(6), 599.

Schwartz, A. (2009, January 28). New sign of brain damage in N.F.L. *New York Times,* p.B11.

Seager, M. A., Johnson, L. D., Chabot, E. S., Asaka, Y., & Berry, S. D. (2002). Oscillatory brain states and learning: Impact of hippocampal theta-contingent training. *Proceedings of the National Academy of Sciences, USA, 99*(3), 1616–1620.

Shipstead, Z., Hicks, K. L., & Engle, R. W. (2012). Cogmed working memory training: Does the evidence support the claims? *Journal of Applied Research in Memory and Cognition, 1*(3), 185–193.

Shipstead, Z., Redick, T. S., & Engle, R. W. (2012). Is working memory training effective? *Psychological Bulletin, 138*(4), 628–654.

Stellar, E. (1980). Brain mechanisms and hedonic processes. *Acta Neurobiologiae Experimentalis, 40*(1), 313–324.

Tang, Y. Y., Ma, Y., Wang, J., Fan, Y., Feng, S., Lu, Q., . . . Posner, M. I. (2007). Short-term meditation training improves attention and self-regulation. *Proceedings of the National Academy of Sciences, 104*(43), 17152–17156.

Thurman, D., Alverson, C., Dunn, K., Guerrero, J., & Sniezek, J. (1999). Traumatic brain injury in the United States: A public health perspective. *Journal of Head Trauma and Rehabilitation, 14*(6), 602–615.

Toglia, J., Johnston, M. V., Goverover, Y., & Dain, B. (2010). A multicontext approach to promoting transfer of strategy use and self regulation after brain injury: An exploratory study. *Brain Injury, 24*(4), 664–677.

Toglia, J. P. (1991). Generalization of treatment: A multicontext approach to cognitive perceptual impairment in adults with brain injury. *American Journal of Occupational Therapy, 45*(6), 505–516.

Van Den Heuvel, C., Thornton, E., & Vink, R. (2007). Traumatic brain injury and Alzheimer's disease: A review. *Progress in Brain Research, 161*, 303–316.

van der Oord, S., Ponsioen, A. J. G. B., Geurts, H. M., Ten Brink, E. L., & Prins, P. J. M. (2014). A pilot study of the efficacy of a computerized executive functioning remediation training with game elements for children with ADHD in an outpatient setting: Outcome on parent- and teacher-rated executive functioning and ADHD behavior. *Journal of Attention Disorders, 18*(8), 699–712.

van Velzen, J. M., van Bennekom, C. A., Edelaar, M. J., Sluiter, J. K., & Frings-Dresen, M. H. (2009). How many people return to work after acquired brain injury? A systematic review. *Brain Injury, 23*(6), 473–488.

Vanderploeg, R. D., Curtiss, G., & Belanger, H. G. (2005). Long-term neuropsychological outcomes following mild traumatic brain injury. *Journal of the International Neuropsychological Society, 11*(3), 228–236.

Vasterling, J. J., Bryant, R. A., & Keane, T. M. (2012). *PTSD and mild traumatic brain injury*. New York: Guilford Press.

Vogel, E. K., McCollough, A. W., & Machizawa, M. G. (2005). Neural measures reveal individual differences in controlling access to working memory. *Nature, 438*(7067), 500–503.

Mai, N. (1991). Problem-solving deficits in brain-injured patients: A therapeutic approach. *Neuropsychological Rehabilitation, 1*, 45–64.

Weeks, W. B., Wallace, A. E., West, A. N., Heady, H. R., & Hawthorne, K. (2008). Research on rural veterans: An analysis of the literature. *The Journal of Rural Health, 24*(4), 337–344.

Ylvisaker, M. S., Turkstra, L., & Coelho, C. (2005). Behavioral and social interventions for individuals with traumatic brain injury: A summary of the research with clinical implications. *Seminars in Speech and Language, 26*(4), 256–267.

Yu, W., Ravelo, A., Wagner, T. H., Phibbs, C. S., Bhandari, A., Chen, S., & Barnett, P. G. (2003). Prevalence and costs of chronic conditions in the VA health care system. *Medical Care Research and Review, 60*(3 Suppl.), 146S–167S.

# 13

# Incorporating Neuroimaging into Cognitive Assessment

## Erin D. Bigler

All traditional neuropsychological assessment techniques emerged in an era prior to modern neuroimaging. In fact, question-answer/paper-and-pencil test origins that gained traction[1] with Alfred Binet in 1905 remain the same core techniques today. Indeed, Binet's efforts began the era of standardized human metrics designed to assess a broad spectrum of cognitive, emotional, and behavioral functions and abilities. During the early part of the 20th century, the concept of an intellectual quotient expressed as a standard score with a mean of 100 and a standard deviation of 15 also initiated the era of quantitative descriptions of mental and emotional functioning (Anastasi, 1968; Stern, 1912). Other descriptive statistical metrics were applied to human measurement, including scaled, percentile, T-score, and z-score statistics. Statistical measures became part of the assessment lexicon and each possessed strength as well as weakness for descriptive purposes, but together proved to be immensely effective for communicating test findings and inferring average and above or below the norm performances. In turn, descriptive statistical methods became the cornerstone for describing neuropsychological findings, typically reported by domain of functioning (memory, excutive, language, etc.; Cipolotti & Warrington, 1995; Lezak, Howieson, Bigler, & Tranel, 2012).

As much as psychology and medicine have incorporated descriptive statistics into research and clinical application, a major focus of both disciplines also has been binary classification—normal versus abnormal. This dichotomization recognizes some variability and individual differences within a test score or laboratory procedure, but at some point the clinician makes the binary decision of normal or abnormal. In the beginnings of neuroimaging, which are discussed more thoroughly below, interpretation of computed tomographic (CT) or magnetic resonance imaging (MRI) scans mostly was approached in this manner. Although lots of information was available from CT and MRI images, if nothing obviously abnormal was seen, the radiological conclusion merely stated in the Impression section, "Normal CT (or MRI) of the brain," with no other qualification (or quantification) of why the findings were deemed normal other than the image appeared that way. Until recently, quantification of information in an image required hand editing and was excruciatingly time consuming. Surprisingly, not until recently has there been a push for quantification. However, once automated technology established a variety of techniques for neuroimaging quantification, the field of neuroimaging rapidly embraced quantitative methods (Raji et al., 2015; Saykin et al., 2015; Weiskopf, Mohammadi, Lutti, & Callaghan, 2015; Wilde et al., 2015).

Embracing technology changes a field of study, as has been the case with neuroimaging. Parallel with the psychological assessment era initiated by Binet, equipped with the aforementioned descriptive statistical methods, medicine continued its quest to measure essentially every anatomical and physiological variable possible with the technology of the day to establish normative databases, deviation from which permitted diagnosis as well as study of disease and pathological processes. Taking a patient's temperature and finding a fever represents a simple but well understood example of such a quest. Assessing body temperature began with feeling a patient's skin, and if it was "warm" to the touch (i.e., a just noticeable difference), that was considered a sign of potential fever. The discovery that mercury was temperature sensitive and that by encasing and sealing it in glass, both air as well as body temperature could be measured, were remarkable advances during the Renaissance (McGee, 1988). Temperature metrics had to be established, leading to the well-known Celsius and Fahrenheit debates. With the advent of thermometers for use in humans and an acceptable scaling (see review by Pearn, 2012), body temperatures could be recorded; however, the measurements were analog and the thermometer had to be inserted into the patient and then had to be visually examined for the reading of the temperature. Once it was read, if the temperature needed to be permanently recorded, it had to be written/recorded by hand. The next advancements involved digital temperature displays (Houdas & Ring, 1982; Nisbet, 1971), followed by thermally sensitive probes which could take temperatures within the ear canal or via a swabbing action across the forehead (Jensen, Jensen, Madsen, & Lossl, 2000). Although the temperature output was now digitally displayed, initially all of the output still required hand recording. With further technological advancements to fully digital, integrated temperature-measurement devices were developed that automatically recorded temperature. Currently, infrared thermography can measure skin temperature via noncontact and noninvasive methods (Rossignoli, Benito, & Herrero, 2015). At each stage, a technological advancement supplanted its predecessor. Numerous analogies from standard of care diagnostic medicine show how new technological advances supplant accepted methods of assessment. Indeed, a physician of Binet's era (circa early 1900s) would be astonished at the technological advances in medicine, most of which would be unrecognizable to him.

Despite the digital revolution of the 20th and 21st centuries, much of neuropsychological assessment has not embraced any transition to the digital world whatsoever. While the latest version of nationally standardized measures of cognitive assessment may permit some digital data entry, the findings are still mostly hand entered by the examiner. Some tests have started to interface with computerized presentations, but they are not universally used, standardization issues remain, and digital assessment tests have only limited clinical utility at this time (Canini et al., 2014). Possibly, concussion management is where the most use of computerized neuropsychological assessment methods occur, but this is not without controversy (Iverson & Schatz, 2015).

Although the intact brain processes all sensory stimuli with millisecond precision, traditionally administered neuropsychological tests, except for some reaction-time tasks, measure processing speed in seconds to minutes, not in milliseconds. The measures still require the examiner to issue "start" and "stop" commands and to use a handheld stopwatch. Questions are still asked by the examiner, rather than in an interactive virtual assessment environment that would mimic real-world cognitive and behavioral tasks, as discussed elsewhere in this volume. The National Institutes of Health has sponsored a common data elements approach to neuropsychological assessment with the development of the NIH Toolbox Cognition Battery (Casaletto et al., 2015; Heaton et al., 2014; Mungas et al., 2014) to address some of these deficiencies, but the NIH Toolbox remains a research tool that, as of this writing, has not transitioned into a clinical assessment method. More of these technological limitations are reviewed in this volume in other chapters.

## Historical Note and Current Status of Neuroimaging in Service of Neuropsychology

As discussed above, clinical neuropsychology has been slow to capitalize on the electronic and digital advances of the 20th and 21st centuries. Of course, a basic old-style thermometer still accurately measures temperature despite all of the digital advances. It may be that traditional neuropsychological assessment methods will retain their role as established techniques for assessing human cognition and behavior as well. Nevertheless, given all that has accompanied the technological advances of the digital era, the intent of this chapter is to provide some context for where the field is now and to establish a potential framework for future undertakings to bring the digital (quantitative) world of neuroimaging to clinical neuropsychology. As outlined in the recent review by Sullivan and Bigler (2015), current neuroimaging should be in the service of neuropsychology.

Continuing with the historical contrasts between neuropsychological assessment and neuroimaging, the modern era of brain imaging began in 1973 with Hounsfield's publications of what was then called computerized axial tomography (or CAT) scanning (Ambrose & Hounsfield, 1973; Hounsfield, 1973, 1980). (Hounsfield received the Nobel Prize in 1979 for his revolutionary contributions to brain imaging.) The discovery of CAT scanning set into motion rapid improvements in what was to become computed tomography (CT), from which nuclear medicine developed positron emission tomography (PET) and single photon emission computed tomographic (SPECT) imaging. Capitalizing on the insights afforded by tomographic imaging, but using powerful magnetic fields, radiofrequency waves, and image reconstruction algorithms, by the early 1980s what was originally called nuclear magnetic resonance imaging was on the verge of becoming the imaging method for even greater identification of anatomical and pathological detail of the human brain (Marx, 1980). Thus, in a very short time, incredible gains were made in brain imaging. As an example of this, Figure 13.1 shows how magnetic resonance (MR) diffusion tensor imaging (DTI) tractography of a healthy human brain depicts all of the aggregate major pathways of the brain visible in the living individual (via data extracted from an MRI).

Contrast this with neuropsychological test development during the same time. Wechsler introduced the Block Design subtest in 1939, as a standard manipulative task in the first edition of the intellectual test that bears his name (see Wechsler, 1950), which by 1981 had been twice updated (Bornstein & Matarazzo, 1984). The Block Design measure is essentially unchanged in the manner in which it is administered and scored today, even with the newest edition. For someone who trained in the early to mid 1970s, as did this author, the core aspects of neuropsychological assessment have changed very little in 40+ years. In comparison, Figure 13.2 from Ecker, Bookheimer, and Murphy (2015) shows what has emerged in image quantification of the brain just in the first 15 years of the 21st century.

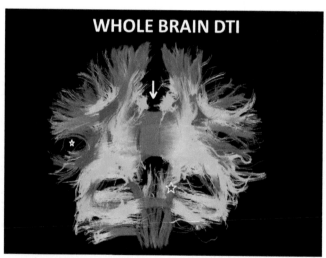

FIGURE 13.1 *Anterior view of diffusion tensor imaging (DTI) tractography depicting the major tracts in the human brain, where the colors represent directionality of the aggregate fiber tracts: Blue (vertically oriented), warm colors (lateral or side-to-side) or green (anterior–posterior). Downward arrow points to the corpus callosum, the left star sits with a U-fiber connection, and the blue star with white outline sits in the region of the corticospinal tract (CST).*

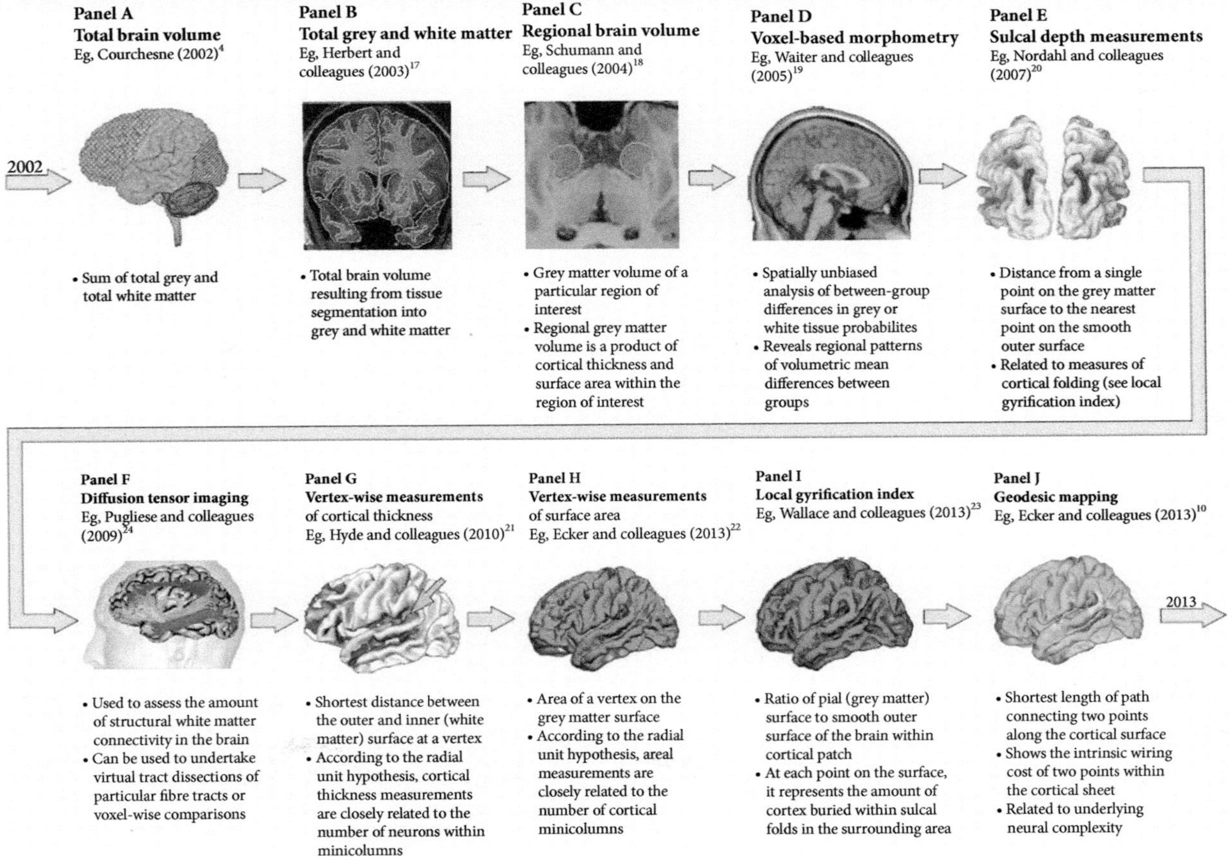

**Panel A**
**Total brain volume**
Eg. Courchesne (2002)[4]

- Sum of total grey and total white matter

**Panel B**
**Total grey and white matter**
Eg, Herbert and colleagues (2003)[17]

- Total brain volume resulting from tissue segmentation into grey and white matter

**Panel C**
**Regional brain volume**
Eg, Schumann and colleagues (2004)[18]

- Grey matter volume of a particular region of interest
- Regional grey matter volume is a product of cortical thickness and surface area within the region of interest

**Panel D**
**Voxel-based morphometry**
Eg, Walter and colleagues (2005)[19]

- Spatially unbiased analysis of between-group differences in grey or white tissue probabilities
- Reveals regional patterns of volumetric mean differences between groups

**Panel E**
**Sulcal depth measurements**
Eg, Nordahl and colleagues (2007)[20]

- Distance from a single point on the grey matter surface to the nearest point on the smooth outer surface
- Related to measures of cortical folding (see local gyrification index)

**Panel F**
**Diffusion tensor imaging**
Eg, Pugliese and colleagues (2009)[34]

- Used to assess the amount of structural white matter connectivity in the brain
- Can be used to undertake virtual tract dissections of particular fibre tracts or voxel-wise comparisons

**Panel G**
**Vertex-wise measurements of cortical thickness**
Eg. Hyde and colleagues (2010)[21]

- Shortest distance between the outer and inner (white matter) surface at a vertex
- According to the radial unit hypothesis, cortical thickness measurements are closely related to the number of neurons within minicolumns

**Panel H**
**Vertex-wise measurements of surface area**
Eg, Ecker and colleagues (2013)[22]

- Area of a vertex on the grey matter surface
- According to the radial unit hypothesis, areal measurements are closely related to the number of cortical minicolumns

**Panel I**
**Local gyrification index**
Eg, Wallace and colleagues (2013)[23]

- Ratio of pial (grey matter) surface to smooth outer surface of the brain within cortical patch
- At each point on the surface, it represents the amount of cortex buried within sulcal folds in the surrounding area

**Panel J**
**Geodesic mapping**
Eg, Ecker and colleagues (2013)[10]

- Shortest length of path connecting two points along the cortical surface
- Shows the intrinsic wiring cost of two points within the cortical sheet
- Related to underlying neural complexity

FIGURE 13.2   *The progression of brain imaging technology as reviewed by Ecker et al. (2015). All of the procedures have become more and more automated and provide considerable anatomical and functional information about the brain with immense potential to inform neuropsychology.*

Without doubt, as shown in Figure 13.2, neuroimaging has taken advantage of the digital era, computerization, and the ability to image the brain, whereas neuropsychological assessment practices have remained static. However, this is not the only limitation. As a result of how neuropsychological test measures were developed, along with nosological attempts at classification, various cognitive domains have evolved and been specified, but most of the classification occurred prior to contemporary neuroimaging. Conceptualizations of brain function in the early to mid 20th century, when most of the tests in current use were introduced, is hardly the current theory of brain function in the 21st century. To illustrate, two of the most frequently written about domains in neuropsychology are executive functioning (EF) and memory. In reality, it is impossible to separate EF and memory function, because every EF task is somewhat dependent on holding information at least in working memory while a solution is being worked out to complete the task. As EF task complexity increases, so does memory load. Likewise, memory and attention guide cognitive processes throughout any multistep process. So these functions are intertwined and are not separable from a traditional neuropsychological assessment perspective. Furthermore, all cognitive processing begins with sensory input, so EF and memory functioning also require fast and efficient sensory processing along with some kind of motor output for execution of the task.

The EF term did not become a common part of the neuropsychological lexicon until publications in the mid to late 20th century (see Weinberger, 1993), with a clear reference to the so-called frontal lobe disorders and studies earlier in the 20th century (Glees, 1947; McKenzie & Proctor, 1946; Negrin, 1953a, 1953b). Before neuroimaging it was largely assumed that classic neuropsychological measures of EF like card sorting tasks and novel learning/decision making tasks or impairments associated with inhibition were *sine qua non* indicators of "frontal pathology." Using 20th century neuropsychological terminology, neuropsychological reports would often make statements that findings of EF impairment were indicative of frontal "damage" or "frontal impairment." In an era still flirting with lesion-localization theory of brain function (see Catani et al., 2012), it seemed simple and straightforward that "impaired executive functioning" meant frontal pathology of some sort and vice versa.

So it was surprising to researchers in the 1990s that solid neuroimaging measures of cortical integrity, like SPECT imaging, failed to show relations between traditional neuropsychological measures of EF (card sorting, word fluency, Tower of London measures, associate learning tasks) and SPECT radiotracer uptake or lack thereof (see Goldenberg, Oder, Spatt, & Podreka, 1992). Some patients with significant frontal pathology clearly demonstrated by emerging neuroimaging technologies had no demonstrable neuropsychological deficit on tradition EF measures (Bigler, 1988).

Today, we understand that EF requires more than frontal lobe integrity, because the EF network is a complex array of cortical and subcortical structures working in concert. Figure 13.3 is from Raichle (2011) and it shows the multifaceted EF network and associated networks involved in cognitive EF. The illustration is from the culmination of cognitive neuroscience research studies, mostly using functional MRI (fMRI) techniques, showing brain activity at rest compared to cortical activation occurring during task engagement. Note that, in the EF network overviewed in Figure 13.3, there is as much nonfrontal involvement as frontal. Indeed, in a meta-analysis of EF and neuroimaging correlates, Nowrangi, Lyketsos, Rao, and Munro (2014) demonstrated the complex networks that underlie EF and that EF functioning cannot be isolated independent of other networks, most importantly the attentional and working memory networks. This meta-analysis, as well as numerous other studies (see Parks & Madden, 2013; Shaw, Schultz, Sperling, & Hedden, 2015), shows the dependence of EF networks on memory networks and vice versa. The anatomical challenge for neuropsychology and neuroimaging is that the memory network is just as complex as the EF network (see Figure 13.4, from Moscovitch et al., 2005).

Keeping in mind the above discussion, we have to ask: if a neuropsychological assessment finds EF or memory impairment, what does the impairment indicate in the way of brain pathology? Given the complexity and diversity of EF and memory networks, without neuroimaging, traditional neuropsychological approaches cannot answer the question.

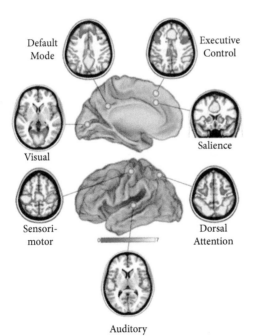

Default Mode

Executive Control

Visual

Salience

Sensori-motor

Dorsal Attention

Auditory

FIGURE 13.3 *Different brain networks derived from functional neuroimaging (Raichle, 2011).*

Schematic of the Memory Network

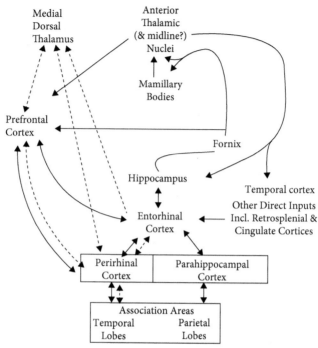

FIGURE 13.4  *The complexity of the memory network is shown in this schematic from Moscovitch et al. (2005). Used with permission.*

If neuropsychology is going to move in the direction of describing how memory and/or EF impairments in neuropsychological findings actually relate to brain structure and function, it will require using contemporary neuroimaging methods. If there is a neuropsychological test finding suggestive of a deficit, what are the corresponding anatomical regions affected? And, with all of the advancements in neuroimaging, why would a 21st century neuropsychological report implicate EF or memory impairment (or any other cognitive dysfunction) without exploring neuroanatomical and neuropathological correlates?

As outlined in Figures 13.3 and 13.4, the major anatomical players in EF and memory are known, so why not report the neuroanatomical and neuropathological findings related to cognitive, motor, sensory, visual-perceptual, emotional, and behavioral domains in conjunction with the neuropsychological test findings? Why not provide a normative neuroimaging database that can integrate with the neuropsychological test findings?

Clearly, neuropsychology without neuroimaging is stuck in a traditional approach that has not kept pace with advances in the clinical and cognitive neurosciences; however, there is a remedy available and that is to integrate structural neuroimaging findings with neuropsychology (Bigler, 2015; Sullivan & Bigler,

2015), in a way that can be automated and used across multiple platforms (Iscan et al., 2015). This chapter focuses on just the structural side of neuroimaging, but the real future, which is briefly addressed at the end of the chapter, is a fully integrated structural and functional neuroimaging methodology integrated with clinically meaningful neuropsychological measures.

The hippocampus, a key brain region involved in both memory and EF (Godsil, Kiss, Spedding, & Jay, 2013), with an enduring history in neuropsychology and neuroimaging, is used here as a model for what can currently be done. Hippocampal morphometrics began with simple hand tracing methods (Jack et al., 1989) but can now be computed with automated techniques (Ochs, Ross, Zannoni, Abildskov, & Bigler, 2015). Strangman and colleagues (2010) showed in cases of traumatic brain injury (TBI) the anatomical correlation of temporal lobe and cingulate gyrus atrophy with traditional memory assessment using paper-and-pencil neuropsychological tasks. An approach like this reports not just simply memory scores from a neuropsychological battery, but memory scores in the context of hippocampal and cingulate gyrus volumetric measures.

Enormously complex issues are associated with image acquisition and the technology for neuroimaging analyses, all of which are beyond the scope of this chapter. The chapter does not review basics of neuroimaging, which can be found elsewhere (Bigler, 2015b; Wilde, Hunter, & Bigler, 2012). What has revolutionized neuroimaging analysis has been automatization (Fischl, 2012). Pathoanatomical information from a scan can be derived with fully automated and reliable techniques and with minimal operator involvement, as is described in the following sections.

## What Can Contemporary Neuroimaging Do for Neuropsychology?

Figure 13.5 is an axial view of the author's brain when he was 65 years old, matched to a postmortem and histologically stained section from a younger individual who succumbed to a nonneurological illness. While it is singularly impressive that by using neuroimaging technology one can examine one's own brain, it is even more impressive that neuroimaging quality matches gross anatomy and everything in an image like Figure 13.5 can be quantified using the NIH-funded and open access software FreeSurfer (freesurfer-software.org/). The fundamentals of quantification begin with what is straightforwardly visible and identifiable in the gray-scale image, where gray-scale differences define tissue types and boundaries. As seen in Figure 13.6, brain tissue, referred to as parenchyma, can be divided into either gray or white matter, with both tissue types visibly distinctive from one another and cerebrospinal fluid (CSF)-filled spaces. In this T1-weighted MRI, again of the author's brain, the first step is to separate the different tissue and CSF boundaries as well as to remove the meninges and any skull, a

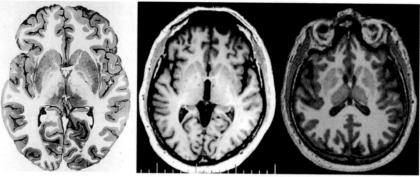

FIGURE 13.5 *(Left) Postmortem brain with gray matter Nissl staining with clear demarcation of white and gray matter. (Middle) Author's MRI at age 65 at a somewhat similar level, which shows how MRI has the ability to depict gross brain structure. (Right) Segmentation of the author's brain showing the cortical gray matter ribbon in darker flesh tone, putamen in light pink, globus pallidus in blue, thalamus in green, and caudate nucleus in orange-yellow.*

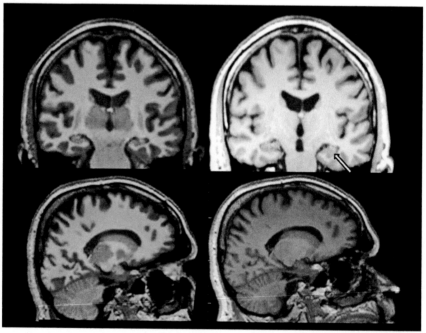

FIGURE 13.6 *Coronal and sagittal views of the author's segmented brain with the same color-coded schema as presented for the axial view in Figure 13.5. The images were generated from FreeSurfer. The arrow points to the hippocampus.*

procedure referred to as skull stripping and tissue segmentation, followed by image classification. The segmentation process uses gray-scale pixel intensity to define boundaries, literally to segment or separate white matter (WM), gray matter (GM), and CSF from one another. After tissue segmentation, then, as a result of some exceedingly elaborate image-analysis algorithms, the images are classified according to well-defined/known boundaries, such as the different lobes, gyri, or brain structures like the hippocampus. Once the image is classified and color coded, as shown in Figure 13.6, every region of interest (ROI) has a separate color, including the hippocampus (white arrow in the upper right coronal T1 image, yellow in the classified coronal image in the upper left). Next, using the parameters of MRI slice thickness and distance between slices, the volume can be calculated for each identified structure. Note that, in this image, both cortical and subcortical regions are segmented.

Accordingly, all cortical and subcortical regions can be identified and quantified. Furthermore, cortical surface area (gyrification), cortical volume, and cortical thickness can be computed, along with the shape of any ROI, as is shown in Figure 13.7.

The next step is to compare the individual values to a normative sample. In our Brain Imaging and Behavior Laboratory at Brigham Young University, we have developed an interactive quantitative three-dimensional imaging analysis method that utilizes the FreeSurfer volumetric findings obtained by running scans from the open source brain-imaging database referred to as the Open Access Series of Imaging Studies (OASIS—see http://www.oasis-brains.org/) through FreeSurfer. The OASIS database consists of a cross-sectional collection of 416 subjects aged 18 to 96. For each subject, three or four individual T1-weighted MRI scans obtained

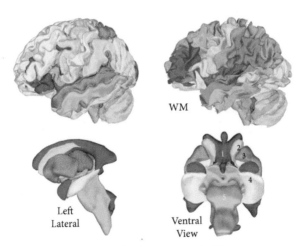

FIGURE 13.7 *From FreeSurfer cortical volume, cortical white matter volume and subcortical volumes can be computed for every brain. (1) ventricle, (2) caudate, (3) putamen, (4) hippocampus and the red blob above is the amygdala, (5) brainstem. These are three-dimensional FreeSurfer-generated outputs of the author's brain.*

in single scan sessions are included. The subjects are all right-handed and include both men and women. One hundred of the included subjects over the age of 60 have been clinically diagnosed with very mild to moderate Alzheimer's disease (AD). Currently, there are two major approaches to volumetric image quantification using FreeSurfer, one referred to as the Desikan approach (Desikan et al., 2006, 2009) and the other as the Destriuex approach (Destrieux, Fischl, Dale, & Halgren, 2010). Figure 13.8 shows a schematic where cortical gyri are divided into "parcels," resulting in the "parcellation" of the cerebral cortex into universally accepted ROIs. Figure13. 8 (from Desikan et al., 2009) shows the major cortical gyri and their parcellations. As a result, from the FreeSurfer analyses, accurate

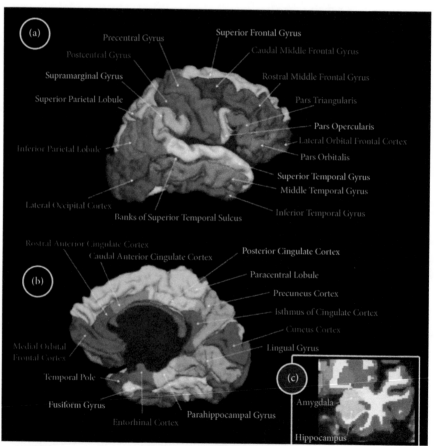

FIGURE 13.8 *Three-dimensional representations of all 34 ROIs that can be derived from FreeSurfer (only one hemisphere is shown). All of the neocortical ROIs visible in (A) lateral and (B) medial views of the gray matter surface and (C) the two nonneocortical regions (i.e., the hippocampus and amygdala) visible in the coronal view of a T1-weighted MRI image. (From Desikan et al., 2009; used with permission.)*

output of patient volume for each of the brain regions is performed using automated methods.

Figure 13.9 is a spreadsheet comparing the author's FreeSurfer volumes generated by the "aparc" file from the Destrieux atlas as well as the "aseg" file from the Desikan atlas to the OASIS database for other men between 63 and 67 years old, run through the same FreeSurfer processing pipeline. In this interactive program, the clinician can control how conservative or liberal a cut-point may be established, which in the illustration is set at 1.5 standard deviations from

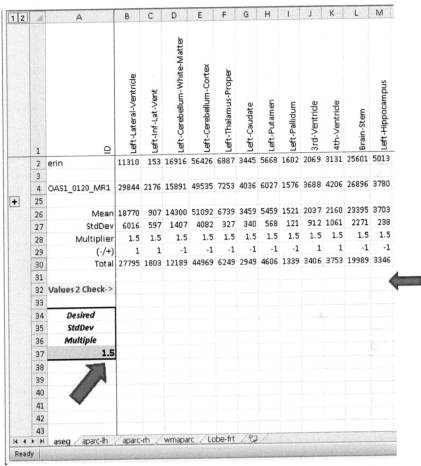

FIGURE 13.9 *A standard Excel spread that reflects the normative values from the FreeSurfer output from analyzing all of the scans in the OASIS database and then the author's FreeSurfer volumetric values. The left blue arrow points to the standard deviation setting, which for these comparisons was set at 1.5. The right blue arrow points to the line where a check would be registered if a value deviated from the normative sample. The bottom tabs show which file from FreeSurfer is being used. In this case it is the aseg. File and the label at the top of its row identifies the brain structure being assessed.*

the mean (large blue arrow in the figure). As visualized, all brain variables as measured in volume are within the average range of the normative sample (i.e., within the set standard deviation boundaries). What is learned very quickly from scanning the numeric anatomical findings in Figure 13.9 is that, from a quantitative volumetric standpoint, coarse brain anatomy was within normal limits at the time of this writing (lucky for the author!).

Next, a clinical case demonstrates the utility of this approach. The patient (approximately 62 years old), presented in Figure 13.10, had sustained a mild traumatic brain injury along with orthopedic injuries (leg fracture) and soft tissue and internal injuries in a high-speed motor vehicle accident several months before neuroimaging and neuropsychological evaluation. Since the accident, memory problems have persisted. This individual had a college degree and a professional-level position in the workforce, so reportedly premorbid history suggested above-average ability. The patient had a complicated medical history, including diabetes mellitus, and had received counseling in the past for depression and marital problems. A psychiatrist had recently diagnosed depression, had started the patient on antidepressant medication, and had made the referral for neuroimaging and neuropsychological consultation. The patient still had residual pain associated with the orthopedic injuries and was taking various pain medications at the time of testing. On neuropsychological assessment, memory performance was consistently observed to hover around a standard deviation below the normative mean for tests like the California Verbal Learning Test (CVLT), Wechsler Memory Scale-IV, and Rey-Complex Figure.

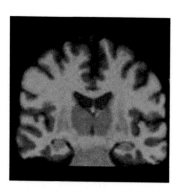
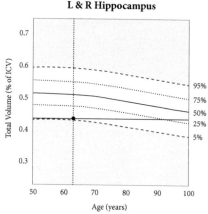

FIGURE 13.10  *This color-classified image in the coronal plane from NeuroQuant shows a patient's brain from which hippocampal volume was obtained and plotted to a normative sample. Hippocampal atrophy is documented. The context of hippocampal atrophy in light of documented deficits in memory function on neuropsychological assessment implicates pathology of a neurodegenerative nature and establishes baseline information for future monitoring.*

In this patient's case, the commercially available automated image analysis method referred to as NeuroQuant (http://www.cortechslabs.com) was used. NeuroQuant methods of image analysis are comparable to FreeSurfer (Ochs et al., 2015) and therefore what was said above about FreeSurfer applies to NeuroQuant. Currently, NeuroQuant provides quantitative comparisons with an age-adjusted normative sample only for the hippocampus and temporal horn (an omnibus measure of temporal lobe integrity, where larger temporal horn volume relates to temporal lobe atrophy). NeuroQuant also performs a right versus left hemisphere comparison for forebrain parenchyma, cortical gray matter, lateral ventricle, temporal horn, hippocampus, amygdala, caudate, putamen, pallidum, thalamus, and cerebellum. Since the two hemispheres should mirror one another, there should be a minimal percentage difference if neither the right nor left hemisphere is selectively damaged. In this approach, patients serve as their own controls for right and left hemisphere comparisons. In this patient's case, quantitative analyses revealed hippocampal volume to be reduced and approximately 1.5 standard deviations below normative value for her age (see Figure 13.10). Temporal horn was within the average range for age, so the volume loss appeared to be most specific to the hippocampus and not the temporal lobe in general. Furthermore, right versus left hemisphere comparisons revealed no significant asymmetry, with the majority of differences below 5%, which is within expected variation for the norm and age. Hippocampal volume loss, history of head injury, and neuropsychological confirmation of reduced memory performance suggest a neuropathological basis for the patient's complaints and symptoms of memory difficulties. The NeuroQuant and neuropsychological measures establish baseline clinical information that can provide a comparison for future follow-up, which will help address whether an early degenerative disorder is emerging or there are more static changes attributable to neuropsychiatric history, diabetes, and/or head injury.

Recently, Tanner, Mellott, Dunne, and Price (2015) showed how quantitative neuroimaging may be incorporated into the neuropsychological assessment process in cases of dementia and neurodegenerative disease using this type of integrated approach.

Since the NeuroQuant is FDA approved and commercially available for clinical application, with a straightforward method for formatting and report output, the technique is ready for clinical application. Neuropsychology merely needs to link with radiology and the proper acquisition of MRI with a thin slice volume. Other, similar technologies are on the horizon (see Brain Reader at brainreader.net).

Also, these techniques can be used when substantial lesions are present (Bigler et al., 2010). Figure 13.11 shows a child with major frontal pathology from a traumatic brain injury. The figure shows not only the brain pathology but also its quantification. As shown in this single image, the left frontal focal defect and its relation to the rest of the brain can be seen. Furthermore, using another image-analysis technique referred to as Advanced Normalization Tools, or ANTs (Avants, Tustison, Wu, Cook, & Gee, 2011; Tustison et al., 2014) the patient's brain can be warped to a template of control subjects, which now reflects where there

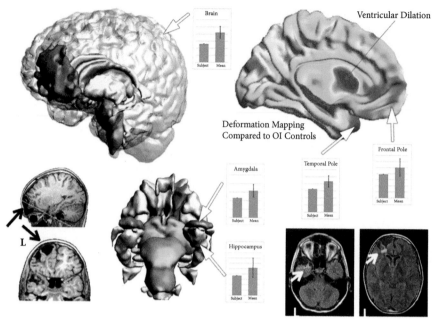

FIGURE 13.11  *Three-dimensional rendered image based on FreeSurfer analyses depicting the large area of focal frontal pathology. The red area represents the focal area of encephalomalacia also noted by the bottom black arrow as depicted in the T1 images. The top black arrow in the T1 images shows the lower left hemisphere lesion. The upper right image is a surface rendering from the advanced normalization tools (ANTs; Avants et al., 2011; Tustison et al., 2014) method following deformation analysis comparing an individual with traumatic brain injury (TBI) to a normative data set matched for age and sex. "Cold colors" (blue colors) reflect significant volume reductions, in contrast to "warm colors" that indicate a significant increase in volume. Histograms are from FreeSurfer-derived volumes for whole brain, amygdala, hippocampus, temporal pole, and frontal pole. Note in each case a substantial and significant reduction in volume has occurred. Lower right shows the FLAIR sequence depicting white matter signal abnormalities in the frontal and temporal lobe regions, with left (L) now on the viewer's left, since the images are three-dimensional. These depictions and quantifications of brain anatomy in a child with TBI provide additional information about brain structure and integrity that can be integrated with neuropsychological findings.*

are substantial volume differences, with blue areas reflecting parenchymal loss from the brain injury. Note that in this illustration, every anatomical feature and ROI can be quantified, shown in three dimensions, and referenced to a normative neuroimaging database.

## Functional Neuroimaging

There are still major issues with fMRI and its clinical application because of a variety of technical issues that need to be worked out, but tremendous progress has been and is being made toward that objective and the clinical implementation of fMRI (Bick, Mayer, & Levin, 2012; Jack et al., 2015; Small et al., 2008; Sugarman et al., 2012; Tomasi, Shokri-Kojori, & Volkow, 2015; Vitali, Di Perri, Vaudano, Meletti, & Villani, 2015). Currently, an imaging center may have appropriate experience with a particular fMRI protocol to assess a specific cognitive function and have a sufficient normative database for making comparisons. Problems arise across platforms and different labs, where generalization from one neuroimaging center to another may not be replicated. Nonetheless, based on what is currently available, some forecasting about how functional imaging may be incorporated into the neuropsychological examination of the future is given at the end of this chapter.

## What Neuropsychology Needs from Functional Neuroimaging

Those involved in bringing functional neuroimaging to the forefront of clinical application in neuropsychology and medicine know there are several fundamental impediments (as introduced above) that need to be overcome before there is universal application of the techniques. First, cognitive probes must be agreed upon and established. At this point in time, fMRI clinical applications are far beyond proof of concept, but what measures to use, validation, normative data, and reporting standards, etc., are still required (McAndrews, 2014; Sundermann, Herr, Schwindt, & Pfleiderer, 2014). No universally accepted cognitive probes have been accepted for widespread clinical use. Second, cross-platform issues described above must be resolved so that imaging centers have common quantitative metrics that are universally accepted (Bigler, 2015a). Regardless of what memory test is used by a neuropsychologist, if the findings are reported as being more than two standard deviations below average and the test is nationally standardized with appropriate norms and validity indices, describing the findings statistically is a universal language understood by all clinicians and researchers. Third, however, just like traditional neuropsychological methods, there are likely to be significant age, sex, educational attainment, ethnic, and cultural differences that potentially affect the MR signal and the clinical implications of any neuroimaging finding (Gess, Fausett, Kearney-Ramos, Kilts, & James, 2014). Fourth, unique patterns of disease and how injury or disease may influence neuroimaging findings at different stages of progression or recovery need to be established (Rocca et al., 2015).

Currently, traditional neuropsychological tests have been effectively adapted to be used in fMRI investigations (Allen & Fong, 2008a, 2008b; Arenth, Russell, Scanlon, Kessler, & Ricker, 2012; Sowell et al., 2007; Thermenos et al., 2004). These are necessary steps but are not designed to capitalize on all of the advances that are taking place in network theory of brain function (Bernhardt, Hong, Bernasconi, & Bernasconi, 2013; Gleichgerrcht, Fridriksson, & Bonilha, 2015; O'Callaghan, Shine, Lewis, Andrews-Hanna, & Irish, 2015; Vertes & Bullmore, 2015), including the clinical implementation of resting-state connectivity mapping and quantitative neuroimaging analysis (Bigler, 2015a). Remember, traditional neuropsychological tests currently in use evolved during the lesion-localization era and the modularity view of cortical function as the guiding principles for brain-behavior relations.

Figure 13.12 demonstrates a potential approach to address these issues. The example is simple and utilizes motor function, since the motor network is well known and less complex than cognitive and behavioral networks. Finger tapping (FT, also referred to as the finger oscillation test) and strength of grip (SOG) tests are well-established neuropsychological measures of basic motor function and the integrity of the corticospinal tract (CST; Lezak et al., 2012). A simple finger movement and/or SOG task performed in the MRI scanner during fMRI activates contralateral motor cortex and anatomically is dependent on CST intactness, as is shown in Figure 13.12 (lower left image). FT and SOG measures are well suited for fMRI and have been appropriately used to define and assess motor cortex and motor networks (Roessner et al., 2013; Rosso et al., 2013; Specogna et al., 2012). Notably, the CST readily can be defined using DTI, as already depicted in Figure 13.1 (star) as well as in Figure 13.12. Importantly, CST integrity assessed with the DTI-derived fractional anisotropy (FA) metric, (also depicted in Figure 13.12) is associated with finger tapping speed scores (Travers et al., 2015).

FreeSurfer provides automated volumetric findings of motor cortex, and resting state addresses connectivity strength between the two motor cortices and other regions within the motor network, as shown in Figure 13.12 (Rehme & Grefkes, 2013). In resting state, the synchronicity of the blood oxygen level dependent (BOLD) MR signal is used to infer connectivity. As depicted in Figure 13.13, two points in homologous occipital regions are examined for how synchronized and in phase the BOLD signal is. The correlation can be visually plotted with a color activation map that highlights the regions at rest that are connected. The same principle can be applied by specifically examining a particular ROI within one hemisphere and, in turn, examining what is in phase in the opposite hemisphere. As an example, in Figure 13.13 (right image), when one motor cortex is used as the "seed point" (left hemisphere in the dorsal surface rendering of the brain on the right), the area in the other hemisphere that shows connectivity is, indeed, just the motor cortex. In other words, when the in-phase oscillation of the BOLD signal in one brain region exhibits similar correlated BOLD activity in another, the assumption is that synchronicity between brain regions indicates that they are connected. In resting state, fMRI BOLD synchronicity implies connectivity.

Currently, *all* that neuropsychology can do is report FT and SOG performance findings on an individual patient compared to some normative standard and then make an "inference" about the integrity of the individual's motor network. With the current state of computational and quantitative neuroimaging, this traditional approach does not utilize the available information that directly

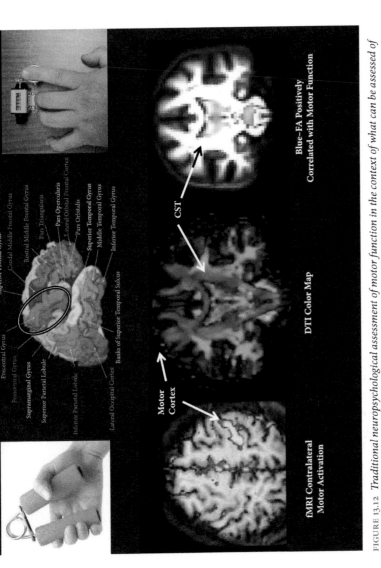

**FIGURE 13.12** *Traditional neuropsychological assessment of motor function in the context of what can be assessed of motor areas with neuroimaging. Upper left depicts measuring strength of grip (SOG), with the upper right illustration showing the finger tapping (TP) task. The upper middle illustration has motor cortex circled on an image from FreeSurfer, indicating that motor cortex volume may be computed. Lower left shows fMRI activation during contralateral FT or SOG assessment, with the bottom middle and right depicting where the corticospinal tract is located using DTI and how fractional anisotropy (FA) is positively correlated with motor function. If all of these assessment tools were used in evaluating a patient, not only would there be motor performance information, but it would be integrated with neuroimaging to provide a more complete picture of motor functioning. The FA plots are from Travers et al. (2015).*

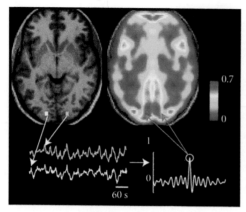
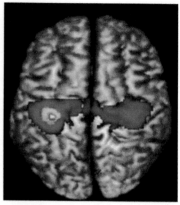

FIGURE 13.13   *(Left) The yellow and blue squares are positioned within the homologous occipital regions of each hemisphere, with their respective patterns of fluctuations in blood oxygen level dependent (BOLD) signal assessed at rest by merely having the subject lie in the scanner. Note the similar rhythmic fluctuations between the two hemispheres, which can be correlated and placed on a T1 co-registered image showing which areas are most in phase, indicating connectivity. (From Anderson et al., 2011; used with permission from Oxford University Press.) (Right) The image on the right also demonstrates at-rest connectivity but with a different technique. In this case, motor cortex in one hemisphere was used as a seed point, with functional connectivity mapping performed in the other hemisphere to determine where BOLD signal was most in phase. As can be seen in the illustration, the two motor cortices are most correlated. These kinds of techniques can be used to assess which brain regions are most connected and connectivity strength between two regions. (From Rehme & Grefkes, 2013; used with permission.)*

addresses anatomical integrity of the motor system and that could be integrated with neuroimaging findings. As shown in Figures 13.12 and 13.13, a multimodality approach could be used to integrate the neuropsychological ST and SOG findings with neuroimaging, so that the integrity of the motor network can be measured and assessed behaviorally, motorically, and anatomically. With such an integrated approach, the traditional behavioral motor performance of the patient is reported in reference to a standard normative database, but likewise the anatomical integrity and connectivity of motor ROIs are volumetrically and functionally compared to an anatomical database involving both fMRI activation and resting-state studies. Finally, tracts that are part of the network could be identified and assessed.

In this demonstration, the example in Figure 13.12 involved only the motor system, but similar discrete cognitive probes for major domains of function could also be developed. Potentially, one very viable approach to achieve this goal is the NIH Toolbox for cognitive assessment. Part of the toolbox development was specifically designed so that some of the cognitive probes could be adapted to fMRI (Gershon et al., 2013). If such a goal is achieved, then using the motor system analogy as described above will allow functional neuroimaging to assist in defining networks as outlined in Figure 13.3 with ROI volumetric and tract-based studies that will assess anatomical integrity. In this scenario, neuropsychological findings would not be presented in isolation, but always integrated with neuroimaging.

## The Brain at Rest and Why It Is so Important for Neuropsychology

As introduced above, resting-state (rs)· functional connectivity (fc) MRI or rs-fcMRI has major implications for neuropsychology. It has the potential to reveal networks and connectivity strength with the patient merely lying in the scanner at rest (Chen & Glover, 2015b; Duchek et al., 2013; Posner, Park, & Wang, 2014; Vogel, Power, Petersen, & Schlaggar, 2010). The rs-fcMRI sequence can be obtained at the end of a routine set of image sequences used for volumetric, anatomical, and pathological studies, with all of the rs-fcMRI analyses done during postprocessing of the images. Interestingly, studying the brain at rest is not limited to fMRI techniques: electroencephalography (EEG) and magnetoencephalography (MEG; see de Pasquale, Penna, Sporns, Romani, & Corbetta, 2015; Engels et al., 2015) can be similarly used to derive brain networks.

Neuropsychology uses assessment techniques that actively engage brain function (Lezak et al., 2012). All current measures of neurocognitive functioning require the participant/patient's involvement in a task and measure a behavioral response. However, neuropsychology has no standardized measures of brain function at rest. Simply observing a patient at rest does not permit the neuropsychologist to make any kind of statement about brain function or neural integrity other than the patient "appears" to be "resting."

Nonetheless, functional neuroimaging and electrophysiological techniques that permit network extraction undertaken while the patient is not engaging in any cognitive or behavioral test and appears to just be at rest, although there are limits on whether the patient is truly at rest (see Barkhof, Haller, & Rombouts, 2014), can be integrated with current neuropsychological methods. It may be that advanced neuroimaging and/or physiological indices of brain networks and connectivity are identified first. Once a network deficit is identified, then, depending on where in the brain and which networks are affected, neuropsychological tests explore cognitive and behavioral domains that may be relevant.

On the other hand, if neuropsychological assessment test findings are obtained prior to neuroimaging and implicate a particular network as damaged/dysfunctional, such findings could, in turn, direct where in the brain resting-state connectivity is examined. Such an approach would assist neuropsychology in relating abnormal test findings to where neural pathology may reside in the individual patient. If neuropsychology integrates its findings with neuroimaging, then much more could be said about the intactness of brain systems or where pathology may reside that is disrupting neurocognitive or neurobehavioral functioning.

Additionally, resting-state functional connectivity mapping can provide connectivity network diagrams that show the degree to which network connections are typical or atypical at rest, which in turn permits exploration of network integrity based on DTI metrics (Ribeiro, Lacerda, & Ferreira, 2015), or what is referred to as structural covariance, that examines the symmetry/similarity of gray matter structures (Zielinski et al., 2012).

Currently, MEG, EEG and event-related potentials extracted from EEG during a cognitive task can be displayed on topographic representations of the brain, which can also be examined in the context of certain neuropsychological tasks, in particular error processing (Logan, Hill, & Larson, 2015; Vigliocco, Vinson, Druks, Barber, & Cappa, 2011). What is important in today's technological world is that all of these techniques may be integrated with, and superimposed on, three-dimensional imaging using MRI to show where normal and/or abnormal activation patterns occur (Gevins, 1998; Nowell et al., 2015). Space does not permit discussion of the advances in physiological monitoring relevant to this topic but what is particularly important about quantitative EEG methods is that they are inexpensive and don't have any of the limitations of MRI. Suffice it to say that integrated physiological monitoring techniques, in addition to MRI and fMRI, assimilated with network theory and analysis of brain function may provide the best approach to interpreting neurocognitive disorders (Sharp, Scott, & Leech, 2014). EEG-based neurocognitive assessment techniques include the ability to measure processing speed with millisecond precision (Clawson, Clayson, South, Bigler, & Larson, 2015) and to be integrated with neuroimaging (Nishida et al., 2015; van Graan, Lemieux, & Chaudhary, 2015). Dennis et al. (2015) and Ellis et al. (2016) have used this approach in assessing children with TBI, specifically demonstrating that the electrophysiological indices of interhemispheric transfer times integrated with quantitative neuroimaging provide superior information about intact and damaged neural systems in brain injury.

## Multimodal Multidimensional Presentation of Neuroimaging and Neuropsychological Findings—The Future

Fagerholm, Hellyer, Scott, Leech, and Sharp (2015) provide a rationale for how to assess imaging studies in the service of neuropsychological outcome, as shown in Figure 13.14. In their study, which involved individuals with TBI, ROI segmentation was used to identify start points that allowed identification of WM interhemispheric connectivity, combined with methods to assess tract FA as a marker of tract health (an aggregate regional indicator of axonal integrity). From this, a WM connectivity matrix could be generated to serve two purposes—patient classification and prediction of neuropsychological outcome.

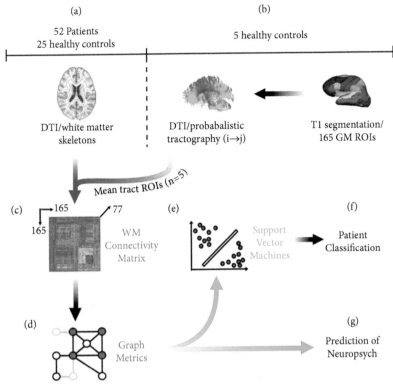

(a)

52 Patients
25 healthy controls

(b)

5 healthy controls

DTI/white matter
skeletons

DTI/probabalistic
tractography (i→j)

T1 segmentation/
165 GM ROIs

Mean tract ROIs (n=5)

(c) 165 77

165

(e)

WM
Connectivity
Matrix

Support
Vector
Machines

(f)

Patient
Classification

(d)

Graph
Metrics

(g)

Prediction of
Neuropsych

FIGURE 13.14 *(A) Tract-based spatial statistics (TBSS) is a method for group analysis of the fractional anisotropy (FA) metric from DTI. The green lines reflect midpoints in white matter tracts, referred to as a skeleton. In this manner, large data comparisons can be automated for analyzing DTI findings. The illustration also shows how additional anatomical and DTI information can be incorporated into developing a connectivity matrix (plotting findings from one hemisphere with the other). The information is then used to differentiate individuals with TBI from uninjured controls and to relate to neuropsychological outcome. While the illustration demonstrates a group approach, the approach can be adapted for assessing the individual. (Image from Fagerholm et al., 2015; used with permission from Oxford University Press.)*

Even more complicated connectivity matrices may be developed if resting-state fMRI data are included (Chen & Glover, 2015a). Irimia, Chambers, Torgerson, and Van Horn (2012) provide a first-step graphic on how best to display connectivity findings, as is presented in Figure 13.15. This is referred to as a connectogram.

The connectogram provides a nice graphical display of where connectivity is present, along with connectivity strength. Exactly how to integrate the neuropsychological finding with the connectogram is what is missing at this time. However, as the neuropsychological relations of brain networks and function become established, it seems a straightforward next step to integrate the neuropsychological with a connectogram or connectogram-like presentation.

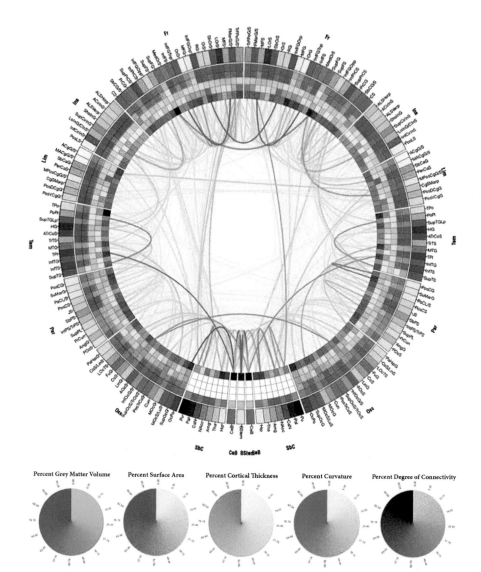

FIGURE 13.15 *A connectogram—which integrates volumetric, thickness, surface area, shape, and strength of connectivity by utilizing multiple neuroimaging data points. What has not been integrated is how to show neuropsychological test correlates, but something along these lines will likely be a future method for showing neuroimaging findings in individual patients that graphically includes complex morphometric data. From Irimia et al. (2012); used with permission.*

# Conclusion

In a recent interview in *Science* (July 17, 2015, Volume 349, issue 6245), Albert "Skip" Rizzo, Ph.D., who has been at the forefront of providing healthcare information and psychotherapy via a computer-based virtual human interface (see Rizzo et al., 2011), is quoted as stating that technological advances are "dragging clinical psychology kicking and screaming into the 21st century" (p. 251). This chapter lodges the same claim about neuropsychology. Clinical psychology and neuropsychology cannot ignore the avalanche of technology that is descending on the field. This chapter provides a potential roadmap for how the integration of neuroimaging and neuropsychology can proceed. As reviewed, the tradition in neuropsychology has been to administer behavioral tests and make inferences about brain function, without necessarily directly measuring any aspect of brain anatomy or physiology. In light of current technology, that approach cannot be sustained.

# Note

1. Actually Francis Galton and his book *Human Faculty and its Development* in 1883 was the first, but his assessment methods were unsuccessful (see Burbridge, D. (2001). Francis Galton on twins, heredity and social class. *British Journal for the History of Science 34* (3), 323–340. doi:10.1017/S0007087401004332).

# References

Allen, M. D., & Fong, A. K. (2008a). Clinical application of standardized cognitive assessment using fMRI. I. Matrix reasoning. *Behavioural Neurology, 20*(3), 127–140. doi:10.3233/BEN-2008-0223

Allen, M. D., & Fong, A. K. (2008b). Clinical application of standardized cognitive assessment using fMRI. II. Verbal fluency. *Behavioural Neurology, 20*(3), 141–152. doi:10.3233/BEN-2008-0224

Ambrose, J., & Hounsfield, G. (1973). Computerized transverse axial tomography. *The British Journal of Radiology, 46*(542), 148–149.

Anastasi, A. (1968). *Psychologcal testing,* (3rd Ed). Macmillan Psychological Testing, Oxford: England.

Anderson, J. S., Druzgal, T. J., Froehlich, A., DuBray, M. B., Lange, N., Alexander, A. L., ... Lainhart, J. E. (2011). Decreased interhemispheric functional connectivity in autism. *Cerebral Cortex, 21*(5), 1134–1146. doi:10.1093/cercor/bhq190

Arenth, P. M., Russell, K. C., Scanlon, J. M., Kessler, L. J., & Ricker, J. H. (2012). Encoding and recognition after traumatic brain injury: Neuropsychological and functional magnetic resonance imaging findings. *Journal of Clinical and Experimental Neuropsychology, 34*(4), 333–344. doi:10.1080/13803395.2011.633896

Avants, B. B., Tustison, N. J., Wu, J., Cook, P. A., & Gee, J. C. (2011). An open source multivariate framework for n-tissue segmentation with evaluation on public data. *Neuroinformatics*, 9(4), 381–400. doi:10.1007/s12021-011-9109-y

Barkhof, F., Haller, S., & Rombouts, S. A. (2014). Resting-state functional MR imaging: A new window to the brain. *Radiology*, 272(1), 29–49. doi:10.1148/radiol.14132388

Bernhardt, B. C., Hong, S., Bernasconi, A., & Bernasconi, N. (2013). Imaging structural and functional brain networks in temporal lobe epilepsy. *Frontiers in Human Neuroscience*, 7, 624. doi:10.3389/fnhum.2013.00624

Bick, A. S., Mayer, A., & Levin, N. (2012). From research to clinical practice: implementation of functional magnetic imaging and white matter tractography in the clinical environment. *Journal of the Neurological Sciences*, 312(1–2), 158–165. doi:10.1016/j.jns.2011.07.040

Bigler, E. D. (1988). Frontal lobe damage and neuropsychological assessment. *Archives of Clinical Neuropsychology: The Official Journal of the National Academy of Neuropsychologists*, 3(3), 279–297.

Bigler, E. D. (2015a). Structural image analysis of the brain in neuropsychology using magnetic resonance imaging (MRI) techniques. *Neuropsychology Review*, 25(3):224–249. doi:10.1007/s11065-015-9290-0

Bigler, E. D. (2015b). Structural neuroimaging. *Neuropsychology Review*, 25(3), 224–249.

Bigler, E. D., Abildskov, T. J., Wilde, E. A., McCauley, S. R., Li, X., Merkley, T. L., . . . Levin, H. S. (2010). Diffuse damage in pediatric traumatic brain injury: A comparison of automated versus operator-controlled quantification methods. *NeuroImage*, 50(3), 1017–1026. doi:10.1016/j.neuroimage.2010.01.003

Bornstein, R. A., & Matarazzo, J. D. (1984). Relationship of sex and the effects of unilateral lesions on the Wechsler Intelligence Scales. Further considerations. *The Journal of Nervous and Mental Disease*, 172(12), 707–710.

Canini, M., Battista, P., Della Rosa, P. A., Catricala, E., Salvatore, C., Gilardi, M. C., & Castiglioni, I. (2014). Computerized neuropsychological assessment in aging: Testing efficacy and clinical ecology of different interfaces. *Computational and Mathematical Methods in Medicine*, 2014, 804723. doi:10.1155/2014/804723

Casaletto, K. B., Umlauf, A., Beaumont, J., Gershon, R., Slotkin, J., Akshoomoff, N., & Heaton, R. K. (2015). Demographically corrected normative standards for the English version of the NIH Toolbox Cognition Battery. *Journal of the International Neuropsychological Society: JINS*, 21(5), 378–391. doi:10.1017/S1355617715000351

Catani, M., Dell'acqua, F., Bizzi, A., Forkel, S. J., Williams, S. C., Simmons, A., . . . Thiebaut de Schotten, M. (2012). Beyond cortical localization in clinico-anatomical correlation. *Cortex; A Journal Devoted to the Study of the Nervous System and Behavior*, 48(10), 1262–1287. doi:10.1016/j.cortex.2012.07.001

Chen, J. E., & Glover, G. H. (2015). Functional magnetic resonance imaging methods. *Neuropsychol Review*. doi:10.1007/s11065-015-9294-9

Cipolotti, L., & Warrington, E. K. (1995). Neuropsychological assessment. *Journal of Neurology, Neurosurgery, and Psychiatry*, 58(6), 655–664.

Clawson, A., Clayson, P. E., South, M., Bigler, E. D., & Larson, M. J. (2015). An electrophysiological investigation of interhemispheric transfer time in children and adolescents with high-functioning autism spectrum disorders. *Journal of Autism and Developmental Disorders*, 45(2), 363–375. doi:10.1007/s10803-013-1895-7 de Pasquale, F., Penna, S. D., Sporns, O., Romani, G. L., & Corbetta, M. (2016). A dynamic core network and global efficiency in the resting human brain. *Cerebral Cortex, 10*, 4015–4033.doi:10.1093/cercor/bhv185

Dennis, E. L., Ellis, M. U., Marion, S. D., Jin, Y., Moran, L., Olsen, A., . . . Asarnow, R. F. (2015). Callosal function in pediatric traumatic brain injury linked to disrupted white matter integrity. *The Journal of Neuroscience: The Official Journal of the Society for Neuroscience, 35*(28), 10202–10211. doi:10.1523/JNEUROSCI.1595-15.2015

Desikan, R. S., Cabral, H. J., Hess, C. P., Dillon, W. P., Glastonbury, C. M., Weiner, M. W., . . . Fischl, B. (2009). Automated MRI measures identify individuals with mild cognitive impairment and Alzheimer's disease. *Brain:A Journal of Neurology, 132*(Pt. 8), 2048–2057. doi:10.1093/brain/awp123

Desikan, R. S., Segonne, F., Fischl, B., Quinn, B. T., Dickerson, B. C., Blacker, D., . . . Killiany, R. J. (2006). An automated labeling system for subdividing the human cerebral cortex on MRI scans into gyral based regions of interest. *NeuroImage, 31*(3), 968–980. doi:10.1016/j.neuroimage.2006.01.021

Destrieux, C., Fischl, B., Dale, A., & Halgren, E. (2010). Automatic parcellation of human cortical gyri and sulci using standard anatomical nomenclature. *NeuroImage, 53*(1), 1–15. doi:10.1016/j.neuroimage.2010.06.010

Duchek, J. M., Balota, D. A., Thomas, J. B., Snyder, A. Z., Rich, P., Benzinger, T. L., . . . Ances, B. M. (2013). Relationship between Stroop performance and resting state functional connectivity in cognitively normal older adults. *Neuropsychology, 27*(5), 516–528. doi:10.1037/a0033402

Ecker, C., Bookheimer, S. Y., & Murphy, D. G. (2015). Neuroimaging in autism spectrum disorder: Brain structure and function across the lifespan. *The Lancet. Neurology, 14*(11), 1121–1134. doi:10.1016/S1474-4422(15)00050-2

Ellis, M. U., Marion, S. D., McArthur, D. L., Babikian, T., Giza, C. C., Kernan, C. L., . . . Asarnow, R. F. (2016). The UCLA study of children with moderate to severe traumatic brain injury: Event-related potential measure of interhemispheric transfer time. *Journal of Neurotrauma, 33*(11), 990–996. doi:10.1089/neu.2015.4023

Engels, M. M., Stam, C. J., van der Flier, W. M., Scheltens, P., de Waal, H., & van Straaten, E. C. (2015). Declining functional connectivity and changing hub locations in Alzheimer's disease: An EEG study. *BMC Neurology, 15*, 145. doi:10.1186/s12883-015-0400-7

Fagerholm, E. D., Hellyer, P. J., Scott, G., Leech, R., & Sharp, D. J. (2015). Disconnection of network hubs and cognitive impairment after traumatic brain injury. *Brain: A Journal of Neurology, 138*(Pt. 6), 1696–1709. doi:10.1093/brain/awv075

Fischl, B. (2012). FreeSurfer. *NeuroImage, 62*(2), 774–781. doi:10.1016/j.neuroimage.2012.01.021

Gershon, R. C., Wagster, M. V., Hendrie, H. C., Fox, N. A., Cook, K. F., & Nowinski, C. J. (2013). NIH toolbox for assessment of neurological and behavioral function. *Neurology, 80*(11 Suppl. 3), S2–S6. doi:10.1212/WNL.0b013e3182872e5f

Gess, J. L., Fausett, J. S., Kearney-Ramos, T. E., Kilts, C. D., & James, G. A. (2014). Task-dependent recruitment of intrinsic brain networks reflects normative variance in cognition. *Brain and Behavior, 4*(5), 650–664. doi:10.1002/brb3.243

Gevins, A. (1998). The future of electroencephalography in assessing neurocognitive functioning. *Electroencephalography and Clinical Neurophysiology, 106*(2), 165–172.

Glees, P. (1947). The significance of the frontal lobe connections in mental diseases. *Experientia, 3*(10), 394–397.

Gleichgerrcht, E., Fridriksson, J., & Bonilha, L. (2015). Neuroanatomical foundations of naming impairments across different neurologic conditions. *Neurology, 85*(3), 284–292. doi:10.1212/WNL.0000000000001765

Godsil, B. P., Kiss, J. P., Spedding, M., & Jay, T. M. (2013). The hippocampal-prefrontal pathway: The weak link in psychiatric disorders? *European Neuropsychopharmacology: The Journal of the European College of Neuropsychopharmacology, 23*(10), 1165–1181. doi:10.1016/j.euroneuro.2012.10.018

Goldenberg, G., Oder, W., Spatt, J., & Podreka, I. (1992). Cerebral correlates of disturbed executive function and memory in survivors of severe closed head injury: A SPECT study. *Journal of Neurology, Neurosurgery, and Psychiatry, 55*(5), 362–368.

Heaton, R. K., Akshoomoff, N., Tulsky, D., Mungas, D., Weintraub, S., Dikmen, S., . . . Gershon, R. (2014). Reliability and validity of composite scores from the NIH Toolbox Cognition Battery in adults. *Journal of the International Neuropsychological Society: JINS, 20*(6), 588–598. doi:10.1017/S1355617714000241

Houdas, Y., & Ring, E. F. J. (1982). *Human body temperature.* New York: Springer.

Hounsfield, G. N. (1973). Computerized transverse axial scanning (tomography). 1. Description of system. *The British Journal of Radiology, 46*(552), 1016–1022. doi:10.1259/0007-1285-46-552-1016

Hounsfield, G. N. (1980). Computed medical imaging. Nobel lecture, December 8, 1979. *Journal of Computer Assisted Tomography, 4*(5), 665–674.

Irimia, A., Chambers, M. C., Torgerson, C. M., & Van Horn, J. D. (2012). Circular representation of human cortical networks for subject and population-level connectomic visualization. *NeuroImage, 60*(2), 1340–1351. doi:10.1016/j.neuroimage.2012.01.107

Iscan, Z., Jin, T. B., Kendrick, A., Szeglin, B., Lu, H., Trivedi, M., . . . DeLorenzo, C. (2015). Test-retest reliability of Freesurfer measurements within and between sites: Effects of visual approval process. *Human Brain Mapping, 36*(9), 3472–3485. doi:10.1002/hbm.22856

Iverson, G. L., & Schatz, P. (2015). Advanced topics in neuropsychological assessment following sport-related concussion. *Brain Injury, 29*(2), 263–275. doi:10.3109/02699052.2014.965214

Jack, C. R., Jr., Barnes, J., Bernstein, M. A., Borowski, B. J., Brewer, J., Clegg, S., . . . Weiner, M. (2015). Magnetic resonance imaging in Alzheimer's Disease Neuroimaging Initiative 2. *Alzheimer's & Dementia: The Journal of the Alzheimer's Association, 11*(7), 740–756. doi:10.1016/j.jalz.2015.05.002

Jack, C. R., Jr., Twomey, C. K., Zinsmeister, A. R., Sharbrough, F. W., Petersen, R. C., & Cascino, G. D. (1989). Anterior temporal lobes and hippocampal formations: Normative volumetric measurements from MR images in young adults. *Radiology, 172*(2), 549–554. doi:10.1148/radiology.172.2.2748838

Jensen, B. N., Jensen, F. S., Madsen, S. N., & Lossl, K. (2000). Accuracy of digital tympanic, oral, axillary, and rectal thermometers compared with standard rectal mercury thermometers. *The European Journal of Surgery (Acta Chirurgica), 166*(11), 848–851. doi:10.1080/110241500447218

Lezak, M. D., Howieson, D. B., Bigler, E. D., & Tranel, D. (2012). *Neuropsychological assessment.* New York: Oxford University Press.

Logan, D. M., Hill, K. R., & Larson, M. J. (2015). Cognitive control of conscious error awareness: Error awareness and error positivity (Pe) amplitude in moderate-to-severe traumatic brain injury (TBI). *Frontiers in Human Neuroscience, 9,* 397. doi:10.3389/fnhum.2015.00397

Marx, J. L. (1980). NMR opens a new window into the body. The use of nuclear magnetic resonance for medical diagnosis hovers on the brink of practical application. *Science, 210*(4467), 302–305.

McAndrews, M. P. (2014). Memory assessment in the clinical context using functional magnetic resonance imaging: A critical look at the state of the field. *Neuroimaging Clinics of North America, 24*(4), 585–597. doi:10.1016/j.nic.2014.07.008

McGee, T. D. (1988). *Principles and methods of temperature measurement.* New York: Wiley.

McKenzie, K. G., & Proctor, L. D. (1946). Bilateral frontal lobe leucotomy in the treatment of mental disease. *Canadian Medical Association Journal, 55*(5), 433–441.

Moscovitch, M., Rosenbaum, R. S., Gilboa, A., Addis, D. R., Westmacott, R., Grady, C., . . . Nadel, L. (2005). Functional neuroanatomy of remote episodic, semantic and spatial memory: A unified account based on multiple trace theory. *Journal of Anatomy, 207*(1), 35–66. doi:10.1111/j.1469-7580.2005.00421.x

Mungas, D., Heaton, R., Tulsky, D., Zelazo, P. D., Slotkin, J., Blitz, D., . . . Gershon, R. (2014). Factor structure, convergent validity, and discriminant validity of the NIH Toolbox Cognitive Health Battery (NIHTB-CHB) in adults. *Journal of the International Neuropsychological Society: JINS, 20*(6), 579–587. doi:10.1017/S1355617714000307

Negrin, J., Jr. (1953a). Frontal lobe syndrome in thrombosis of the internal carotid artery. *The Journal of Nervous and Mental Disease, 118*(6), 559–560.

Negrin, J., Jr. (1953b). Frontal lobe syndrome in thrombosis of the internal carotid artery. *A.M.A. Archives of Neurology and Psychiatry, 70*(4), 530–532.

Nisbet, W. (1971). Digital display of temperature using copper constantan thermocouples. *The Journal of Physiology, 217*(Suppl.), 2P–3P.

Nishida, K., Razavi, N., Jann, K., Yoshimura, M., Dierks, T., Kinoshita, T., & Koenig, T. (2015). Integrating different aspects of resting brain activity: A review of electroencephalographic signatures in resting state networks derived from functional magnetic resonance imaging. *Neuropsychobiology, 71*(1), 6–16. doi:10.1159/000363342

Nowell, M., Rodionov, R., Zombori, G., Sparks, R., Winston, G., Kinghorn, J., . . . Duncan, J. (2015). Utility of 3D multimodality imaging in the implantation of intracranial electrodes in epilepsy. *Epilepsia, 56*(3), 403–413. doi:10.1111/epi.12924

Nowrangi, M. A., Lyketsos, C., Rao, V., & Munro, C. A. (2014). Systematic review of neuroimaging correlates of executive functioning: Converging evidence from different clinical populations. *The Journal of Neuropsychiatry and Clinical Neurosciences, 26*(2), 114–125. doi:10.1176/appi.neuropsych.12070176

O'Callaghan, C., Shine, J. M., Lewis, S. J., Andrews-Hanna, J. R., & Irish, M. (2015). Shaped by our thoughts—A new task to assess spontaneous cognition and its associated neural correlates in the default network. *Brain and Cognition, 93,* 1–10. doi:10.1016/j.bandc.2014.11.001

Ochs, A. L., Ross, D. E., Zannoni, M. D., Abildskov, T. J., & Bigler, E. D. (2015). Comparison of automated brain volume measures obtained with NeuroQuant® and FreeSurfer. *Journal of Neuroimaging: Official Journal of the American Society of Neuroimaging, 25*(5), 721–727. doi:10.1111/jon.12229

Parks, E. L., & Madden, D. J. (2013). Brain connectivity and visual attention. *Brain Connectivity, 3*(4), 317–338. doi:10.1089/brain.2012.0139

Pearn, J. (2012). Sir George Shuckburgh Evelyn (1751–1804): Precision in thermometry. *Journal of Medical Biography, 20*(1), 42–46. doi:10.1258/jmb.2011.011005

Posner, J., Park, C., & Wang, Z. (2014). Connecting the dots: A review of resting connectivity MRI studies in attention-deficit/hyperactivity disorder. *Neuropsychol Review, 24*(1), 3–15. doi:10.1007/s11065-014-9251-z

Raichle, M. E. (2011). The restless brain. *Brain Connectivity, 1*(1), 3–12. doi:10.1089/brain.2011.0019

Raji, C. A., Eyre, H., Wei, S. H., Bredesen, D. E., Moylan, S., Law, M., . . . Vernooij, M. W. (2015). Hot topics in research: Preventive neuroradiology in brain aging and cognitive decline. *AJNR. American Journal of Neuroradiology, 36*(10), 1803–1809. doi:10.3174/ajnr.A4409

Rehme, A. K., & Grefkes, C. (2013). Cerebral network disorders after stroke: Evidence from imaging-based connectivity analyses of active and resting brain states in humans. *The Journal of Physiology, 591*(Pt. 1), 17–31. doi:10.1113/jphysiol.2012.243469

Ribeiro, A. S., Lacerda, L. M., & Ferreira, H. A. (2015). Multimodal Imaging Brain Connectivity Analysis (MIBCA) toolbox. *PeerJ, 3,* e1078. doi:10.7717/peerj.1078

Rizzo, A. A., Lange, B., Buckwalter, J. G., Forbell, E., Kim, J., Sagae, K., . . . Kenny, P. (2011). An intelligent virtual human system for providing healthcare information and support. *Studies in Health Technology and Informatics, 163,* 503–509.

Rocca, M. A., Amato, M. P., De Stefano, N., Enzinger, C., Geurts, J. J., Penner, I. K., . . . Filippi, M. (2015). Clinical and imaging assessment of cognitive dysfunction in multiple sclerosis. *The Lancet. Neurology, 14*(3), 302–317. doi:10.1016/S1474-4422(14)70250-9

Roessner, V., Wittfoth, M., August, J. M., Rothenberger, A., Baudewig, J., & Dechent, P. (2013). Finger tapping-related activation differences in treatment-naive pediatric Tourette syndrome: A comparison of the preferred and nonpreferred hand. *Journal of Child Psychology and Psychiatry, and Allied Disciplines, 54*(3), 273–279. doi:10.1111/j.1469-7610.2012.02584.x

Rossignoli, I., Benito, P. J., & Herrero, A. J. (2015). Reliability of infrared thermography in skin temperature evaluation of wheelchair users. *Spinal Cord, 53,* 243–248. doi:10.1038/sc.2014.212

Rosso, C., Valabregue, R., Attal, Y., Vargas, P., Gaudron, M., Baronnet, F., . . . Samson, Y. (2013). Contribution of corticospinal tract and functional connectivity in hand motor impairment after stroke. *PloS One, 8*(9), e73164. doi:10.1371/journal.pone.0073164

Saykin, A. J., Shen, L., Yao, X., Kim, S., Nho, K., Risacher, S. L., . . . Alzheimer's Disease Neuroimaging Initiative. (2015). Genetic studies of quantitative MCI and AD phenotypes in ADNI: Progress, opportunities, and plans. *Alzheimer's & Dementia: The Journal of the Alzheimer's Association, 11*(7), 792–814. doi:10.1016/j.jalz.2015.05.009

Sharp, D. J., Scott, G., & Leech, R. (2014). Network dysfunction after traumatic brain injury. *Nature Reviews. Neurology, 10*(3), 156–166. doi:10.1038/nrneurol.2014.15

Shaw, E. E., Schultz, A. P., Sperling, R. A., & Hedden, T. (2015). Functional connectivity in multiple cortical networks is associated with performance across cognitive domains in older adults. *Brain Connectivity, 5*(8), 505–516. doi:10.1089/brain.2014.0327

Small, G. W., Bookheimer, S. Y., Thompson, P. M., Cole, G. M., Huang, S. C., Kepe, V., & Barrio, J. R. (2008). Current and future uses of neuroimaging for cognitively impaired patients. *The Lancet. Neurology, 7*(2), 161–172. doi:10.1016/S1474-4422(08)70019-X

Sowell, E. R., Lu, L. H., O'Hare, E. D., McCourt, S. T., Mattson, S. N., O'Connor, M. J., & Bookheimer, S. Y. (2007). Functional magnetic resonance imaging of verbal learning in children with heavy prenatal alcohol exposure. *Neuroreport, 18*(7), 635–639. doi:10.1097/WNR.0b013e3280bad8dc

Specogna, I., Casagrande, F., Lorusso, A., Catalan, M., Gorian, A., Zugna, L., . . . Cova, M. A. (2012). Functional MRI during the execution of a motor task in patients with multiple sclerosis and fatigue. *La Radiologia Medica, 117*(8), 1398–1407. doi:10.1007/s11547-012-0845-3

Stern, W. (1912). *Psychologische Methoden der Intelligenz-Pnufung.* Leipzig: Barth.

Strangman, G. E., O'Neil-Pirozzi, T. M., Supelana, C., Goldstein, R., Katz, D. I., & Glenn, M. B. (2010). Regional brain morphometry predicts memory rehabilitation outcome after traumatic brain injury. *Frontiers in Human Neuroscience, 4*, 182. doi:10.3389/fnhum.2010.00182

Sugarman, M. A., Woodard, J. L., Nielson, K. A., Seidenberg, M., Smith, J. C., Durgerian, S., & Rao, S. M. (2012). Functional magnetic resonance imaging of semantic memory as a presymptomatic biomarker of Alzheimer's disease risk. *Biochimica et Biophysica Acta, 1822*(3), 442–456. doi:10.1016/j.bbadis.2011.09.016

Sullivan, E. V., & Bigler, E. D. (2015). Neuroimaging's role in neuropsychology: Introduction to the special issue of *Neuropsychology Review* on neuroimaging in neuropsychology. *Neuropsychology Review, 25*(3), 221–223. doi:10.1007/s11065-015-9296-7

Sundermann, B., Herr, D., Schwindt, W., & Pfleiderer, B. (2014). Multivariate classification of blood oxygen level-dependent FMRI data with diagnostic intention: A clinical perspective. *AJNR. American Journal of Neuroradiology, 35*(5), 848–855. doi:10.3174/ajnr.A3713

Tanner, J. J., Mellott, E., Dunne, E. M., & Price, C. C. (2015). Integrating neuropsychology and brain imaging for a referral of possible pseudodementia: A case report. *The Clinical Neuropsychologist, 29*(2), 272–292. doi:10.1080/13854046.2015.1008047

Thermenos, H. W., Seidman, L. J., Breiter, H., Goldstein, J. M., Goodman, J. M., Poldrack, R., . . . Tsuang, M. T. (2004). Functional magnetic resonance imaging during auditory verbal working memory in nonpsychotic relatives of persons with schizophrenia: A pilot study. *Biological Psychiatry, 55*(5), 490–500. doi:10.1016/j.biopsych.2003.11.014

Tomasi, D., Shokri-Kojori, E., & Volkow, N. D. (2015). High-resolution functional connectivity density: Hub locations, sensitivity, specificity, reproducibility, and reliability. *Cerebral Cortex.* doi:10.1093/cercor/bhv171

Travers, B. G., Bigler, E. D., Tromp do, P. M., Adluru, N., Destiche, D., Samsin, D., . . . Lainhart, J. E. (2015). Brainstem white matter predicts individual differences in manual motor difficulties and symptom severity in autism. *Journal of Autism and Developmental Disorders, 45*(9), 3030–3040. doi:10.1007/s10803-015-2467-2469

Tustison, N. J., Cook, P. A., Klein, A., Song, G., Das, S. R., Duda, J. T., . . . Avants, B. B. (2014). Large-scale evaluation of ANTs and FreeSurfer cortical thickness measurements. *NeuroImage, 99*, 166–179. doi:10.1016/j.neuroimage.2014.05.044

van Graan, L. A., Lemieux, L., & Chaudhary, U. J. (2015). Methods and utility of EEG-fMRI in epilepsy. *Quantitative Imaging in Medicine and Surgery, 5*(2), 300–312. doi:10.3978/j.issn.2223-4292.2015.02.04

Vertes, P. E., & Bullmore, E. T. (2015). Annual research review: Growth connectomics— The organization and reorganization of brain networks during normal and abnormal development. *Journal of Child Psychology and Psychiatry, and Allied Disciplines, 56*(3), 299–320. doi:10.1111/jcpp.12365

Vigliocco, G., Vinson, D. P., Druks, J., Barber, H., & Cappa, S. F. (2011). Nouns and verbs in the brain: A review of behavioural, electrophysiological, neuropsychological and imaging studies. *Neuroscience and Biobehavioral Reviews, 35*(3), 407–426. doi:10.1016/j.neubiorev.2010.04.007

Vitali, P., Di Perri, C., Vaudano, A. E., Meletti, S., & Villani, F. (2015). Integration of multimodal neuroimaging methods: A rationale for clinical applications of simultaneous EEG-fMRI. *Functional Neurology, 30*(1), 9–20.

Vogel, A. C., Power, J. D., Petersen, S. E., & Schlaggar, B. L. (2010). Development of the brain's functional network architecture. *Neuropsychol Review, 20*(4), 362–375. doi:10.1007/s11065-010-9145-7

Wechsler, D. (1950). Historical bases for psychological tests. *Proceedings of the Annual Meeting of the American Psychopathological Association*, Discussion 39–44.

Weinberger, D. R. (1993). A connectionist approach to the prefrontal cortex. *The Journal of Neuropsychiatry and Clinical Neurosciences, 5*(3), 241–253.

Weiskopf, N., Mohammadi, S., Lutti, A., & Callaghan, M. F. (2015). Advances in MRI-based computational neuroanatomy: From morphometry to in-vivo histology. *Current Opinion in Neurology, 28*(4), 313–322. doi:10.1097/WCO.0000000000000222

Wilde, E. A., Bouix, S., Tate, D. F., Lin, A. P., Newsome, M. R., Taylor, B. A., . . . York, G. (2015). Advanced neuroimaging applied to veterans and service personnel with traumatic brain injury: State of the art and potential benefits. *Brain Imaging and Behavior, 9*(3), 367–402. doi:10.1007/s11682-015-9444-y

Wilde, E. A., Hunter, J. V., & Bigler, E. D. (2012). A primer of neuroimaging analysis in neurorehabilitation outcome research. *NeuroRehabilitation, 31*(3), 227–242. doi:10.3233/NRE-2012-0793

Zielinski, B. A., Anderson, J. S., Froehlich, A. L., Prigge, M. B., Nielsen, J. A., Cooperrider, J. R., . . . Lainhart, J. E. (2012). scMRI reveals large-scale brain network abnormalities in autism. *PloS One, 7*(11), e49172. doi:10.1371/journal.pone.0049172

# 14

# Multimodal Biomarkers
# to Discriminate Cognitive State

Thomas F. Quatieri, James R. Williamson,

Christopher J. Smalt, Joey Perricone, Tejash Patel,

Laura Brattain, Brian Helfer, Daryush Mehta, Jeffrey Palmer,

Kristin Heaton, Marianna Eddy, and Joseph Moran

Multimodal biomarkers based on behavioral, neurophysiological, and cognitive measurements have recently increased in popularity for the detection of cognitive stress and neurologically based disorders. Such conditions significantly and adversely affect human performance and quality of life in a large fraction of the world's population. Example modalities used in detection of these conditions include speech, facial expression, physiology, eye tracking, gait, and electroencephalography (EEG). Toward the goal of finding simple, noninvasive means to detect, predict, and monitor cognitive stress and neurological conditions, MIT Lincoln Laboratory is developing biomarkers that satisfy three criteria. First, we seek biomarkers that reflect core components of cognitive status, such as working memory capacity, processing speed, attention, and arousal. Second, and as importantly, we seek biomarkers that reflect timing and coordination relations both within components of each modality and across different modalities. This is based on the hypothesis that neural coordination across different parts of the brain is essential in cognition. An example of timing and coordination within a modality is the set of finely timed and synchronized physiological components of speech production, whereas an example of coordination across modalities is the timing and synchrony that occur between speech and facial expression during speaking. Third, we seek multimodal biomarkers that contribute in a complementary fashion under various channel and background conditions.

In this chapter, as an illustration of the biomarker approach, we focus on cognitive stress and the particular case of detecting different cognitive load levels. We also briefly show how similar feature-extraction principles can be applied to a neurological condition through the example of major depressive disorder (MDD). MDD is one of several neuropsychiatric disorders where multimodal biomarkers based on principles of timing and coordination are important for detection (Cummins et al., 2015; Helfer et al., 2014; Quatieri & Malyska, 2012; Trevino, Quatieri, & Malyska, 2011; Williamson, Quatieri, Helfer, Ciccarelli, & Mehta, 2014; Williamson et al., 2013, 2015; Yu, Quatieri, Williamson, & Mundt, 2014). In our cognitive load experiments, we use two easily obtained noninvasive modalities, speech and facial expression, and show how these two modalities can be fused to perform comparably to more difficult-to-obtain "gold-standard" EEG measurements. Speech and facial expression are also used in our MDD case study. Our current focus in both application areas is timing and coordination relations within components of each modality.

The ease of obtaining vocal and facial features (e.g., via mobile tablets or smartphones) greatly increases global accessibility to an automated method for cognitive assessment. Certain vocal and facial features have been shown to change with a subject's mental and emotional state under numerous conditions, including cognitive load and neurological conditions. For speech, the features include characterizations of prosody (e.g., fundamental frequency and speaking rate), spectral representations (e.g., mel-cepstra), and glottal excitation flow patterns, such as flow shape, timing jitter, amplitude shimmer, and aspiration (Canter, 1963, 1965a, 1965b; Darby, Simmons, & Berger, 1984; Dejonckere & Lebacq, 1996; Fava & Kendler, 2000; France, Shiavi, Silverman, Silverman, & Wilkes, 2000; Greden & Carroll, 1981; Logemann, Fisher, Boshes, & Blonsky, 1978; Orozco-Arroyave, Arias-Londoño, Vargas-Bonilla, González-Rátiva, & Nöth, 2014; Ozdas, Shiavi, Silverman, Silverman, & Wilkes, 2004). For facial expression, the features include spectral representations and facial action units (FAUs; Ekman, Freisen, & Ancoli, 1980; Gaebel & Wölwer, 1992). There are many examples of each of the three modalities being used to detect cognitive stress (Boril, Sadjadi, Kleinschmidt, & Hansen, 2010; Khawaja, Ruiz, & Cheng, 2008; Le, Epps, Choi, & Ambikairajah, 2010; Lively, Pisoni, Van Summers, & Bernacki, 1993; Yap, 2011; Yin & Chen, 2007; Yin, Chen, Ruiz, & Ambikairajah, 2008; Zarjam et al., 2011a, 2011b, 2015) and of speech or facial expression modalities being used to detect a variety of neurological conditions, such as depression and Parkinson's disease (Canter, 1963, 1965a, 1965b; Darby et al., 1984; Dejonckere & Lebacq, 1996; Fava & Kendler, 2000; France et al., 2000; Greden & Carroll, 1981; Logemann et al., 1978; Moore, Clements, Peifer, & Weisser, 2003; Mundt, Snyder, Cannizzaro, Chappie, & Geralts, 2007; Orozco-Arroyave et al., 2014; Ozdas et al., 2004). Speech has been used in cognitive load by Yin and colleagues (Yin & Chen, 2008; Yin et al., 2007), who achieved 77% accuracy using standard vocal features (e.g., mel-cepstra, delta-delta mel-cepstra, and shifted mel-cepstra) to discriminate three cognitive load levels in a read story and several questions about the story, and in the Stroop test. FAUs have been used to predict neuropsychiatric disorders (Schmidt, Bhattacharya, & Denlinger, 2009; Wang et al., 2008), whereas EEG entropy and power have been used to discriminate multiple cognitive load levels by Zarjam et al. (2011a, 2011b, 2015).

For all modalities, we use an approach that deviates from convention. While we begin with standard "low-level" features, we build upon them to obtain "high-level" timing- and coordination-based features. For speech, the low-level features are phoneme boundaries, formant (vocal tract resonance) tracks, delta mel-cepstra coefficients (spectral dynamics), and creakiness (vocal-fold period irregularity). For facial expression, the features are FAUs (Littlewort et al., 2011). For EEG, following standard artifact removal, the low-level features are bandpass-filtered signals in the time domain and spectral power features in the frequency domain computed in five frequency bands.

The high-level timing features include (from speech) phoneme-based measures of rate, duration, pitch dynamics, and pause information, and (from facial expression) measures of FAU rate. The high-level coordination features for all modalities are based on eigenspectra analysis of covariance, correlation, and coherence matrices that are constructed from sets of low-level features. Various subsets of these features have been used at MIT Lincoln Laboratory in cognitive stress (Quatieri et al., 2015) and neurocognitive contexts, such as in detection of depression, Parkinson's disease, cognitive impairment, and traumatic brain injury (Cummins et al., 2015; Helfer et al., 2014; Quatieri & Malyska, 2012; Trevino, Quatieri, & Malyska, 2011; Williamson et al., 2013, 2014, 2015; Yu et al., 2014), thus perhaps forming a common feature basis for neurocognitive change.

Detection of cognitive load is used as a case study. However, the algorithms described provide a more general framework for detection of neurocognitive changes from multiple sensing modalities.

The discussion on design of a multimodal platform for cognitive load opens with a novel cognitive load data-collection protocol that taxes auditory working memory by eliciting sentence and digit span recall under varying levels of cognitive load. Then we describe our signal-processing methodology for vocal, facial expression, and EEG feature extraction for detection of cognitive load under this protocol, including approaches to reduce feature dimensionality to reduce the possibility of overfitting to small multimodal datasets. The next section summarizes cognitive load detection results using a Gaussian classifier. Then we show how we can use our principles of timing and coordination to detect MDD from vocal and facial expression signals. The chapter closes with conclusions and projections toward future work.

## Design of a Multimodal Platform for Cognitive Load

Cognitive load is defined loosely as the mental demand experienced for a particular task. Demand can increase or decrease depending on the task and the degree of working memory required (Lively et al., 1993; Yin et al., 2008). Efficient and effective methods are needed to monitor cognitive load under cognitively and physically stressful situations. In many scenarios, environmental and occupational stressors can produce cognitive overload, thereby degrading task performance and endangering safety. Examples of mental stressors are repetitive and/or intense cognitive tasks, psychological stress, and lack of sleep. Physical stressors include intense, long-duration operations and/or heavy loads. Both stressors can cause cognitive load, and often contribute simultaneously to load. Applications for cognitive load assessment include individualized detection of cognitive load in an ambulatory, field, or clinical setting. In clinical applications, the objective is often to find and measure the specific causes of load. In operational settings, the objective is often to quickly assess cognitive ability and readiness under loaded conditions, regardless of their etiology. In designing a multimodal speech/face/EEG database protocol that reflects typical cognitive load conditions, we employed the hypothesis that speech, and the corresponding facial movements that occur in speaking, are complex motor activities requiring precise neural timing and coordination and that manipulating cognitive load level systematically alters this complex motor activity.

Subjects gave informed consent to our working memory–based protocol, which was approved by the MIT Committee on the Use of Humans as Experimental Subjects (COUHES). Audio data were collected with a DPA acoustic lapel microphone (with a Roland Octa-Capture audio interface), facial video with a Canon high-definition video camera, and EEG signals with a 64-element Neuroscan device. The collection platform is shown in Figure 14.1.

Following setup and training, each subject engages in the primary task of verbally recalling sentences with varying levels of cognitive load, as determined by the number of digits being held in working memory (Hansberger, Wright, & Pisoni, 2008; Le, Ambikairajah, Choi, & Epps, 2009). Specifically, a single trial of the auditory working memory task comprises the following: the subject's hearing a string of digits, then hearing a sentence, then waiting for a tone eliciting spoken recall of the sentence, followed by another tone eliciting recall of the digits. This task is administered with three difficulty levels, involving 108 trials per level. The same set of 108 sentences is used in each difficulty level. The order of trials (sentences and difficulty level) is randomized. The entire protocol, approximately 2 hours long, is illustrated in Figure 14.2. The multitalker PRESTO sentence database is used for sentence stimuli (Park, Felty, Lormore, & Pisoni, 2010). We recorded 17 subjects but used 11 subjects from whom robust recordings were obtained in all three modalities.

The working memory task is split into a training and a testing phase. During training, the maximum number of digits a subject can recall is estimated using an adaptive tracking algorithm (Levitt, 1971). This number, nmax, is used to determine the three difficulty levels in the test phase, which were typically set as: {ceil(nmax), ceil(nmax)−1, ceil(nmax)−2}. Despite some minor protocol changes among early subjects, this common load assessment test was used for most subjects and was used in 10 of the 11 subjects analyzed in this chapter. Later we define a binary detection problem of discriminating high load (max number)

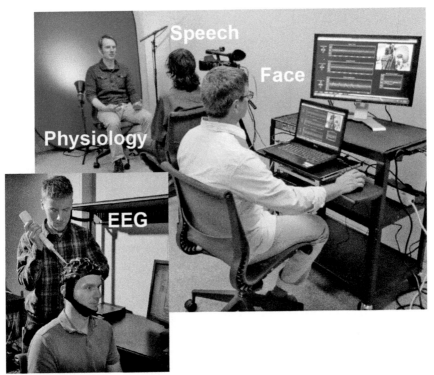

FIGURE 14.1 *Platform for recording speech, facial expression, EEG, and physiological signals.*

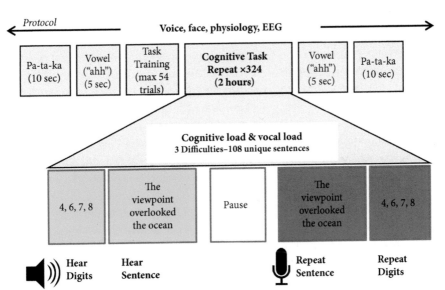

FIGURE 14.2 *Auditory working memory protocol. Audio and video are analyzed during sentence recall while the EEG is analyzed during the pause interval to avoid motion and muscle artifacts.*

from low load (max number minus two). The range of digit spans across all sub-jects was 2 to 5 for low load and 4 to 7 for high load.

Finally, as seen in Figure 14.1, with our protocol we also measure skin con-ductance, temperature, and pulse oxygenation level. These are not a focus of the present study but pave the way to investigating a broader suite of multimodal biomarkers.

## Feature Extraction and Selection

Biomarkers for detecting and monitoring cognitive stresses, as well as neuropsy-chiatric disorders, comprise behavioral, physiological, and cognitive modalities. Three particular modalities that are gaining popularity are speech, facial expres-sion, and EEG signals. The effectiveness of predicting cognitive load from these modalities is based on the hypothesis that manipulating cognitive load level sys-tematically alters the underlying neural motor activation required in speech pro-duction and facial expression due to a competition for mental resources between motor activity and working memory. This neural activation is reflected in the EEG measurement, which is sometimes considered a gold standard in viewing the effect of working memory demand (Zarjam et al., 2011a, 2011b, 2015).

Our features from the three modalities (speech, facial expression, EEG) are based on principles of timing and coordination within components of each modality. In each case, we extract first low-level (standard) features, followed by high-level (novel) features as functions of the low-level features. For speech, feature vectors are extracted only from the single spoken sentence component of each trial in the test phase of the auditory memory task. Low-level vocal features comprise measures of phoneme and pseudosyllable durations, pitch dynamics, spectral (formant) dynamics, and vocal-fold period irregularity (creak). We con-struct high-level features that capture timing and interrelationships across the low-level features. The feature sets are derived under the hypothesis that differ-ences in cognitive load produce detectable changes in speech production timing and coordination within and across articulatory and vocal-fold components. For facial expression, analyzed during the same time interval as audio, the extracted low-level features are FAUs (Ekman et al., 1980; Gaebel & Wölwer, 1992; Littlewort et al., 2011), which are followed by correlation-based measures as high-level fea-tures. For the EEG, during the sentence listening and pause intervals to avoid motion and muscle artifacts, we perform preprocessing to extract low-level EEG signals free of many typical artifacts, followed by frequency-dependent covari-ance, coherence, and power measures.

In this section, we describe key details of the feature extraction methods for each modality. The suite of low- and high-level features, which provides a general foundation for cognitive state estimation, is illustrated using case studies in cog-nitive load detection and depressive disorder estimation. In both applications, feature extraction produces high-dimensional feature vectors from relatively small datasets, requiring dimensionality reduction techniques to avoid statistical model overfitting. Therefore, we conclude the secton by overviewing our dimensionality reduction approaches and discussing strategies for achieving robust generalization to novel test sets.

## Speech Features

We describe below a broad suite of speech features that are used in detection of cognitive load and in detection of depression, as well as other cognitive stress and neurological disorders (Cummins et al., 2015; Darby et al., 1984; Helfer et al., 2014; Moore et al., 2003; Mundt et al., 2007; Ozdas et al., 2004; Quatieri et al., 2015; Quatieri & Malyska, 2012; Trevino, Quatieri, & Malyska, 2011; Williamson et al., 2013, 2014, 2015; Yu et al., 2014).

### LOW-LEVEL SPEECH FEATURES

This section introduces a set of low-level speech features that are used in the cognitive load study and the depression estimation study. We exploit dynamic variation and interrelationships across speech production systems by computing features that reflect complementary aspects of the speech voice source, vocal tract system, and prosody (Quatieri, 2002). These features are also widely used in our other cognitive load and neurological detection efforts (Cummins et al., 2015; Helfer et al., 2014; Quatierri et al., 2015; Quatieri & Malyska, 2012; Trevino et al., 2011; Williamson et al., 2013, 2014, 2015; Yu et al., 2014).

The voice source is primarily characterized by three measures: harmonics-to-noise ratio (HNR), cepstral peak prominence (CPP), and probability of a creaky voice quality. A spectral measure of HNR was performed using a periodic/noise decomposition method that employs a comb filter to extract the harmonic component of a signal (Jackson & Shadle, 2000, 2001). The HNR is the ratio, in decibels, of the power of the decomposed harmonic signal and the power of the decomposed speech noise signal, and was computed every 10 milliseconds. Several studies have reported strong correlations between CPP and overall dysphonia perception (Dejonckere & Lebacq, 1996; Heman-Ackah et al., 2003; Maryn, Corthals, Van Cauwenberge, Roy, & De Bodt, 2010), breathiness (Heman-Ackah, Michael, & Goding, 2002; Hillenbrand & Houde, 1996), and vocal fold kinematics. CPP is defined as the difference, in decibels, between the magnitude of the highest peak and the noise floor in the power cepstrum for quefrencies greater than 2 milliseconds (corresponding to a range minimally affected by vocal tract–related information) and was computed every 10 milliseconds. The cepstrum is defined as the Fourier transform of the log-spectrum with quefrency being the time axis of the cepstrum (Quatieri, 2002). A creaky voice quality (vocal fry, irregular pitch periods, glottalization, etc.), is characterized using acoustic measures of low-frequency/damped glottal pulses (Gerratt & Kreiman (2001). The creak measure builds on metrics of short-term power, intraframe periodicity, interpulse similarity (Ishi, Skakibara, Ishiguro, & Hagita, 2008), and two measures of the degree of subharmonic energy (reflecting the presence of secondary glottal pulses) and the temporal peakiness of glottal pulses (Kane, Drugman, & Gobl, 2013). These values are input into an artificial neural network (http://tcts.fpms.ac.be/~drug-man/Toolbox/) to yield creak posterior probabilities on a frame-by-frame basis every 10 milliseconds.

The vocal tract system is characterized by vocal tract resonant (formant) frequencies and mel-frequency cepstral coefficients (MFCCs) (Quatieri, 2002). A Kalman filter technique is used to characterize formant dynamics by smoothly tracking the first three formant frequencies, while also smoothly coasting through nonspeech regions (Mehta, Rudoy, & Wolfe, 2012). Sixteen delta MFCCs are used to characterize velocities of vocal tract spectral magnitudes, typical in speech-related recognition applications (Reynolds, Quatieri, & Dunn, 2000). MFCCs are computed similarly to the cepstrum but with an approximately constant-Q filterbank in place of the Fourier transform. Delta MFCCs are computed using regression with the two frames before and after a given frame (Quatieri, 2002).

Speech properties related to prosody include the detection of phonemes, pseudosyllables, and fundamental frequency contours. Using an automatic phoneme-recognition algorithm (Shen, White, & Hazen, 2010), phonetic boundaries are detected, with each segment labeled with one of 40 phonetic speech classes (see Figure 14.15). Vocal syllable-like patterns are also detected based on the concept of a pseudosyllable (PS; Rouas, 2007). The automatic phoneme-recognition system detects vowels (v) and consonants (c), which are combined into PS segments. For example, "v," "cv," and "ccv" are all valid PSs. The fundamental frequency contour was estimated using, every 1 millisecond, a time-domain autocorrelation over 40-millisecond Hanning windows (Quatieri, 2002).

HIGH-LEVEL SPEECH FEATURES

Our high-level features are designed to characterize properties of timing and coordination from the low-level features. Structure of correlation reflects relations across components of a single low-level feature type, e.g., across vocal tract formants, as well as across different low-level feature types, e.g., formant tracks and creak.

Measures of the correlation structure among low-level speech features have been applied in the estimation of depression (Williamson et al., 2013, 2014) and Parkinson's disease (Williamson et al., 2015), the detection of age-related cognitive decline (Yu et al., 2014) and cognitive changes associated with mild traumatic brain injury (Helfer et al., 2014), and in the detection of cognitive load

(Quatieri et al., 2015). The mathematical details for this signal-analysis approach are in Williamson et al. (2012), where the method was first introduced for analysis of EEG signals for epileptic seizure prediction.

Channel-delay correlation and covariance matrices are computed from multiple time series channels of vocal parameters. Each matrix contains correlation or covariance coefficients between the channels at multiple time delays. Changes over time in the coupling strengths among the channel signals cause changes in the eigenvalue spectra of the channel-delay matrices. The matrices are computed at multiple "time scales" corresponding to separate subframe spacings. Features at each time scale consist of the eigenvalue spectra of channel-delay correlation matrices, as well as summary covariance-based features: the covariance power (logarithm of the trace) and entropy (logarithm of the determinant) from channel-delay covariance matrices. This methodology is illustrated in Figure 14.3 with the generation of formant track correlation matrices.

In the cognitive load application, parameters were used to extract correlation structure features from three different low-level speech sources: formant frequency tracks, creak probabilities, and delta MFCCs. Subframe spacings of 1, 3, and 7 are used and, due to the 10-millisecond frame interval of the low-level features, these correspond to time spacings of 10, 30, and 70 milliseconds, respectively. Each matrix (for each scale) is constructed using 15 time delays. The number of correlation-based eigenvalue features is the number of signal channels times the number of scales (i.e., number of subframe spacings) times the number of time delays (15) per time scale. The number of summary covariance-based features is the number of time scales (entropy features) plus one log power feature, as power is invariant across scale. Parameters are similar to those of previous studies (Cummins et al., 2015; Helfer et al., 2014; Williamson et al., 2013, 2014, 2015; Yu et al., 2014). Additional specifics are given in the discussion below on the use of these features for cognitive load detection. An example comparison of formant-based correlation matrices for low and high cognitive loads for one subject is shown in Figure 14.4, indicating more complexity in the high-load correlation matrix. The matrix eigenvalues obtained from these matrices, ordered from largest to smallest, are shown at right for the low-load (blue) and high-load (red) examples. Observe that the high-load condition results in more power in the low-rank eigenvalues (i.e., the eigenvalues with high index values).

The differences in eigenspectra patterns due to high versus low cognitive loads, illustrated in Figure 14.4, provide indications about the effect of load on speech. In Figure 14.5, we show that these differences are robust by plotting averages across all subjects of normalized ($z$-scored) eigenvalues from formant, creak, and delta-MFCC speech features. Once again, the eigenvalues are ordered from largest to smallest. Average normalized eigenvalues are plotted in blue for low loads and in red for high loads. The curves are symmetrical because there are the same number of low-load and high-load trials. For all three feature types, there is greater power in the medium-level eigenvalues during higher cognitive load.

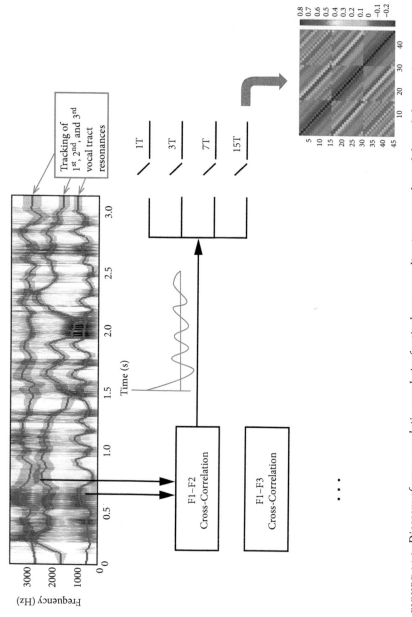

FIGURE 14.3 *Diagram of cross-correlation analysis of articulatory coordination, as performed through formant-based features using channel-delay correlation matrices at multiple delay scales. A channel-delay correlation matrix from one scale is shown.*

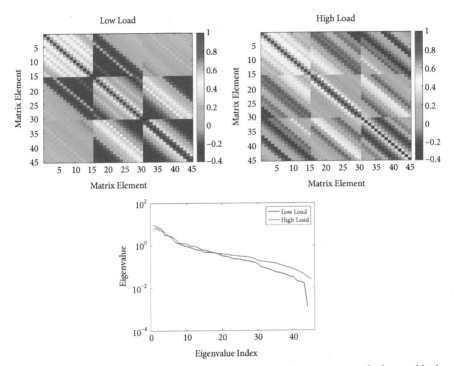

FIGURE 14.4 *Example comparison of formant-based correlation matrices for low and high cognitive load for one subject. Matrix eigenvalues from the matrices are shown (bottom).*

This indicates greater dynamical complexity in formant frequencies, creak, and some of the spectral content during higher cognitive load. The normalized eigenvalues are plotted in standard units, with the distance between lines indicating the Cohen's *d* effect size between the two load classes.

We have also introduced a feature set that characterizes the structure of signal coherence and power at multiple frequency bands. The coherence between channels, indicating the amount of cross-channel power in a frequency band relative to the amount of within-channel power, provides a measure of how closely related the signals are within a frequency band. The power and cross-power are computed among three formant frequency tracks at three different frequency bands (0.25–1.0 Hz, 1.0–2.0 Hz, and 2.0–4.0 Hz), with a 3 × 3 coherence matrix constructed for each band. The eigenspectra of the coherence matrices indicate the structure of coherence across the formant frequency tracks.

The differences in coherence and power features due to high versus low cognitive load provide indications about the effect of load on speech. In Figure 14.6 (left), averages across all subjects of normalized coherence eigenvalues from the middle frequency band (1.0–2.0 Hz) are shown for low load (blue) and high load (red). As before, the eigenvalues are ordered from largest to smallest. Similar to the correlation structure results shown in Figure 14.5, the results in Figure 14.6

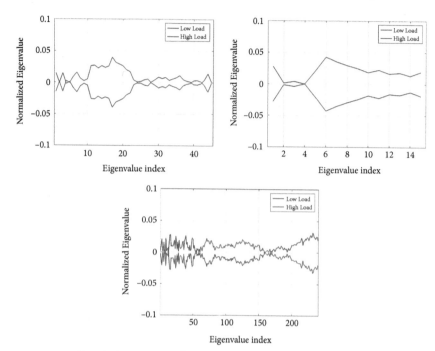

FIGURE 14.5  *Correlation structure features: Average normalized eigenvalues from all subjects for low and high cognitive loads, based on formant frequencies (top left), creak (top right), and delta mel-cepstra (lower).*

indicate greater power in the mid-level eigenvalue for the higher load condition. In Figure 14.6 (right), it is also shown that the higher load condition is associated with more power (i.e., variability) in all three formant tracks. The normalized eigenvalues and power features are plotted in units of standard deviation.

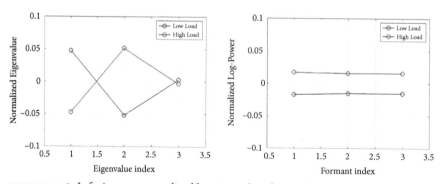

FIGURE 14.6  *Left: Average normalized log eigenvalues from coherence matrix at frequency band 1.0–2.0 Hz for low and high cognitive loads from formant frequencies. Right: Normalized log power for the three formant frequency tracks at frequency band 1.0–2.0 Hz.*

Based on the phoneme- and PS-based boundaries introduced above as low-level features, we find that computing high-level phoneme- and PS-specific characteristics, rather than the more typical average measures, such as average speaking rate, can reveal stronger relationships with the severity of a condition (Trevino, Quatieri, & Malyska, 2011). Example high-level phoneme- and PS-specific features include average phoneme and PS durations, as well as pitch and formant slopes across each segment type, and frequency and count of phonemes and PSs. As described below, further postprocessing of these feature types can provide strong discrimination across condition level.

## Video Features

### LOW-LEVEL VIDEO FEATURES

Although FAUs provide a formalized method for identifying changes in facial expression frame by frame (Ekman et al., 1980), their extraction in large quantities of data has been impeded by the need for trained annotators to mark individual frames of a recorded video session. For this reason, the University of California San Diego has developed a computer expression recognition toolbox (CERT) for the automatic identification of FAUs from individual video frames (Wang et al., 2008). Table 14.1 lists the 20 FAUs from CERT used for the video-based facial expression analysis.

Each FAU feature is converted from a support vector machine (SVM) hyperplane distance to a posterior probability using a logistic model trained on a separate database of video recordings (Lucey et al., 2010). Henceforth, the term FAU refers to these frame-by-frame estimates of FAU posterior probabilities. Frames are removed if they are marked as invalid by CERT or if we automatically classify any of the 20 FAU features in that frame as an outlier. If the duration of the remaining "stitched" FAU time series is either less than 30 s or less than 40% of

TABLE 14.1 The 20 Facial Action Units from CERT

| Facial Action Unit | Description | Facial Action Unit | Description |
|---|---|---|---|
| 1 | Inner Brow Raise | 11 | Lip Stretch |
| 2 | Outer Brow Raise | 12 | Cheek Raise |
| 3 | Brow Lower | 13 | Lids Tight |
| 4 | Eye Widen | 14 | Lip Pucker |
| 5 | Nose Wrinkle | 15 | Lip Tightener |
| 6 | Lip Raise | 16 | Lip Presser |
| 7 | Lip Corner Pull | 17 | Lips Part |
| 8 | Dimpler | 18 | Jaw Drop |
| 9 | Lip Corner Depressor | 19 | Lips Suck |
| 10 | Chin Raise | 20 | Blink/Eye Closure |

the original passage duration, then the entire set of FAUs for that recording is not used.

### HIGH-LEVEL VIDEO FEATURES

Our high-level features are designed to characterize properties of timing and coordination from the low-level features. Facial coordination features are obtained by applying the correlation structure technique to the FAU time series using the same parameters that were used to analyze the vocal-based features. Because of the 30 Hz FAU frame rate, the spacings that are used in the three time scales, of 1, 3, and 7 data points, correspond to time sampling in increments of approximately 33, 100, and 234 milliseconds, respectively. Examples of correlation matrices for low and high loads (for one of the 11 subjects) are shown in Figure 14.7 (left and center) while average (across all 11 subjects) normalized eigenvalues from all subjects' trials are shown in Figure 14.7 (right). Once again, more power is found in the middle-level eigenvalues during high cognitive load.

An alternative FAU-based feature set, the facial activation rate, can be obtained by computing mean FAU values (an estimate of percent time present via posteriori probabilities) over each passage and combining several of these into a fused

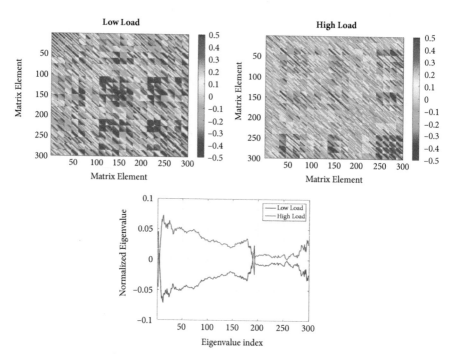

FIGURE 14.7 *Example correlation matrix for low-load (top left) and high-load (top right) condition. Average normalized eigenvalues for correlation matrix for FAU features (bottom).*

FAU rate measure. These features represent changes due to cognitive load in the probability of occurrence of a set of FAUs.

## EEG Features

### LOW-LEVEL EEG FEATURES

EEG signals were measured at a sampling frequency of 500 Hz with a 64-element Neuroscan system, followed by high-pass filtering and standard artifact removal. Measurements were made during the sentence listening and pause region of the protocol (Figure 14.2) to avoid motion and muscle artifacts during speaking. We decompose the EEG signals into five frequency bands that have been implicated in working memory (delta, theta, alpha, beta, and gamma), with associated band ranges (0–4 Hz, 4–8 Hz, 8–16 Hz, 16–32 Hz, and 32–49 Hz, respectively) (Zarjam et al., 2015). In the time domain, we compute bandpass-filtered signals at each channel in each frequency band. In the frequency domain, we compute auto- and cross-channel power at each frequency.

### HIGH-LEVEL EEG FEATURES

For EEG analysis, our guiding principles are that successful cognition requires coordinated neural activations in brain networks linking multiple brain regions, and that these networks communicate using oscillatory codes operating over a wide range of frequencies. Based on these principles, our high-level feature approach is to use measures of neural coordination based on EEG connectivity at each frequency band. We use two connectivity measures: pairwise channel coherence and covariance. Coherence measures cross-channel power relative to within-channel power, whereas covariance measures cross-channel correlation weighted by within-channel power. These coordination features are invariant to the channel identities of EEG signals. We also compute measures of EEG channel-dependent band power, which may provide complementary information.

Example beta band covariance matrices for the low and high conditions from one subject are shown in Figure 14.8 (upper), and average normalized eigenvalues across all subjects' trials in Figure 14.8 (lower). Average normalized EEG coherence eigenvalues and channel log-power at the beta frequency band (16–32 Hz) are shown in Figure 14.9. As with the speech and facial expression biomarkers above, greater relative power is found in the middle to small EEG eigenvalues in the high-load condition. Unlike the formant power features in Figure 14.7, we find that high load is associated with lower levels of EEG power. Because covariance is a measure that combines correlation and power, the average normalized eigenvalues in Figure 14.8 (lower) combine with the properties in Figure 14.7, namely, greater overall power for low load and greater relative power in middle and small eigenvalues for high load.

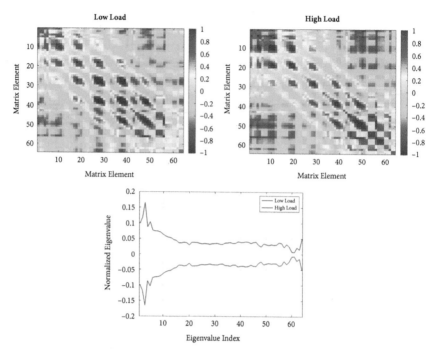

FIGURE 14.8  *Example comparison of EEG covariance matrices in the beta band for low and high cognitive load for one subject. Average normalized eigenvalues for covariance features in the beta band (lower).*

## Dimensionality Reduction

As seen above, our vocal, facial, and EEG feature extraction approaches create high-dimensional feature vectors. Machine learning applied directly to such high-dimensional features risks the possibility of overfitting of statistical

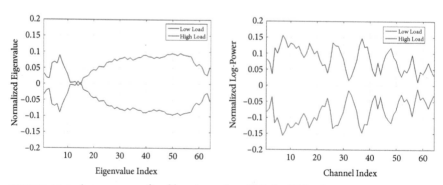

FIGURE 14.9  *Average normalized log eigenvalues (left) for EEG coherence matrices and channel log power (right) at the beta frequency band (16–31 Hz) for low and high cognitive loads.*

models, particularly when the underlying dataset is small. In order to obtain robust statistical models that aim to generalize well to novel test data, we employ dimensionality reduction prior to their construction. For the correlation structure, coherence structure, and power features, we have found that the unsupervised approach of using principal component analysis (PCA), which maximally preserves feature variability for a given projection dimensionality, consistently works well. Despite large variation in the dimensionality of our feature vectors from different feature types, we have found surprisingly little variation in the best performing number of principal components, which typically ranges from two to six. In the cognitive load study, to further mitigate the possibility of overfitting, we use a uniform number of four principal components for each feature type, with the exception that we use three components for three-dimensional feature vectors. These parameter selections are furthered detailed in the discussion of results for cognitive load and the MDD case study.

For our phoneme- and PS-dependent features, a different approach first introduced in Trevino, Quatieri, and Malyska (2011) is preferred. In cognitive stress and neuropsychiatric conditions, our high-level features are based on aggregations of phoneme (or PS) counts, phoneme durations, and phoneme-dependent pitch slopes. The aggregations of these features across the 40 phoneme or 18 PS classes are performed using linear combinations of subsets of phonemes or PSs, based on supervised feature selection and weighting of features due to their associations with output variables. For the binary classification problem of cognitive load detection, we use weights equal to discrimination indices (Cohen's $d$) between the two output classes for each phoneme or PS. For depression estimation, we use weights based on correlation coefficients between each phoneme or PS and the output depression score (Williamson et al., 2014).

Because the phoneme- and PS-dependent feature selection and weighting approach is supervised, how the training data are chosen is an important consideration. If feature selection/weighting is done independently within each cross-validation fold, as opposed to once over the entire training set, then it will result in a more robust estimate of generalization performance. In our previous cognitive load study (Quatieiri et al., 2015), the combination weights were obtained once over the entire data set, resulting in estimates of strong load classification performance in subsequent cross-validation testing. Subsequent re-analysis with the feature selection done independently in each cross-validation loop resulted in weaker classification performance, such that the phoneme- and PS-dependent features did not improve upon performance obtained by the correlation structure, coherence structure, and power features outlined above. The lack of improvement from phonemes and PSs may be due to the fact that the single-sentence data segments in which they are obtained are of such short duration (~6 s). Therefore, we do not include results obtained using phoneme- and PS-based features for cognitive load detection, even though phoneme-based features are used for depression estimation in the MDD case study.

## Results for Cognitive Load

Our goal is to detect differences in cognitive load from speech and facial expression measurements and compare them with EEG signal analysis. To evaluate detection performance, for each subject the 108 feature vectors (one vector per spoken sentence and load condition) from the max-digit condition are assigned to the high-load class, and the 108 vectors from the max-digit-minus-two condition are assigned to the low-load class. Leave-one-subject-out cross-validation is used, with a classifier trained on the data from 10 held-out subjects used to discriminate between high and low load on a test subject.

A key processing step is individualized feature normalization. This involves, for each subject (whether in the training or test set), subtracting the mean from each feature across both load conditions. This processing step is done to remove intersubject feature variability, and implies that the ability to discriminate load conditions requires some knowledge of a subject's baseline features.

Load discrimination is done with a Gaussian classifier (GC), where the Gaussians are centered on the two class means, and a common covariance matrix is used based on the data across both load conditions. In each trial, the GC produces a load score (log-likelihood ratio of high versus low load). A receiver operating characteristic (ROC) curve is obtained by varying a detection threshold to characterize the sensitivity/specificity tradeoff. For each subject, 216 scores are obtained (108 for each load). A single ROC curve derived from scores of all 11 subjects characterizes total performance, with the area under the curve (AUC) serving as a summary statistic.

### AUC AS A SUMMARY STATISTIC: SINGLE TRIAL CASE

Vectors comprising our correlation-, covariance- and coherence-based eigenspectra, as well as covariance-based entropy and power, are projected using PCA into lower-dimensional representations. To reduce the possibility of overfitting, we use the same number of principal components (four) for each feature vector, with the exception that we use three principal components for the three-dimensional coherence- and power-based features derived from formant tracks at different frequency bands.

For EEG, feature vectors of the same type derived from different frequency bands belong to the same feature set. For audio, correlation- and covariance-based features from the same speech-derived modality (e.g., formant frequencies, delta-MFCCs, and creak) belong to the same feature sets, as do coherence- and

TABLE 14.2   Summary of Area Under ROC Curve (AUC) Results for Detecting High Cognitive Load from a Single Trial for the EEG Modality

| Feature sets | Description[a] | AUC |
|---|---|---|
| 1 | Covariance structure | 0.59 |
| 2 | Coherence structure | 0.54 |
| 3 | Channel power | 0.59 |
| **Combined** | | **0.60** |

[a]Coherence and channel features cover five frequency bands: delta, theta, alpha, beta, and gamma.

power-based features derived from analysis of formant tracks in different frequency bands. For video, there is a single feature set comprising correlation- and covariance-based features. Fusion of features within the same feature set is done by concatenating principal component feature vectors from the different feature types in that set. Fusion across different feature sets is done by multiplying classifier likelihoods.

Tables 14.2 to 14.4 list the number of features used by the GC for each feature set, and the AUC results. We see that the EEG modality achieves AUC = 0.60, outperforming audio (with AUC = 0.56) and video (with AUC = 0.55). Table 14.5 summarizes various combinations of the features. The best overall performance, AUC = 0.62, is obtained by combining (via class fusion) all of the feature sets.

TABLE 14.3   Summary of Area Under ROC Curve (AUC) Results for Detecting High Cognitive Load from a Single Trial for the Audio Modality

| Feature sets | Description[a] | AUC |
|---|---|---|
| 1 | Covariance and correlation structure of formants | 0.52 |
| 2 | Covariance and correlation structure of delta-MFCC | 0.54 |
| 3 | Covariance and correlation structure of creak | 0.52 |
| 4 | Coherence structure | 0.53 |
| 5 | Channel power | 0.52 |
| **Combined** | | **0.56** |

[a]Coherence and channel features are applied to formant tracks at three frequency bands: 0.25–1.0 Hz, 1.0–2.0 Hz, and 2.0–4.0 Hz.

TABLE 14.4   Summary of Area Under ROC Curve (AUC) Results for Detecting High Cognitive Load from a Single Trial for the Video Modality

| Feature sets | Description | AUC |
|---|---|---|
| 1 | Covariance and correlation structure | **0.55** |

TABLE 14.5  Summary of Area Under ROC Curve (AUC)
Results for Detecting High Cognitive Load from a Single
Trial for the Various Feature Combinations from Audio,
Video, and EEG Modalities

| Feature combinations | AUC |
| --- | --- |
| Audio + Video | 0.57 |
| EEG + Audio | 0.61 |
| EEG + Video | 0.61 |
| EEG + Audio + Video | 0.62 |

### DETECTION VERSUS FALSE-ALARM RESULTS

Our protocol involves feature processing of data from a single trial: listening to a single sentence followed by a 2-s pause (EEG) and speaking the sentence (audio and video). The ability to detect load after fusing evidence across multiple trials can be assessed by combining the GC scores from the trials, provided that they involve the same load condition. This is done by randomly

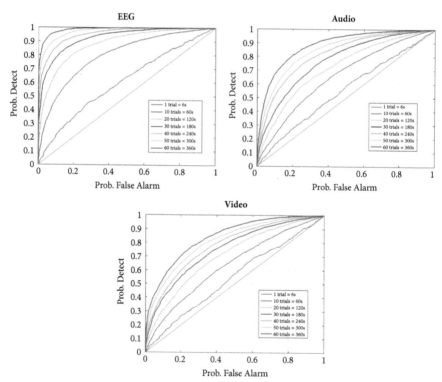

FIGURE 14.10  *Probability of detection versus false alarm for EEG, audio, and video modalities. Each panel gives ROCs as a function of increasing number of trials from 1 to 360, corresponding to 6 s to 360 s (6 min) for low and high cognitive loads.*

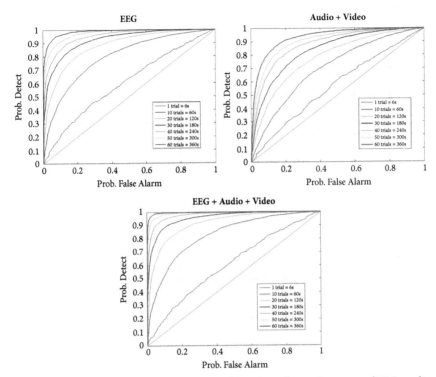

FIGURE 14.11 *Probability of detection versus false alarm for combinations of EEG, audio, and video modalities. Each panel gives ROC curves as a function of increasing number of trials from 1 to 60, corresponding to 6 s to 360 s (6 min) for low and high cognitive loads.*

selecting, from the same subject, a number of trials of either high load or low load, and summing their GC scores. For each subject, load condition, and combination number, 400 randomly chosen sets of trials are used to determine the fused scores across multiple trials. Figures 14.10 and 14.11 summarize the ROC results (detection versus false alarm) for each modality alone and in combination, respectively. Figure 14.10 shows a comparison of ROCs across each modality alone. We observe that the EEG-based detector converges to AUC = 0.99 after 60 trials. The AUC for audio and video modalities converge more slowly to 0.89 and 0.84 individually, and 0.93 in combination. Finally, combining all three modalities converges to near perfect performance, with AUC ~ 1.00.

## ANALYSIS OF CONVERGENCE

Figure 14.12 contains box plots (25th–75th percentile ranges) summarizing AUC values for the 11 subjects within each modality, given combinations of 1, 10, 20, . . . 60 trials. The median AUC value, plotted in red, increases as a function of the number of trials, with EEG detection accuracy converging toward 100%

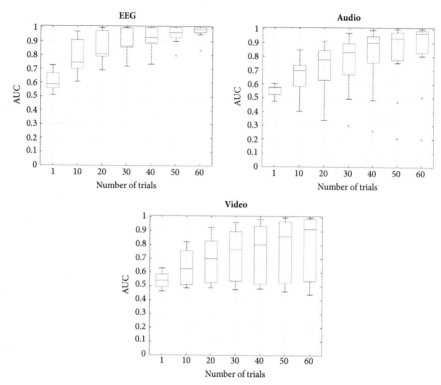

FIGURE 14.12  *AUC results across 11 subjects as a function of number of combined trials with same load for each modality.*

for all 11 subjects, and audio and video converging more slowly and less reliably. Figure 14.13 contains boxplots comparing the EEG AUC values with two combined-modality results, which correspond to the ROC plots of Figure 14.11. Observe that load remains undetected in two of 11 subjects in the audio modality, and in one of 11 subjects in the audio plus video modalities. Red crosses indicate performance for the outlier subjects, which are not included in calculation of the box plots.

## Timing- and Coordination-Based Multimodal Features in Other Conditions: Major Depressive Disorder Case Study

In individuals with MDD, neurophysiological changes often alter motor control and thus affect the mechanisms controlling speech production and facial expression. These changes are typically associated with psychomotor retardation, a condition marked by slowed neuromotor output that is behaviorally manifested as altered coordination and timing across multiple motor-based properties. As with cognitive load, changes in motor outputs can be inferred from vocal acoustics

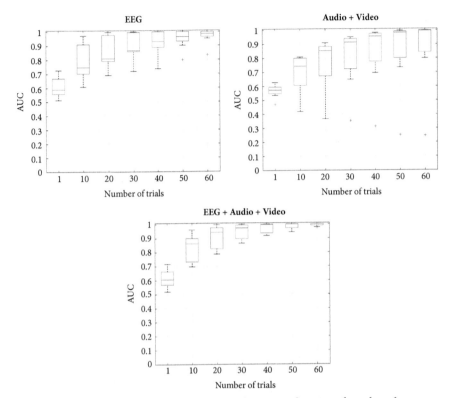

FIGURE 14.13 *AUC variance results across 11 subjects as a function of number of combined trials with same load for EEG, audio + video, and audio + video + EEG modalities.*

and facial movements as individuals speak. Correspondingly, our novel multi-scale correlation structure and timing feature sets from audio-based vocal features and video-based FAUs have been shown to be effective. The feature sets enable detection of changes in coordination, movement, and timing of vocal and facial gestures that are potentially symptomatic of depression. Combining complementary features in Gaussian mixture model (GMM) and extreme learning machine classifiers, our multivariate regression scheme predicts self-reported Beck Depression Inventory (BDI) ratings (over 0–60 range) with a root mean square error of 8.12 and mean absolute error of 6.31 using a dataset from the 2014 Audio-Video Emotion Challenge (Valstar et al., 2014; Williamson et al., 2014). In this section, we briefly summarize use of our principles of timing and coordination in vocal and facial expression.

## AUDIO-VISUAL AVEC DEPRESSION DATABASE

AVEC 2014 is the fourth challenge for comparing different methods of audiovisual analysis. AVEC 2014 includes a depression subchallenge with a depression corpus containing audio and video recordings of subjects with depression performing a human–computer interaction task (Valstar et al., 2014). Data were collected from 84 German subjects, with a subset of subjects recorded during multiple sessions: 31 subjects were recorded twice and 18 subjects were recorded three times. The subjects' ages varied between 18 and 63 years, with a mean of 31.5 years and a standard deviation of 12.3 years.

Subjects performed two speech tasks in the German language: reading a phonetically balanced passage and replying to a free-response question. The read passage (NW) was an excerpt from the fable *Die Sonne und der Wind* (*The North Wind and the Sun*). The free speech section (FS) asked the subjects to respond to one of a number of questions (prompted in written German), such as "What is your favorite dish?" "What was your best gift, and why?" and "Discuss a sad childhood memory." The NW passage ranged in duration from 31 s to 1 min and 29 s, and the FS passage from 6 s to 3 min and 50 s.

Video of the subject's face was captured using a webcam at 30 frames per second and a spatial resolution of 640 x 480 pixels. Audio was captured with a headset microphone connected to a laptop soundcard at sampling rates of 32 kHz or 48 kHz using the AAC codec. For each session, the self-reported BDI score was available (see Figure 14.14). The BDI assessment scores range from 0 to 60 with 60 being the highest depression severity. The recorded sessions were split into three parts (training, development, and test) with 50 recordings in each set. We combined the training and development sets into a single 100-session data set, which is henceforth termed the Training Set. In the AVEC 2014 depression subchallenge, the objective was to predict the BDI scores of the Test Set, which was not provided to participants.

### FEATURE EXTRACTION

As with the cognitive load problem, our high-level speech and facial expression features are designed to characterize properties of coordination and timing from the low-level features. The measures of coordination use assessments of the multiscale structure of correlations among the low-level features. As before, this approach is motivated by the observation that auto- and cross-correlations of measured signals can reveal hidden parameters in the stochastic-dynamical systems that generate the time series. For vocal-based timing features, we use cumulative phoneme-dependent durations and pitch slopes, obtained using estimated phoneme boundaries. For facial-based timing features, we use FAU rates obtained from their estimated posterior probabilities.

### Speech Features

As described in the discussion of feature extraction and selection, low-level speech features selected are based on articulatory (formant) correlations, source (vocal-fold period irregularity) correlations, and articulatory-to-source

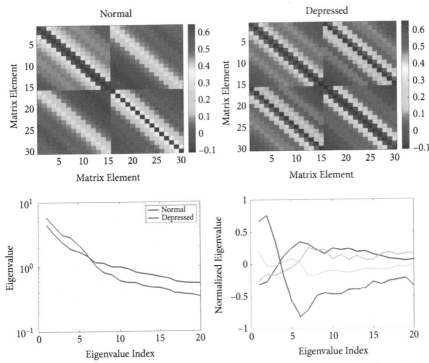

FIGURE 14.14  *CPP–HNR correlation features. Top: Channel-delay correlation matrices from NW passage for a normal and a depressed subject. Bottom: Eigenvalues for these subjects (left) and average normalized eigenvalues for four BDI assessment ranges in the training set (right). The BDI ranges are: 0–8 (blue), 9–18 (cyan), 19–28 (green), and 29–45 (red).*

correlations. As an example, Figure 14.14 shows the correlation structure matrix for the source correlation of cepstral peak prominence and harmonic-to-noise ratio (CPP–HNR). The matrix is based on vectors that consist of 88 elements (two channels, four scales, 15 delays per scale, and two covariance features per scale) comparing one control and depressed subject. Figure 14.14 also shows the top 20 eigenvalues per scale corresponding to these subjects and the average normalized eigenvalues across all subjects for four different depression severity ranges. Similar correlation structures and eigenvalue spreads are found for formant correlation features, delta MFCC correlation features, and formant-CPP (articulatory-to-source) features.

Based on phoneme boundaries (introduced as low-level features above), we find that computing phoneme-specific characteristics, rather than the more typical average measures of speaking rate, can reveal stronger relationships between speech rate and depression severity (Trevino, Quatieri, & Malyska, 2011; Williamson et al., 2014). Figure 14.15 shows the example of average phoneme durations, which can be used themselves as features or as a basis for other features, such as when those most highly correlating with a disorder assessment are combined.

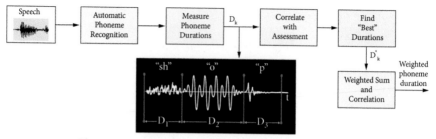

FIGURE 14.15  *Phoneme recognizer provides boundaries. In one feature set, average pho-*
*neme durations are correlated against severity of a disorder and are combined according to*
*the highest correlations.*

From the pitch estimate above, within each phoneme segment, a linear fit is
made to the pitch values, yielding also a pitch slope feature ($\Delta$Hz/s) associated
with each instance of phonemic speech units. As with phoneme durations, these
average values can be used themselves as features or as a basis for other features,
such as when the phoneme-dependent pitch slopes that are most highly correlating with a disorder are combined.

Based on estimated average durations for each phoneme, the summed average durations of certain phonemes are linearly combined to yield fused phoneme duration measures. A subset of phonemes whose summed durations are
highly correlated with BDI scores on the Training Set are selected to create these
fused measures, with weights based on the strength of their individual correlations. Table 14.6 lists the selected phonemes for the North Wind (NW) passage (left) and the first six of the ten selected phonemes for the Free Speech
(FS) passage (right), along with their individual BDI correlations. The correlations of the fused measures for each passage are shown at the bottom. The

TABLE 14.6  Pearson's Correlation Coefficients ($R$, $p < 0.01$) Between
Fused[a] Phoneme Durations and BDI Scores in the Training Set

| North Wind | | Free Speech | |
|---|---|---|---|
| Phoneme | R | Phoneme[b] | R |
| 'l' | 0.50 | 'ng' | 0.38 |
| 'ah' | 0.45 | 't' | 0.34 |
| 'n' | 0.41 | 'hh' | 0.33 |
| 'ih' | 0.34 | 'ey' | 0.32 |
| 'b' | 0.34 | 'ow' | 0.28 |
| 'ow' | 0.34 | 'er' | 0.27 |
| **Fused** | **0.54** | **Fused** | **0.57** |

[a] Fusion is done using linear combinations of phoneme durations.
[b] Only six of the ten Free Speech phonemes are shown.

linear combination used to obtain the fused measures is more fully described in Williamson et al. (2014).

A fused phoneme-dependent pitch slope measure is also obtained using essentially the same procedure as described above. For each phoneme, we compute the sum of valid pitch slopes across all instances of that phoneme. Invalid slopes are those with absolute value greater than eight, resulting in the exclusion of most slopes that are computed from discontinuous pitch contours. For each passage, the set of phonemes with the highest correlating summed pitch slopes are then selected. The summed pitch slopes are combined to obtain fused measures for the NW and FS passages. Using 20 phonemes for NW and 15 phonemes for FS, these fused measures have BDI correlations of $R = 0.63$ (NW) and $R = 0.51$ (FS), respectively.

## Video Features

As described in the discussion of feature extraction and selection, features related to facial correlation structure are obtained by applying the correlation technique to the FAU time series using the same parameters that were used to analyze the vocal-based features. Because of the 30-Hz FAU frame rate, spacing for the four time scales corresponds to time sampling in increments of approximately 33, 100, 234, and 500 milliseconds. Figure 14.16 (top) shows example FAU channel-delay matrices at a single time scale from the same normal and depressed subjects who were used for illustration in Figure 14.14. These matrices are derived from the FS passage. As with the correlation-based speech features, Figure 14.16 (bottom left) shows that the eigenspectra of the depressed subjects contain less power in the small eigenvalues. This effect is observed across a spectrum of BDI scores in all 83 free-response Training Set recordings with valid FAU features. The facial-based eigenvalue differences are similar to those found in the correlation-based speech features.

We also used FAU rate as described above. Weights are based on FAU correlations with BDI scores using the same correlation-based combination rule described for phonemes above (Williamson et al., 2014) using Pearson's correlation coefficient ($R$) between mean FAU posterior probabilities and BDI in the Training Set ($p < 0.05$ for all $|R| \geq 0.21$). Fusion is done using linear combinations of the mean FAU posterior probabilities.

## Dimensionality Reduction

The correlation feature vectors typically contain highly correlated elements. To obtain lower-dimensional uncorrelated feature vectors for machine-learning techniques, we apply PCA. Table 14.7 lists the number of principal components we chose for each correlation feature type, along with phonetic and FAU rate features. The number of principal components in each case was determined empirically by cross-validation performance.

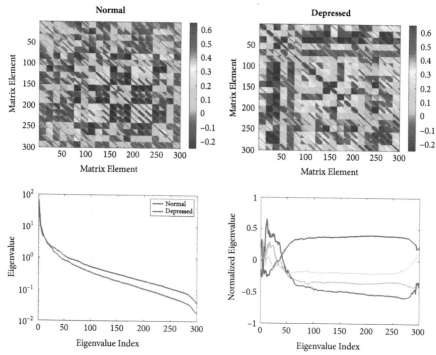

FIGURE 14.16 *FAU correlation features. Top: Channel-delay correlation matrices from FS passage for a normal and a depressed subject. Bottom: Eigenvalues for the subjects (left) and average normalized eigenvalues for four BDI ranges in Training Set (right). The BDI ranges are: 0–8 (blue), 9–18 (cyan), 19–28 (green), and 29–45 (red).*

TABLE 14.7 Total Number of Dimensions (# Dim.) and Number of Dimensions Selected after Principal Component Analysis (PCA #) for Each of the Eight Feature Sets

| Feature Set | Data | Feature Type[a] | # Dim. | PCA # |
|---|---|---|---|---|
| 1 | NW | Format–CPP *xcorr* | 248 | 4 |
| | NW | CPP–HNR *xcorr* | 88 | 2 |
| | NW | Delta MFCC *xcorr* | 968 | 5 |
| 2 | NW | Phoneme duration | 1 | 1 |
| 3 | NW | Pitch slope | 1 | 1 |
| 4 | NW | FAU rate | 1 | 1 |
| 5 | FS | FAU *xcorr* | 1208 | 6 |
| 6 | FS | Phoneme rate | 1 | 1 |
| 7 | FS | Pitch slope | 1 | 1 |
| 8 | FS | FAU rate | 1 | 1 |

[a]*xcorr* = cross-correlation features.

## MULTIVARIATE FUSION AND PREDICTION

Our next step involves mapping the features described in "Feature Extraction" into univariate scores that can be easily mapped into BDI predictions. To do this, we use both generative GMMs, which have been widely used for automatic speaker recognition (Reynolds et al., 2000) and have recently been extended to speech-based depression classification (Williamson et al., 2013, 2014), and discriminative extreme learning machines, a single-layer feedforward neural network architecture with randomly assigned hidden nodes (Huang, Zhou, Ding, & Zhang, 2012; Huang, Zhu, & Siew, 2006).

### Gaussian Staircase

To train the generative GMMs, we utilize the Gaussian staircase approach, in which each GMM is comprised of an ensemble of GCs (Williamson et al., 2013, 2014). The ensemble is derived from six partitions of the training data into different ranges of depression severity for low (Class 1) and high (Class 2) depression. Given a BDI range of 0 to 45, the Class 1 ranges for the six GCs are: 0–4, 0–10, 0–17, 0–23, 0–30, and 0–36, with the Class 2 ranges being the complement of these. The GCs comprise a single, highly regularized GMM classifier, with feature densities that smoothly increase in the direction of decreasing (Class 1) or of increasing (Class 2) levels of depression. Additional regularization of the densities is obtained by adding 0.1 to the diagonal elements of the normalized covariance matrices.

### Subject-Based Adaptation

Individual variability in the relationships between features and BDI are partially accounted for within the GMMs using Gaussian-mean subject-based adaptation. Motivated by GMM adaptation methods in automatic speaker recognition (Reynolds et al., 2000), if one or more sessions in the Training Set have the same subject ID as the Test subject and are in the same BDI-based partition, the mean of the Gaussian for that partition is assigned to the mean of the data from that subject only, rather than the mean of the data from all subjects within the partition (Williamson et al., 2013, 2014).

### Fusion

A separate GMM classifier is used for each Feature Set, outputting a log-likelihood ratio score for Class 1 (Normal) and Class 2 (Depressed) (Williamson et al., 2014). Separate ELM classifiers are used for Feature Sets 1 and 2. Initial BDI predictions are obtained from the three Predictors 1, 2, 3, which use different combinations of the eight Feature Sets and two types of classifiers. Within each Predictor, the classifier outputs from Feature Sets are summed together. Following this, a univariate regression model is created from the Training Set and is applied to the classifier output from the Test data. The resulting univariate regression output is the initial BDI score prediction from each Predictor. For Predictors 1 and 2, subject-based adaptation is then applied to adjust the initial prediction by correcting for consistent biases seen in the BDI Training Set predictions of the same subject. If there are any Training sessions from a given Test subject, then the average Training Set error from that subject is used to adjust the prediction. Details of our fusion methodology are described in Williamson et al. (2014).

## RESULTS

The prediction system described above was used in our winning system in the AVEC 2014 competition, with test root mean square error (RMSE) = 8.12 and mean absolute error (MAE) = 6.31. These results are an improvement on our winning submission in the AVEC 2013 competition, which was test RMSE = 8.50 and MAE = 6.52. The 2013 result was obtained using speech only and a read passage (*Homo Faber*) that was much longer than the NW passage made available in 2014. Introduction of vocal and facial features helped improve performance in 2014 despite the relative lack of data in this challenge. A different perspective on these results is shown in Figure 14.17, giving the ROC curve for both the AVEC 2013 and 2014 databases. In this binary detection problem, the two classes are mild/moderate (a BDI score range of 0-19) and moderate/severe severity (a BDI score range of 20 and higher). . With significantly less data using speech and facial expression (2014), performance is comparable to a speech-only system (2013).

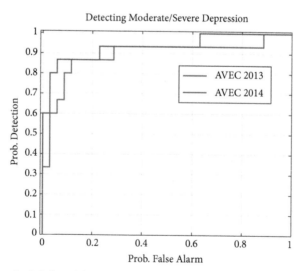

FIGURE 14.17  *Probability of detection versus false alarm of depression using AVEC 2013 and 2014 databases. With significantly less data using voice and face (2014), performance is comparable to a voice-only system (2013).*

# Conclusion and Discussion

In this chapter, we demonstrate the power of a multimodal approach using speech and facial features to discriminate between high and low cognitive load conditions, and illustrate its generality to cognitive disorders using a case study in MDD. Our vocal features capture timing and interrelationships among phoneme durations, pitch dynamics, articulation, spectral dynamics, and creak, while facial features capture relations and rate of FAUs underlying facial muscle activity. In our cognitive load study, as a reference, we extracted EEG features that reflect relations across EEG channels. Using a database consisting of audio, video, and EEG from 11 subjects and recalled sentences and pauses prior to recalling a digit span, we effectively applied classification models of cognitive load and explored tradeoffs with audio and video in comparison with the EEG gold standard. We found that merging audio and video brought us close to EEG-based performance, thus providing a simple noninvasive alternative to a complex 64-channel EEG. In illustrating an extension of our timing and coordination features to neurological disease, we described a predictor of depression state based on speech and facial modalities using the AVEC 2014 dataset. Finally, we briefly overviewed our approaches to feature dimensionality reduction, and the importance of unbiased methodologies for estimating generalization ability.

Future work will involve refining our timing and coordination features from speech and facial modalities, but also expanding them to include other observable behaviors, such as physiologic and motor responses, and generalizing from the current approach of extracting within-modality relations to the extraction of cross-modality components, thereby enabling the capture of vocal and facial relations in fine detail. An objective is a rich set of features derived from noninvasive, accessible behavioral measurements. The required algorithmic simplicity and modularity will promote access to large populations through mobile-device technology, and will allow us to validate our proposed algorithms beyond the current small datasets. Another important aspect of our validation will involve investigating specificity, as well as sensitivity, of our multimodal features, as well as the importance of confounding conditions. Finally, we are collaborating with the MIT McGovern Institute in brain imaging and neural computational modeling of neuropsychiatric disorders to aid in our goal of understanding the neural basis for current biomarkers so that we can both refine our current biomarkers and also develop the next generation of behavioral biomarkers.

# Disclaimer

The acknowledgement must be added to cover all three affiliations: "DISTRIBUTION STATEMENT A. NSREC OPSEC# U17-036. Approved for public release: distribution unlimited. This material is based upon work supported by the Assistant Secretary of Defense for Research and Engineering under Air Force Contract No. FA8721-05-C-0002 and/or FA8702-15-D-0001. Any opinions, findings, conclusions or recommendations expressed in this material are those of the author(s) and do not necessarily reflect the views of the Assistant Secretary of Defense for Research and Engineering."

# References

Boril, H., Sadjadi, O., Kleinschmidt, T., & Hansen, J. (2010). Analysis and detection of cognitive load and frustration in drivers' speech. *Proceedings of the Annual Conference of the International Speech Communication Association* (pp. 502–505).

Canter, G. J. (1963). Speech characteristics of patients with Parkinson's disease: I. Intensity, pitch, and duration. *J. Speech Hear. Disord, 28*(3), 221–229.

Canter, G. J. (1965a). Speech characteristics of patients with Parkinson's disease: II. Physiological support for speech. *J. Speech Hear. Disord, 30*(1), 44–49.

Canter, G. J. (1965b). Speech characteristics of patients with Parkinson's disease: III. Articulation, diadochokinesis, and over-all speech adequacy. *J. Speech Hear. Disord, 30*(3), 217–224.

Cummins, N., Scherer, S., Krajewski, J., Schnieder, S., Epps, J., & Quatieri, T. F. (2015). A review of depression and suicide risk assessment using speech analysis. *Speech Communication, 71*, 10–49.

Darby, J. K., Simmons, N., & Berger, P. A. (1984). Speech and voice parameters of depression: A pilot study. *Journal of Communication Disorders, 17*(2), 75–85.

Dejonckere, P., & Lebacq, J. (1996). Acoustic, perceptual, aerodynamic and anatomical correlations in voice pathology. *Journal for Oto-Rhino-Laryngology, 58*(6), 326–332.

Dejonckere, P., & Lebacq, J. (1996). Acoustic, perceptual, aerodynamic and anatomical correlations in voice pathology. *Annals of Otology Rhinology and Laryngology, 58*(6), 326–332.

Ekman, P., Freisen, W. V., & Ancoli, S. (1980). Facial signs of emotional experience. *Journal of Personality and Social Psychology, 39*(6), 1125.

Fava, M., & Kendler, K. S. (2000). Major depressive disorder. *Neuron, 28*(2), 335–341.

France, D. J., Shiavi, R. G., Silverman, S., Silverman, M., & Wilkes, D. M. (2000). Acoustical properties of speech as indicators of depression and suicidal risk. *IEEE Transactions on Biomedical Engineering, 47*(7), 829–837.

Gaebel, W., & Wölwer, W. (1992). Facial expression and emotional face recognition in schizophrenia and depression. *European Archives of Psychiatry and Clinical Neuroscience, 242*(1), 46–52.

Gerratt, B. R., & Kreiman, J. (2001). Toward a taxonomy of nonmodal phonation. *Journal of Phonetics, 29*(4), 365–381.

Greden, J. F., & Carroll, B. J. (1981). Psychomotor function in affective disorders: An overview of new monitoring techniques. *The American Journal of Psychiatry.*

Harnsberger, J. D., Wright, R., & Pisoni, D. B. (2008). A new method for eliciting three speaking styles in the laboratory. *Speech Communication, 50*(4), 323–336.

Helfer, B. S., Quatieri, T. F., Williamson, J. R., Keyes, L., Evans, B., Greene, W. N., Palmer, J., & Heaton, K. (2014). Articulatory dynamics and coordination in classifying cognitive change with preclinical mTBI. *Proceedings of the Annual Conference of the International Speech Communication Association.*

Heman-Ackah, Y. D., Heuer, R. J., Michael, D. D., Ostrowski, R., Horman, M., Baroody, M. M., . . . Sataloff, R.T. (2003). Cepstral peak prominence: A more reliable measure of dysphonia. *Annals of Otology Rhinology and Laryngology, 112*(4), 324–333.

Heman-Ackah, Y. D., Michael, D. D., & Goding, G. S., Jr. (2002). The relationship between cepstral peak prominence and selected parameters of dysphonia. *Journal of Voice, 16*(1), 20–27.

Hillenbrand, J., & Houde, R. A. (1996). Acoustic correlates of breathy vocal quality dysphonic voices and continuous speech. *Journal of Speech, Language, and Hearing Research, 39*(2), 311–321.

Huang, G. B., Zhou, H., Ding, X., & Zhang, R. (2012). Extreme learning machine for regression and multiclass classification. *IEEE Transactions on Systems, Man, and Cybernetics, Part B (Cybernetics), 42*(2), 513–529.

Huang, G. B., Zhu, Q. Y., & Siew, C. K. (2006). Extreme learning machine: Theory and applications. *Neurocomputing, 70*(1–3), 489–501.

Ishi, C. T., Sakakibara, K. I., Ishiguro, H., & Hagita, N. (2008). A method for automatic detection of vocal fry. *IEEE Transactions on Audio, Speech, and Language Processing, 16*(1), 47–56.

Jackson, P. J., & Shadle, C. H. (2000). Performance of the pitch-scaled harmonic filter and applications in speech analysis. *Proceedings of EEE International Conference on Acoustics, Speech, and Signal Processing* (pp. 1311–1314).

Jackson, P. J., & Shadle, C. H. (2001). Pitch-scaled estimation of simultaneous voiced and turbulence-noise components in speech. *IEEE Transactions on Speech and Audio Processing, 9*(7), 713–726.

Kane, J., Drugman, T., & Gobl, C. (2013). Improved automatic detection of creak. *Computer, Speech and Language, 27*(4), 1028–1047.

Khawaja, M. A., Ruiz, N., & Cheng, F. (2008, December). Think before you talk: An empirical study of relationship between speech pauses and cognitive load. *Proceedings of Annual Conference for the Computer-Human Interaction Special Interest Group, December 8–12.*

Le, P. N., Ambikairajah, E., Choi, H. C., & Epps, J. (2009). A non-uniform sub-band approach to speech-based cognitive load classification. *Proceedings of International Conference on Information and Communication Systems.*

Le, P., Epps, J., Choi, H. C., & Ambikairajah, E. (2010). A study of voice source- and vocal tract-based features in cognitive load classification. *Proceedings of International Conference on Pattern Recognition* (pp. 4516–4519).

Levitt, H. (1971). Transformed up-down methods in psychoacoustics. *The Journal of the Acoustical Society of America, 49,* 467–477.

Littlewort, G., Whitehill, J., Wu, T., Fasel, I., Frank, M., Movellan, J., & Bartlett, M. (2011). The computer expression recognition toolbox (CERT). *IEEE International Conference on Automatic Face & Gesture Recognition and Workshops* (pp. 298–305).

Lively, S. E., Pisoni, D. B., Van Summers, W., & Bernacki, R. H. (1993). Effects of cognitive workload on speech production: Acoustic analyses and perceptual consequences. *The Journal of the Acoustical Society of America, 93*(5), 2962–2973.

Logemann, J. A., Fisher, H. B., Boshes, B., & Blonsky, E. R. (1978). Frequency and co-occurrence of vocal tract dysfunctions in the speech of a large sample of Parkinson patients. *J. Speech Hear. Disord. 43*(1), 47.

Lucey, P., Cohn, J. F., Kanade, T., Saragih, J., Ambadar, Z., & Matthews, I. (2010). The Extended Cohn-Kanade Dataset (CK+): A complete dataset for action unit and emotion-specified expression. *IEEE Computer Society Conference on Computer Vision and Pattern Recognition Workshops* (pp. 94–101).

Maryn, Y., Corthals, P., Van Cauwenberge, P., Roy, N., & De Bodt, M. (2010). Toward improved ecological validity in the acoustic measurement of overall voice quality: Combining continuous speech and sustained vowels. *Journal of Voice, 24*(5), 540–555.

Mehta, D. D., Rudoy, D., & Wolfe, P. J. (2012). Kalman-based autoregressive moving average modeling and inference for formant and antiformant tracking. *The Journal of the Acoustical Society of America, 132*(3), 1732–1746.

Moore, E., Clements, M., Peifer, J., & Weisser, L. (2003). Analysis of prosodic variation in speech for clinical depression. *Proceedings of the Annual International Conference of Engineering in Medicine and Biology* (pp. 2925–2928).

Mundt, J. C., Snyder, P. J., Cannizzaro, M. S., Chappie, K., & Geralts, D. S. (2007). Voice acoustic measures of depression severity and treatment response collected via interactive voice response (IVR) technology. *Journal of Neurolinguistics, 20*(1), 50–64.

Orozco-Arroyave, J., Arias-Londoño, J., Vargas-Bonilla, J., González-Rátiva, M., & Nöth, E. (2014). New Spanish speech corpus database for the analysis of people suffering from Parkinson's disease. *Proceedings of International Conference on Language Resources and Evaluation* (pp. 342–347).

Ozdas, A., Shiavi, R. G., Silverman, S. E., Silverman, M. K., & Wilkes, D. M. (2004). Investigation of vocal jitter and glottal flow spectrum as possible cues for depression and near-term suicidal risk. *IEEE Transactions on Biomedical Engineering, 51*(9), 1530–1540.

Park, H., Felty, R., Lormore, K., & Pisoni, D. B. (2010). PRESTO: Perceptually robust English sentence test: Open-set—Design, philosophy, and preliminary findings. *The Journal of the Acoustical Society of America, 127*(3), 1958–1958.

Quatieri, T. F. (2002). *Discrete-time speech signal processing: Principles and practice.* Pearson Education.

Quatieri, T. F., & Malyska, N. (2012). Vocal-source biomarkers for depression: A link to psychomotor activity. *Proceedings of Annual Conference of the International Speech Communication Association.*

Quatieri, T. F., Williamson, J. R., Smalt, C. J., Patel, T., Perricone, J., Mehta, D. D., . . . Moran, J. (2015). Vocal biomarkers to discriminate cognitive load in a working memory task. *Proceedings of Annual Conference of the International Speech Communication Association.*

Reynolds, D. A., Quatieri, T. F., & Dunn, R. B. (2000). Speaker verification using adapted Gaussian mixture models. *Digital Signal Processing, 10*(1), 19–41.

Rouas, J. (2007). Automatic prosodic variations modeling for language and dialect discrimination. *IEEE Transactions on Audio, Speech, and Language Processing, 15*(6), 1904–1911.

Schmidt, K. L., Bhattacharya, S., & Denlinger, R. (2009). Comparison of deliberate and spontaneous facial movement in smiles and eyebrow raises. *Journal of Nonverbal Behavior, 33,* 35–45.

Shen, W., White, C., & Hazen, T. J. (2010). A comparison of query-by-example methods for spoken term detection. *Proceedings of the IEEE International Conference on Acoustics Speech and Signal Processing.*

Trevino, A., Quatieri, T. F., & Malyska, N. (2011). Phonologically-based biomarkers for major depressive disorder. *EURASIP Journal on Advances in Signal Processing: Special Issue on Emotion and Mental State Recognition from Speech, 42,* 2011–2042.

Valstar, M., Schuller, B., Smith, K., Almaev, T., Eyben, F., Krajewski, J., . . . Pantic, M. (2013). AVEC 2014, 3D dimensional affect and depression recognition challenge. *Proceedings of the 3rd ACM International Workshop on Audio/visual Emotion Challenge (AVEC).*

Wang, P., Barrett, F., Martin, E., Milonova, M., Gurd, R. E., Gur, R. C., . . .Verma, R. (2008). Automated video-based facial expression analysis of neuropsychiatric disorders. *Journal of Neuroscience Methods, 168,* 224–238.

Williamson, J. R., Bliss, D. W., Browne, D. W., & Narayanan, J. T. (2012). Seizure prediction using EEG spatiotemporal correlation structure. *Epilepsy & Behavior, 25*(2), 230–238.

Williamson, J. R., Quatieri, T. F., Helfer, B. S., Ciccarelli, G., & Mehta, D. D. (2014). Vocal and facial biomarkers of depression based on motor incoordination and timing. *Proceedings of the 4th ACM International Workshop on Audio/Visual Emotion Challenge (AVEC)* (pp. 65–72).

Williamson, J. R., Quatieri, T. F., Helfer, B. S., Horwitz, R., Yu, B., & Mehta, D. D. (2013). Vocal biomarkers of depression based on motor incoordination. *Proceedings of the 3rd ACM International Workshop on Audio/visual Emotion Challenge (AVEC)* (pp. 41–48).

Williamson, J. R., Quatieri, T. F., Helfer, B. S., Perricone, J., Ghosh, S. S., Ciccarelli, G., & Mehta, D. D. (2015). Segment-dependent dynamics in predicting Parkinson's disease. *Proceedings of the Annual Conference of the International Speech Communication Association.*

Yap, T. F. (2011). *Speech production under cognitive load: Effects and classification* (Doctoral thesis, The University of New South Wales School of Electrical Engineering and Telecommunications Sydney, Australia).

Yin, B., & Chen, F. (2007). Towards automatic cognitive load measurement from speech analysis. *Human-computer interaction: Interaction design and usability* (pp. 1011–1020). Berlin Heidelberg: Springer.

Yin, B., Chen, F., Ruiz, N., & Ambikairajah, E. (2008). Speech-based cognitive load monitoring system. *Proceedings of EEE International Conference on Acoustics, Speech, and Signal Processing.*

Yu, B., Quatieri, T. F., Williamson, J. W., & Mundt, J. (2014). Prediction of cognitive performance in an animal fluency task based on rate and articulatory markers.

*Proceedings of the Annual Conference of the International Speech Communication Association.*

Zarjam, P., Epps, J., et al. (2011a). Spectral EEG features for evaluating cognitive load. *Proceedings of the 33rd EMBS Conference* (pp. 3841–3844).

Zarjam, P., Epps, J., et al. (2011b). Evaluation of working memory load using EEG signals. *Proceedings of the 2nd APSIPA Conference* (pp. 715–719).

Zarjam, P., Epps, J., & Lovell, N. H. (2015). Beyond subjective self-rating: EEG signal classification of cognitive workload. *IEEE Transactions on Autonomous Mental Development, 7*(4), 301–310.

# 15

# Integrating Technologies in the Study of Attentional Networks
## Michael I. Posner

## Computerized Testing

The literature supports the idea that attention is not a unified concept, but involves separate mechanisms that support its varied functions (Petersen & Posner, 2012). One common taxonomy involves three such functions: obtaining and maintaining the alert state, orienting to sensory stimuli, and resolving conflict among competing responses. Each of the functions has a long history and has spawned tests designed to measure individual differences in attention.

Many individual tests and batteries of tests are designed to measure attention. Tests of vigilance usually involve maintaining attention over long periods of time, originally simulating the job of scanning radar returns for low-probability targets (Mackworth, 1969; Parasuraman, 1985). Another approach is to require responses to infrequent events, as in the continuous performance test (Rosvold et al., 1956) or the serial response test (Manly et al., 1999). Vigilance varies with the diurnal rhythm and vigilance can be reduced by sleep deprivation. Collectively, the tests of performance during continuous tasks are often called measures of tonic alertness, which is thought to change rather slowly.

It is also possible to cause phasic shifts of the level of alertness by the use of warning signals (Nickerson, 1967). A warning signal can bring a person from a relatively relaxed state to one fostering the very best performance within less than half a second. Recent fMRI studies have defined a default state in which a person is off task (Raichle, 2009). It seems likely that scalp electrodes recording direct current shifts following warning signals called the contingent negative variation (CNV) capture the shift from the default to the alert state.

The most frequently studied area in attention research involves orienting to a sensory source that contains a target. For example, in a visual search, a target may be defined as a red triangle. If it appears in a field that contains other colored triangles and red forms other than triangles, one can ensure that the field is carefully searched until the target is found. If the distractors are all blue squares, the target will pop out without any evident search (Treisman & Galade, 1980).

Studies of fMRI and of patients with lesions of the parietal lobe have given evidence of a common network that is the source of an orienting effect, regardless of the sensory modality involved (Petersen & Posner, 2012).

The ability to resolve conflict has been most frequently studied by using the Stroop effect, in which a color word (e.g., "red") is printed in colored ink that might be congruent or incongruent with the word (Macleod, 1991). Studies using fMRI and EEG with the Stroop effect have revealed a network of brain areas involved in detecting and resolving conflict. The areas include the anterior cingulate, anterior insula, and links to the striatum (Petersen & Posner, 2012). The Stroop task has versions appropriate for animals, young children, or patients and has been studied many hundreds of times. Another task that has been used for studies involving the resolution of conflict involves surrounding the target (which might be an arrow or word) with flankers that signal either the same or opposite response. Versions of the flanker task can be used with young children.

The Attention Network Test (ANT) (Fan et al., 2002) measures all three functions by using cues that indicate the location where the target will occur or that serve as a warning that a target will follow shortly. The target has congruent or incongruent flankers (see Figure 15.1). While the reliability of the original version

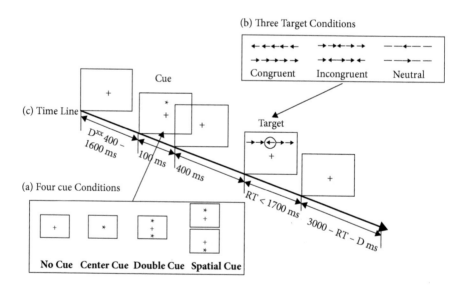

FIGURE 15.1 (a) Cues used in the Attention Network Test (ANT). (b) Target types in the ANT. (c) Time line of events in the ANT. Bottom of figure are subtraction to obtain alerting, orienting, and conflict (executive) network scores. Adapted from Fan et al. (2002).

of the ANT was weak for orienting and alerting, revisions that make the orienting cue valid only 80% of the time and using an auditory warning signal have both improved reliability. Moreover, in an analysis of many neuropsychological tests that could serve to document neglect of contralesional space after cortical lesions, the use of a partly valid cue followed by a target (cued detection task) proved best in allowing neglect to be assessed and followed over many months following the lesion (Rengachary et al., 2009).

## Functional MRI

The ANT can be studied during fMRI by having participants perform the task while undergoing MRI (Fan et al., 2005). The fMRI studies have shown that each of the three networks has several cortical nodes, mostly confirming findings with individual tests and with patients showing that the networks have substantially independent anatomy (see Figure 15.2).

Niogi and McCandliss (2009) were able to show correlations between scores for alerting, orienting, and executive networks (see Figure 15.1) and the efficiency of white matter as measured by diffusion tensor imaging. Fractional anisotropy (FA) measures the degree to which water molecules diffuse in a particular direction, marking the white matter pathways. Higher FA scores indicate more efficient white matter connections.

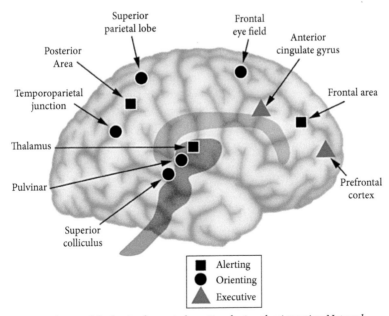

FIGURE 15.2 *Areas of the brain shown to be active during the Attention Network Test (ANT).*

Resting-state MRI (Dosenbach et al., 2007; Fair et al., 2009) has been used to reveal brain areas correlated when not performing any task. Among the brain areas found to be correlated during rest are areas of the lateral frontal and parietal cortex related to the orienting network and medial frontal areas (cingulo-opercular network), including the anterior cingulate and anterior insula, related to the executive network.

The resting-state method has been used to study the development of brain networks from infancy to adulthood since it is unnecessary to define a task in order to study the networks (Fair et al., 2009; Gao et al., 2012). Among the many findings is that the orienting network is present in infancy in nearly its adult form, while anterior cingulate activity is also present during infancy (Berger, Tzur, & Posner, 2006; Gao et al., 2012), but it only slowly becomes connected to the motor, sensory, and limbic areas that it controls. Behavioral and EEG data show that while the anterior cingulate cortex (ACC) activates in detecting error at 7 months of age, the ability to act on the error to slow subsequent performance does not occur until after 3 years of age (Jones, Rothbart, & Posner, 2003). The use of resting-state MRI, together with EEG and behavioral data, gives promise of greater understanding of the neural basis for the changes in control of behavior and emotion that mark the transition from infancy and beyond.

## EEG-MEG

The use of scalp electrodes to record electrical activity or superconducting coils for magnetic activity complements MRI by allowing acquisition of more precise temporal information (Luck, 2014). This is particularly useful where re-entrant activity, as in many cognitive tasks, is common. For example, activation of prestriate areas may be involved in the original intake of sensory information or may occur as the result of attention processes in, for example, creating a visual image. To distinguish the activities, it is important to be able to know when exactly the input occurs. While some temporal information can be obtained from the MRI signal, EEG and MEG can provide precise information, millisecond by millisecond. Often it is important to know in what order a series of activation occurs. Figure 15.3 indicates a possible time course of the several attentional, representational, and motoric events that mark the interpretation of a visually presented phrase or sentence (see Figure 15.3).

The EEG signal can be broken down by a power analysis to reveal the energy in various frequency bands. This can provide very important information. For example, neurons in the posterior parietal lobe can oscillate in the gamma frequency band (30-100 Hz) and be synchronized with activity in the ventral extrastriate areas to amplify the input signal there (Womelsdorf, Fries, Mitra, & Desimone; 2006).

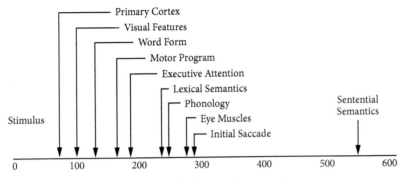

FIGURE 15.3 *Time course of activity related to reading a word or sentence.*

## Lesions

### PATIENTS

A study in a neurological care facility used the ANT to test 110 stroke patients and 62 controls (Rinne et al., 2013). The investigators found that, compared to controls, patients had slower reaction times, and one set of patients showed an alerting deficit, mainly associated with lesions of the anterior thalamus, while another set presented with an orienting deficit, due to lesions in the right pulvinar and temporoparietal cortex, and a third set presented with executive deficits, due mainly to lesions involving bilateral white matter tracts associated with the anterior cingulate.

All three of the patient groups fit well with previous imaging findings, as illustrated in Figure 15.2. The thalamic norepinephrine system is central to the alert state. Lesions of the right temporoparietal junction produce neglect of space opposite the lesion. The observation that lesions of the anterior corona radiata disrupt executive control fits with the finding that the executive network correlated with the efficiency of this pathway in diffusion tensor imaging studies (Niogi & McCandliss, 2009). While imaging studies indicate whether a particular brain area or white matter tract is involved in the network, the lesion data add to the evidence that these areas are critical for the efficient operation of the networks.

### TRANSCRANIAL MAGNETIC STIMULATION (TMS)

The clinical ANT study discussed above indicates that brain areas common to imaging and lesion effects are necessary in order to achieve particular attentional functions. While the use of neurological patients forms a natural experiment, the lesions involved may be too large and complex to test particular theories.

TMS enlarges the scope of lesion studies by rendering areas of the brain near the site of stimulation ineffective for a brief period of time. Although such studies are mostly effective for lateral brain areas, the experimenter can have the area function or not function depending on the TMS site of stimulation. TMS also can achieve temporal precision in controlling exactly when the area is rendered inoperative. As an example, in the orienting network, a cue at a particular location will attract attention and improve reaction time (RT) to targets at that location. When attention is summoned away from the cued location, that location becomes less effective in returning attention, and therefore targets at that cued location have longer reaction times than comparable areas that have not been cued (inhibition of return(IOR); Posner & Cohen, 1984). Ro, Farne, and Chang (2003) found that a brief TMS pulse to the scalp above the frontal eye fields eliminates inhibition of return. This implicates the frontal eye fields in the reduced reaction time to stimuli that occurs at a previously attended location. While this is a new finding, the role of the eye movement system in general and the superior colliculus in particular in inhibition of return(IOR) has been known from both behavioral and patient studies (Posner & Cohen, 1984; Sapir et al., 1999).

## Cellular Activity

A number of tools are available for recording from depth electrodes in human neurosurgery patients (Sheth et al., 2012) and in animals. These methods have been used both to confirm and to enlarge some of the results discussed above and to allow tests of microcircuits that involve areas impossible for fMRI and EEG/MEG to resolve. Many of these techniques involve recording electrical activity from individual neurons or summed activity among several neurons.

It has now become possible to use light to control the onset and offset of particular classes of neurons through a method called optogenetics. This method has begun to reveal important new pathways for information from the executive attention network to reach brain areas related to memory (Xu & Sudhoff, 2013). Little was known about the pathways by which attention interacted with the hippocampus. Studies on rodents have shown that the anterior cingulate is critical to the recall of information stored for a month or more (Weible, 2013). The ACC connection to the hippocampus pathway in mice appears to be critical for the rodent to obtain the proper level of generalization. After being conditioned to a shock in one context, mice with intact ACC generalize to similar, but not to dissimilar, contexts. However, those with inactivated ACC show overgeneralization, and respond with fear to dissimilar contexts (Xu & Sudhof, 2013). The authors argue that the ACC and mid prefrontal cortex control the degree of generalization of memory via links to the hippocampus.

## Neurochemical and Genetic Differences

The association of attentional networks with particular neuromodulators (Marrocco & Davidson, 1998) has led to identification of candidate genes that are expected to relate to each network. The results were summarized by Green et al. (2009), but a number of other results that have qualified the view are shown in Table 15.1. It seems clear that serotonin as well as dopamine can influence the executive attention network (Reuter et al., 2007), and that there are interactions between dopaminergic and cholinergic genes at the molecular level that modify the degree of independence between them (Markett et al., 2010). Nonetheless, the scheme in Table 15.1 provides a degree of organization and prediction that is often lacking in studies of genetic influence on cognition and behavior. It supports the distinction between the three separate networks by showing dissociations at the neurochemical and genetic levels. Table 15.1 also points the way to studies that help our understanding of how genes lead to the development of specific networks.

TABLE 15.1  Brain Attention Networks—Anatomy, Dominant Modulators, and Genetic Alleles

| Network | Modulator | Genes |
|---|---|---|
| **Alerting** | Norepinephrine | *ADRA2A* |
| Locus ceruleus | | *NET* |
| Right frontal cortex | | |
| Right parietal cortex | | |
| **Orienting** | Acetylcholine | *CHRNA4* |
| Frontal eye fields | | *APOE* |
| Superior parietal lobe | | |
| Temporoparietal junction | | |
| Superior colliculus | | |
| Pulvinar | | |
| **Executive** | Dopamine | *DRD4, DAT1, COMT* |
| Anterior cingulate | | *MAOA, DBH* |
| Anterior insula | Serotonin | *TPH2, 5HTT* |
| Frontal cortex | | |
| Striatum | | |

Adapted from Green et al., 2008.

# Conclusion

A large toolkit of technology is available for the detailed study of the human brain. The technologies may be employed together to trace the time course of localized brain activation and to determine their causal effects. Within the field of attention, a great deal of progress has been made by skillful joint employment of the technologies to determine the separation and overlap of brain networks that carry out different attentional functions. We need more effort to integrate the technologies in order to answer the many outstanding questions in the field and to apply them to the many cognitive domains that remain to be studied in detail.

# Acknowledgment

This research was supported by NIH grant 060563 to Georgia State University. The author is grateful to Prof. Mary K. Rothbart for help in writing.

# References

Berger, A., Tzur, G., & Posner, M. I. (2006). Infant brains detect arithmetic errors. *Proceedings of the National Academy of Sciences of the United States of America, 103*(33), 12649–12653.

Dosenbach, N. U. F., Fair, D. A., Miezin, F. M., Cohen, A. L., Wenger, K. K. R., Dosenbach, A. T., . . . Petersen, S. E. (2007). Distinct brain networks for adaptive and stable task control in humans. *Proceedings of the National Academy of Sciences of the United States of America, 104*, 1073–1078.

Fair, D. A., Cohen, A. L., Power, J. D., Dosenbach, N. U. F., Church, J. A., Miezin, F. M., . . . Petersen, S. E. (2009). Functional brain networks develop from a "local to distributed" organization. *PLoS Computational Biology, 5*, e1000381. doi:10.1371/journal.pcbi.100038

Fan, J., McCandliss, B. D., Fossella, J., Flombaum, J. I., & Posner, M. I. (2005). The activation of attentional networks. *Neuroimage 26*, 471–479.

Fan, J., McCandliss, B. D., Sommer, T., Raz, M., & Posner, M. I. (2002). Testing the efficiency and independence of attentional networks. *Journal of Cognitive Neuroscience, 3*(14), 340–347.

Gao, W., Gilmore, J. H., Shen, D., Smith, J. K., Zhu, H., & Lin, W. (2013). The synchronization within and interaction between the default and dorsal attention networks in early infancy. *Cerebral Cortex, 23*/3, 594–603. doi:10.1093/cercor/bhs043

Gao, W., Zhu, H., Giovanello, K. S., Smith, J. K., Shen, D., Gilmore, J. H., & Lin, W. (2009). Evidence on the emergence of the brain's default network from 2-week-old to 2-year-old healthy pediatric subjects. *Proceedings of the National Academy of Sciences USA, 106*, 6790–6795. doi:10.1073/pnas.0811221106

Green, A. E., Munafo, M. R., DeYoung, C. G., Fossella, J. A., Fan, J., & Gray, J. R. (2008). Using genetic data in cognitive neuroscience: From growing pains to genuine insights. *Nature Review Neuroscience, 9*, 710–720.

Jones, L. B., Rothbart, M. K., & Posner, M. I. (2003). Development of executive attention in preschool children. *Developmental Science, 6*(5), 498–504.

Luck, S. J. (2014). *Introduction to the event potential technique.* Cambridge, MA:MIT Press.

Mackworth, J. F. (1969). *Vigilance and habituation.* London, England: Penguin.

Macleod, C. M. (1991). Half a century of research on the Stroop effect: An integrative review. *Psychological Bulletin, 109,* 163–203.

Manly, T., Robertson, I. H., Galloway, M., & Hawkins, K. (1999) The absent mind: Further investigations of sustained attention to response. *Neuropsychologia, 37*(6), 661–670.

Markett, S.A., Montag, C., & Reuter, M. (2010). The association between dopamine DRD2 polymorphisms and working memory capacity is modulated by a functional polymorphism on the nicotinic receptor gene *CHRNA4. Journal of Cognitive Neuroscience, 22*(9), 1944–1954.

Marrocco, R. T., & Davidson, M. C. (1998). Neurochemistry of attention. In R. Parasuraman (Ed.), *The attentive brain* (pp. 35–50). Cambridge, MA: MIT Press.

Nickerson, R. S. (1967). Expectancy, waiting time and the psychological refractory period. *Acta Psychologica, 27,* 23–34.

Niogi, S., & McCandliss, B. D. (2009). Individual differences in distinct components of attention are linked to anatomical variations in distinct white matter tracts. *Frontiers in Neuroanatomy, 3,* 21.

Parasuraman, R. (1985). Sustained attention: A multifactorial approach. In M. I. Posner & O. M. Marin (Eds.), *Attention and performance XI.* Hillsdale NJ: Erlbaum.

Petersen, S. E., & Posner, M. I. (2012). The attention system of the human brain: 20 years after. *Annual Review of Neuroscience 35,* 71–89.

Posner, M. I., & Cohen, Y. (1984). Components of attention. In H. Bouma & D. Bowhuis (Eds.), *Attention and performance X* (pp. 531–556). Hillsdale NJ: Erlbaum.

Raichle, M. E. (2009). A paradigm shift in functional imaging. *Journal of Neuroscience, 29,* 12729–12734.

Rengachary, J., d'Avossa, J., Sapir, A., Shulman, G. L., & Corbetta, M. (2009). Is the Posner Reaction Time Test more accurate than clinical tests in detecting left neglect in acute and chronic stroke? *Archives of Physical Medicine and Rehabilitation, 90*(12), 2081–2088.

Reuter, M., Ott, U.,Vaitl, D., & Hennig, J. (2007). Impaired executive control is associated with a variation in the promoter region of the tryptophan hydroxylase 2 gene. *Journal of Cognitive Neuroscience, 19*(3), 401–408. doi:10.1162/jocn.2007.19.3.401

Rinne, P., Hassan, M., Goniotakis, D., Chohan, K., Sharma, P., Langdon, D., Soto, D., & Bentley, P. (2013). Triple dissociation of attention networks in stroke according to lesion location. *Neurology, 81,* 812–820.

Ro, T., Farne, A., & Chang, E. (2003). Inhibition of return and the human frontal eye fields. *Experimental Brain Research, 150*(3), 290–296.

Rosvold, H. E., Mirsky, A. F., Sarason, I., Bransome, E. D., & Beck, L. H. (1956). A continuous performance test of brain damage. *Journal of Consulting Psychology, 20,* 343–350.

Sapir, A., Soroker, N., Berger, A., & Henik, A. (1999). Inhibition of return in spatial attention: Direct evidence of collicular generation. *Nature Neuroscience, 2,* 1053–1054.

Sheth, S. A., Mian, M. K., Patel, S. R., Asaad, W. F., Williams, Z. M., Dougherty, D. D., . . . Eskander, E. N. (2012). Human dorsal anterior cingulate cortex neurons mediate ongoing behavioural adapation. *Nature, 488,* 218. doi:10.1038/nature11239

Treisman, A. M., & Galade, G. (1980). A feature integration theory of attention. *Cognitive Psychology, 12,* 97–136.

Weible, A. P. (2013). Remembering to attend: The anterior cingulate cortex and remote memory. *Behavioural and Brain Resarch, 245,* 63–75.

Womelsdorf, T., Fries, P., Mitra, P. P., & Desimone, R. (2006). Gamma-band synchronization in visual cortex predicts speed of change detection. *Nature, 439,* 733–736.

Xu, W., & Sudhof, T. C. (2013). A neural circuit for memory specificity and generalization. *Science, 339*(6125), 1290–1295.

{ PART V }

# Conclusion

# 16

# Advanced Technology and Assessment: Ethical and Methodological Considerations

## Shane S. Bush and Philip Schatz

The role of technology in neuropsychological practice has expanded dramatically in recent years, and its presence and evolving nature provide both exciting opportunities and sizeable risks that challenge practitioners ethically. Computerized test administration, scoring, and interpretation are now so common that is it hard to imagine a neuropsychologist's practice that does not incorporate some combination of these technologies. Some of the most commonly used measures have become so complex or offer so many variables to consider that their scoring and interpretation would be extremely difficult, if not prohibitive, without the use of technology. Additionally, assessment of some cognitive constructs, such as sustained attention or response time, typically requires a computer for administration. Without computers for assessing such constructs, the understanding of the test taker's cognitive abilities would be limited, and the decision to forgo use of such measures would not be consistent with optimal practice. Some referral sources, particularly in forensic contexts, specifically require the use of measures that are computer-administered, scored, and/or interpreted. Finally, computers, or other technologic devices, such as tablets, are now widely used by practitioners for completing and storing reports and other documentation, and telecommunications like email are commonly used for transmitting reports. Thus, technology now permeates the practice of clinical neuropsychology and will likely continue to do so forever.

Even practitioners who prefer to limit use of technology must accept that it is here and is here to stay. This is not a bad thing. There are many advantages to the use of digital assessment and data storage. As Wahlstrom (in press) stated:

> After decades of incremental technological advancements, neuropsychology is beginning to see a rapid expansion of digital applications available to clinicians. In the short-term, these applications promise to replace paper materials and will make testing more efficient, accurate, and engaging for both the examinee and examiner. In the long-term, technology will likely revolutionize the practice of forensic neuropsychology similar to how it has

other industries, whether through advanced data analytics, the creation of new tests that change the constructs used to understand examinees, or completely new environments that replace the traditional testing setting.

In this context, failure to utilize technology when it offers the best method of assessing a cognitive construct in a particular examinee may be inconsistent with best practices.

Appropriate use of technology can promote effective, ethical neuropsychological services, as well as pose risks to ethical practice. Understanding the ethical issues associated with the use of technology in neuropsychological assessment prepares practitioners to provide quality services while helping protect themselves, test takers, referral sources, and the public from the limitations and possible misuses inherent in the application of technology in clinical practice. The primary goal of this chapter is to present the relevant ethical issues and potential challenges (see Box 16.1) and to offer recommendations for avoiding ethical dilemmas and for addressing challenges when they occur.

## Resources and Priorities

The individual practitioner is not alone in attempting to determine the ethical implications of using technology in neuropsychological practice. Numerous resources exist to guide neuropsychologists in their efforts to employ technology in an ethical manner. Some resources, such as the *Ethical Principles of Psychologists and Code of Conduct* (Ethics Code; American Psychological Association [APA], 2010) are not specific to technology and in fact address it only minimally, but the principles and standards that apply to psychological services more generally are also applicable to the use of technology and can guide neuropsychologists in their practices.

Similarly, valuable resources for promoting ethical practice in psychological specialties in which neuropsychologists apply their knowledge and skills provide little guidance specific to technology, but their content nevertheless remains

---

BOX 16.1  Primary ethical challenges in the use of technology in neuropsychological practice

- Attaining and maintaining professional competence in the use of technology
- Selecting and using appropriate technological assessment measures, including platform and scoring and interpretation programs
- Identifying and negating threats to the validity of test data
- Identifying and negating threats to the accuracy of conclusions and diagnoses
- Maintaining privacy and confidentiality
- Maintaining test and data security

informative for the application of technology in neuropsychological assessment. For example, although the *Specialty Guidelines for Forensic Psychology* (APA, 2013) do not specifically mention technology, and only mention computerized scoring and interpretation once (Guideline 10.02, Selection and Use of Assessment Procedures), many of the guidelines offer information about forensic practice that can be readily applied to the use of technology.

As with the *Specialty Guidelines for Forensic Psychology*, technology and computerized assessment are addressed in only one guideline (Guideline 8, which covers the use of psychometric instruments) of the *Guidelines for the Evaluation of Dementia and Age-Related Cognitive Change* (APA, 2012), but the guidelines remain a valuable source of information in the context of neuropsychological assessment with technology. Compared to those guidelines, the *Standards for Educational and Psychological Testing* (American Educational Research Association [AERA], APA, & National Council on Measurement in Education [NCME], 2014) provide more coverage of the use of technology. The standards address computer administration of tests, computer adaptive testing, and automated test scoring and interpretation.

In contrast to resources that were developed for more general purposes or for related specialties, some are more specific to the use of technology in neuropsychological assessment. The *Guidelines for the Practice of Telepsychology* (Joint Task Force for the Development of Telepsychology Guidelines for Psychologists, 2013) address issues that are relevant to the use of technology in psychological practice overall, rather than only telepsychology, and an entire guideline (Guideline 7) is devoted to testing and assessment. Additional guidelines on computer-based and Internet-delivered testing target an international audience of practitioners, test developers, test publishers, test takers, and other interested parties (International Test Commission, 2005). In addition to formal guidelines and codes, scholarly works like articles and book chapters devoted to this specific topic are excellent resources, as are colleagues who are experienced in this type of practice. Finally, but by no means least important, jurisdictional laws (both where the service is provided and where it is received, if different), institutional regulations, and other policies governing the practice of neuropsychology must be understood and followed.

Efforts to engage in ethical practice range from risk management, which is essentially the avoidance of ethical misconduct, to the pursuit of ethical ideals. The pursuit of ethical ideals can require time and effort beyond that required for basic risk management, but outcomes that are better for individual patients, the profession, and society can result. Each neuropsychologist must decide how invested he or she is in attaining and maintaining high standards of ethical practice. Although disagreements can and do exist about specific decisions or actions that reflect ethical ideals, choosing not to strive for high standards of ethical practice does a disservice to consumers of neuropsychological services and reflects poorly on neuropsychology as a profession.

## Professional Competence

Possessing the knowledge and skills to competently execute the professional activities that are being performed positions neuropsychologists to assist patients or other clients without harming them, which is consistent with the general bioethical principles of beneficence and nonmaleficence. The Ethics Code explains that professional competence is established through "education, training, supervised experience, consultation, study, or professional experience" (Ethical Standard 2.01, Boundaries of Competence). This requirement is easier to satisfy when using tools or procedures that existed when one was originally educated or trained but is more challenging to satisfy when new measures and methods emerge rapidly during one's career. Although neuropsychologists understand the need to maintain competence throughout their careers (Ethical Standard 2.03), keeping pace with the emergence of new technology can be extremely challenging. It is not just a matter of keeping one's skills sharp; it is a matter of continuously trying to remain informed about new products and applications and to evaluate their effectiveness compared to existing measures or methods. Such challenges cannot be overstated, given that new technology-based products often emerge and are brought into common use before extensive research, including studies by those without a vested interest in the product, can be undertaken, particularly with specialty populations, and published.

The *Guidelines for the Practice of Telepsychology* (Joint Task Force for the Development of Telepsychology Guidelines for Psychologists, 2013) list "Competence of the Psychologist" as the first guideline, which seems to emphasize its importance. The guideline acknowledges that sometimes technology precedes research and advises clinicians as follows: "Research may not be available in the use of some specific technologies, and clients/patients should be made aware of those telecommunication technologies that have no evidence of effectiveness. However, this, in and of itself, may not be grounds to deny providing the service to the client/patient. Lack of current available evidence in a new area of practice does not necessarily indicate that a service is ineffective" (p. 794). While seemingly reasonable in theory, it is difficult to imagine applying this advice with a patient. Informing the client that the methods about to be used have no, or minimal, research to support their use, seems completely inconsistent with the strong emphasis on evidence-based practice that permeates healthcare in general and psychology specifically (APA Presidential Task Force on Evidence-Based Practice, 2006).

Although the lack of supporting evidence does not indicate that the service is ineffective, it certainly does not comply with ethical requirements to base one's work "upon established scientific and professional knowledge of the discipline" (Ethical Standard 2.04, Bases for Scientific and Professional

Judgments). Additionally, Ethics Code (Ethical Standard 9.02, Use of Assessments), states:

(a) Psychologists administer, adapt, score, interpret, or use assessment techniques, interviews, tests, or instruments in a manner and for purposes that are appropriate in light of the research on or evidence of the usefulness and proper application of the techniques.

If no such research or evidence exists, neuropsychologists cannot meet the requirements of the standard. The information presented in Guideline 1 also seems inconsistent with information provided in Guideline 7 of the same document, which states that for assessment procedures "conducted via telepsychology, psychologists are encouraged to ensure that the integrity of the psychometric properties of the test or assessment procedure (e.g., reliability and validity) and the conditions of administration indicated in the test manual are preserved when adapted for use with such technologies" (p. 798). Together, Guidelines 1 and 7 state that it may be acceptable to provide services that are lacking empirical support while also ensuring that empirical support exists for the services provided. Inconsistent professional guidelines and requirements like this challenge practitioners who are invested in understanding and following the highest standards of ethical behavior.

Best practices indicate that despite inconsistencies in some of the available guidelines, neuropsychologists have a primary obligation to avoid harming patients, such as through use of unsupported assessment measures that could lead to inaccurate diagnoses and inappropriate recommendations. The *Standards for Educational and Psychological Testing* (AERA, APA, & NCME, 2014) state, "Test takers have the right to be assessed with tests that meet current professional standards" (p. 131), which may include preferential use of digital measures over traditional measures, although either administration method may be used if both meet current professional standards.

## COMPETENCE OF INTERDISCIPLINARY COLLEAGUES

It is likely that most neuropsychologists personally know or are aware of colleagues in other healthcare disciplines who are using technologically based cognitive assessment measures, and often question the manner in which they are being used. While neuropsychologists have long been concerned about this practice with traditional cognitive measures, the ease with which computerized measures can be obtained and used seems to have increased this concern exponentially.

For example, it is common practice in some areas for "concussion specialists," who may be orthopedic surgeons by training, to have assistants or subordinates with no training in psychometrics or brain–behavior relationships place a patient in front of a brief self-administered computer program that generates a report that the concussion specialist then uses diagnostically and for decisions about return to school or some other activity or as the basis for a medication. Such clinicians are typically not trained to integrate information regarding premorbid cognitive functioning, performance validity, emotional factors, environmental distractions, or the myriad other issues that neuropsychologists routinely take into account. Such practices, at best, are not helpful. Best practices, in contrast, involve neuropsychologists' attempting to educate interdisciplinary colleagues about the complexity of the issues involved and the potential for interdisciplinary collaboration or referral, so that each professional's strengths can be used for the benefit of the patient. Educating not just the colleague in question but also others in the area can promote competent practices more broadly. Of course, such efforts will not be enthusiastically received by those driven solely by greed, but patients and society are best served when neuropsychologists try.

## Selection and Use of Technological Assessment Measures

Technological advances offer opportunities and advantages not available with traditional measures. A primary advantage is the ability to reduce human error. However, while technology has the potential to reduce human error, human error in the use of technology can have severe consequences (Bush, Naugle, & Johnson-Greene, 2002). Perhaps the most significant mistake that practitioners make in their use of technology is in its noncritical acceptance. The loudest criticism heard about technology-based assessment typically involves the cost. Heard less commonly and less loudly are concerns about the platform used or the scoring and interpretation programs, likely because those are less well understood by practitioners. For example, it is probably fairly common for practitioners to have little understanding of the basis of computer-generated narrative reports. The International Guidelines (International Test Commission, 2005) advise users of computer-based tests (CBTs) and Internet-administered tests to "Review and understand the rules underlying the scoring of the CBT/Internet test" and "Know how the statements in the CBTI (computer-based test interpretations) are derived and be aware of the limitations such methods may have" (p. 13). Standard 9.10 of the *Standards for Educational and Psychological Testing* (AERA, APA, & NCME, 2014) states, "The user of automatically generated scoring and reporting services has the obligation to be familiar with the principles on which such interpretations were derived" (p. 144). Additionally, Standard 10.17 states, "Those who use computer-generated interpretations of test data should verify that the quality of the evidence of validity is sufficient for the interpretations" (p. 168), including reviewing the normative data on which the interpretations are based for their relevance and appropriateness for a given examinee. The

British Psychological Society (2002) also recommended that users of computerized tests understand the principles underlying the scoring of the measures. Selection and use of assessment measures should be evidence based (Ethical Standard 9.02):

(b) Psychologists use assessment instruments whose validity and reliability have been established for use with members of the population tested. When such validity or reliability has not been established, psychologists describe the strengths and limitations of test results and interpretation.

It is difficult to make generalizations regarding the reliability, validity, or equivalence of digital tests because, where such research does exist, methodology varies substantially between studies (Wahlstrom, in press). An established evidence base for a test administered in the traditional manner does not automatically transfer to the same test administered with technology. Some measures, such as the Wisconsin Card Sorting Test, specifically have been found to produce different results depending on the method of administration (Steinmetz et al., 2010), and mixed results have been found for some Wechsler measures (Daniel, 2012; Daniel et al., 2014; Wahlstrom, in press).

Practitioners who use of technology-based assessment strive to use test norms derived from technology-based administration when possible (APA, 2013). The International Guidelines direct test publishers to evaluate and provide the evidence of equivalence of the CBT/Internet and traditional versions of tests, particularly when the norms from the manual versions are to be used with the computerized versions (p. 13). Practitioners must also consider equality of access and appropriateness for all test takers. Persons with sensory or motor deficits may be able to demonstrate strengths and weaknesses more or less accurately by using technology, depending on their limitations and the features of the technology. Similarly, the abilities of persons with limited exposure to technology may not be accurately reflected in the scores of computer-administered tests. Best practices suggest that, for each evaluation, the neuropsychologist must consider the advantages and disadvantages of proceeding with the new technology given what is known about its usefulness for the specific patient and the purpose of the assessment.

### INFORMED CONSENT

The right of examinees to be informed about proposed evaluation methods and procedures, including foreseeable risks and benefits, is well established. This right is based on the general bioethical principle of respect for patient autonomy and is reflected in the Ethics Code (ES 3.10, Informed Consent; ES 9.03, Informed Consent in Assessments) and most other guidelines for psychological assessment. Competent adult examinees also have the right to consent to or to decline the proposed services, with the exception of persons mandated for evaluation who face consequences if they refuse. Examinees who report being, or appear to be, uncomfortable with technology should be informed about alternative assessment options, as well as the advantages and disadvantages of both approaches, and should be allowed to choose the method for being assessed. Standard 8.3 of the *Standards for Educational and Psychological Testing* (AERA, APA, & NCME, 2014) states:

> When the test taker is offered a choice of test format, information about the characteristics of each format should be provided. . . . Test takers need to know the characteristics of each alternative that is available to them so that they can make an informed choice. (p. 134)

## Threats to the Validity of Test Data

Accurate data are required to make accurate diagnoses and offer meaningful opinions and recommendations. However, numerous factors related to technology, both within and beyond the assessment setting, threaten the validity of test data. Within a clinical practice, a variety of technology-related interferences can occur, such as cell phones ringing or buzzing (despite prior assurances from patients that they have turned off all devices), computer or software glitches, and power outages. Additionally, patient familiarity and comfort with technology vary, often according to cohort, and some patients with sensory or motor impairments may not be able to participate or interact fully in digital assessment. These issues can influence whether a patient's test performance accurately reflects the construct of interest. To help ensure that the patient's test performance reflects that abilities of interest, clinicians should assess patients' comfort levels with, and ability to fully engage in, the planned digital assessment process and make any changes necessary, including shifting to more traditional measures or administration formats where feasible.

Assessments performed via teleneuropsychology offer many advantages for examinees residing in rural areas where access to a neuropsychologist is limited, or those who are too frail, lack transportation, or are otherwise unable to present to the clinician's office. However, the success of the assessment may depend on the specific parameters of the teleneuropsychological assessment, including the training of those involved on the user's end, the examinee's comfort with the technology, the degree of control over the testing environment, and the reliability of the technology. The primary psychometric concern is whether the initial psychometric properties that were established in traditional assessment contexts are retained when the same measures are administered in a teleneuropsychology context. In their review of the literature on neuropsychological assessment performed with telemental health (TMH), Yoder and Turner (2014) determined that early investigations have shown promising results. They concluded that "The vast majority of procedures and measures, including standardized tests, used in mental health in-person settings are appropriate for use via TMH" (p. 164). Grosch et al. (2011) offered guidelines for the practice of teleneuropsychology, and subsequent publications have confirmed its value and acceptability (Cullum et al., 2014; Parikh et al., 2013).

Technology-based observation and/or the recording of neuropsychological evaluations can affect the examinee's performance. As with having a third party present during an evaluation, the presence of a video camera or auditory recording device during a neuropsychological evaluation affects test performance and skews the results (Constantinou, Ashendorf, & McCaffrey, 2002, 2005), and thus should be avoided in routine clinical and forensic contexts.

Outside of the assessment setting, examinees and anyone else who is interested can obtain electronic access to specific information about assessment measures and procedures and in some instances view or download copies of test materials (Bauer & McCaffrey, 2006). Such advance preparation for a neuropsychological evaluation invalidates the results of the evaluation and in the process wastes both the time of all involved and valuable resources. Neuropsychologists in some instances may be well served by asking examinees if they have researched or been coached about how to best respond to items on neuropsychological tests, or strategies for performing to the best (or in the case of malingering, the worst) of one's ability.

## TEST AND DATA SECURITY

Widespread or uncontrolled dissemination of information and materials can occur quickly and relatively easily via electronic means. Such dissemination threatens the privacy of individual examinees and the usefulness of the measures for future evaluations, and it can result in harmful effects for individuals whose materials are misused or misinterpreted by untrained persons. Neuropsychologists have an obligation to examinees, the profession, and society to safeguard test data and materials (Bush & Lees-Haley, 2006; Bush & Martin, 2006; Bush, Rapp, & Ferber, 2010). Consistent with the general bioethical principle of nonmaleficence, neuropsychologists strive to prevent harm from occurring as a result of their professional actions. Encryption technologies and passwords offer some protection from unauthorized access to test data and materials stored and used by neuropsychologists. Use of such security methods in the context of transmitting data is supported by the *Standards for Educational and Psychological Testing* (AERA, APA, & NCME, 2014). Standard 8.6 states, "If facsimile or computer communication is used to transmit test responses to another site for scoring or if scores are similarly transmitted, reasonable provisions should be made to keep the information confidential, such as encrypting the information" (p. 135).

## Threats to the Accuracy of Conclusions and Diagnoses

Automated test scoring and interpretation have the potential to help maximize accuracy of assessment conclusions and diagnoses, and thus recommendations. Reducing human error and receiving general interpretative statements from test developers, who are typically among the leaders in the field in their given areas of specialty, can, when combined with additional information and clinical judgment, result in sound conclusions and accurate diagnoses. Providing referral sources accurate information about an examinee is consistent with the bioethical principle of beneficence. The primary risk comes from noncritical acceptance of automated interpretations. General interpretive statements may not apply to a specific examinee.

> Although interpretation accuracy may be increased with patients who are similar to the standardization sample, many of the populations with whom neuropsychologists work have not traditionally been well represented in the standardization samples of commonly used tests. Therefore, the use of computerized interpretation may not accurately reflect the neuropsychological status of those with compromised neurological functioning" (Bush, Naugle, & Johnson-Greene, 2002, p. 539).

An automated report may accurately reflect the neuropsychological status of a given examinee but should not be automatically accepted without consideration of the examinee's history and other relevant information, which should all be included in the clinician's analysis. Whether cutting and pasting computer-generated reports into clinical reports is acceptable or good practice is a topic worthy of consideration from clinical, ethical, and legal perspectives. More than 16 years ago, less than half (42%) of surveyed respondents believed that cutting and pasting computerized narratives into reports raises ethical concerns (McMinn et al., 1999). However, the nature, sophistication, and use of automated reports have evolved substantially in the intervening years, and a recent review of ethical resources found no prohibition against such practice (Bush, 2014). While some automated materials are protected by copyright laws, some computer-generated reports are explicitly intended by test publishers to be used as provided (for a comprehensive review of this topic, see Bush, 2014). The primary consideration, as described in the Ethics Code (Standard 9.09c, Test Scoring and Interpretation Services) is that "psychologists retain responsibility for the appropriate application, interpretation, and use of assessment instruments, whether they score and interpret such tests themselves or use automated or other services." In making determinations about exact wording from automated reports in clinical reports, neuropsychologists must consider clinical relevance and permissions or restrictions provided by the test publishers. Bush (2014, p. 508) concluded: "if a clinician with the requisite expertise determines that (a) a computer-generated interpretation accurately reflects a patient's psychological status and (2) use of the wording is not prohibited by the test publisher, then use of the exact wording of the interpretation in the clinical report can be appropriate."

In the interest of expediency, some clinicians dictate reports using voice recognition software. Misinterpretation of speech by a software program can result in wording errors that misrepresent otherwise accurate and meaningful patient information and assessment results. Clinicians using voice recognition software must be sure to proof read reports before signing and disseminating them.

## Privacy and Confidentiality

Neuropsychologists have ethical and legal responsibilities to retain reports and other records for specified lengths of time (ES 6.01 and 6.02; also APA, 2007). In addition to the requirements posed by APA, state and federal laws, such as the Health Insurance Portability and Accountability Act and Health Information Technology for Economic and Clinical Health Act, govern the maintenance and security of records. A distinction is made between "data at rest," which refers to data on hard drives, and "data in transit," which refers to data that are being sent from one place to another. Data at rest are much more vulnerable to data breach or compromised systems than data in transit, for which cyber attacks are uncommon. Neuropsychologists should strive to safeguard test materials and data. However, there may not always be an awareness of how digital programs transmit and store information. Personal and test data that are transmitted to remote servers or databases for normative referencing or automated report generation must be protected from corruption and security intrusion, but clinicians may little understand how, or the extent to which, such protection occurs.

Neuropsychologists should strive to attain at least a basic understanding of data transfer and maintenance issues and know where to find additional information if needed. As previously noted, encryption technologies and passwords offer some protection from unauthorized access. Free encryption services available online may help meet the digital security needs of some practitioners. Although digital records are easily stored in perpetuity, deletion of old records consistent with time frames established by laws and professional guidelines prevents the loss of the materials through unauthorized access or accidental transmission.

## Conclusion

Advanced technology has much to offer the clinical neuropsychologist and, by extension, recipients of neuropsychological services. Competent use of technology is increasingly becoming required for good clinical and sound ethical neuropsychological practice, but it is not without its risks. An understanding of general bioethical principles and familiarity with relevant guidelines and related resources positions neuropsychologists to integrate technology into clinical activities in a manner that promotes patient care while reducing the risks of harmful outcomes. It is certain that use of advanced technology in neuropsychological practice in general and assessment in particularly will continue to increase. The pursuit of high standards of ethical practice requires that neuropsychologists attain and maintain competence in the use of technological applications in neuropsychological assessment, despite its rapid proliferation and evolution; the consumers of our services count on it.

# References

American Educational Research Association, American Psychological Association, & National Council on Measurement in Education. (2014). *Standards for educational and psychological testing*. Washington, DC: Author.

American Psychological Association. (2007). Record keeping guidelines. *American Psychologist, 62,* 993–1004. www.apa.org/practice/recordkeeping.pdf.

American Psychological Association. (2010). *Ethical Principles of Psychologists and Code of Conduct: 2010 Amendments*. Retrieved 2/17/11 from www.apa.org/ethics/code/index.aspx.

American Psychological Association. (2012). Guidelines for the assessment of dementia and age-related cognitive change. *American Psychologist, 67,* 1–9.

American Psychological Association. (2013). Specialty guidelines for forensic psychology. *American Psychologist, 68,* 7–19.

American Psychological Association Presidential Task Force on Evidence-Based Practice. (2006). Evidence-based practice in psychology. *American Psychologist, 61,* 271–285.

Bauer, L., & McCaffrey, R. J. (2006). Coverage of the Test of Memory Malingering, Victoria Symptom Validity Test, and Word Memory Test on the Internet: Is test security threatened? *Archives of Clinical Neuropsychology, 21,* 121–126.

British Psychological Society. (2002). *Guidelines for the development and use of computer-based assessments*. Leicester, UK: Author.

Bush, S. S. (2014). Ethical, legal, and professional considerations in the psychological assessment of veterans. In S. S. Bush (Ed.), *Psychological assessment of veterans* (pp. 494–513). New York NY: Oxford University Press.

Bush, S. S., & Lees-Haley, P. R. (2005). Threats to the validity of forensic neuropsychological data: Ethical considerations. *Journal of Forensic Neuropsychology, 4,* 45–66.

Bush, S. S., & Martin, T. A. (2006). The ethical and clinical practice of disclosing raw test data: Addressing the ongoing debate. *Applied Neuropsychology, 13,* 115–124.

Bush, S., Naugle, R., & Johnson-Greene, D. (2002). The interface of information technology and neuropsychology: Ethical issues and recommendations. *The Clinical Neuropsychologist, 16,* 536–547.

Bush, S. S., Rapp, D. L., & Ferber, P. S. (2010). Maximizing test security in forensic neuropsychology. In A. M. Horton, Jr., & L. C. Hartlage (Eds.), *Handbook of forensic neuropsychology* (2nd ed., pp. 177–195). New York NY: Springer Publishing Co.

Constantinou, M., Ashendorf, L., & McCaffrey, R. J. (2002). When the third-party observer of a neuropsychological evaluation is an audio-recorder. *The Clinical Neuropsychologist, 16*, 407–412.

Constantinou, M., Ashendorf, L., & McCaffrey, R. J. (2005). Effects of a third party observer during neuropsychological assessment: When the observer is a video camera. *Journal of Forensic Neuropsychology, 4*(2), 39–47.

Cullum, C. M., Hynan, L. S., Grosch, M., Parikh, M., & Weiner, M. F. (2014). Teleneuropsychology: Evidence for video teleconference-based neuropsychological assessment. *Journal of the International Neuropsychological Society, 20*, 1028–1033.

Daniel, M. H. (2012). Equivalence of Q-interactive administered cognitive tasks: WISC®–IV (Q-interactive Technical Report 2). Bloomington, MN: Pearson.

Daniel, M. H., Wahlstrom, D., & Zhang, O. (2014). Equivalence of Q-interactive® and paper administrations of cognitive tasks: WISC®-V. (Q-interactive Technical Report 8). Bloomington, MN: Pearson.

Grosch, M. C., Gottlieb, M. C., & Cullum, C. M. (2011). Initial practice recommendations for teleneuropsychology. *The Clinical Neuropsychologist, 25*, 1119–1133.

International Test Commission. (2005). *International guidelines on computer-based and Internetdelivered testing* (Version 2005). Author.

Joint Task Force for the Development of Telepsychology Guidelines for Psychologists. (2013). Guidelines for the practice of telepsychology. *American Psychologist, 68*, 791–800.

McMinn, M.R., Ellens, B.M., & Soref, E. (1999). Ethical perspectives and practice behaviors involving computer-based test interpretation. *Assessment, 6*, 71-77.

Parikh, M., Grosch, M. C., Graham, L. L., Hynan, L. S., Weiner, M., Shore, J. H., & Cullum, C. M. (2013). Consumer acceptability of brief videoconference-based neuropsychological assessment in older individuals with and without cognitive impairment. *The Clinical Neuropsychologist, 27*, 808–817.

Steinmetz, J., Brunner, M., Loarer, E., & Houssemand, C. (2010). Incomplete psychometric equivalence of scores obtained on the manual and the computer version of the Wisconsin Card Sorting Test? *Psychological Assessment, 22*, 199–202.

Wahlstrom, D. (in press). Technology and computerized assessments: Current state and future directions. In S. S. Bush, G. J. Demakis, & M. Rohling (Eds.), *APA handbook of forensic neuropsychology*. Washington, DC: American Psychological Association.

Yoder, M. S., & Turner, T. H. (2014). Assessment via telemental health technology. In S. S. Bush (Ed.), *Psychological assessment of veterans* (pp. 159–173). New York NY: Oxford University Press.

# 17

# Computational Neuropsychology: Current and Future Prospects for Interfacing Neuropsychology and Technology

Thomas D. Parsons and Robert L. Kane

Other chapters in this volume focus on the use of technology to enhance and expand the field of neuropsychology. Some of the enhancements are natural outgrowths of trends present in society at large and involve updating the assessment process to make it more efficient and reliable. Computerized approaches to assessment frequently use off-the-shelf technology, in some cases to administer traditional style tests, while in others to present tasks not readily accomplished with test booklets and paper (see Section II of this book on "Beyond Paper-and-Pencil Assessment"). The computer has also permitted the implementation of new testing paradigms such as scenario-based assessment and the use of virtual reality (see Section III: "Domain and Scenario-based Assessment").

The use of the computer has also made possible efforts to expand access to care through the development of efficient test batteries and telemedicine-based assessment (see Chapter 5 on Teleneuropsychology). The use of computers, the ability to implement life-like scenarios in a controlled environment, and telemedicine will also expand available approaches to cognitive remediation with cellphones augmenting the ability of individuals to engage in self-monitoring. The integration of neuroimaging into the assessment process was clearly presented in the chapter in this volume by Erin Bigler (see also Section IV of this book on "Integrating Cognitive Assessment with Biological Metrics"). An additional role for neuroimaging is the use of its ever evolving techniques and methods to model neural networks and to refine our understanding of how the brain works and how best to conceptualize cognitive domains. Both neuroimaging to model neural networks and the role of neuroinformatics will be discussed in the remaining sections of this chapter on some prospects for a future computational neuropsychology.

# Technology for Change in Neuropsychology

## NEUROIMAGING

Technological advances in neuroimaging of brain structure and function offer great potential for revolutionizing neuropsychology (Bilder, 2011). While neuro-imaging has taken advantage of advances in computerization and neuroinformatics, neuropsychological assessments are outmoded and reflect nosological attempts at classification that occurred prior to contemporary neuroimaging (see Chapter 13 in this volume). This lack of development in neuropsychological assessment makes it very difficult to develop clinical neuropsychological models. The call for advances in neuropsychological assessment is not new. Twenty years ago, Dodrill (1997) argued that neuropsychologists had made much less progress than would be expected, in both absolute terms and in comparison with the progress made in other clinical neurosciences. Dodrill pointed out that clinical neuropsychologists are using many of the same tests that they were using 30 years ago (in fact close to 50 years ago). If neuroradiologists were this slow in technological development, then they would be limited to pneumoencephalography and radioisotope brain scans—procedures that are considered primeval by current neuroradiological standards. According to Dodrill, the advances in neuropsychological assessment (e.g., Weschler scales) have resulted in new tests that are by no means conceptually or substantively better than the old ones. The full scope of issues raised by Dodrill becomes more pronounced when he compares progress in clinical neuropsychology to that in other neurosciences. For example, clinical neuropsychologists have historically been called upon to identify focal brain lesions. When one compares clinical neuropsychology's progress with that of clinical neurology, it is apparent that while the difference may not have been that great prior the appearance of CT scanning (in the 1970s), the advances since then (e.g., magnetic resonance imaging) have given clinical neurologists a dramatic edge.

While neuropsychological assessment measures remain static, advances in systems neuroscience have resulted in conceptual and methodological developments that are contributing to a changing paradigm in the study of psychopathology (Menon, 2011). New neuropsychological measures and models are needed that emphasize the ways in which the human brain produces cognition via its large-scale organization (Bressler & Menon, 2010). Given the human brain's complex patchwork of interconnected regions, network approaches have become increasingly useful for understanding how functionally connected systems prompt and restrain neurocognitive functions (Menon & Uddin, 2010). Furthermore, large-scale brain network approaches provide new insights into aberrant brain organization in several psychiatric and neurological disorders. Neuroimaging studies into psychopathology have increasingly focused on understanding the way in which disturbances in large-scale networks contribute to neurocognitive and affective dysfunction.

Vinod Menon at Stanford University's Institute for Neuro-Innovation and Translational Neurosciences has proposed a triple network model of aberrant saliency mapping and cognitive dysfunction in psychopathology (Menon, 2011). Menon's triple network model focuses on three intrinsic connectivity networks that have turned out to be particularly important for understanding higher cognitive function, and dysfunction: the central executive network, the default-mode network, and the salience network. First, the brain's central executive network (key nodes include the dorsolateral prefrontal cortex and posterior parietal cortex) handles high-level neurocognitive functions, such as planning, decision making, and the control of attention and working memory (Sridharan, Levitin, & Menon, 2008). Next, the default-mode network plays an important role in monitoring the person's internal mental landscape (Qin & Northoff, 2011). Finally, the salience network is involved in detecting and orienting to salient external stimuli and internal events. The salience network plays a key role in both the attentional capture of neurobiologically relevant events and in the subsequent engagement of frontoparietal systems for working memory and higher-order cognitive control (Menon & Uddin, 2010; Seeley et al., 2007). Whereas the central executive network and salience network typically reveal increases in activation during stimulus-driven neurocognitive and affective information processing, the default-mode network reveals decreased activation during tasks in which self-referential and stimulus-independent memory recall is not crucial (Raichle, 2015). The Menon model proposes that deficits in engagement and disengagement of these three core networks play a significant role in many psychiatric and neurological disorders. A key aspect of Menon's model is that inappropriate assignment of saliency to external stimuli or internal mental events can be found in dysfunctional processing.

## NEW NEUROPSYCHOLOGICAL ASSESSMENTS THAT TAP INTO LARGE-SCALE BRAIN NETWORKS

Where does neuropsychology fit into the developing understanding of large-scale brain networks? We argue that neuropsychologists can use neuroimaging to develop new frameworks for neuropsychological testing that are rooted in the current evidence base on large-scale brain system interactions. This will allow for traditional assessment of discrete areas of neurocognitive functioning (e.g., memory, attention) to be brought in line with recent findings that highly nuanced relations exist between cortical and subcortical processes (Koziol et al., 2014a, 2014b). Furthermore, the new findings from systems neuroscience may allow for the development of neuropsychological assessments with greater accuracy and increased targeted testing.

In addition to serving as an example of progress in neurology and the clinical neurosciences, neuroimaging reflects a technology that changed the way clinical neuropsychologists answered referral questions. By the 1990s, neuropsychologists were experiencing a shift in referrals from lesion localization to assessment of everyday functioning (Sbordone & Long, 1996). With the advent and development of advanced technologies in the clinical neurosciences, there was decreased need for neuropsychological assessments to localize lesions and an increased need for neuropsychologists to describe behavioral manifestations of neurological disorders. Clinical neuropsychologists were increasingly being asked to make prescriptive statements about everyday functioning (Sbordone & Long, 1996). Hence, future development of neuropsychological tests should involve enhanced understandings of large-scale brain networks and approaches that assess activities of daily living.

## BRAIN RESEARCH THROUGH ADVANCING INNOVATIVE NEUROTECHNOLOGIES

Recent growth in the human neurosciences has been spurred in part by the U.S. government's designation of the 1990s as "The Decade of the Brain," the National Institute of Mental Health's Research Domain Criteria framework for studying mental disorders, and the White House's BRAIN (Brain Research through Advancing Innovative Neurotechnologies) Initiative. First, the Decade of the Brain (1990 to the end of 1999) was an interagency effort that sponsored various activities (e.g., publications and programs) aimed at introducing cutting-edge research on the brain and encouraging public dialogue on the ethical, philosophical, and humanistic implications of the emerging discoveries.

The National Institute of Mental Health's Research Domain Criteria (RDoC) is a research framework for developing and implementing novel approaches to the study of mental disorders. The RDoC integrate multiple levels of information to enhance understanding of basic dimensions of functioning underlying the full range of human behavior from normal to abnormal. The RDoC framework consists of a matrix with rows that represent particular functional constructs (i.e., concepts that represent a specified functional behavior dimension) categorized in aggregate by the genes, molecules, circuits, etc., used to measure dimensions of observable behavior. In turn, the constructs are grouped into higher-level domains of functioning that reflect current knowledge of the major systems of cognition, affect, motivation, and social behavior (see Insel et al., 2010).

The BRAIN Initiative represents an ambitious but achievable set of goals for advances in science and technology. Since the announcement of the BRAIN Initiative, dozens of leading academic institutions, scientists, technology firms, and other important contributors to neuroscience have responded to the call. A group of prominent neuroscientists have developed a 12-year research strategy for the National Institutes of Health to achieve the goals of the initiative. The BRAIN Initiative may do for neuroscience what the Human Genome Project did for genomics. It supports the development and application of innovative technologies to enhance our understanding of brain function. Moreover, the BRAIN

Initiative endeavors to aid researchers in uncovering the mysteries of brain disorders (e.g., Alzheimer's, Parkinson's, depression, and traumatic brain injury). It is believed that the initiative will accelerate the development and application of new technologies for producing dynamic imaging of the brain that expresses the ways in which individual brain cells and complex neural circuits interact at the speed of thought.

## Computerized Neuropsychological Assessment

Occurring in parallel and acting as a significant facilitator of neuroinformatic research have been the many advances in computer technology. Inexpensive and powerful advances in hardware and software allow for relational knowledge bases, Internet-accessible databases, server–client computer architectures, and visualization and simulation software.

### COMPUTER-AUTOMATED NEUROCOGNITIVE ASSESSMENTS

The ability to capture highly accurate response times is one of the important capabilities of computer-based tests. In addition, computers also log scores in a uniform manner (e.g., all tests produce a similar series of scores). Each individual test can be used to produce a data file with a unique file extension. The resulting uniform sets of raw scores allow for straightforward importing of the data into databases. Furthermore, separation of data files for each neuropsychological measure is important for various database/query-driven intertest comparisons. The logging and coding of raw data into a compatible format allow for more complex sets of data fields. As a result, there is substantial potential for querying functions that allow the neuropsychologist to observe the data in various permutations. Furthermore, the neuropsychologist can perform queries to sift out or analyze data based on particular criteria. With such robust database abilities, computers make it possible to aggregate large data sets, to develop algorithms to enhance diagnosis and test interpretation, and to increase our understanding of cognitive deficit patterns associated with neurological and psychiatric disorders. Data from these databases can be used to facilitate the development of tests with multiple forms for repeated administration. Also, computerized measures can facilitate group testing, not only by standardizing task administration but also through enhanced data management.

### WEB-BASED NEUROCOGNITIVE ASSESSMENTS

Some neuropsychologists are calling for greater inclusion of Internet-based neuropsychological assessments as a method for enhancing the development of meaningful data sets (Bilder, 2011; Jagaroo, 2009). The exponential increase in access to computers and the Internet across the lifespan allows for interactive web-based neuropsychological assessments (Bart, Raz, & Dan, 2014; Raz, Bar-Haim, Sadeh, & Dan, 2014). While some neuropsychologists have concerns that web-based neuropsychological assessments will somehow replace human neuropsychologists, it is important to note that web-based tests are just tools for enhanced presentation and logging of stimuli. Online neuropsychological assessment may enhance dissemination of testing, because tests could be administered in a variety of settings (e.g., office, home, school), at different times of the day, and to multiple persons at the same time. When properly used, web-based neuropsychological assessments can greatly enhance the assessment in terms of precision and rapid implementation of adaptive algorithms. Furthermore, web-based testing allows for enhanced database development and knowledge sharing.

The timing precision offered by computers allows for the enactment of procedures from the human neurosciences that rely on more refined task operations and trial-by-trial analyses that may be more sensitive and specific to individual differences in neural system function. A caveat is that there are technical challenges to capturing precise response times with web-based testing that have to be addressed. However, web-based computerized assessments also have the capacity for adaptive testing strategies that are likely to multiply efficiency in construct measurement (Bilder, 2011). In one study, Gibbons and colleagues (Gibbons et al., 2008) found that use of a computerized adaptive test resulted in a 95% average reduction in the number of items administered. The potential of adaptive web-based neurocognitive assessment protocols can be seen in the capacity to sample a large number of participants in relatively short periods of time. While there may be concerns that the neuropsychologist cannot be sure of the identity of the test-takers or that they are performing tasks as instructed, validity indicators, on-line video surveillance, and anthropometric identifiers can be included to remove these concerns. For example, algorithms can be implemented that allow for item-level response monitoring and automated consistency checks. Further, neuroinformatics algorithms are available that will allow for detection of outlying response patterns of uncertain validity.

WebNeuro is a widely used web-based neuropsychology battery that includes a number of neuropsychological measures: sensorimotor, memory, executive planning, attention, and emotion perception (Mathersul et al., 2009; Silverstein et al., 2007; Williams et al., 2009). In addition to neuropsychological measures, the WebNeuro battery includes measures of emotion recognition and identification: immediate explicit identification followed by implicit recognition (within a priming protocol). The WebNeuro protocol was developed as a web-based version of the IntegNeuro computer-automated neuropsychological assessment battery. IntegNeuro was developed by a consortium of scientists interested in establishing a standardized international database called Brain Resource International Database (BRID; Gordon, 2003; Gordon, Cooper, Rennie, & Williams, 2005; Paul et al., 2005). The BRID project aims to move beyond outdated approaches to aggregating neuropsychological data and to develop standardized testing approaches that facilitate the integration of otherwise independent sources of data (genetic, neuroimaging, psychophysiological, neuropsychological, and clinical). These platforms allow for data to be acquired internationally using a centralized database infrastructure for storage and manipulation of neuropsychological assessment (and other neuroinformatic) data. The data from WebNeuro are linked to a standardized and integrative international database (see www.BrainResource. com; www.BRAINnet.com). The data are aggregated with data from genetic, neuroimaging, psychophysiological, and other clinical markers. The data can be incorporated into databases as new marker discoveries emerge from personalized medicine.

## VIRTUAL REALITY-BASED NEUROPSYCHOLOGICAL ASSESSMENTS

The issue of ecological validity in psychological assessment has been expressed a number of times over the years via discussions of the limitations of generalizing sterile laboratory findings to the processes normally occurring in people's everyday lives. One methodology that has potential for a laboratory versus everyday functioning rapprochement is virtual reality (Parsons, 2015). Recent advances in virtual reality technology allow for enhanced computational capacities for administration efficiency, stimulus presentation, automated logging of responses, and data-analytic processing (Bohil, Alicea, & Biocca, 2011). Since virtual environments provide experimental control and dynamic presentation of stimuli in ecologically valid scenarios, they allow for controlled presentations of emotionally engaging background narratives to enhance affective experience and social interactions (Diemer, Alpers, Peperkorn, Shiban, & Mühlberger, 2015; Gorini, Capideville, DeLeo, Mantovani, & Riva, 2011).

Virtual environments (VEs) represent a special case of computerized neuropsychological assessment. VEs are able to present and control dynamic perceptual stimuli in a manner that provides for ecologically valid assessments that combine the veridical control and rigor of laboratory measures with a verisimilitude that reflects real-life situations (Sanchez-Vives & Slater, 2005; Tarr & Warren, 2002). Additionally, the enhanced computation power allows for increased accuracy in the recording of neurobehavioral responses in a perceptual environment that systematically presents complex stimuli. Such simulation technology appears to be distinctively suited for the development of ecologically valid environments, in which three-dimensional objects are presented in a consistent and precise manner (Parsons, 2015; Parsons, Carlew, Magtoto, & Stonecipher, 2015). VE-based neuropsychological assessments can provide a balance between naturalistic observation and the need for exacting control over key variables (Campbell et al., 2009). Virtual reality permits patients to be presented with lifelike scenarios that capture how they perform in situations, and not just how they do tasks.

## Consilience in Neuropsychological Concepts and Measurements

### NEUROINFORMATICS FOR NEUROPSYCHOLOGISTS

A growing interest in the human neurosciences is found in the potential of neuroinformatics to develop knowledge bases traversing genomics, gene expression, and proteomics (Bilder, 2011). The interface between neuroinformatics and clinical neuropsychology practice is largely an uncharted area (Jagaroo, 2009). Neuropsychology's lack of technological sophistication in neuroinformatics separates it from neuroimaging and clinical electrophysiology. Neurophysiological assessments, unlike clinical neuropsychological assessments, take data from electroencephalography and evoked potentials and analyze it using computational and neuroinformatic tools. There is promise for integrating computerized neuropsychological assessment of brain injury for computational modeling using a neuroinformatic approach.

E. O. Wilson (Wilson, 1998, 1999) called for a consilience of knowledge via the linking of facts and fact-based theories across disciplines to construct a common ground of explanation. An important growth area for neuropsychology is the capacity for sharing knowledge gained from neuropsychological assessments with related disciplines. Before this can happen, though, neuropsychologists need to formalize neuropsychological concepts into ontologies that offer formal descriptions of content domains.

### FORMALIZING NEUROPSYCHOLOGICAL CONSTRUCTS

Data from clinical neuropsychological assessments often involve interrelated dimensional constructs that refer to a hypothetical cognitive resource whose existence is inferred from research findings (Burgess et al., 2006). For example, the cognitive construct *working memory* is not a unitary concept. Instead, working memory is a latent construct that is estimated in a given study by performance on one or more neuropsychological measures. Sabb et al. (2008) examined 478 articles to evaluate the relationship among estimates of heritability, behavioral measures, and component constructs of executive function. They applied a phrase search algorithm to isolate key terms that are regularly used in the neuropsychology literature. Next, they selected the term *cognitive control* and four phrases based on their frequency of co-occurrence with the term cognitive control: "working memory," "task switching," "response inhibition," and "response selection." High internal consistency was found among these phrases for their indicators and associated heritability measures. Hence, they may effectively capture distinct components of executive functions. However, Sabb and colleagues (Sabb et al., 2008) also found that the same indicators associated with the term "cognitive control" had also been associated with the other constructs. While this may reflect shared neural systems that can be important in establishing distinct cognitive constructs (Lenartowicz, Kalar, Congdon, & Poldrack, 2010), there is also the possibility that the neuropsychological measures themselves may be a confound. For some measures, there was good consistency across studies in the use of a specific indicator (e.g., digit span backwards used only one indicator: correct recall of digits). However, other measures had substantial variation in the specific indicator used (e.g., each of three studies reporting Go/No-Go performance used different indicators and versions of the test). This suggests an inconsistency that significantly decreases the potential for pooling data and interpreting results across studies. Nevertheless, the work of Sabb and colleagues (Sabb et al., 2008) does offer a potential roadmap for developing ontologies.

## CLINICAL NEUROPSYCHOLOGY ONTOLOGIES

In addition to shared definitions of neuropsychological constructs, the development of ontologies enables systematic aggregation of neuropsychological knowledge into shared databases. The term *ontology* in neuroinformatics reflects the formal specification of entities that exist in a domain and the relations among them (Lenartowicz et al., 2010). A given ontology contains designations of separate entities along with a specification of ontological relations among entities that can include hierarchical relations (e.g., "is-a" or "part-of") or spatiotemporal relations (e.g., "preceded-by" or "contained-within"). These knowledge structures allow for consistent representations across models, which can facilitate communication among domains by providing an objective, concise, common, and controlled vocabulary. This consistency also allows for enhanced interoperability and provision of links among levels of analysis. Such ontologies have become central within many areas of neuroscience.

While ontologies abound in other biomedical disciplines, neuropsychological assessment lags in its development of formal ontologies (Bilder, 2011; Jagaroo, 2009). That said, there are attempts to develop cognitive ontologies for neuropsychology. For example, the Consortium for Neuropsychiatric Phenomics (www. phenomics.ucla.edu) aims to enable more effective collaboration, and facilitation of knowledge sharing about cognitive phenotypes, with other levels of biological knowledge (Bilder, 2011). A technological advance that enhances the potential for developing cognitive ontologies from neuropsychological assessment data is the Internet. Web 2.0 represents a trend in open platform Internet use that incorporates user-driven online networks and knowledge bases. While there are no large Internet-based repositories for neuropsychological data, efforts have been made to allow users to input individual test scores via a web portal (www. neuropsychnorms.com) and obtain immediate reports comparing a patient's neuropsychological data to published findings (Mitrushina, Boone, Razani, & D'Elia, 2005). In addition to these, the Cognitive Atlas (http://www.cognitive-atlas.org/) project describes the "parts" and processes of cognitive functioning in a manner similar to descriptions of the cell's component parts and functions in gene ontology.

In sum, the growing interest in the human neurosciences to develop collaborative knowledge bases traversing genomics, gene expression, and proteomics offers exciting potential for neuropsychology (Bilder, 2011). While the interface between neuroinformatics and clinical neuropsychology practice is largely an uncharted area (Jagaroo, 2009), the development of cognitive ontologies could allow neuropsychologists to develop a common language for knowledge sharing and neuroinformatics. The inclusion of cognitive ontologies and technological advances in the development of neuropsychological assessments would allow for amalgamation with biomarker data for analysis with computational and neuroinformatic tools. There is promise for integrating computerized neuropsychological assessment of brain injury for computational modeling using a neuroinformatic approach.

## Conclusion

This book presents ways we believe technology will shape the future practice of neuropsychology. Implementing technology goes beyond establishing face validity and credibility when testing persons born into the modern age. Rather, it has to do with thoughtfully implementing current and emerging capabilities to refine and expand the assessment process. As noted throughout this work, in some cases the increased capabilities are incremental and permit the implementation of traditional measures in a more efficient manner. The ability to assess clinically relevant cognitive domains with computerized measures will expand with advances in voice and language recognition and data analytics. Computers have also opened new paradigms for assessment in analyzing emotion, in implementing virtual scenario-based assessment, and in integrating cognitive with physiological measures, and by offering methods to aggregate data to better understand cognitive constructs and clinical presentations associated with disease entities. It is impossible to predict all the ways in which technology will add capabilities and drive the assessment process. What is clear is that neuropsychology has little choice but to adopt technological advances and to keep pace with the developments being made in other areas of neuroscience.

## References

Bart, O., Raz, S., & Dan, O. (2014). Reliability and validity of the Online Continuous Performance Test among children. *Assessment, 21*(5), 637–643.

Bilder, R. M. (2011). Neuropsychology 3.0: Evidenced-based science and practice. *Journal of the International Neuropsychological Society, 17*(1), 7–13.

Bohil, C. J., Alicea, B., & Biocca, F. A. (2011). Virtual reality in neuroscience research and therapy. *Nature Reviews Neuroscience, 12*(12), 752–762.

Bressler, S. L., & Menon, V. (2010). Large-scale brain networks in cognition: Emerging methods and principles. *Trends in Cognitive Sciences, 14*(6), 277–290.

Burgess, P. W., Alderman, N., Forbes, C., Costello, A., Coates, L. M., Dawson, D. R., . . . Channon, S. (2006). The case for the development and use of "ecologically valid" measures of executive function in experimental and clinical neuropsychology. *Journal of the International Neuropsychological Society, 12*(2), 194–209.

Campbell, Z., Zakzanis, K. K., Jovanovski, D., Joordens, S., Marz, R., & Graham, S. J. (2009). Utilising virtual reality to improve the ecological validity of clinical neuropsychology: An fMRI case study elucidating the neural basis of planning by comparing the Tower of London with a three-dimensional navigation task. *Applied Neuropsychology, 16*, 295–306.

Diemer, J. E., Alpers, G. W., Peperkorn, H. M., Shiban, Y., & Mühlberger, A. (2015). The impact of perception and presence on emotional reactions: A review of research in virtual reality. *Frontiers in Psychology, 6*(26), 1–9.

Dodrill, C. B. (1997). Myths of neuropsychology. *The Clinical Neuropsychologist, 11*, 1–17.

Gibbons, R. D., Weiss, D. J., Kupfer, D. J., Frank, E., Fagiolini, A., & Grochocinski, V. J. (2008). Using computerized adaptive testing to reduce the burden of mental health assessment. *Psychiatric Services, 59*(4), 361–368.

Gordon, E. (2003). Integrative neuroscience. *Neuropsychopharmacology, 28*(Suppl. 1), 2–8.

Gordon, E., Cooper, C., Rennie, D., & Williams, L. M. (2005). Integrative neuroscience: The role of a standardized database. *Clinical EEG and Neuroscience, 36*(64–75).

Gorini, A., Capideville, C. S., DeLeo, G., Mantovani, F., & Riva, G. (2011). The role of immersion and narrative in mediated presence: The virtual hospital experience. *Cyberpsychology, Behavior, and Social Networking, 14*, 99–105.

Insel, T., Cuthbert, B., Garvey, M., Heinssen, R., Pine, D. S., Quinn, K., . . . Wang, P. (2010). Research domain criteria (RDoC): Toward a new classificaion framework for research on mental disorders. *American Journal of Psychiatry, 167*(7), 748–751.

Jagaroo, V. (2009). Obstacles and aids to neuroinformatics in neuropsychology. *Neuroinformatics for neuropsychology* (pp. 85–93). New York NY: Springer.

Koziol, L. F., Barker, L. A., Hrin, S., & Joyce, A. W. (2014a). Large-scale brain systems and subcortical relationships: Practical applications. *Applied Neuropsychology: Child, 3*(4), 264–273.

Koziol, L. F., Barker, L. A., Joyce, A. W., & Hrin, S. (2014b). Large-scale brain systems and subcortical relationships: The vertically organized brain. *Applied Neuropsychology: Child, 3*(4), 253–263.

Lenartowicz, A., Kalar, D. J., Congdon, E., & Poldrack, R. A. (2010). Towards an ontology of cognitive control. Topics in Cognitive Science. *Cognitive Science, 2*(4), 678–692.

Mathersul, D., Palmer, D. M., Gur, R. C., Gur, R. E., Cooper, N., Gordon, E., & Williams, L. M. (2009). Explicit identification and implicit recognition of facial emotions: II. Core domains and relationships with general cognition. *Journal of Clinical and Experimental Neuropsychology, 31*(3), 278–291.

Menon, V. (2011). Large-scale brain networks and psychopathology: A unifying triple network model. *Trends in Cognitive Sciences, 15*(10), 483–506.

Menon, V., & Uddin, L. Q. (2010). Saliency, switching, attention and control: A network model of insula function. *Brain Structure & Function, 214*, 655–667.

Mitrushina, M. N., Boone, K. B., Razani, J., & D'Elia, L. F. (2005). *Handbook of normative data for neuropsychological assessment.* New York NY: Oxford University Press.

Parsons, T. D. (2015). Virtual reality for enhanced ecological validity and experimental control in clinical, affective, and social neurosciences. *Frontiers in Human Neuroscience, 9,* 1–19.

Parsons, T. D., Carlew, A. R., Magtoto, J., & Stonecipher, K. (2015). The potential of function-led virtual environments for ecologically valid measures of executive function in experimental and clinical neuropsychology. *Neuropsychological Rehabilitation, 11,* 1–31.

Paul, R. H., Lawrence, J., Williams, L. M., Richard, C. C., Cooper, N., & Gordon, E. (2005). A new computerized battery of neurocognitive tests. *International Journal of Neuroscience, 115*(11), 1549–1567.

Qin, P., & Northoff, G. (2011). How is our self related to midline regions and the default-mode network? *Neuroimaging, 57*(3), 1221–1233.

Raichle, M. E. (2015). The brain's default mode network. *Annual Review of Neuroscience, 38,* 433–447.

Raz, S., Bar-Haim, Y., Sadeh, A., & Dan, O. (2014). Reliability and validity of the online continuous performance test among young adults. *Assessment, 21*(1), 108–118.

Sabb, F. W., Bearden, C. E., Glahn, D. C., Parker, D. S., Freimer, N., & Bilder, R. M. (2008). A collaborative knowledge base for cognitive phenomics. *Molecular Psychiatry, 13*(4), 350–360.

Sanchez-Vives, M. V., & Slater, M. (2005). From presence to consciousness through virtual reality. *Nature Reviews Neuroscience, 6*(4), 332–339.

Sbordone, R. J., & Long, C. J. (1996). *Ecological validity of neuropsychological testing.* Boca Raton, FL: CRC Press.

Seeley, W. W., Menon, V., Schatzberg, A. F., Keller, J., Glover, G. H., Kenna, H., . . . Greicius, M. D. (2007). Dissociable intrinsic connectivity networks for salience processing and executive control. *The Journal of Neuroscience, 27,* 2349–2356.

Silverstein, S. M., Berten, S., Olson, P., Paul, R., Williams, L. M., Cooper, N., & Gordon, E. (2007). Development and validation of a World-Wide-Web-based neurocognitive assessment battery: WebNeuro. *Behavior Research Methods, 39*(4), 940–949.

Sridharan, D., Levitin, D. J., & Menon, V. (2008). A critical role for the right fronto-insular cortex in switching between central-executive and default-mode networks. *Proceedings of the National Academy of Sciences, 105*(34), 12569–12574.

Tarr, M. J., & Warren, W. H. (2002). Virtual reality in behavioral neuroscience and beyond. *Nature Neuroscience, 5,* 1089–1092.

Williams, L. M., Mathersul, D., Palmer, D. M., Gur, R. C., Gur, R. E., & Gordon, E. (2009). Explicit identification and implicit recognition of facial emotions: I. Age effects in males and females across 10 decades. *Journal of Clinical and Experimental Neuropsychology, 31*(3), 257–277.

Wilson, E. O. (1998). Integrated science and the coming century of the environment. *Science, 279*(5359), 2048–2049.

Wilson, E. O. (1999). *Consilience: The unity of knowledge* (Vol. 31): Vintage Books, New York, NY.

# { INDEX }

Page numbers followed by *b, f,* or *t* indicate boxes, figures, or tables, respectively. Numbers followed by n indicate notes.

The role of technology in
clinical neuropsychology